Manual *for* Pharmacy Technicians

FOURTH EDITION

Manual *for* Pharmacy Technicians

FOURTH EDITION

Bonnie S. Bachenheimer, PharmD

Drug Information Clinical Specialist
Advocate Lutheran General Hospital
Park Ridge, Illinois

AMERICAN SOCIETY OF HEALTH-SYSTEM PHARMACISTS®
Bethesda, Maryland

Any correspondence regarding this publication should be sent to the publisher, American Society of Health-System Pharmacists, 7272 Wisconsin Avenue, Bethesda, MD 20814, attention: Special Publishing.

Director, Special Publishing: Jack Bruggeman

Acquisitions Editor: Rebecca Olson

Senior Editorial Project Manager: Dana Battaglia

Developmental Editor: Nancy Peterson

Production Editor: Publication Services

Design: Publication Services

ISBN 978-1-58528-207-4

Dedication

This *Manual* is dedicated to the pharmacy technicians I have worked with who are such valuable partners in patient care; their knowledge and dedication to the profession allow us to perform at the highest level possible.

This *Manual* is also dedicated to future pharmacy technicians and their educators, who must be fearless in using their curiosity and creativity to push the boundaries of current practice so that we can continue to move the profession forward.

Bonnie S. Bachenheimer, PharmD

Acknowledgments

I would like to acknowledge the following groups and individuals for their contributions to this book:

The Illinois Council of Health-System Pharmacists (ICHP), for giving me the opportunity to be editor of this edition of the *Manual*.

Linda Fred, for all of her hard work as editor and contributor of the previous editions.

The support staff at the American Society of Health-System Pharmacists (ASHP), especially Dana Battaglia and Rebecca Olson for their patience, encouragement, and assistance throughout the process.

Nancy Peterson for her great ideas and thorough development of the book.

Katy Thompson from Publication Services for always being organized and keeping everything and everyone on track.

All of the contributing authors and reviewers. Their efforts are the main reason that this book is such a high quality and highly respected reference book.

My colleagues at Advocate Lutheran General Hospital for their advice and enthusiasm regarding the book and for sharing my passion for the profession of pharmacy.

I am grateful to my husband Eric, and my children, Sara, Ben, and Max for their love, support, and understanding throughout the publication of this book.

Bonnie S. Bachenheimer, PharmD

Contents

Preface

This is an exciting time to be in the profession of pharmacy! Pharmacists continue to be more involved in direct patient care, drug therapy continues to become more complex, and ensuring appropriate and safe medication use continues to be a major focus of our profession. Pharmacists rely on the support of pharmacy technicians to be able to provide quality patient care, and technicians are valued members of the healthcare team. Technicians are assuming more responsibilities and are taking on more leadership roles. As their roles continue to expand and evolve, it is imperative that pharmacy technicians be well-trained. Many states are passing laws that mandate technician certification as a minimum requirement for all technicians.

This manual has been updated to reflect the changing role of pharmacy technicians and of the profession. The *Manual, Workbook*, and *Practice Exam Guide* were constructed as instructional manuals for pharmacy technicians enrolled in formal training programs, for those wishing to achieve certification, and for training purposes at the workplace. This manual and additional Web content will also appeal to instructors of formal and informal pharmacy technician training programs.

If you are familiar with previous editions of the *Manual*, you will notice significant changes in its appearance, organization, and content. This edition was developed to meet the current and future needs of pharmacy technicians and their educators. The look of the *Manual* has been given a make-over that includes more color, more figures, and additional features to stimulate students interest and inspire instructors.

Organization and Chapter Content

The order of the chapters has changed from the previous edition to follow the structure of most curriculums and to complement the ASHP model curriculum. The Manual is now divided into four parts:

1. **Introduction to Pharmacy Practice.** This section introduces the practice of pharmacy and the most common practice settings, including a new chapter on "Specialty Pharmacy."
2. **Foundation Knowledge and Skills.** This section highlights the important foundation knowledge and skills that are necessary to understand the basics of medication use. A new chapter on "Communication and Teamwork" is included in this section.
3. **Practice Basics.** This section includes the chapters directly related to processing prescriptions and medication orders.

4. **Business Applications.** This section includes the chapters related to the business end of the practice of pharmacy. There are two new chapters in this section: "Durable and Nondurable Medical Equipment, Devices, and Supplies," and "Billing and Reimbursement."

Appendixes. A glossary of key terms can be found at the end of the book. Several appendixes have been added as important resources:

Appendix A: Medical Terminology and Abbreviations
Appendix B: Confused Drug Names
Appendix C: Glossary

Organization within the Chapters:

The beginning of each chapter contains an **outline of the chapter** and **key terms** with definitions. Key terms are also bolded within the text for reinforcement.

Learning outcomes help the student understand what they need to learn from the chapter.

An **introduction** explains what the student will learn in the chapter and why it is important.

A **summary** at the end of each chapter briefly reiterates the chapter's key topics and learning outcomes and why they are important.

References and a listing of **resources,** such as suggested books, journals, Web sites, and other media, is included at the end of each chapter.

Self-Assessment questions help students test their knowledge of the content and evaluate their learning outcomes. The **Self-Assessment answers** include a rationale for the correct answers.

Explanation of New Features:

A number of new pedagogical features in the chapters have been added to this edition:

Key Points are highlighted in the chapter as in the example below:

✔The qualifications for pharmacy technician registration or licensure generally include a minimum age, high school graduation or the equivalent, completion of a training program, including pharmacy employer training programs, and an examination.

Rx for Success boxes include practice tips, pearls, and words of wisdom. They provide additional insight into important topics with the goal of helping the reader achieve success on the job and in their career. An example is shown below:

Rx for Success

Technicians who are able to identify patients with these types of special needs and can effectively communicate these concerns with the pharmacist and other health care professionals are invaluable in patient care.

Safety First boxes stress prevention, identification, and management of drug-related problems and point out alerts and cautions relating to the safe use of medications. An example is shown below:

Safety First

The patient's name and some other identifying information (e.g., date of birth, address, phone number) must be verified to ensure that the correct medication is being given to the correct patient.

Technology Topics boxes highlight technology, as in the example below. The previous edition had a chapter on Technology, but this edition integrates the latest technology into individual chapters both within the text and by using this feature.

TECHNOLOGY TOPICS

"Smart pumps" are equipped with IV medication error prevention software. These devices have specific drug libraries, dose calculators, programming limits, and remote communication capabilities.

Updated Content:

All of the chapters from the previous edition were revised and updated. Several new chapters were created, including:

Specialty Pharmacy Practice. This chapter includes information on Nuclear Pharmacy, Specialty Compounding, and Veterinary Pharmacy Practice.

Communication & Teamwork. This chapter was specifically requested by pharmacy technicians and technician educators since effective communication skills and working well as a team are so important in the workplace.

Durable and Nondurable Medical Equipment, Devices and Supplies. This chapter describes commonly used durable medical equipment (DME) and non-DME devices and supplies, since many pharmacies provide them for their patients.

Billing and Reimbursement. Pharmacy technicians are often involved in pharmacy billing and reimbursement; therefore, this chapter was added to provide a broad overview of the topic.

Web Content. Additional Web content includes links to the Top 200 Drugs, ASHP Technical Assistance Bulletins, and Practice Guidelines. There will be Web content for instructors including powerpoint presentations and additional sample problems with answers that will be available for downloading for teaching and testing purposes. Web content can be found at: www.ashp.org/techmanual.

Pharmacy Technician Certification: Review and Exam Guide

The Pharmacy Technician Certification Review and Practice Exam, third edition, is a self-study guide designed as a companion to the *Manual for Pharmacy Technicians*. While the Manual is designed to provide a broad overview of essential knowledge and skills, the goal of the Exam Guide is to prepare technician students for the Pharmacy

Technician Certification Exam offered by the Pharmacy Technician Certification Board (PTCB), as well as other certification exams.

The Exam Guide contains chapters focused on each section of the PTCE exam, as well as a thorough calculations review, a section on commonly prescribed medications, and important test-taking tips and strategies. In addition to the practice exam and numerous review questions throughout the text, a CD packaged with the book allows users to build multiple practice exams. We recommend using this book in conjunction with the Manual as a helpful study aid in preparing for certification.

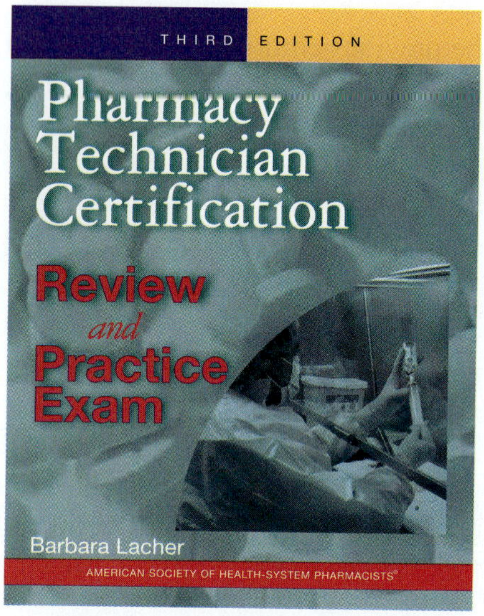

New! Workbook for the Manual for Pharmacy Technicians

The *Workbook for the Manual for Pharmacy Technicians* helps technician students master the concepts and skills discussed in the *Manual*. By asking students to apply their knowledge, the exercises in the Workbook reinforce key points and allow for targeted assessment. Chapters in the Workbook complement those in the Manual, so that instructors and students can easily work between both books. Each chapter includes a wide range of exercises, such as multiple-choice, true/false, fill in the blank, concept and key term matching, short answer, and activity questions. Where appropriate, calculation, conversion, and visual identification questions are included. We recommend using this book alongside the Manual to enhance learning.

A lot of hard work, time and energy have gone into making this Manual a valuable resource for pharmacy technicians and their educators. We hope that you are as excited about this new edition as we are!

Bonnie S. Bachenheimer, PharmD
Editor

Contributors

Bonnie S. Bachenheimer, PharmD
Clinical Pharmacist, Drug Information
Advocate Lutheran General Hospital
Park Ridge, Illinois

Karen E. Bertch, PharmD, FCCP
Director, Formulary Development
Medication Management Group
Premier, Inc.
Lisle, Illinois

Susan P. Bruce, PharmD, BCPS
Associate Professor and Chair
Pharmacy Practice
Colleges of Medicine and Pharmacy
Northeastern Ohio Universities
Rootstown, Ohio

Margaret Byun, PharmD, MS
Assistant Director, Finance
and Administration
Ambulatory Care Pharmacy Department
Clinical Assistant Professor of
Pharmacy Practice
University of Illinois at Chicago
College of Pharmacy
Chicago, Illinois

Diane L. Darvey, PharmD, JD
Alexandria, Virginia

Thomas C. Dowling, PharmD, PhD, FCP
Associate Professor
Vice Chair, Department of Pharmacy
Practice and Science
University of Maryland School of Pharmacy
Baltimore, Maryland

Sandra F. Durley, RPh, PharmD
Associate Director, Ambulatory Care
Pharmacy Department
Clinical Assistant Professor
University of Illinois at Chicago
College of Pharmacy
Chicago, Illinois

John F. Falkenholm, PharmD
Pharmacy Manager
Advocate Lutheran General Hospital
Park Ridge, Illinois

Alice J. A. Gardner, BSc, PhD
Associate Professor of Pharmacology
School of Pharmacy–Worcester
Massachusetts College of Pharmacy and
Health Sciences
Worcester, Massachusetts

David R. Karls, RPh, MBA
Community Pharmacist
Fuquay Varina, North Carolina

Jacqueline Z. Kessler, MS, FASHP
Clinical Pharmacist
Advocate Lutheran General Hospital
Park Ridge, Illinois

Thomas E. Kirschling, PharmD, MS
Manager, Pharmacy Operations
University of Pittsburg Medical Center Presbyterian
Pittsburgh, Pennsylvania

Jane E. Krause, BS Pharm, MS, RPh
Clinical Associate Professor of Pharmacy Practice
Purdue University College of Pharmacy
West Lafayette, Indiana

Christopher M. Kutza, PharmD
Pharmacy Manager
Advocate Lutheran General Hospital
Park Ridge, Illinois

Steven Lundquist, PharmD
Clinical Director
Cardinal Health, Pharmacy Solutions
Marco Island, Florida

Scott M. Mark, PharmD, MS, MEd, MBA, MPH, FASHP, FACHE
Director of Pharmacy
Director, Pharmacy Practice Management Residency
University of Pittsburgh Medical Center
Associate Professor and Vice Chair of Pharmacy Systems
University of Pittsburgh School of Pharmacy
Pittsburgh, Pennsylvania

Mary B. McHugh, PharmD
Director, Pharmacy Technology
University of Montana College of Technology
Missoula, Montana

Jerrod Milton, Bsc Pharm, RPh
Vice President, Operations
Children's Hospital
Aurora, Colorado

Bertram A. Nicholas Jr., BS, MS, EdD, RPh
Assistant Dean for Experiential Education
Saint Joseph College School of Pharmacy
West Hartford, Connecticut

Michele F. Shepherd, PharmD, MS, BCPS, FASHP
Pharmacy Coordinator for Medical Education and Anticoagulation Services
Abbott Northwestern Hospital
Minneapolis, Minnesota

Miriam A. Mobley Smith, BS Pharm, PharmD
Interim Dean
Chicago State University College of Pharmacy
Chicago, Illinois

Daphne E. Smith-Marsh, PharmD, CDE
Clinical Assistant Professor/Clinical Pharmacist
University of Illinois at Chicago College of Pharmacy
Chicago, Illinois

Sheri Stensland, PharmD, AE-C, FAPhA
Associate Professor, Pharmacy Practice
Midwestern University–Chicago College of Pharmacy
Downers Grove, Illinois

JoAnn Stubbings, RPh, MHCA
Manager, Research and Public Policy
Clinical Associate Professor
Center for Pharmacoeconomic Research
University of Illinois at Chicago College of Pharmacy
Chicago, Illinois

Kara D. Weatherman, PharmD, BCNP, FAPhA
Clinical Assistant Professor of Pharmacy Practice
Purdue University College of Pharmacy
West Lafayette, Indiana

Reviewers

Larry M. Allen, PhD, MBA, RPh
Academic Coordinator
Pharmacy Technician Program
Arapahoe Community College
Littleton, Colorado

Gail B. Askew, PharmD
Executive Director
Pharmacy Technician Educators Council
Former Director
Pharmacy Technology Program
Santa Ana College
Santa Ana, California

Marlene Lamnin, RPh
Program Director
Pharmacy Technology Department
Carrington College California (formerly Western Career College)
San Leandro, California

Mary B. McHugh, PharmD
Director, Pharmacy Technology
University of Montana College of Technology
Supervisor
Community Medical Center Retail Pharmacy
Missoula, Montana

Part One

Introduction to Pharmacy Practice

This section introduces the practice of pharmacy and the most common practice settings, including community and hospital pharmacies, as well as unique settings, such as Nuclear Pharmacy and Veterinary Pharmacy. It contains a chapter on pharmacy law and an introduction to drug information resources, which applies to all pharmacy practice settings.

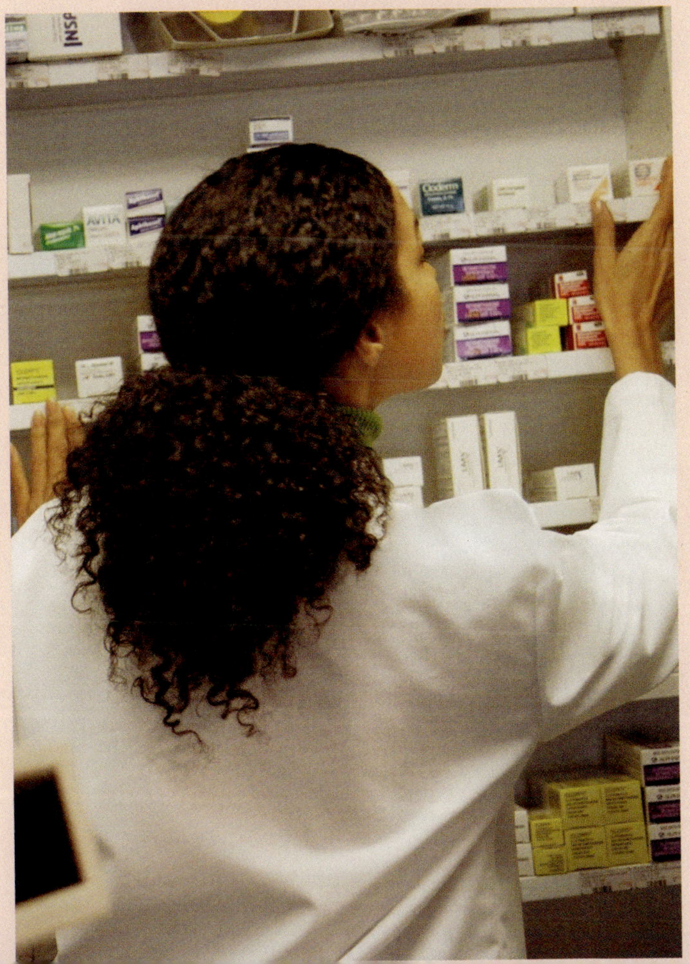

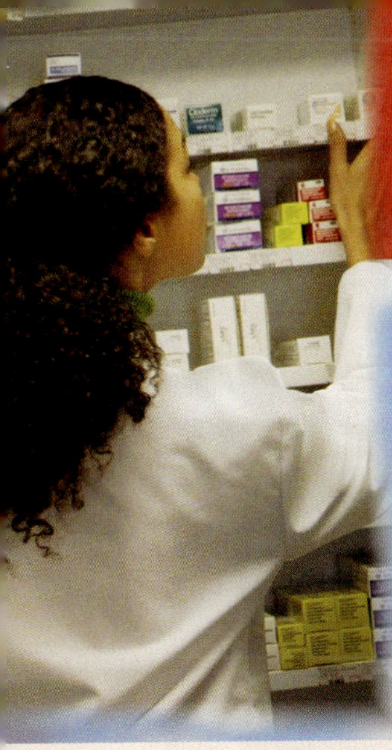

Chapter 1

Introduction to Pharmacy

Michele F. Shepherd

Learning Outcomes

After completing this chapter, you will be able to

- Compare and contrast the responsibilities of pharmacy technicians and pharmacists.
- Outline the differences among licensure, certification, and registration.
- Describe the advantages of formal training for pharmacy technicians.
- Describe the differences between the ambulatory and institutional pharmacy practice settings.
- List two specific examples each of ambulatory and institutional pharmacy practice settings.
- Describe at least six characteristics of a professional.
- List five tasks that pharmacy technicians perform in various pharmacy settings.
- Describe the concept of pharmaceutical care.
- Define medication therapy management.
- Explain why the use of outpatient pharmacy and medical services is increasing.

Key Terms

accreditation The process of granting recognition or vouching for compliance with established criteria (usually in reference to recognition of an institution or program).

certification A voluntary process by which a nongovernmental agency or association grants recognition to an individual who has met certain predetermined qualifications specified by that agency or association. This recognition demonstrates that the certified individual has achieved a certain level of knowledge, skill, or experience.

health-system pharmacy The practice of pharmacy in a practice setting that is part of a health-system. A health-system is two or more health care practice settings (e.g., hospital, home care, ambulatory clinic) that have a working relationship with each other and are managed or owned by the same business entity. Health-systems provide complete health care-related services to the patients they serve.

home health care Physician-ordered health care services provided to a patient in the home or other setting in which the patient lives.

licensure The process by which an agency of the government grants permission to an individual to engage in a given occupation upon finding that the applicant has attained a degree of competency necessary to ensure that public health, safety, and welfare will be protected.

medication therapy management (MTM) A service or group of services that optimize therapeutic outcomes for a patient. Such services include: assessment of a patient's health status; formulation of a medication treatment plan; selection, initiation, modification, or administration of medication therapy; monitoring of a patient's response to therapy; review of medications for medication-related problems; documentation and communication of care; provision of patient education and information to increase patient understanding and appropriate use of medications; and coordination and integration of MTM services into the broader health care services provided to the patient.

pharmaceutical care Direct, responsible provision of medication-related care that achieves outcomes that improve a patient's quality of life. Pharmaceutical care involves cooperation between the pharmacist, the patient, and other health care professionals in designing, implementing, and monitoring a therapeutic medication plan. Such a plan serves to identify potential and actual drug-related problems, resolve actual drug-related problems, and prevent potential drug-related problems.

pharmacist A health care professional licensed by the state to engage in the practice of pharmacy. Pharmacists have advanced training in the pharmaceutical sciences, such as pharmacology (the study of drugs and their actions in the body), pharmacokinetics (the process by which drugs are absorbed, distributed, metabolized, and eliminated in the body), and pharmaceutics (the science of preparing and dispensing drugs).

pharmacy technician A pharmacy technician assists pharmacists by performing routine, day-to-day functions of the practice of pharmacy that do not require the judgment of a pharmacist.

registration The process of making a list or being enrolled in an existing list. A pharmacy technician may be required to be registered with the state board of pharmacy before being legally able to carry out some pharmacy functions.

The pharmacy profession has roots dating back thousands of years and is based on the sciences of mathematics, chemistry, and medicine. Knowledge from these sciences is applied to the development and study of drugs and their actions (pharmacology); the understanding of how drugs are absorbed, distributed, metabolized, and eliminated by the body (pharmacokinetics); and the preparation and dispensing of drugs (pharmaceutics).

The primary responsibility of any employee in the pharmacy profession is to ensure that patients receive optimal drug therapy to maintain or restore their health. To achieve this goal, pharmacy personnel in hospitals, community pharmacies, and other health care settings perform a variety of duties designed to deliver the correct drug in the correct amount to the right patient at all times and in a timely manner. These duties include ordering medications from suppliers, evaluating the appropriateness of each medication based on patient-specific information, distributing medications to patients, and monitoring patients while they are taking medications. Pharmacists are assisted by pharmacy technicians in several capacities to fulfill these obligations.

Pharmacists and pharmacy technicians must be honest and ethical and protect the rights and privacy of patients. To establish and maintain a profession consistent with these goals, state boards of pharmacy enforce pharmacy laws and regulations and require pharmacists to meet minimum education and experience standards. Most state boards of pharmacy also require that pharmacy technicians be registered or certified.

The purpose of this chapter is to describe pharmacy training and education, licensure and certification, aspects of professionalism, various settings in which pharmacy technicians practice, and how technician responsibilities are expanding. It emphasizes the differences between the duties and responsibilities of pharmacy technicians and pharmacists and introduces pharmacy technician competency expectations.

Pharmacy Training and Education

A profession is an occupation or vocation that requires advanced training in a liberal art or science. Pharmacy is a profession in which pharmacists are trained in the pharmaceutical sciences. Technicians are individuals who are skilled in the practical or mechanical aspects of a profession. **Pharmacy technicians** assist pharmacists by performing the routine, day-to-day functions that do not require the judgment of a pharmacist. Although technicians may be capable of functioning efficiently and safely without supervision, pharmacists are ultimately responsible for the technicians' activities and performance. The assistance of pharmacy technicians allows pharmacists more time to engage in activities that require professional judgment. Such assistance includes activities such as repackaging medications and maintaining medication inventory. Educating patients about their medications and suggesting medication alternatives to physicians require a pharmacist's judgment and are not to be performed by pharmacy technicians. Legally, pharmacists are held liable for the performance of technicians and must oversee and approve the technicians' work.

✔Pharmacists are ultimately responsible for the technicians' activities and performance and are legally held liable for the technicians' work.

Pharmacy Technicians

Pharmacy technicians assist pharmacists by completing tasks that do not require the professional judgment of a pharmacist and that can be reviewed for accuracy by a pharmacist. In this way, pharmacy technicians give pharmacists more time to concentrate on clinical services, such as patient consultation and education, physician collaboration, disease and medication management, and other clinical activities.

The Pharmacy Technician Certification Board (PTCB) is a national certification program that administers a nationally accredited pharmacy technician certification examination. The PTCB defines pharmacy technicians as

> individuals working in a pharmacy, who, under the supervision of a licensed pharmacist, assist in pharmacy activities not requiring the professional judgment of a pharmacist. The pharmacy technician is accountable to the supervising pharmacist, who is legally responsible by virtue of state licensure for the care and safety of patients served by the pharmacy. The pharmacy technician performs activities as the result of having certain knowledge and skills.[1]

Training prerequisites for pharmacy technicians vary from state to state and from employer to employer, but most employers require pharmacy technicians to have at least a high school diploma. As the level of responsibility for pharmacy technicians increases, so does the amount of required training or experience. Many employers have established criteria to classify technicians on the basis of their training or experience. For example, a hospital pharmacy technician 1 (PT-1) may be a newly hired technician responsible only for filling automated medication dispensing cabinets (e.g., Pyxis® MedStation™ medication management systems). A pharmacy technician 2 (PT-2) in that same hospital may have five years' job experience and be able to fill automated medication dispensing cabinets, as well as charge and credit patient accounts, compound (mix) intravenous (IV) solutions, and inventory narcotics.

Similar classifications may exist in community pharmacies. There, a PT-1 might receive prescriptions as patients leave them to be filled and check out patients at the cash register when they are ready to pay, whereas a PT-2 may be able to enter data in computerized patient profiles, fill and label prescriptions, and review patient insurance information.

✔Training prerequisites for pharmacy technicians vary from state to state and from employer to employer.

The work that pharmacy technicians perform is becoming more and more demanding. Some states allow technicians to check the work of other technicians (tech-check-tech) under the supervision of a pharmacist. Because most pharmacy practice settings rely heavily on computers and automated technology, technicians frequently are responsible for the day-to-day operations and upkeep of these systems. Computerized narcotic inventory control is one example of a technology that requires a high degree of computer skill, and the preparation and compounding of IV and sterile products is an example of a technician duty that demands a high level of proficiency and competence.

Patient safety is a top priority for all pharmacists and pharmacy technicians. Technicians often perform the first step in dispensing medication to patients. As such, they must be sure that they choose the right drug in the right dose to give to the right patient by the right route at the right time. Technicians may be responsible for preparation of drugs that must be reconstituted, mixed, or otherwise prepared before administration, and they must be sure that no errors occur in this process. Technicians often enter patient information into a computer profile for later verification by a pharmacist. Errors made in any of the steps to get the correct medication to the correct patient can carry through and cause potentially fatal errors. Technicians play a key role in minimizing the risk of such errors happening.

Safety First Patient safety is a top priority for pharmacists and pharmacy technicians. Technicians must be sure to choose the right drug, the right dose, and the right route and must check to make sure that no errors have been made in the drug preparation. Check your work!

Technicians may be trained on the job or by completing a formal program, such as a certificate of completion or associate degree program at a community or technical college.

On-the-Job Training. In some states, employers offer on-the-job training to technicians. Technicians are trained to perform tasks that are specific to the job or position for which they were hired. Usually, technicians are taught only those skills needed to perform the particular job. For example, a technician may be trained on the job to fill prescriptions or automated medication dispensing cabinets, compound IV solutions or medications, or enter prescription information into a computer database. When this type of training is very informal, a pharmacist or technician who is familiar with the job often instructs the trainee. In more structured training situations, the trainee participates in a training course developed by the employer.

Some practice sites offer training courses that consist of classroom teaching combined with hands-on experience that may last from a week to six months. In addition to covering general pharmacy topics, such as aseptic (sterile) technique, pharmaceutical calculations, technician responsibilities, and pharmacy rules and regulations, these courses may cover job-related issues such as patient confidentiality, organizational policies and procedures, and employee responsibilities.

Formal Programs. Community and technical college programs are broader in scope than on-the-job training. These programs are more rigorous and take from six to twenty-four months to complete. They cover the technical duties related to pharmacy, as well as such topics as medical terminology, pharmaceutical calculations, drug distribution systems, IV admixture procedures, and medication packaging techniques. In these programs, student technicians gain skills, knowledge, and experience by attending classes and completing clerkships (educational training in actual practice settings such as local hospitals or community pharmacies). After completion of many of these programs, students earn associate degrees or pharmacy technician certificates. Most programs offer full-time, part-time, and night classes, as well as financial assistance to those individuals who qualify. Some are available as online distance learning programs.

Pharmacists

Pharmacists are professionals who have had advanced training in the pharmaceutical sciences.

When filling prescriptions or medication orders, pharmacists depend on their education, experience, and professional judgment to determine whether the prescription is appropriate for each patient. Often, answers are not black and white, so they rely on their education, experience, and judgment to make the best decision. They are obliged to verify that the medication is appropriate for a patient's condition, that the dosage is correct, that the patient is not allergic to the drug, and that the prescribed medication will not interact with other medications the patient is taking. They must also educate the patient on how to take the medication properly and alert the patient to possible side effects of the drug. Pharmacists perform these functions every time a prescription or medication order is filled.

In all states, pharmacists must be licensed by the state's board of pharmacy before they can practice pharmacy and must follow the board of pharmacy regulations as they practice. Licensed pharmacists supervise the activities of technicians and are held accountable for the technicians' performance.

Pharmacists are required to earn a college or university degree in pharmacy to take the licensing examination offered by their state boards of pharmacy. To be qualified for enrollment in a college pharmacy degree program, students must have completed a minimum of two years of college course work that includes prerequisite classes for pharmacy school. While earning a pharmacy degree, would-be pharmacists learn how to use medical information to evaluate health care-related situations safely and effectively.

The first professional college degree that pharmacists graduating today usually earn is a doctor of pharmacy (PharmD), although some older pharmacists may hold a bachelor of science (BS) in pharmacy. Some schools of pharmacy have also developed "external PharmD" programs for pharmacists with BS degrees who wish to earn a PharmD Using advanced communication technology such as videoconferencing and the Internet, pharmacists can take classes from a school of pharmacy located any distance away, continue to work a full-time job, and maintain their family lives while fulfilling the requirements of a PharmD degree. Pharmacists who choose this option are often those who have several years of experience working as pharmacists and desire to advance their education but have other obligations that make it impractical for them to return to college full-time.

Many pharmacists have also completed one- or two-year postgraduate training programs called residencies. Residencies provide the opportunity to gain clinical experience, usually in hospital, ambulatory, or community settings, after earning a degree. Fellowships, usually two to three years long, also provide postgraduate training but focus on pharmacy research rather than clinical pharmacy practice.

Licensure and Certification

Before learning about licensure and certification for pharmacy technicians and pharmacists, it is important to know some key terminology. The American Society of Health-System Pharmacists (ASHP) Task Force on Technical Personnel in Pharmacy has provided these definitions:

- **Accreditation**—The process of granting recognition or vouching for conformance with established criteria (usually refers to recognition of an *institution*).[2]
- **Certification**—A voluntary process by which a nongovernmental agency or association grants recognition to an *individual* who has met certain predetermined qualifications specified by that agency or association. This recognition demonstrates to the public that the certified individual has achieved a certain level of knowledge, skill, or experience.[2]
- **Credentialing**—The process by which an organization or institution obtains, verifies, and assesses a pharmacist's qualifications to provide patient care.[2,3]
- **Licensure**—The process by which an agency of government grants permission to an individual to engage in a given occupation upon finding that the applicant has attained the minimal degree of competency necessary to ensure that the public health, safety, and welfare will be reasonably well protected.[2]
- **Registration**—The process of making a list or being enrolled in an existing list. Registration of pharmacy technicians by state boards may be required to legally carry out some functions.[4]

Pharmacy Technicians

Successful completion of an accredited pharmacy technician program or certification examination helps assure pharmacy employers and patients that pharmacy technicians have met a predefined set of standards and possess an established set of skills and knowledge. Some states and employers may require one or the other, but even if they don't, pharmacy technicians who are certified or who have completed an accredited training program may have an advantage in terms of job responsibilities, salary, and seniority over technicians who are not certified or who have not completed such a program.

Pharmacy Technician Certification. In 1994, several professional organizations, including the ASHP, the American Pharmaceutical Association (APhA, now known as the American Pharmacists Association), the American Association of Colleges of Pharmacy (AACP), and the National Association of Boards of Pharmacy (NABP), completed a joint endeavor named the Scope of Pharmacy Practice Project. The objective of the project was to perform a validated task analysis of the functions, responsibilities, and tasks of pharmacists and technicians. This analysis documented what pharmacy technicians actually do and what knowledge they need to effectively perform those tasks.

Participants in the Scope of Pharmacy Practice Project identified the need for a national technician recognition program to replace the various state programs that then existed. In 1995, APhA, ASHP, the Illinois Council of Hospital Pharmacists (ICHP, now known as the Illinois Council of Health System Pharmacists), and the Michigan Pharmacists Association (MPA) established the Pharmacy Technician Certification Board (PTCB). The PTCB was created to develop a voluntary national pharmacy technician certification program.[5]

Some states require registration of pharmacy technicians, whereas other states require certification; still others are considering the matter. There is no national requirement for certification at this time. However, a 2007 consumer survey conducted by the PTCB revealed that 73% of the public believes that "pharmacy technicians are required by law to be trained and certified before they can help prepare prescriptions." Most consumers (91%) felt that employers should hire only certified pharmacy technicians.[6] Given this strong public opinion, it may be only a matter of time before certification is mandated by law.

✔Most consumers believe that all pharmacy technicians have been trained and certified before they are allowed to prepare prescriptions.

Technicians who wish to become certified may take the national Pharmacy Technician Certification Examination (PTCE) offered by the PTCB. The first such examination was held in 1995. To take the examination, candidates must have earned a high school diploma or a graduate equivalency diploma (GED or foreign diploma) and submit the appropriate application form, fee, and supporting documents. Candidates are not eligible if they have been convicted of a drug- or pharmacy-related felony, or have had any felony convictions any time during the five years before applying for the PTCE.

The PTCE is a two-hour, closed-book, computer-based examination consisting of eighty multiple-choice questions plus an additional ten non-scored questions. The non-scored questions are pretest questions and are not used in calculating the candidate's score, but provide information for possible use on future examinations. Each question has four possible answers from which to choose, with only one being the best, or correct, answer. The score is based on the number of correctly answered questions.

The questions are written to assess the knowledge and skills that are deemed necessary to perform the work of pharmacy technicians. The exam divides these activities into three function areas:

I. *Assisting the pharmacist in serving patients*, including activities related to dispensing prescriptions, distributing medications, and collecting and organizing information
II. *Maintaining medication and inventory control systems* pertaining to activities related to purchasing medications and supplies, controlling inventory, and storing, preparing, and distributing medications according to policies and procedures
III. *Participating in the administration and management of pharmacy practice,* including administrative activities that deal with such issues as operations, human resources, facilities and equipment, and information systems

Of the scored questions on the examination, 66% of the examination tests the candidate on topics in function area I, 22% on topics in function area II, and the remaining 12% on topics in function area III. Candidates who pass the exam may use the designation *CPhT* (certified pharmacy technician) after their names.

To maintain the certification, technicians must recertify every two years by completing at least twenty hours of continuing education. A maximum of ten hours may be earned at the technician's workplace under the direct supervision of a pharmacist. These hours must be special assignments or training; regular work hours do not apply. At least one hour of continuing education must be related to pharmacy law. Several references are available to assist candidates preparing for the examination. Refer to the PTCB Web site to verify current eligibility requirements and test specifics (www.ptcb.org).

In 2005, the Institute for the Certification of Pharmacy Technicians (ICPT) also began offering a national certification examination, called the Exam for the Certification of Pharmacy Technicians (ExCPT). It is offered in an on-demand, computer-based format; pharmacy technicians may take the examination at any time at any one of over 600 supervised test centers throughout the United States. After completing the ExCPT, and before leaving the testing center, technicians are immediately given the examination results.

Eligibility requirements to take the ExCPT are similar to those of the PTCE. The ExCPT is a two-hour test with 110 multiple-choice questions (of which 10 are not counted in the score) examination. Questions are categorized into three areas:

1. *Regulations and Technician Duties* (25% of the examination), which includes questions about technician duties and general information, controlled substances, and other laws and regulations
2. *Drugs and Therapy* (23% of the examination), which contains questions about drug classification and most frequently prescribed medications
3. *Dispensing Process* (52% of the examination), which relates to areas such as prescription information, preparing/dispensing prescriptions, calculations, sterile products, and unit dose and repackaging

Pharmacy technicians must recertify every two years by completing twenty hours of continuing education, with at least one hour related to pharmacy law. Refer to the ICPT Web site to verify current eligibility requirements and test specifics (http://www.nationaltechexam.org/excptinfo.html). Check with your state's board of pharmacy to determine which certification examination is required or accepted for pharmacy technicians in your state.

Rx for Success

Whether or not your state requires technician certification, becoming certified and maintaining the certification is advantageous. The knowledge and skills that are tested by either the PTCE or the ExCPT are pertinent to any technician working in any pharmacy practice setting. Becoming certified demonstrates a commitment to your profession and to your career.

The National Pharmacy Technician Association (NPTA) offers further certification in two specialty areas: sterile products and compounding. To obtain these additional certifications, candidates must complete several home-study modules and pass module exams before attending a two-day training institute in Texas. While attending the training institute, candidates get hands-on teaching and experience. Upon completion, a certificate of validated training is awarded to candidates.

Pharmacy Technician Training Program Accreditation. Currently, the ASHP is the only organization that specifically accredits pharmacy technician training programs. Many ASHP-accredited programs are offered by vocational, technical, and community colleges, although some hospitals, chain drug stores, and military branches also have ASHP-accredited programs. Accreditation standardizes the formal training that pharmacy technicians receive; it also provides institutions that offer a technician training program with guidelines on how to train competent pharmacy technicians. Pharmacy technician training programs must meet minimum requirements, or criteria, set by ASHP to earn accreditation.[4]

The goals of ASHP accreditation are to upgrade and standardize technician training, assist and recognize such training programs, provide criteria for technician trainees as they choose a technician training program, provide pharmacies with a yardstick with which to measure the level of competency of pharmacy technicians, and assist in the advancement and professional development of pharmacy technicians. Other organizations also offer guidelines for pharmacy technician training: for example, the APhA offers guidelines for nuclear pharmacy technician training programs.[7]

Pharmacists

After earning a PharmD degree, pharmacy graduates must pass examinations as required by their state's board of pharmacy. These examinations test pharmacy skills, knowledge, and pharmacy law. A board of pharmacy includes pharmacists and members of the public who have been appointed to the board by the state governor or state legislature. The members of a state board of pharmacy are responsible for protecting the citizens of their state. The board does so by passing pharmacy rules and regulations to be followed in addition to the laws enacted by the state legislature. Once candidates have fulfilled their state's board of pharmacy requirements, they become registered pharmacists (R.Ph.) and are allowed to practice pharmacy in that state.

Some pharmacists also choose to become certified as pharmacotherapy specialists. After passing a certification examination, they earn the title of board-certified pharmacotherapy specialist and may add the initials BCPS to their credentials. These pharmacists must still comply with the requirements of their state's board of pharmacy. There are also certification examinations for nutrition support, nuclear pharmacy, psychiatric pharmacy, oncology, and, most recently, ambulatory care. Other specialty certification examinations are under consideration. Pharmacists who have expertise in a specialty area may submit portfolios that outline their education and experience in the area for review. If the portfolios meet the requirements, these pharmacists may add the term "added qualification" to their credentials. Currently, the approved added qualifications are cardiology and infectious diseases.

Professionalism

As members of the profession of pharmacy, pharmacists and pharmacy technicians are expected to practice and act in a professional manner at all times. Professionalism is actively demonstrating the attitudes, qualities, and behaviors of a person well educated in an area of specialized knowledge. An important aspect of acting professionally is putting the needs of others before one's own. Professionalism also refers to the way in which members of a profession present themselves and communicate with others.

For pharmacy technicians, a good place to start when discussing professionalism is the Code of Ethics for Pharmacy Technicians (box 1–1). This code outlines ten guiding principles that pharmacy technicians are encouraged to follow.[4] To these ethical principles, ASHP adds ten characteristics of a professional (box 1–2).[8] These characteristics are equally applicable to pharmacy technicians. Violation of these values and qualities not only is unprofessional but also may be against federal or state law.

Practical examples of professional conduct include respect for patients' privacy and keeping patient information confidential, participation in continuing education courses and seminars, and cultivating an honest, conscientious attitude while performing job-related activities. Asking a sports celebrity for an autograph while he or she is hospitalized is not professional behavior. Neither

Box 1-1. Code of Ethics for Pharmacy Technicians[4]

Preamble

Pharmacy Technicians are health care professionals who assist pharmacists in providing the best possible care for patients. The principles of this code, which apply to pharmacy technicians working in any and all settings, are based on the application and support of the moral obligations that guide the pharmacy profession in relationships with patients, healthcare professionals, and society.

Principles

- A pharmacy technician's first consideration is to ensure the health and safety of the patient, and to use knowledge and skills to the best of his or her ability in serving patients.
- A pharmacy technician supports and promotes honesty and integrity in the profession, which includes a duty to observe the law, maintain the highest moral and ethical conduct at all times, and uphold the ethical principles of the profession.
- A pharmacy technician assists and supports pharmacists in the safe and efficacious and cost-effective distribution of health services and health care resources.
- A pharmacy technician respects and values the abilities of pharmacists, colleagues, and other healthcare professionals.
- A pharmacy technician maintains competency in his or her practice and continually enhances his or her professional knowledge and expertise.
- A pharmacy technician respects and supports the patient's individuality, dignity, and confidentiality.
- A pharmacy technician respects the confidentiality of a patient's records and discloses pertinent information only with proper authorization.
- A pharmacy technician never assists in dispensing, promoting, or distribution of medication or medical devices that are not of good quality or that do not meet the standards required by law.
- A pharmacy technician does not engage in any activity that will discredit the profession, and will expose, without fear or favor, illegal or unethical conduct of the profession.
- A pharmacy technician associates with and engages in the support of organizations that promote the profession of pharmacy through the utilization and enhancement of pharmacy technicians.

Originally published in American Society of Health System Pharmacists. White paper on pharmacy technicians 2002: Needed changes can no longer wait. Am J Health-Syst Pharm. 2003;60:37–51.

Box 1-2. Ten Characteristics of a Professional[8]

1. Knowledge and skills of the profession
2. Commitment to self-improvement of skills and knowledge
3. Service orientation
4. Pride in and service to the profession
5. Covenantal relationship with the patient
6. Creativity and innovation
7. Conscience and trustworthiness
8. Accountability for his or her work
9. Ethically sound decision making
10. Leadership

is adding an extra two weeks to a medication's expiration date in order to "use it all up."

Pharmacy technicians must remember that "patients are people first" and treat them with courtesy and respect. Depending on the practice setting, a pharmacy technician may be the first person with whom a patient has contact, and it is important that the technician interact with the patient in a competent and professional manner. As in any profession, good customer (patient) service is the mark of a professional and provides the patient with a sense of confidence in the service that the technician, and other health care providers, offer.

Communicating and interacting in a professional manner is equally important among coworkers. Maintaining self-control and a professional attitude when solving work problems creates a more professional and efficient work environment (see Chapter 8, Communication and Teamwork).

Personal appearance communicates a message as well. It is important for pharmacy technicians, whether wearing scrubs or a lab coat, to project a professional image. Neatness in appearance is an easy way to build professional behavior. A professional appearance conveys a serious attitude about the work.

Another way that a pharmacy technician can become more professional is to join a membership organization such as the NPTA or the American Association of Pharmacy Technicians (AAPT). These types of organizations offer members benefits and services that support pharmacy technician professionalism. These services include continuing education opportunities, job placement services, subscriptions to pharmacy technician journals and newsletters, and online discussion groups and networks. Many national and state pharmacist organizations also offer membership to technicians or sponsor technician sections within their organizations.

Rx for Success

Become an active member of your local pharmacy technician organization; regularly read pharmacy technician-related publications, such as newsletters and journals; and find opportunities for continuing education.

Pharmacy Practice Settings

The profession of pharmacy is practiced in many environments, which are commonly divided into *ambulatory care* and *institutional* settings. Ambulatory care, or outpatient, settings serve patients living in their own homes or similar situations and include community (ambulatory) clinics, home care, and mail order. Institutional or inpatient settings are those in which patients reside in a facility where they receive long- or short-term care from health professionals. The two primary institutional settings are long-term care and hospitals. Other examples of pharmacy practice settings include pharmacy benefit managers and managed care, hospice care, research facilities, educational centers, and the pharmaceutical industry.

Often, two or more of these practice settings—for example, a hospital, an outpatient surgery center, home care services, and an ambulatory clinic—may have a working relationship with each other and may even be managed or owned by the same business entity. These settings may then be "packaged" together as a **health-system**. Health systems are intended to provide complete health care–related services to the patients they serve. Although the specific pharmacy activities of practice settings may vary, the primary goal of each remains the same: to ensure that patients receive optimal drug therapy to maintain or restore their health.

Community Pharmacy

The community pharmacy is the corner drugstore or the local retail or grocery store pharmacy. Community pharmacies can be members of a chain of pharmacies or can be independently owned. Usually, patients are customers who are treated as outpatients by doctors and who come into the store with prescriptions. Generally, these patients live in their own homes, under their own care.

Technicians in community settings often prepare prescription labels for checking by a pharmacist, order and maintain drug inventory, process insurance claims, and operate a cash register. In some states, pharmacy technicians may fill prescriptions to be later checked by a pharmacist. Pharmacy technicians must be familiar with brand and generic names, dosage forms, and therapeutic uses of common prescription and over-the-counter medications. Good communication skills, including telephone etiquette and the ability to interpret nonverbal body language, are critical for community pharmacy technicians, because they have a lot of direct patient interaction.

Additional information about community and ambulatory care pharmacy practice is found in Chapter 3.

Mail-Order Pharmacy

Pharmacists and technicians also work in mail-order facilities, through which patients have their prescriptions filled and refilled through the mail. The major difference between mail-order and community pharmacies is the lack of face-to-face contact with patients. Technicians' duties in a mail-order pharmacy are similar to those in the community setting and require the same amount of competence. Mail-order pharmacists must use their professional judgment, just as in community and institutional settings.

Pharmacy Benefit Managers and Managed Care

A pharmacy benefit manager (PBM) oversees prescription medication programs and processes and pays prescription medication insurance claims. A PBM also develops and maintains a medication formulary, or list of approved prescription medications, from which physicians may prescribe for the PBM's patient members. Because a PBM has a large number of members, it can negotiate with drug manufacturers for medication discounts and rebates and may contract with pharmacies for their services. By doing so, a PBM is able to offer prescription medications at lower prices to its members. Pharmacists and pharmacy technicians who work in a PBM environment usually do not have direct patient contact but instead manage drug therapy on a global scale by collecting information from patients' computerized medication profiles and pooling it into a large database. Prescription drug use and physician prescribing patterns are analyzed for trends that indicate optimal or suboptimal medication therapy. Pharmacists subsequently try to minimize drug costs and improve patient outcomes or results through the development of medication formularies and disease-specific medication therapy guidelines. Pharmacy technicians who work for a PBM may collect data, research information, and assist pharmacists in writing reports.

A managed care program is a type of health insurance program that allows patients to pay a blanket fee for their health care services rather than by the traditional fee-for-service system. Managed care programs attempt to improve the quality of health care delivery and patient outcomes. One definition of a managed care prescription program is "the application of management principles to achieve maximum health outcomes at the lowest cost."[9] Managed care programs often operate ambulatory clinics and hospitals from which their patient members obtain their health care.

Hospital Pharmacy

Patients are admitted to hospitals for short-term, supervised medical care by health care professionals in a structured, formal manner. Pharmacists are directly involved with patient care and have daily interactions with physicians, nurses, and other caregivers. They develop plans of pharmaceutical care and medication management and, with the other caregivers, monitor the patients' drug therapy. Depending on the size of the hospital, some pharmacists provide specialized services in areas such as pediatrics, oncology, infectious diseases, nutrition support, and drug information.

In addition to providing direct patient care, pharmacists evaluate trends in medication use and physician prescribing, develop guidelines for medication use, educate patients and health care professionals, and implement and maintain drug distribution systems. They also work with nurses, physicians, and other members of hospital committees and workgroups, both within and outside the pharmacy department.[10]

Pharmacy technicians in hospitals work with pharmacists to accomplish many of the pharmacy's goals. Generally, technicians may enter physician medication orders into the pharmacy computer system, prepare IV drug admixtures, repackage and label unit dose medications, restock automated dispensing cabinets, deliver medications, and complete paperwork for quality assurance or billing purposes. In some hospitals, pharmacy technicians may dispense medications from a preapproved list or even administer some types of medications.

Additional information about hospital pharmacy practice is found in Chapter 4.

Part 1

Home Health Care

Home health care is defined as "physician ordered services provided to patients at their residences, be it their own homes or any other setting in which the patients live."[11] Such services may include personal care, hospice and respite care, shopping assistance, drug and infusion therapy, and speech, physical, and occupational therapy.[11,12] Home care pharmacists assess the patient for the appropriateness of home medication administration and develop a medication management plan to educate and monitor the patient. Medications administered in the home setting may be as simple as oral tablets or capsules or as complex as continuous infusions of pain medications or total parenteral nutrition (TPN).

Technician duties in a home care setting may include preparing sterile injectable products, maintaining computerized patient profiles, and delivering medications and supplies to a patient's home.

Additional information about home care pharmacy practice is found in Chapter 5.

Long-Term Care

Long-term care facilities are those institutions where patients stay for extended periods. They include nursing homes, psychiatric or behavioral health institutions, intermediate care facilities for mentally disabled patients, and skilled nursing facilities. Patients in these settings require professional care, but not to the same degree as hospitalized patients. Most of these facilities do not have pharmacies on site but contract with local community pharmacies for pharmacy services; pharmacists and pharmacy technicians thus do not have direct patient interaction. However, pharmacists and technicians in long-term care practices perform many of the same functions as those in other settings.

Hospice care is care that is given to those patients with incurable diseases who are generally not expected to live more than six months. Hospice care may be offered in long-term care settings, hospitals, or patients' own homes. The aim of hospice care is not to cure the disease, but to provide dying patients with the best possible quality of life for the remainder of their lives. Pharmacist and pharmacy technician activities in hospice settings focus on the relief of symptoms (e.g., pain, nausea, vomiting, anxiety) rather than on treating disease.

Specialty Pharmacy Services

Some areas of pharmacy practice, such as nuclear pharmacy and veterinary pharmacy, require very specific knowledge and expertise. Just as pharmacists may choose to specialize in an area of pharmacy (e.g., ambulatory care, cardiology, infectious diseases, nutrition, oncology, organ transplantation, or pediatrics), so may technicians. Technicians may specialize in areas such as inventory purchasing and management, sterile product preparation, surgical pharmacy, nuclear pharmacy, veterinary pharmacy, and nonsterile (extemporaneous) compounding.

Additional information about specialty pharmacy practice is found in Chapter 6.

Expansion of Technician Responsibilities

Rx for Success

To perform duties in a competent manner, technicians must develop the ability to determine the best course of action in a specific situation. Applying critical thinking skills allows pharmacy technicians to prioritize, problem-solve, and troubleshoot issues that arise that may not require the judgment of a pharmacist but that still call for careful attention.

Table 1–1 lists some of the functions that pharmacy technicians perform in community and institutional pharmacy settings.[13] Some of the listed functions are not routinely performed by all technicians in all inpatient or outpatient pharmacies. Most pharmacy technicians perform routine activities such as answering telephone calls, obtaining patient information, and updating patient profiles. Technicians with advanced skills and knowledge may perform more sophisticated functions, such as checking the work of another technician, dispensing medications from an approved list, or even administering medications.[14–18]

As the demand for cost-effective health care increases, pharmacy technicians with well-developed critical thinking skills may find themselves assuming responsibilities previously assigned to pharmacists. In some situations, after gaining the right experience and expertise, some technicians may even assume managerial duties and be promoted to supervisory positions once held by pharmacists. The role of pharmacy technicians will continue to change and develop as the profession of pharmacy evolves to meet the changing health care needs of the public.

Rx for Success

Demonstrating an eagerness to learn and take on more responsibilities can help advance your career.

Trends in Pharmacy Practice

The profession of pharmacy involves much more than counting tablets and filling prescriptions. Pharmacists and pharmacy technicians are important members of a patient's health care team. They contribute specialized medication knowledge and expertise to the team. Integration of the technicians' knowledge with that of other team members (e.g., pharmacists, nurses, physicians, social workers, etc.) may be described by concepts known as pharmaceutical care and medication therapy management.

Pharmaceutical Care and Medication Therapy Management

The concept of pharmaceutical care was introduced in the early 1990s. **Pharmaceutical care** is defined as "the direct, responsible provision of medication-related care for the purpose of achieving definite outcomes that improve a patient's quality of life."[19]

Pharmaceutical care involves cooperation between a pharmacist, patient, and other health care professionals

Table 1–1. Tasks Typically Performed by Certified Pharmacy Technicians (as allowed by individual state law)[13]

This list is based on the results of a survey conducted in 2005 of 4,000 certified pharmacy technicians wherein survey respondents were asked to rate elements of their job functions, responsibilities, and knowledge.

Ambulatory Care Pharmacies	■ Accept electronic refill authorizations from prescribers ■ Assist the pharmacist in obtaining patient information such as diagnosis, desired therapeutic outcome, disease state, and medication history ■ Assess prescription or medication order for completeness, accuracy, authenticity, legality, and reimbursement eligibility ■ Update the medical record or patient profile ■ Assist the patient in choosing the best payment assistance plan ■ Select the appropriate product for dispensing (e.g., brand names; generic substitutes) ■ Assemble patient information materials ■ Check for accuracy during processing of the prescription or medication order ■ Provide medication and supplemental information to the patient ■ Communicate with third-party payers to determine or verify coverage and to obtain prior authorizations ■ Communicate with third-party payers and patients or to rectify rejected third-party claims ■ Identify and resolve problems with rejected claims ■ Direct patient or patient's representative to pharmacist for counseling ■ Maintain required inventories and records ■ Update and maintain patient information ■ Perform billing and accounting functions for products and services
Institutional Pharmacies	■ Package finished dosage forms ■ Assemble equipment and supplies necessary for compounding prescriptions or medication orders ■ Perform calculations required for preparation of compounded IV admixtures ■ Compound medications for dispensing according to prescription and compounding guidelines ■ Prepare sterile products ■ Record medication preparation and ingredients ■ Place medications in dispensing system ■ Deliver medications to patient care unit ■ Record distribution of controlled substances ■ Receive pharmaceuticals, medical equipment, devices, and supplies, and verify against purchase orders ■ Place pharmaceuticals, medical equipment, devices, and supplies in inventory under proper storage conditions while incorporating error-prevention strategies ■ Perform non–patient-specific preparation, distribution, and maintenance of pharmaceuticals, medical equipment, devices, and supplies while incorporating error-prevention strategies ■ Maintain required inventories and records ■ Repackage finished dosage forms for dispensing ■ Perform and record routine sanitation, maintenance, and calibration of equipment
Ambulatory and Institutional Pharmacies	■ Affix labels and auxiliary labels to containers ■ Prepare prescriptions and medication orders for final check by pharmacist

Table 1-1. Tasks Typically Performed by Certified Pharmacy Technicians (as allowed by individual state law)[13] (continued)

	■ Store medication prior to distribution ■ Remove from inventory expired, discontinued, slow-moving, overstocked, and recalled pharmaceuticals, medical equipment, devices, and supplies ■ Coordinate written, electronic, and oral communications throughout the practice setting (e.g., route telephone calls, faxes, and oral and written refill authorizations; disseminate policy and procedure changes) ■ Update, maintain, and use job-related manual or electronic information systems ■ Coordinate and participate in staff training and continuing education
Quality Assurance	■ Multiple-point checking ■ Assist pharmacist in monitoring patient outcomes (e.g., collect patient-specific data) ■ Inventory control (e.g., separation of medications; bar code scanning; process verification; system updates) ■ Coordinate written, electronic, and oral medication error communications throughout the practice setting (e.g., unapproved abbreviations; look-alike and sound-alike medications) ■ Education, training, and certification ■ Review discrepancies and billing and fraud errors

in designing, implementing, and monitoring a therapeutic medication plan. It consists of three major functions:

1. Identification of potential and actual drug-related problems
2. Resolution of actual drug-related problems
3. Prevention of potential drug-related problems

Pharmaceutical care makes the pharmacist directly responsible to the patient for the quality of the patient's care. The basic goals, processes, and relationships of pharmaceutical care are the same regardless of practice setting.[19]

More recently, **medication therapy management (MTM)** has become the pharmacy practice model. In 2003, the Medicare Modernization Act was signed into federal law. Under this act, Medicare prescription drug providers are required to establish MTM programs that improve medication use and reduce adverse events.

Medication therapy management has been defined as "a distinct service or group of services that optimize therapeutic outcomes for individual patients. Medication therapy management services are independent of, but can occur in conjunction with, the provision of a medication product."[20] These services include assessment of a patient's health status; formulation of a medication treatment plan; selection, initiation, modification, or administration of medication therapy; monitoring of the patient's response to therapy; review of medications for medication-related problems; documentation and communication of care; provision of patient education and information to increase patient understanding and appropriate use of medications; and coordination and integration of MTM services into the broader health care services provided to the patient.[20]

Increasing Impact of Technology

Technical advances are changing the practice of pharmacy. Computers, bar coding, and robotic systems have been developed to dispense medications and monitor medication use more accurately, timely, and cost-effectively. Because advanced computer systems collect and store patient information, information is more accurate and easier to access. Checks and balances (e.g., checks for drug interactions, patient allergies, and duplicate therapy) are built into computer systems and result in fewer errors. Automation of these checks and balances and other traditional functions allows pharmacists more time for activities that require their professional judgment and expertise. In turn, pharmacists are relying more than ever on technicians to operate and maintain these new systems.

TECHNOLOGY TOPICS

Automated dispensing technology is more accurate and faster than manual dispensing.

The major advantage of automated dispensing technology is that it is more accurate and faster than humans and makes the dispensing process safer for patients. However, technology and machines can—and do—fail, so it is still necessary for a human to check the work of a machine. Many medication-related errors occur when pharmacists and pharmacy technicians assume that technology functions correctly 100% of the time. As an example, a bar code label could be damaged so that a bar code scanner either does not read the label or reads it incorrectly, causing the wrong medication to be dispensed to a patient. It is the duty of the pharmacy technician working with the scanner to identify and correct the malfunction and error before the medication even leaves the pharmacy.

Safety First Technology and machines can fail or malfunction, so it is still necessary for a human to oversee their use.

Machines are programmed to perform their jobs the exact same way every time. They do not have the ability to use judgment. Pharmacists and pharmacy technicians must still apply judgment when checking the work of a machine. For example, an IV pump may be programmed to allow a certain medication to be infused at a rate no faster than 50 mL/hour. But a certain patient who is critically ill might need the medication infused at 100 mL/hour. A pharmacist must use judgment to determine whether or not to override the IV pump's programming and to allow the medication to infuse at that faster rate.

Increasing Use of Outpatient Services

More and more, patients are cared for and treated as outpatients. This is a result of the need to contain the skyrocketing costs of health care. Patients who would have been admitted to the hospital a day or two before surgery are now admitted on the day of the procedure and discharged earlier. Many hospitals have established outpatient surgery centers that admit patients for surgery and release them hours later. For many diagnostic tests, patients are no longer admitted to a hospital but are seen as outpatients, and return home shortly after the tests.

The practice of pharmacy is changing to adapt to the new health care environment. Some clinics and outpatient centers have pharmacists and pharmacies available on site. In these settings, pharmacists have less time to gather patient information and thus depend more on technicians to assist them in providing optimal pharmaceutical care.[21]

Summary

Pharmacy technicians are key professionals who may be found in virtually all pharmacy practice settings. They perform their jobs with a high degree of professionalism and are critical to the successful operation of any pharmacy. Pharmacy technicians now commonly review and fill medication orders or prescriptions that are then checked by a pharmacist. Technicians also do most of the IV admixture and sterile compounding. More and more computer-entry functions, such as patient billing and order entry, are also the responsibility of technicians. In some settings, technicians may check each other's work, dispense medications from a preapproved list, or administer medications.

Given the changes occurring in the pharmacy profession, the roles of pharmacy technicians in all settings are expanding, and more is expected from technicians than in the past. Increasingly, technicians are primarily responsible for the mechanical and routine aspects of pharmacy practice; they are also called upon to develop and use critical thinking skills and to prioritize activities, make timely decisions, and solve problems. As a team, pharmacists and pharmacy technicians work to improve patient care, avoid medication errors, and optimize medication use.

Self-Assessment Questions

1. Which of the following is true of certification?
   a. Certification is granted by a governmental agency to an institution in recognition that the institution has met predetermined requirements.
   b. Certification is a voluntary process whereby a person who has met defined requirements established by a nongovernmental agency or association is recognized by that agency or association as having met those requirements.
   c. Certification is a mandatory process whereby a person who has met requirements established by a governmental agency is endorsed by that agency as having met established criteria.
   d. Certification is a process whereby a governmental agency allows a person to perform the duties associated with an occupation after that person has demonstrated the minimum acceptable degree of competency in that occupation.
2. Tekno Technical College has a new pharmacy technician training program. The administration wants to show that the program meets the national standards for pharmacy technician education. Which type of recognition will the program seek?
   a. Accreditation
   b. Certification
   c. Licensure
   d. Registration
3. From a legal standpoint, who is ultimately responsible for a pharmacy technician's activities and performance?
   a. The technician who performs the activity
   b. The patient's physician
   c. The technician with the most experience and seniority
   d. The supervising pharmacist
4. How can a pharmacy technician become certified?
   a. By submitting the proper application and documentation to the state board of pharmacy
   b. By working as a pharmacy technician for the number of years specified by the state medical board
   c. By passing a national examination that evaluates the technician's knowledge and skills needed to perform the work of pharmacy technicians
   d. By passing a test offered by the National Association of Boards of Pharmacy that assesses the technician's knowledge of drug therapy and pharmacokinetics
5. Which of the following activities is a typical pharmacy technician duty?
   a. Recommending an antibiotic to treat an ear infection in an infant to a physician
   b. Filling an automated medication dispensing cabinet in a nursing home
   c. Giving a nurse an order for an alternative medication to morphine for a patient who has had an allergic reaction to morphine in the past
   d. Filling in for a pharmacist when she is on her lunch break
6. What is medication therapy management?
   a. Proper storage and handling of medication
   b. Medication-related advertising that is directed to consumers from drug manufacturers
   c. Medication-related information provided to physicians and other health care professionals by pharmacists
   d. A service or group of services that optimize therapeutic outcomes for individual patients
7. A(n)______________ pharmacy practice setting is one in which pharmacists care for patients in their own places of residence.
   a. Home health care
   b. Institutional
   c. Acute care
   d. Ambulatory
8. Which of the following statements is false?
   a. Technicians must conduct themselves in a professional manner when performing their job duties.
   b. Pharmacists are solely responsible for assuring patient medication safety.
   c. A characteristic of a professional includes pride in his or her chosen profession.

Self-Assessment Questions

d. Even after completion of a training program, technicians should still participate in continuing education programs.

9. As a pharmacy technician, you may perform all of the following activities except which?
   a. Entering orders into a computer or patient profile
   b. Performing mathematical calculations
   c. Checking the work of other technicians
   d. Changing the dose of a prescribed medication on the basis of a patient's poor kidney function
10. A pharmacy technician's job duties ________.
    a. Are the same as a pharmacist's, but the technician's work must be checked by a pharmacist
    b. Are the same for each technician position within a practice setting
    c. Include routine tasks that require professional judgment
    d. May include medication preparation, inventory management, and training of other technicians

Self-Assessment Answers

1. b. Certification is a *voluntary* process granted by a *nongovernmental* agency to an *individual* and recognizes that the individual has met certain requirements set forth by that agency. Therefore, choices a, c, and d are incorrect.
2. a. Certification is associated with personal achievement of standard criteria, while accreditation is associated with organizational achievement. Licensure is a governmental recognition of the right to perform a specific occupation. Registration is a listing function.
3. d. While the physician may be ultimately responsible for a patient's care, the pharmacist is ultimately responsible for the actions of technicians working under his or her supervision.
4. c. Certification is offered by an independent organization and is not affiliated with either the State Boards of Pharmacy or the National Association of Boards of Pharmacy. Although working as a technician for a number of years might increase the likelihood of passing the certification exam, it is not sufficient to earn certification.
5. b. All the other answers are tasks that must be done by a pharmacist.
6. d. Medication storage and handling, as well as both consumer and professional information, may be parts of medication therapy management, but the more comprehensive definition of a service or group of services that optimize therapeutic outcomes for individual patients is the best answer.
7. a. Home health care pharmacists serve patients in their own homes. Institutional and acute care pharmacists generally work in hospitals or long-term care facilities. Ambulatory pharmacists generally see patients in an outpatient setting but do not serve patients directly in their homes.
8. b. While pharmacists are ultimately responsible for assuring patient medication safety, technicians also play a critical role. The remaining statements are all true.
9. d. The other functions listed are acceptable for technicians to perform, but a pharmacist must do all dose adjustments.
10. d. Pharmacists usually do not have the same job duties as technicians. Technician duties may be the same for each technician position within a practice setting or may vary based on the job assignment and expected activities. Technicians perform routine tasks that do *not* require professional judgment; those that do are carried out by pharmacists.

Resources

More information about the PTCE pharmacy certification examination may be obtained from the Pharmacy Technician Certification Board at 1100 15th Street, NW, Suite 730, Washington, DC, 20005-1707, or at (800) 363–8012 or www.ptcb.org. Specifics about the exam may be found in the *Guidebook to Certification* at www.ptcb.org/AM/Template.cfm?Section=Guidebook_to_Certification&Template=/CM/HTMLDisplay .cfm&ContentID=2952.

More information about the ExCPT pharmacy certification examination may be obtained from the Institute for the Certification of Pharmacy Technicians at 2536 South Old Highway 94, Suite 214, St. Charles, MO, 63303, or at (314) 442–6775 or www.nationaltechexam.org/home.html. Specifics about the exam may be found in the *Candidates' Guide—2008*, at www.nationaltechexam.org/excptinfo.html.

American Association of Pharmacy Technicians: www.pharmacytechnician.com.

American Society of Health-System Pharmacists (pharmacy technician page): www.ashp.org/technicians.

National Pharmacy Technician Association: www.pharmacytechnician.org.

Links to each state's board of pharmacy may be found on the National Association of Boards of Pharmacy Web site: www.nabp.net.

Criteria for pharmacy technician training programs for accreditation by the American Society of Health-System Pharmacists may be found on the ASHP Web site: www.ashp.org/s_ashp/docs/files/RTP_TechStandards.pdf.

References

1. Pharmacy Technician Certification Board. What is a pharmacy technician? Available at: www.ptcb.org/AM/Template.cfm?Section=Learn&Template=/CM/ContentCombo.cfm&NavMenuID=565&ContentID=2729. Accessed November 19, 2009.
2. The Council on Credentialing in Pharmacy. Credentialing in pharmacy. *Am J Health-Syst Pharm.* 2001;58:69–76.
3. Galt KA. Credentialing and privileging for pharmacists. *Am J Health-Syst Pharm.* 2004;61:661–670.
4. American Society of Health-System Pharmacists. White paper on pharmacy technicians 2002: Needed changes can no longer wait. *Am J Health-Syst Pharm.* 2003;60:37–51.
5. Zellmer WA. Pharmacy technicians, part 1: National certification. *Am J Health-Syst Pharm.* 1995; 52:918. Editorial.
6. TCB. Survey Shows Broad Support Among Americans For Pharmacy Technician Certification. Available at: https://www.ptcb.org/AM/Template.cfm?Section=Press_Releases1&CONTENTID=2752&TEMPLATE=/CM/ContentDisplay.cfm. Accessed November 19, 2009.
7. American Pharmacists Association. Guidelines for nuclear pharmacy technician training programs. Available at: www.pharmacist.com/AM/Template.cfm?Section=Search1&section=APPM&template= /CM/ContentDisplay.cfm&ContentFileID=214. Accessed November 19, 2009.
8. American Pharmacists Association. Ten characteristics of a professional. *J Am Pharm Assoc.* 2003; 43(1):93–104.
9. Schafermeyer KW. Overview of pharmacy in managed health care. In: Ito SM, Blackburn S, eds. *A Pharmacist's Guide to Principles and Practices of Managed Care Pharmacy.* Alexandria, VA: Foundation for Managed Care Pharmacy; 1995:15–26.
10. American Society of Health-System Pharmacists. ASHP guidelines: Minimum standard for pharmacies in hospitals. *Am J Health-Syst Pharm.* 1995;52:2711–2717.
11. Catania PN. Introduction to home health care. In: Catania PN, Rosner MM, eds. *Home Health Care Practice*, 2nd ed. Palo Alto, CA: Health Markets Research; 1994:1–11.
12. American Society of Hospital Pharmacists. ASHP guidelines on the pharmacist's role in home care. *Am J Hosp Pharm.* 2000;57:1252–1257.
13. Muenzen PM, Corrigan MM, Smith MA, et al. Updating the Pharmacy Technician Certification Examination: A practice analysis study. *Am Journal Health-Syst Pharm.* 2005;62:2542–2546.
14. Andersen SR, St Peter JV, Macres MG, et al. Accuracy of technicians versus pharmacists in checking syringes prepared for a dialysis program. *Am J Health-Syst Pharm.* 1997;54:1611–1613.
15. Ambrose PJ, Saya FG, Lovett LT, et al. Evaluating the accuracy of technicians and pharmacists in checking unit dose medication cassettes. *Am J Health-Syst Pharm.* 2002;59:1183–1188.
16. Kalman MK, Witkowski DE, Ogawa GS. Increasing pharmacy productivity by expanding the role of pharmacy technicians. *Am J Hosp Pharm.* 1992;49:84–89.
17. Scala SM, Schneider PJ, Smith GL, et al. Activity analysis of pharmacy directed drug administration technicians. *Am J Hosp Pharm.* 1986;43:1702–1706.
18. Fillmore AD, Schneider PJ, Bourret JA, et al. Costs of training drug administration technicians. *Am J Hosp Pharm.* 1986;43:1706–1709.
19. Hepler CD, Strand LM. Opportunities and responsibilities in pharmaceutical care. *Am J Hosp Pharm.* 1990;47:533–543.
20. Medication therapy management services definition and program criteria. Available at: www.amcp.com/docs/positions/misc/MTMDefn.pdf. Accessed December 18, 2009.
21. American Society of Health-System Pharmacists. ASHP guidelines: Minimum standard for pharmaceutical services in ambulatory care. *Am J Health-Syst Pharm.* 1999; 56:1744–1753.

22. American Pharmacists Association. Pharmacy technician education and training: Background prepared for the 2007–08 APhA Policy Committee. Available at: www.pharmacist.com. Accessed June 10, 2008.
23. American Society of Hospital Pharmacists. ASHP accreditation standard for pharmacy technician training programs. Available at: www.ashp.org/s_ashp/docs/files/RTP_TechStandards.pdf. Accessed November 19, 2009.
24. American Society of Hospital Pharmacists. ASHP regulations on accreditation of pharmacy technician training programs. Available at: www.ashp.org/s_ashp/docs/files/RTP_TechRegulations.pdf. Accessed November 19, 2009
25. American Society of Hospital Pharmacists. ASHP statement on pharmaceutical care. *Am J Hosp Pharm.* 1993;50: 1720–1723.
26. American Society of Health-System Pharmacists. History of ASHP activities for technicians. Available at: http://www.ashp.org/Import/MEMBERCENTER/Technicians/AboutUs/History.aspx. Accessed November 19, 2009.
27. American Society of Health-System Pharmacists. *Model curriculum for pharmacy technician training*, 2nd ed. Bethesda, MD; 2001. Available at: www.ashp.org/Import/ACCREDITATION/TechnicianAccreditation/StartingaTrainingProgram/ModelCurriculum.aspx. Accessed November 19, 2009.
28. Blake KM. How to achieve teamwork between pharmacists and technicians: A technician's perspective. *Am J Hosp Pharm.* 1992;49:2133, 2137.
29. Knapp DA. Pharmacy practice in 2040. *Am J Hosp Pharm.* 1992;49:2457–2461.
30. McFarland HM. How to achieve teamwork between pharmacists and technicians: A pharmacist's perspective. *Am J Hosp Pharm.* 1992;49:1665–1666.
31. United States Department of Labor; Bureau of Labor Statistics (Pharmacy Technicians). *Occupational Outlook Handbook, 2008–09 Edition*. Available at: www.bls.gov/oco/ocos252.htm. Accessed November 19, 2009.
32. American Society of Health-System Pharmacists. ASHP statement on professionalism. *Am J Health-Syst Pharm.* 2008;65:172–174.

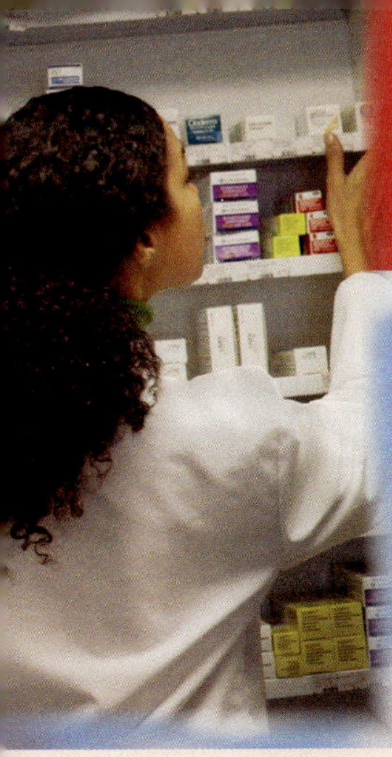

Chapter 2

Pharmacy Law

Diane L. Darvey

Learning Outcomes

After completing this chapter, you will be able to

- Understand how the practice of pharmacy is regulated by federal and state laws and regulations and the role of state boards of pharmacy.
- Discuss state pharmacy laws and regulations that govern pharmacy technicians, including permitted functions and the requirements for pharmacy technician registration or licensure.
- Discuss the laws that regulate controlled substances, special requirements for pharmacy ordering and dispensing controlled substances, and the role of state prescription monitoring programs.
- Describe the restrictions on the sales of products containing pseudoephedrine and ephedrine.
- Describe the FDA approval process for drugs and the differences between brand name and generic drugs.
- Discuss generic drug substitution and the means for prescribers to indicate if substitution is not authorized.
- Discuss the difference between prescription drug inserts for prescribers and for patients.
- Discuss patient privacy in the pharmacy and the federal law that governs privacy of protected health information.

Key Terms

biennial inventory DEA-registered pharmacies are required by law to take an initial inventory of all controlled substances on hand upon commencing operations or upon change in ownership, with subsequent inventories conducted every two years thereafter.

child-resistant packaging Child-resistant packaging is special packaging used for hazardous products such as prescription and over-the-counter drugs and household products to reduce the risk of children ingesting dangerous items by adding caps that children will have difficulty opening. Child-resistant packaging must pass federal tests to assure that it meets the federal requirements.

controlled substances Drugs or chemical substances whose possession and use are regulated under the Federal Controlled Substances Act and by state controlled substance laws and regulations. Controlled substances are subject to stricter controls than other prescription and nonprescription drugs.

Drug Enforcement Administration (DEA) The federal agency that administers and enforces federal laws for controlled substances such as narcotics and other dangerous drugs and illegal substances. The DEA is part of the U.S. Department of Justice.

initial inventory The inventory a pharmacy takes of its stock of controlled substances upon beginning the dispensing or distribution of controlled substances.

legend drug A drug that is required by federal law to be dispensed by prescription only. It is the older term for drugs that are now identified as "Rx Only."

practice of pharmacy The practice of pharmacy is regulated by each state through its pharmacy laws and regulations. The state laws and regulations establish the scope of the practice of pharmacy in the particular state, meaning the responsibilities that pharmacists are permitted to perform in the state.

prescription monitoring programs State prescription drug monitoring programs are programs implemented by the states pursuant to state laws and regulations to collect, review, and analyze information received from pharmacies about controlled substance prescriptions dispensed in the state. The programs provide information that may be reviewed by state law enforcement and regulatory agencies to assist in identifying and investigating potential improper prescribing, dispensing, and use of prescription drugs.

regulations (or rules) Regulations (or rules) are issued by an administrative or governmental agency that establish the requirements that must be followed by the regulated persons or entities. For example, a state board of pharmacy issues regulations for pharmacy technicians to establish the qualifications that pharmacy technicians must meet in order to work as a pharmacy technician in a state.

The practice of pharmacy is extensively regulated by a number of laws and regulations. These laws and regulations cover essentially all aspects of pharmacy practice and establish permitted and prohibited conduct for pharmacies, pharmacists, and pharmacy technicians. States require pharmacies and pharmacists to be licensed. Many states have laws or regulations that require pharmacy technicians to be licensed or registered and meet other requirements, such as specific training and education, certification, and criminal history background checks. Pharmacy practice is also covered by ethical principles to provide a fundamental framework for interacting with patients. Examples of ethical principles are acting with honesty, integrity, compassion, and respect for patients.

Although states have the primary authority to regulate pharmacy practice, pharmacy is also subject to a number of federal laws. Examples of federal laws include the Food, Drug, and Cosmetics Act (FDCA) that regulates the safety of food, drugs, and cosmetics and the Controlled Substances Act that establishes requirements for the handling and dispensing of narcotics and other controlled substances. Another example is the Omnibus Budget Reconciliation Act of 1990 (commonly called "OBRA '90") that requires pharmacists to provide patient counseling as a condition of reimbursement when dispensing prescriptions to Medicaid patients. Table 2–1 provides a timeline of some of these and other important federal drug laws.

If state and federal laws or regulations differ, both must be followed, including the more stringent requirements, whether federal or state. For example, if a federal law has specific requirements for dispensing controlled substances, and a state pharmacy law has stricter requirements, the state law must be followed in addition to the federal requirements.

✔If the state and federal laws or regulations differ, both laws and regulations must be followed, including the more stringent requirements, whether federal or state.

Ethical Principles

Ethical principles exist in many areas of life. In health care, including pharmacy, they guide the performance of tasks and responsibilities so they fall within an ethical and moral framework. Pharmacy technicians' interactions with patients and other health care professionals should conform to societal values. In simple terms, this equates to "doing the right thing," such as being considerate of patients. Ethical principles include complying with laws and regulations, maintaining competency, and respecting patient privacy and confidentiality. Pharmacy technicians have their own set of ethical principles. The American Association of Pharmacy Technicians (AAPT) has developed a Code of Ethics for Pharmacy Technicians (See box 1–1 in Chapter 1 Introduction to Pharmacy).

State Pharmacy Laws and Regulations

State pharmacy laws and **regulations** set the requirements for pharmacies, pharmacists, pharmacy technicians, and the **practice of pharmacy**. Both laws and regulations are necessary to regulate the practice of pharmacy, including

Table 2-1. A History of the FDA and Drug Regulation in the United States

Year	Act	Purpose
1906	Food and Drug Act	Outlaws states from buying and selling food, drinks, and drugs that have been mislabeled and tainted
1912	Sherley Amendment	Outlaws labeling drugs with fake medical claims meant to trick the buyer
1930	FDA	Food and Drug Administration is named
1938	Federal Food, Drug, and Cosmetic (FDC) Act of 1938	Requires new drugs to be proven safe prior to marketing; starts a new system of drug regulation; requires safe limits for unavoidable poisonous substances; and allows for factory inspections
1951	Durham-Humphrey Amendment	Defines the type of drugs that cannot be used safely without medical supervision and limits the sale to prescription only by medical professionals
1962	Kefauver-Harris Drug Amendments	Requires manufacturers to prove that their drugs are effective prior to marketing
1972	Over-the-Counter Drug Review	Nonprescription medications must be safe, effective, and appropriately labeled
1982	Tamper-Resistant Packaging Regulations	Makes it a crime to tamper with packaged products and requires tamper-proof packaging
1984	Drug Price Competition and Patent Term Restoration Act (Hatch-Waxman Act)	Allowed FDA to approve generic versions of brand-name drugs without repeating research to prove safety and efficacy; allowed brand-name drugs to apply for up to 5 years of additional patent protection for new drugs to make up for time lost while their products were going through the FDA approval process
1988	Prescription Drug Marketing Act	Designed to eliminate diversion of products from legitimate channels of distribution and requires wholesalers to be licensed
1997	Food and Drug Administration Modernization Act	Expands scope of agency activities and moves agency to the Department of Health and Human Services (DHHS)
2003	Medicare Prescription Drug Improvement and Modernization Act of 2003	Includes Medicare Part D which increases access to medications through private insurers

Adapted from U.S. Food and Drug Administration, Center for Drug Evaluation and Research.

pharmacy technicians. State pharmacy laws establish the legal requirements, restrictions, and prohibitions for the practice of pharmacy. State laws are enacted by state legislatures through the legislative process; however, because laws are usually more general, regulations or rules are needed to provide the details to implement the law. While laws are enacted through the state legislative process, regulations or rules are issued and adopted by state regulatory agencies through the regulatory or rule-making process. For pharmacy practice, the pharmacy laws are enacted by the state legislature and regulations are usually adopted through the state board of pharmacy.

Because each state enacts legislation and adopts regulations for pharmacy, the particular requirements may vary from state to state. For example, the requirements for pharmacy technicians vary by state. Nonetheless, an important and universal distinction for pharmacy technicians to understand is that they work under the supervision and direction of pharmacists and may perform only the tasks permitted under state law.

State pharmacy laws and regulations distinguish between the tasks and responsibilities that pharmacists perform and those that pharmacy technicians are permitted to perform. State pharmacy laws do not permit pharmacy technicians to perform pharmacy tasks and responsibilities that are limited to pharmacists and require the professional judgment, education, and training of a pharmacist.

✔State pharmacy laws do not permit pharmacy technicians to perform pharmacy tasks and responsibilities that are limited to pharmacists and require the professional judgment, education, and training of a pharmacist.

State Boards of Pharmacy

State boards of pharmacy are responsible for regulating the practice of pharmacy including pharmacies, pharmacists, pharmacy interns, and pharmacy technicians. The state boards of pharmacy have regulatory authority over a number of areas, such as licensing pharmacies and pharmacists; registering or licensing pharmacy technicians; inspecting pharmacies; issuing rules and regulations; investigating complaints; and disciplinary actions against pharmacies, pharmacists, and pharmacy technicians for violations of pharmacy laws and regulations. Information on the various state boards of pharmacy is available through the National Association of Boards of Pharmacy (NABP) Web site at www.nabp.net.

Pharmacy Licensure

Every state requires pharmacies to have a valid current pharmacy license or permit in order to operate the pharmacy. State pharmacy laws and regulations set the requirements for pharmacy licensure. Pharmacies must satisfy many requirements which include record keeping requirements, security, a pharmacist-in-charge, and a licensed pharmacist on duty while the pharmacy is open. State requirements vary as to whether the pharmacy technicians may or may not remain in the pharmacy during a pharmacist's break period. State boards of pharmacy conduct pharmacy inspections to verify that the pharmacy meets the licensure requirements and also perform periodic pharmacy inspections at other times.

Many states have more than one category of pharmacy license. The different licensure categories that states may identify include retail, community, institutional, hospital, nuclear, mail-order, and long-term care. Some states also use categories for special or limited-use pharmacies and sterile-compounding pharmacies. Another category used by states is for nonresident pharmacies. Most states require pharmacies that are located in another state (i.e., nonresident pharmacies) to be licensed in the state if they mail, ship, dispense, or deliver prescription drugs to residents of the state.

Pharmacy Technicians

Many states have enacted laws and adopted regulations establishing requirements that pharmacy technicians must meet to be able to assist pharmacists. However, the requirements for pharmacy technicians vary from state to state. The state board of pharmacy in each state is the best resource for obtaining the current requirements. Nonetheless, although they are variable, there are several common requirements. These include a requirement for pharmacy technician registration or licensure (and the accompanying qualifications), permitted tasks, and prohibited conduct. Some states require criminal background checks. Regardless of whether licensure or registration is required, these requirements allow states to assure that pharmacy technicians meet certain requirements, to regulate the tasks that pharmacy technicians may perform, and to allow for disciplinary actions against pharmacy technicians for violations of state pharmacy laws and regulations including loss of licensure or registration if appropriate. The qualifications for pharmacy technician registration or licensure generally include a minimum age, high school graduation or the equivalent, completion of a training program including pharmacy employer training programs, and an examination. Some states allow pharmacy technician certification to satisfy the education or training requirements (see Chapter 1 Introduction to Pharmacy for more information on licensure, registration, and certification).

✔The qualifications for pharmacy technician registration or licensure generally include a minimum age, high school graduation or the equivalent, completion of a training program, including pharmacy employer training programs, and an examination.

Many states have established laws and regulations that set a limit on the number of pharmacy technicians who may assist a pharmacist at one time. Other states have no limits on the number of pharmacy technicians who may assist a pharmacist. These limits are known as pharmacy technician ratios. If the ratio is three to one (3:1), one pharmacist may supervise up to three pharmacy technicians at one time. Some states allow a higher pharmacy technician ratio if one or more of the pharmacy technicians meets additional requirements, such as passing a pharmacy technician certification exam. In a few states, all pharmacy technicians are or will eventually be required to be certified by passing a certification examination in addition to meeting the other training and education requirements.

Patient Counseling

State pharmacy laws and regulations set the requirements for patient counseling by pharmacists regarding their prescription medications. Pharmacist counseling involves the pharmacist discussing the patient's medication treatment with the patient or the patient's caregiver. Counseling includes providing the patient with information about his or her medications such as what they are for, when and how much to take, whether to take with food, how to store the medication, and possible side effects. Patient counseling is very important to ensure that patients take their medications correctly.

Nearly every state requires pharmacists to *offer to counsel* patients on new prescriptions. The offer to counsel differs from patient counseling. The offer to counsel occurs when the patient is asked if he or she would like to receive information from the pharmacist about their prescription medication, whereas counseling is providing information to the patient. States vary on whether an offer to counsel is required on refill prescriptions.

An important point for pharmacy technicians is that patient counseling must be provided by the pharmacist. Pharmacy technicians are *not* authorized to counsel patients on their medications. Nevertheless, pharmacy technicians may assist the pharmacist with language translation if they are fluent in the patient's language and such services are needed during the patient counseling process. In some states, pharmacy technicians are permitted to ask patients if they want to receive counseling from the pharmacist (the "offer to counsel"). Many states permit pharmacy interns to provide patient counseling under the supervision of a pharmacist.

✔Patient counseling must be provided by the pharmacist. Pharmacy technicians are not authorized to counsel patients on their medications.

Controlled Substances

Controlled substances are subject to stricter controls through federal and state laws and regulations than other drugs because of their potential for misuse, abuse, diversion, and addiction. Pharmacies, pharmacists, pharmacy technicians, as well as drug manufacturers, drug distributors, physicians, and other health care providers must comply with these additional requirements to avoid penalties and maintain their authorization to handle controlled substances.

The federal law regulating controlled substances is the Controlled Substances Act. The law and its regulations establish comprehensive requirements and controls over the manufacture, import, export, distribution, ordering, dispensing, and prescribing of controlled substances. The definition of controlled substances in the federal law includes drugs and other substances and their immediate precursor chemicals. A precursor is a substance that may be turned into a controlled substance through a chemical reaction.

The federal Controlled Substances Act regulates the distribution and handling of controlled substances including manufacturing, distribution, dispensing, storage and recordkeeping, and other actions involved with the distribution of controlled substances. The federal law includes a number of requirements. Pharmacies, prescribers, wholesale distributors, drug manufacturers, and others must be registered with the **Drug Enforcement Administration (DEA)**. Once registered, a DEA number is assigned. For a physician, the number starts with either the letter A or the letter B followed by the first letter of the physician's last name. An example of the format of a DEA number is AS1234567. On occasion, the pharmacist may instruct the pharmacy technician on how to verify whether the prescriber's DEA number is valid. Some of the requirements for pharmacies include special order forms for ordering Schedule II controlled substances, called DEA Form 222 (see Chapter 19 Purchasing and Inventory). Pharmacists must complete a DEA Form 222 and it must be signed by the pharmacy's authorized pharmacist. Other pharmacy requirements for controlled substances include reporting significant losses, records of dispensing controlled substances, and inventory records. These strict controls for controlled substances guard against abuse, misuse, and diversion of controlled substances throughout their distribution.

States' controlled substance laws and regulations may have stricter controls than federal laws. Pharmacies must comply with both state and federal controlled substance laws. If the state-controlled substance law or regulation has stricter requirements, pharmacies along with others handling controlled substances must comply with the stricter requirements.

✔If a state controlled substance law or regulation has stricter requirements, pharmacies along with others handling controlled substances must comply with the stricter requirements.

Pharmacies are required to keep complete, accurate, and up-to-date records for controlled substances that they purchase, receive, distribute, dispense, or discard. Schedule II records must be kept separately from CIII, IV, and V records. Pharmacies are required to immediately report any theft or significant loss of controlled substances to the DEA using DEA Form 106, "Report of Theft or Loss of Controlled Substances."

Schedules of Controlled Substances

The federal controlled substances law created five schedules (i.e., classifications) for controlled substances numbered I, II, III, IV, and V. A drug is placed into a controlled substance schedule based on certain criteria, such as its potential for abuse or addiction and its medical use. The schedule a drug or substance is placed in determines its level of control. Schedule I is the most restrictive schedule and Schedule V is the least restrictive schedule of controlled substances (table 2–2). Because they have no legally approved medical uses, Schedule I drugs are not available in the pharmacy. Federal regulations allow certain controlled substances to be dispensed *by a pharmacist* without a prescription if specific requirements are met. These requirements include: the substance is not a prescription drug, a pharmacist must approve the sale, the purchaser is at least eighteen years of age, and the pharmacy maintains a record book with information on the sale. The record book should include the purchaser's name and address, the name and quantity of the product purchased, the date of purchase, and the name or initials of the dispensing pharmacist. An example of a controlled substance that may be dispensed by a pharmacist in some states is a Schedule V over-the-counter cough syrup containing a limited amount of codeine. Some states; however, have stricter controlled substances laws and require that all controlled substances be dispensed by prescription only.

Part 1

Table 2–2. Schedules for Controlled Substances

Schedule	Classification characteristics	Examples of controlled substances
Schedule I (CI)	No accepted medical use High potential for abuse Not available by prescription	Heroin and marijuana
Schedule II (CII)	High potential for abuse or misuse High risk of dependence FDA-approved medical uses	Meperidine (Demerol), methadone, morphine, oxycodone (OxyIR, OxyContin), methylphenidate (Ritalin)
Schedule III (CIII)	Moderate potential for abuse, misuse, and dependence	Includes drug products that contain small quantities of controlled substances combined with other noncontrolled drugs such as acetaminophen and codeine (Tylenol #3) and acetaminophen with hydrocodone (Vicodin)
Schedule IV (CIV)	Low potential for abuse and limited risk of dependence	Diazepam (Valium), lorazepam (Ativan), phenobarbital, and other sedatives and hypnotics
Schedule V (CV)	Lower potential for abuse, misuse, or dependence	Cough medications that contain a limited amount of codeine, anti-diarrheal medications containing a limited amount of an opiate, such as diphenoxylate/atropine (Lomotil)

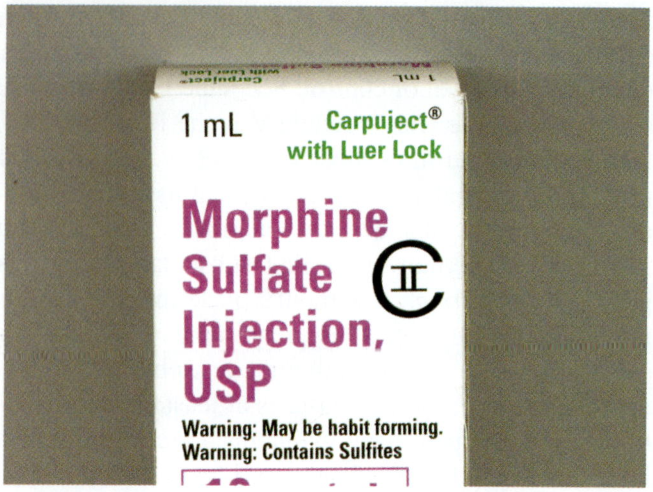

Figure 2–1. CII label for a Schedule II controlled substance.

Labeling of Controlled Substances

Federal law requires that the drug manufacturer's packaging for controlled substances be labeled with a specific symbol to indicate that they are controlled substances. The symbol to indicate a controlled substance is the letter *C* with the appropriate Roman numeral placed inside the *C* symbol. A Schedule II controlled substance is denoted "CII" (figure 2–1). The prescription container labels for dispensing controlled substance prescriptions are not required to contain this symbol; however, federal law requires that pharmacies place a specific caution message on the patient container advising the patient that they may not give the controlled substance to any other person. The required statement is "Caution: Federal law prohibits the transfer of this drug to any person other than the patient for whom it was prescribed."

Dispensing Controlled Substances

Prescribers and pharmacists both have responsibilities to ensure that only legitimate controlled-substance prescriptions are issued and dispensed. For a controlled-substance prescription to be valid, it must be prescribed by a licensed prescriber for a legitimate medical purpose in the normal course of the prescriber's professional practice. The prescribing practitioner must be registered with Drug Enforcement Administration (unless exempt from registration, such as Public Health Service physicians) and be licensed to prescribe controlled substances by the state. Pharmacists have a corresponding responsibility to dispense controlled substances pursuant to a valid prescription issued for a legitimate medical purpose in the course of the prescriber's practice. Prescribing a controlled substance or knowingly filling a controlled-substance prescription in violation of the laws and regulations may result in criminal or civil penalties for violation of the controlled substance laws.

Federal and state laws require specific information for controlled-substance prescriptions. Controlled-substance prescriptions must contain the date issued; the patient's full name and address; the practitioner's name, address, and DEA registration number; the drug name, strength, dosage form, and quantity prescribed; directions for use; the number of authorized refills (if any); and the signature of the prescriber (unless a verbal prescription is permitted). Pharmacists may dispense Schedule II controlled substances only pursuant to a written prescription signed by the practitioner unless an exception applies. For example, in an emergency, the practitioner may telephone or fax the prescription to the pharmacist. The prescriber must still provide the original written signed prescription to the pharmacist within seven days and indicate that it was authorized for emergency dispensing. Some states require specific tamper-resistant or multi-part forms for Schedule II prescriptions (figure 2–2). Federal regulations allow facsimile Schedule II prescriptions in some instances, such as for a patient residing in a long-term care facility or for a hospice patient.

Federal and state laws set specific requirements for refilling and transferring controlled-substance prescriptions. Federal law allows Schedule III and IV prescriptions to be refilled up to five times within six months after the date that the prescription was issued by the prescriber. Schedule V prescriptions may be refilled more than five times, but have a six-month time limit on refills. Schedule II prescriptions may not be refilled and are not transferable between pharmacies. Federal law allows Schedule III, IV, and V prescriptions to be transferred from one pharmacy to another for one refill (if the state law permits). Pharmacies using a real-time online computer system connecting their pharmacies may transfer Schedule III, IV, and V prescriptions up to the maximum number of authorized refills. Pharmacies are required to maintain complete and accurate records for all controlled substances that they purchase, receive, distribute, or dispense. Federal law requires the pharmacy to keep controlled-substance records for two years and have them readily available for DEA inspection if

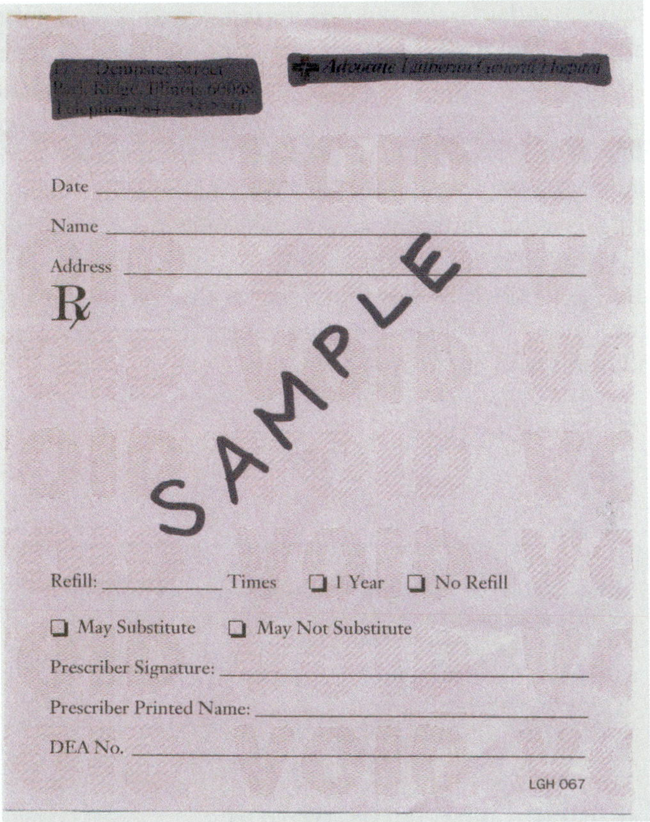

[redacted] [redacted]

Date ______

Name ______

Address ______

℞

SAMPLE

Refill: ______ Times ❑ 1 Year ❑ No Refill

❑ May Substitute ❑ May Not Substitute

Prescriber Signature: ______

Prescriber Printed Name: ______

DEA No. ______

LGH 067

Figure 2-2. Example of a tamper-resistant prescription for a Schedule II drug.

requested. State laws may require pharmacies to keep records for a longer time period. Examples of records that must be kept are invoices or receipts for purchases of controlled substances, inventory records including **initial** and **biennial inventories,** and records of any transfers of controlled substances between pharmacies. Each controlled-substance inventory must be a complete and accurate record of all controlled substances in the pharmacy on the inventory date. A separate inventory is required for each pharmacy location.

State Prescription Monitoring Programs. Many states have enacted laws and regulations to institute **prescription monitoring programs** to monitor prescribing and dispensing of controlled substances. Most state prescription monitoring programs require pharmacies to report information on controlled-substance prescriptions dispensed for drugs in Schedules II, III, IV, and V; however, some programs require reporting for dispensing of Schedules II, III, and IV drugs. These programs require pharmacies to submit information on the controlled-substance prescriptions that they dispense to the designated state authority electronically on a periodic basis (e.g., once or twice a month, or in some states, more frequently). More than thirty-five states have implemented these programs. The information that pharmacies provide to these programs includes patient information, prescriber information, pharmacy identification, and prescription information including the name and quantity of the controlled substance and the date the prescription was dispensed. These programs are used by states to identify potential diversion and abuse of prescription controlled substances by the patient, pharmacy, or prescriber, and to identify potential patients that would benefit from drug abuse treatment programs.

✔Prescription monitoring programs require pharmacies to submit information on controlled-substance prescriptions to help states identify potential diversion and abuse.

Restrictions on Sales of Products Containing Ephedrine or Pseudoephedrine. The sales of over-the-counter drug products containing ephedrine and pseudoephedrine are subject to restrictions on their sales under federal law and laws enacted in many states. The federal law restricting sales of these products is called the Combat Methamphetamine Epidemic Act of 2005 (CMEA). It was enacted due to continuing concerns about the use of over-the-counter (OTC) products to illegally manufacture methamphetamine or amphetamine. Ephedrine and pseudoephedrine, which are the active ingredients in common cough, cold, and allergy products, are precursor chemicals to methamphetamine and amphetamine. The laws limit the amount of these products that a customer may purchase in a single transaction, in a day, or over a 30-day period, and require that the products be locked up or otherwise not available for public access. They also require customers to sign a logbook with details on the drug product and amount purchased. Federal law limits sales of these products to 3.6 grams daily and limits purchasers to 9 grams of these products in a 30-day period. The federal 3.6 gram daily limit for pseudoephedrine hydrochloride 30 mg tablets would be about 146 tablets or about 73 tablets of 60 mg pseudoephedrine hydrochloride. Further information is available from the DEA at http://www.deadiversion.usdoj.gov/meth/trg_retail_081106.pdf.

Purchasers must provide their valid photo identification and sign a logbook with their name, address, and date and time of purchase. The logbooks may be used by law enforcement to identify violations of the law. Many states have also enacted laws restricting the sale and purchase of these OTC products, and some have different requirements and restrictions. The federal law must be followed in all states, and if the state law is stricter, it must also be followed.

Brand Name Drugs and Generic Drugs

The FDA approves all drugs that are available for distribution in the United States to assure that they are safe and effective. Before a new drug is approved, the drug manufacturer must submit a new drug application (NDA) to the FDA. The NDA includes information about the drug, including results from clinical trials in humans, results of animal studies, how the drug acts in the body, and how it is manufactured, processed, and packaged. The FDA reviews the NDA to assess whether the drug is safe and effective for its proposed use(s), if the benefits of the drug outweigh the potential risks, if the proposed labeling is appropriate, and whether the methods used in manufacturing the drug are adequate to ensure the quality of the drug. If the FDA's review of the NDA is favorable and the drug is determined to be safe and effective, the FDA approves the drug for use in the United States.

Most companies market new drugs with a trade or brand name. Lipitor is an example of a brand name for a drug that is manufactured and distributed by the drug manufacturer Pfizer. The generic name for Lipitor is atorvastatin. Pfizer is the company that developed atorvastatin and submitted the NDA to FDA for approval. The FDA approved the drug as safe and effective for use in the United States. Manufacturers that develop new drugs, such as Pfizer in this example, are granted patents for the drug, which give them exclusive rights to market the drug until the patent expires. Typically, patent protection for a drug lasts an average of 11 years. Once the patent expires, other drug manufacturers may seek approval from FDA to market generic equivalents, or copies, of the drug.

Generic equivalents contain the same active ingredients and have the same dosage form, strength, and formulations as their brand name counterparts. Whereas the manufacturer that developed the original version of a drug must submit an NDA to the FDA, generic drug companies must submit abbreviated new drug applications (ANDAs). Generic manufacturers must meet the same standards for manufacturing, quality, and labeling as brand drugs; however, they do not need to repeat the original research. They must show bioequivalence to the brand name drug, which means that the drug will deliver the same amount of the drug to the body in the same amount of time as the brand name drug. Generic drugs have a different appearance than the brand name drug because laws do not allow a generic drug to copy the appearance of the brand name drug. Generic drug companies distribute the drug under the generic name, not the brand name drug.

Rx for Success

Manufacturers of generic drugs can market their drugs at lower prices than their brand name counterparts because they don't have new drug development and research costs that brand name companies have.

Generic Drug Substitution

For drugs that have an FDA-approved generic equivalent, pharmacists are permitted to substitute the generic equivalent drug for the brand name drug unless the prescriber prohibits generic substitution. Generic substitution by pharmacists is regulated by the state generic substitution drug laws and regulations. These laws and regulations set the requirements for when pharmacists may or may not substitute therapeutically equivalent generic drugs for prescribed brand name drugs. State laws and regulations establish different means for prescribers to advise pharmacists that they do not want generic substitution for their patients. Depending on the state, the laws may instruct prescribers to indicate no substitution through various phrases including "dispense as written," "DAW," "no substitution," "do not substitute," "DNS," or words of similar effect. Conversely, if the prescriber wants to permit substitution, state laws may instruct the prescriber to use terms such as "substitution permitted" or words of similar effect. Patients may also ask to have the brand name drug dispensed in place of the generic drug. In some states, pharmacists are required to do generic substitution for certain types of patients, such as all patients with prescription drug coverage paid for by the state medical assistance (Medicaid) program.

The FDA provides a list of generic drugs that the agency has found to be therapeutically equivalent to the brand name drugs in its publication, *"Approved Drug Products with Therapeutic Equivalence Evaluations,"* commonly called the "Orange Book." Pharmacists use the "Orange Book" to find the FDA's determination that a particular manufacturer's generic drug is therapeutically equivalent to the brand name drug. Not all drugs have a generic equivalent. If the drug company still has a patent on the drug, the brand name drug is the only one available.

✔Pharmacists use the "Orange Book" to find the FDA's determination that a particular manufacturer's generic drug is therapeutically equivalent to the brand name

Prescription Drug Labeling and Package Inserts

Prescription drug products are labeled by the drug manufacturer. The prescription drug container label includes standard information such as the name and address of the drug manufacturer, drug name, strength and dosage form, manufacturer's expiration date for the drug, lot number, package size or quantity, DEA schedule (if appropriate), and "Rx Only" to indicate that the drug is for prescription use only (figure 2–3). Prescription drugs are also called **"legend drugs"** due to a federal law enacted in 1951 (the Durham-Humphrey Amendment) that required certain drugs to require a prescription and be labeled with the statement, "Caution: Federal law prohibits dispensing without a prescription." Each product label must include a lot number and expiration date. The lot number is the number used by the drug manufacturer to identify each particular batch of the drug during the manufacturing process and is used to identify drug products that may need to be pulled from distribution in the event of a drug recall. The expiration date is derived from studies conducted by the drug manufacturer on the stability of the drug in the manufacturer's container. The date is used to determine how long the drug product may be used or dispensed to patients. Drugs that have reached their expiration date may not be used or dispensed to patients.

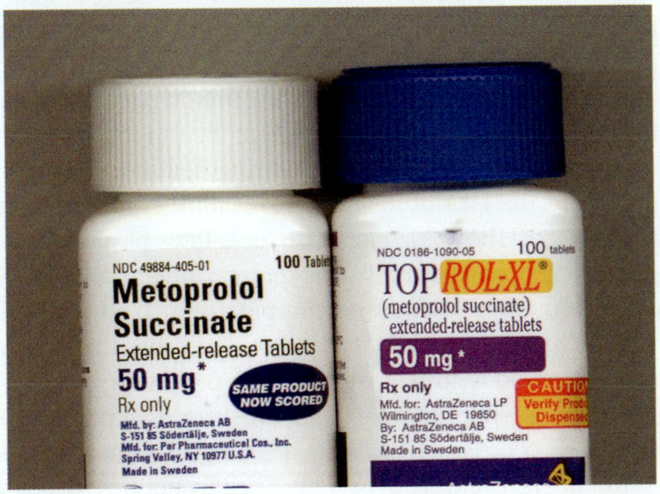

Figure 2–3. Comparison of a brand name (R) and generic (L) equivalent label for the same drug.

Prescription drug products also include a *package insert*. The package insert provides physicians, pharmacists, and other health care professionals with medical and scientific information about the prescription drug. Information in the package insert includes important information about the drug, such as the indications for use, dosage and administration, adverse reactions, warnings, precautions, and contraindications for the drug. The package insert also provides details about how to prepare the drug, proper storage, and the available package sizes with NDC numbers. The prescription drug package insert is not intended for patients.

Prescription Drug Information for Patients. Pharmacists provide patients with different types of written information for their dispensed prescription drugs. Patients are provided with printed information about their dispensed medication called *consumer medicine information* or CMI. In addition, the FDA requires pharmacists to provide patients with a *patient package insert* ("PPI") with the dispensing of *certain* prescription drugs such as estrogens and oral contraceptives. PPIs are written specifically for patient use, whereas, package inserts are developed for use by physicians and pharmacists.

Another type of patient written information used for certain prescription drugs is the *Medication Guide* or *Medguide*. Medication Guides contain FDA-approved information to assist patients with avoiding serious adverse events, to inform patients about known serious side effects, or to promote patient adherence with their treatment. The FDA requires that Medication Guides be provided to patients when certain medications are dispensed. An example of a drug requiring a Medication Guide is zolpidem (Ambien). Medication Guides may be for an individual drug or for a class of drugs. A link to

FDA Medication Guides can be found in the Resources section at the end of this chapter.

Over-the-Counter Drug Labeling. Over-the-counter (OTC) drugs are drugs that the FDA has approved to be safe for use by consumers without a prescription. Because they do not require a prescription, OTC drugs are labeled with information designed to assist consumers in using the medications correctly. The labeling for OTC drug products is intended to sufficiently inform the consumer of the uses for the drug, the recommended dosage, how often to use the drug, who should or should not take the medication, and to provide information on side effects and precautions for using the drug. For example, the container labeling for OTC drugs used for sleep aids would advise the consumer not to drive a car after taking the medication due to the risk of drowsiness. The product labeling also contains the drug name and the total quantity of drugs in the container. OTC products have a specific *Drug Facts* section that lists the active ingredients, uses, warnings, and directions for use (see figure 2–4). OTC drug products, like prescription drug products, are required to be labeled with an expiration date as determined by the drug manufacturer.

Poison Prevention Packaging Act. The federal Poison Prevention Packaging Act requires that hazardous products such as prescription drugs, many OTC drug products, and other products such as household cleaners and furniture polish be sold in **child-resistant packaging**. The packaging must meet a test to show that it will prevent 80% of children from opening the package but allow 90% of adults to open the containers without difficulty. Many OTC products require child-resistant packaging such as products containing aspirin, iron, and ibuprofen.

The law allows consumers or the patient's prescriber to ask the pharmacist to dispense the medication in non-child-resistant packaging. Some prescription drugs are exempt from child-resistant packaging because it is not appropriate, feasible, or practical. Examples of exempt products include sublingual nitroglycerin tablets and oral contraceptives (birth control pills), which are packaged in numbered tablet dispenser packs.

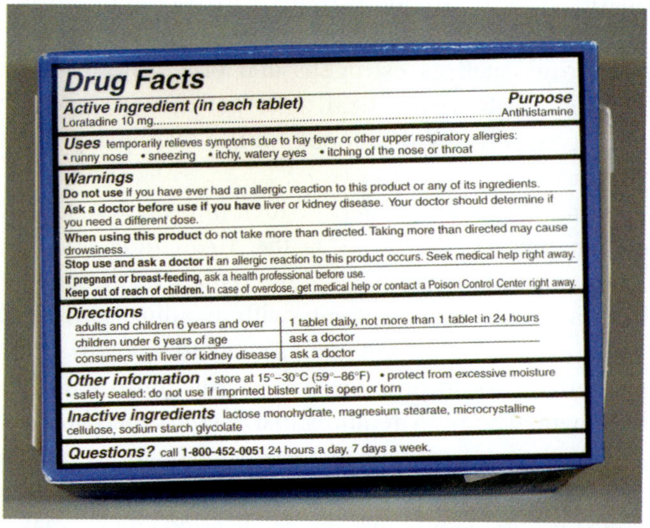

Figure 2–4. Drug Facts section of an OTC label.

Patient Privacy

Pharmacies, including pharmacists and pharmacy technicians, are required by federal and state laws to maintain the required privacy and confidentiality of patient health information. It is important to maintain privacy and confidentiality of patient health information and health records, as failure to comply with the law may subject violators to penalties.

Virtually all pharmacy records contain private patient health information. Examples include prescriptions, computer records, patient profiles, patient prescription containers, written patient information that identifies the patient, patient billing records, and oral conversations regarding patients. Maintaining the privacy and confidentiality of patient health information requires appropriate safeguards for pharmacy patient records. This includes taking care to discard patient information in a secure manner and taking reasonable precautions to maintain privacy of pharmacy conversations about patients.

Both state and federal laws establish requirements for maintaining privacy of patient health information. The primary federal law establishing health information privacy is the Health Insurance Portability and Accountability Act (HIPAA). States also have laws protecting the privacy and confidentiality of patient health and medical information. Due to the complexity of the topic, it is outside of the scope of this section to discuss the various state laws and regulations governing patient privacy.

HIPAA sets national standards for the privacy of medical records. HIPAA is a complex law and the following is a general overview. The law applies to health care providers including pharmacies, physicians, hospitals, nursing homes, and many other entities that handle health information, such as health plans and billing services. HIPAA protects patient's individually identifiable health information, which is known as *"protected health information,"* or *"PHI."* PHI is any health information that identifies the patient or could reasonably be used to identify the person. Examples of pharmacy PHI include pharmacy prescription records, computer records, prescription container labels, and other pharmacy health information records that identify the patient, and oral communications about patients' prescriptions and health care treatment. However, health information that is de-identified, so as not to disclose the identity of the patient, is not PHI. For example, pharmacists and pharmacy technicians discussing a particular drug therapy in general and not in relation to a patient would not be considered PHI.

Pharmacies are permitted to use and disclose patient health information as necessary to provide patient health care services. HIPAA permits certain uses and disclosure of patient health information. HIPAA allows the use and disclosure of PHI for patient care, treatment, and health care operations. Such disclosures are necessary for providing pharmacy services. Examples include dispensing prescriptions, patient treatment, billing for pharmacy services, and managing patient care.

Rx for Success

Pharmacy technicians must maintain the privacy and confidentiality of patients' personal health information. This requires appropriate safeguards for pharmacy patient records, discarding patient information in a secure manner, and taking reasonable precautions to maintain privacy of pharmacy conversations about patients.

Summary

This chapter provides an overview of laws and regulations affecting the practice of pharmacy. It is designed to provide pharmacy technicians with a foundation of the laws that affect the pharmacy profession. Pharmacy technicians who are interested in additional information about the laws and regulations for a particular state and the specific requirements for pharmacy technicians should refer to the resources section and contact their state board of pharmacy.

Disclaimer

This chapter has been prepared by the author for general information purposes only and is not intended to contain all laws and regulations that relate or may relate to the practice of pharmacy, including but not limited to pharmacy technicians. This publication and the information within are not provided in the course of an attorney-client relationship and are not intended to provide legal or other advice. Such advice should be rendered only in reference to the particular facts and circumstances appropriate to each situation by the appropriate legal professionals and/or consultants selected by the person. Any references or links to information or to particular organizations or references are provided as a courtesy and convenience, and are not intended to constitute any endorsement of the linked materials or the referenced organizations or materials by the author or publisher. The content and views on such links and of such organizations are solely their own and do not necessarily reflect those of the author or publisher. The author, Diane L. Darvey, prepared this publication on her own behalf, not as a representative of the National Association of Chain Drug Stores (NACDS). NACDS did not review or approve this publication, and its contents do not necessarily represent the views of NACDS.

Self-Assessment Questions

1. Pharmacy technicians are permitted to do the following
   a. All tasks that pharmacists are permitted to do
   b. Any task that the pharmacist asks them to do
   c. Any tasks that they are permitted to do by the pharmacy laws
   d. Any task that they determine they can safely do
2. Counseling patients about their prescription medications
   a. May be done by the pharmacy technician if he or she believes he or she understands the medication
   b. May be done only by the pharmacist
   c. May be done by the pharmacy technician when the pharmacist is on the telephone or speaking with another patient
   d. May be done by the pharmacy technician if it is only for one drug
3. What is meant by a legend drug?
   a. A drug that is famous
   b. An herbal drug
   c. A drug that can be bought over-the-counter
   d. A drug that can be dispensed only pursuant to a valid prescription
4. Controlled substances are subject to
   a. The same controls as any prescription drug
   b. Stricter controls that other prescription drugs
   c. Stricter controls only in hospital pharmacies
   d. Lesser controls than other prescription drugs
5. Which of the following Schedules of Controlled Substances have the highest abuse potential and an accepted medical use?
   a. Schedule I
   b. Schedule II
   c. Schedule III
   d. Schedule V
6. Products containing ephedrine or pseudoephedrine
   a. May not be sold in pharmacies due to federal restrictions
   b. May be kept in the front of the pharmacy for public access
   c. May only be kept behind the counter and sold in limited amounts
   d. Require a prescription
7. All of the following drugs must be dispensed in a child-resistant container *except*
   a. Sublingual nitroglycerin tablets
   b. Controlled substances
   c. Celecoxib (Celebrex)
   d. Iron-containing multivitamins
8. Which of the following statements is most correct?
   a. The patent holder of a brand name drug is the only company that has the rights to market the drug
   b. Brand name drugs and generic drugs both require an NDA
   c. According to the FDA, generic drugs must look like their brand counterparts
   d. The drug manufacturer determines whether a generic drug can be substituted for its brand name counterpart
9. Who has the authority to sign a DEA Form 222 when ordering Schedule II controlled substances?
   a. Only the owner of the pharmacy
   b. Only the person who signed the application for pharmacy registration with the DEA
   c. Only a pharmacist
   d. The prescribing physician
10. What is the name of the law that requires pharmacists to provide patient counseling as a condition of reimbursement when dispensing prescriptions to Medicaid patients?
    a. Food, Drug, and Cosmetics Act (FDCA)
    b. Omnibus Budget Reconciliation Act of 1990
    c. Durham Humphrey Amendment
    d. The Controlled Substances Act

Self-Assessment Answers

1. c. Pharmacy technicians are allowed to perform only tasks that are permitted by pharmacy laws.
2. b. Patient counseling may be performed only by a pharmacist or a pharmacy intern under the supervision of a pharmacist. In some states, pharmacy technicians are permitted to ask patients if they want to receive counseling from the pharmacist ("offer to counsel").
3. d. A drug is considered "legend" if it has the statement on its label, "Caution: Federal Law Prohibits Dispensing Without a Prescription." Therefore, the drug can't be dispensed without a prescription from an authorized prescriber.
4. b. Controlled substances are subject to stricter controls than other prescription drugs because of their potential for misuse, abuse, diversion, and addiction.
5. b. Schedule I drugs have no accepted medical use. Schedules II-V all have accepted medical uses and have decreasing abuse potential as the numbers increase.
6. c. OTC cough, cold, and allergy products containing ephedrine and pseudoephedrine may be kept only behind the counter and sold in limited amounts. The Combat Methamphetamine Epidemic Act of 2005 (CMEA) is the federal law that restricts sales of these products. It was enacted due to continuing concerns about the use of over-the-counter (OTC) products to illegally manufacture methamphetamine or amphetamine.
7. a. Some drugs, such as sublingual nitroglycerin, oral contraceptives, and other drugs packaged for patient use by the manufacturer, do not require the child-resistant packaging.
8. a. Holding a patent on a drug means no one else can produce or market that drug for the life of the patent. Generic drugs may be bioequivalent to brand name drugs, but may look different. The FDA approves generic drugs and determines whether they are bioequivalent to the branded reference drug. Generic substitutions by pharmacists are regulated by state generic substitution drug laws and regulations.
9. c. The person who signed the application for the pharmacy's registration with the DEA has the authority to sign DEA Form 222. He or she may delegate that authority to another by issuing a power of attorney. You do not have to be a pharmacist to sign a DEA Form 222 as long as you have a valid power of attorney from the registrant.
10. b. Commonly called OBRA '90, the Omnibus Budget Reconciliation Act of 1990 required pharmacists to provide patient counseling as a condition of reimbursement when dispensing prescriptions to Medicaid patients. The Food, Drug, and Cosmetics Act (FDCA) regulates the safety of food, drugs and cosmetics. The Durham-Humphrey Amendment defined the types of drugs that require a prescription and required that prescription drugs be labeled with the statement "Caution: Federal law prohibits dispensing without a prescription." The Controlled Substances Act establishes requirements for handling and dispensing of narcotics and other controlled substances.

Resources

Darvey DL. *Legal Handbook for Pharmacy Technicians*. Bethesda, MD: American Society of Health-System Pharmacists, 2008.

National Association of Boards of Pharmacy (NABP): www.nabp.net

Drug Enforcement Administration (DEA): Office of Diversion Control: www.deadiversion.usdoj.gov/index.html

Food and Drug Administration (FDA) Center for Drug Evaluation and Research: www.fda.gov/drugs/default.htm

Orange Book: *Approved Drug Products with Therapeutic Equivalence Evaluations*: www.accessdata.fda.gov/scripts/cder/ob/default.cfm

Medication Guides: http://www.fda.gov/Drugs/DrugSafety/ucm085729.htm

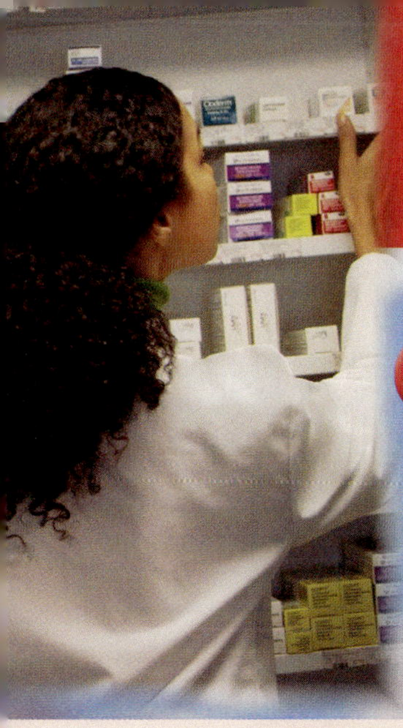

Chapter 3

Community and Ambulatory Care Pharmacy Practice

David R. Karls

Learning Outcomes

After completing this chapter, you will be able to

- Describe the history of community and ambulatory care pharmacy practices.
- Describe the differences among the various types of practice sites in community and ambulatory care pharmacy practice.
- Describe the importance of the pharmacy technician's role in communicating with patients in the community and ambulatory care pharmacy settings.
- Explain the various steps and responsibilities involved in filling a prescription.
- Identify the trends in community and ambulatory care pharmacy practices.
- Describe the evolving role of the pharmacy technician in community and ambulatory care pharmacy practices.

Key Terms

adverse reaction A bothersome or unwanted effect that results from the use of a drug, unrelated to the intended effect of the drug.

ambulatory care pharmacy A pharmacy generally located within or in close proximity to a clinic, hospital, or medical center that provides medication services to ambulatory patients.

brand name drug A drug that is covered by a patent and is therefore available only from a single manufacturer.

chain pharmacy A pharmacy that is part of a large number of corporately owned pharmacies that use the same name and carry similarly branded OTC products.

clinic pharmacy An ambulatory pharmacy located in a clinic or medical center to serve the needs of outpatients.

community pharmacy Generally a stand-alone pharmacy located within a community that provides medication services to ambulatory patients.

copayment (copay) The portion of the cost of a prescription that the patient is responsible for paying, when a part of the cost is covered by a third-party payer.

dispensing The act of preparing a medication for use by a patient as authorized by a prescription.

drug interactions Effects caused by the combined actions of two or more drugs used simultaneously.

formulary A list of drugs and their tiers that a third-party payer will cover.

generic drug A drug that is no longer covered by a patent and is therefore generally available from multiple manufacturers, usually resulting in a significant reduction in cost.

Health Insurance Portability and Accountability Act (HIPAA) Federal legislation enacted to establish guidelines for the protection of patients' private health information.

independent pharmacy A community pharmacy or small group of pharmacies in a limited geographic area that are owned by a single individual or a small number of individuals.

managed care pharmacy An ambulatory care pharmacy that is owned and operated as part of a managed care system such as a health maintenance organization (HMO).

mail-order pharmacy A pharmacy that functions like a warehouse, with pharmacists and technicians who dispense prescriptions that are mailed to (not picked up by) patients.

medication guides Patient information approved by the FDA to help patients avoid serious adverse effects, inform patients about known serious side effects, and provide directions for use to promote adherence to the treatment. These are available for specific drugs or classes of drugs and must be dispensed with the prescription.

National Drug Code (NDC) Number A unique number assigned to each drug, strength, and package size for the purpose of identification.

over-the-counter (OTC) drugs Drugs that are available without a prescription.

patient counseling The act of educating a patient, by a pharmacist, regarding the proper use of a prescribed drug, at the time of dispensing.

prescription The written or verbal authorization, by an authorized prescriber, for the use of a particular pharmaceutical agent for an individual patient. This term also refers to the physical product dispensed.

reimbursement Money that is collected from a third-party payer to cover partial cost or the entire cost of a prescription for a patient.

third-party payer An entity other than the patient that is involved in paying partial cost or the entire cost of prescriptions for a patient.

Community and ambulatory care pharmacies dispense more medications to more patients than any other practice setting. As our country's population continues to age, the number of prescriptions dispensed in these settings continues to rise. Although the number of pharmacies has increased to meet these needs, the number of prescriptions filled in each pharmacy has also continued to rise. This rise in prescription volume, combined with pharmacist shortages in many parts of the country and financial pressures from third-party payers, has increased the importance of the pharmacy technician's role in community and ambulatory pharmacy practice.

This chapter addresses some of the basic operations that are unique to community and ambulatory pharmacy practice, including the technician's responsibilities in this practice setting. Specifically, it provides a brief history of the community and ambulatory care settings, summarizes the different types of community and ambulatory pharmacies, describes the role of technicians in prescription processing, and addresses evolving trends in community and ambulatory pharmacy practice.

History and Evolution of Community and Ambulatory Care Pharmacy Practice

When most people hear the word "pharmacy," they think of a community or ambulatory care pharmacy. **Community pharmacies** were the first pharmacies, and although today's community and **ambulatory care pharmacies** have significantly evolved from the original "corner drug store," they still share the common purpose of providing pharmaceuticals and accessible health information in the community setting for ambulatory patients. Ambulatory care pharmacies evolved from community pharmacies. They still meet the needs of outpatients, but are usually located in close proximity to clinics, hospitals, or medical centers. Whereas community pharmacies often sell items not related to pharmacy, ambulatory pharmacies generally provide only prescription services and possibly a limited number of over-the-counter medications.

In the early part of our country's history, very few medications were manufactured in their final dosage form, as they are today. Pharmaceutical remedies were limited, so pharmacists prepared, or compounded, these remedies, mostly from natural sources and raw chemicals. There were no regulations on drugs and pharmacists were free to prepare and sell almost anything. Physicians would send patients to pharmacists, who would compound remedies based on the patient's evaluation and diagnosis. Pharmacists would also create remedies based on a patient's symptoms or requests.

In 1938, the Food, Drug, and Cosmetics Act (FDCA) was passed, which began to loosely regulate drugs, requiring pre-market approval for new drugs based on safety, and prohibiting false therapeutic claims for drugs. The law also allowed for the designation of a drug to be available only by prescription, but lacked specific guidelines and left it mostly up to the manufacturer.[1]

In 1951, the Durham-Humphrey Amendment to the Food, Drug, and Cosmetics Act was passed, which more precisely defined the previous guidelines for prescription drugs established in 1938 under the original act. Two categories of drugs were established: legend drugs and **over-the-counter (OTC) drugs**. Any drug that was determined to be a legend drug, based on safety and potential for addiction, required authorization from a doctor before a pharmacist could prepare and dispense the product. OTC drugs were considered safe enough for patients' self-administration and could be purchased without a doctor's authorization. The written or verbal authorization and the dispensed product became known as a **prescription**.

As the pharmaceutical industry continued to grow and more and more drugs were being manufactured in their final dosage forms, the focus of the pharmacist's role began to change from making the drug products to repackaging and **dispensing** them. Information about prescriptions was considered to be limited to doctor-patient relationships and it was mostly considered inappropriate for a pharmacist to discuss drug therapy with a patient.

This philosophy began to change in the 1960s and 1970s, as more and more drugs were developed and patients' individual drug therapies began to include medications with increased risks of **drug interactions** and side effects or **adverse reactions**. Whereas, in the past, pharmacists essentially dispensed prescriptions one by one, many pharmacies began maintaining patient profiles that listed all of the drugs each patient was using. This allowed pharmacists to check for potential problems between drugs when new drugs were prescribed or when patients reported problems. These records became much easier to maintain and utilize as computers began to be used more widely for prescription processing.

By the 1980s, the principle of pharmaceutical care was gaining wider acceptance as a standard model for pharmacy practice, beginning the shift toward a more clinical role for pharmacists. Pharmaceutical care essentially encourages the establishment of the pharmacist as the manager of a patient's drug therapy. Guidelines for this level of care include assisting in the selection of drugs, educating patients, and monitoring adverse reactions and outcomes of drug therapy.

Another change taking place was the involvement of **third-party payers** in **reimbursement** for prescriptions. In the past, most patients paid for their prescriptions with cash, but as the costs of health care and drugs increased, third-party payers began to cover some or all of the costs of patients' medications. These third-parties include government employers, government programs such as Medicaid, employers' health insurance policies, and private insurance purchased by individuals. Since then, the most significant influence of third-party payers has been negotiating continually decreasing reimbursement for community and ambulatory pharmacies. To make up for the revenue lost to low reimbursement from third-party payers, pharmacies have had to trim operating costs, which has resulted in such issues as reduced staff, increased prescription volume, and discontinued services, such as free prescription delivery. Third-party payers also play a role in influencing what drugs physicians prescribe for their patients by restricting the drugs they will cover and controlling what portion of the total cost the patient must pay. Today, most prescriptions are covered at least partially by a third-party payer.

In 1990, the U.S. Congress passed the Omnibus Budget Reconciliation Act (OBRA). Part of this law required pharmacists to perform three functions when filling a prescription for a Medicaid recipient:

1. Prospective Drug Utilization Review (DUR)—To review a patient's medication profile to screen for potential problems with the prescribed drug, such as appropriateness of the drug and dose for the patient, drug interactions, or drug duplications.
2. **Patient counseling**—To talk to a patient about his or her prescription and to answer questions.
3. Patient record maintenance—To keep records of each patient, including all of the drugs the patient is taking.

Under the law, states were required to develop specific standards for patient counseling, such as when counseling must be offered (i.e., new prescriptions and/or refills), who may make the offer to counsel (i.e., pharmacist and/or technician), and what types of information should be included during counseling (e.g., what a drug is used for, directions for use, and possible adverse reactions).[2] As these standards were developed, states required them to be applied to all patients' prescriptions, not just Medicaid recipients. Although many of the OBRA requirements were being followed under the principles of pharmaceutical care, OBRA and the subsequent state regulations now require them, by law, to be applied to every prescription and patient.

The role of the pharmacist in community and ambulatory care pharmacies has generally evolved from preparers of drug products, to dispensers of drug products, and to managers of medication therapies. As the pharmacist's role has changed, pharmacy technicians have assumed many of the important technical functions of the processing of prescriptions that were formerly performed by pharmacists. As technicians' roles and responsibilities have increased, so have the professional standards for technician licensure and certification, as described in Chapter 1: Introduction to Pharmacy.

✔The technician's role has become a very important part of delivering pharmaceutical care to patients. The foundation of medication therapy management by pharmacists is the proper handling and preparation of the actual drug product by technicians.

Practice Sites

There are several types of community and ambulatory care pharmacy settings, or practice sites, including community pharmacies, clinic pharmacies, managed care pharmacies, and mail-order pharmacies.

Community Pharmacies

Community pharmacies are generally broken down into two groups: independent and chain pharmacies. **Independent pharmacies** are generally owned and staffed by one or two individual pharmacists. An independent pharmacy owner may own a small number of pharmacies in a limited geographic area, but they are still generally considered to be independent. Originally, all pharmacies were independent, with chain pharmacies beginning to develop in the 20th century.

Chain pharmacies developed when companies began to own larger and larger numbers of pharmacies that all used the same name and logo and carried similarly branded OTC products. As more pharmaceuticals began to be produced by manufacturers, chain pharmacy companies gained a financial advantage by buying in bulk to supply all of their stores. As financial pressures on the pharmacy business have increased, so have the number of chain pharmacies. In fact, although the number of independent pharmacies has been steadily declining, the number of pharmacy chain stores has been steadily increasing. Many independent pharmacies have been sold to chain pharmacies, some of which have combined to form fewer numbers of bigger chains. Chain pharmacies originally were simply large groups of pharmacies, but today other retail chains, such as grocery chains and "big box" retailers, have added pharmacies inside their stores.

Clinic Pharmacies

Clinic pharmacies are ambulatory care pharmacies that are located in clinics or medical centers to serve the needs of outpatients. These pharmacies may be owned and operated by the facility, or owned independently but located in the facility. Clinic pharmacies typically function similarly to community pharmacies, but there is often more direct contact and communication with prescribers and other health care personnel within the facility. As such, clinic pharmacies may be more involved in managing drug therapies and offering other health screening and immunization services. Clinic pharmacies are generally smaller in size and carry a limited amount of OTC medications and other merchandise.

Managed Care Pharmacies

Managed care pharmacies are ambulatory pharmacies that are owned and operated as part of a managed care system, such as a health maintenance organization (HMO). They usually resemble clinic pharmacies but are operated by the managed care company for the patients they serve. As with clinic pharmacies, they would typically be located in proximity to a medical facility. As part of a managed care system, all of the managed care pharmacies within any one organization would likely look similar and offer similar services. There may be even more coordinated communication between managed care pharmacies and other health care professionals in the organization than there would be in clinic pharmacies.

Mail-Order Pharmacies

Although classified as ambulatory pharmacies because they generally serve ambulatory patients, mail-order pharmacies look and operate differently from other types of community and ambulatory care pharmacies. **Mail-order pharmacies** generally fill very large volumes of prescriptions and specialize in maintenance medications. Because of their high prescription volume, the prescription filling process is often highly automated and there is generally less direct contact with patients, except by telephone and electronically via Web sites and the Internet. Mail-order pharmacies are really more like warehouses with pharmacists and technicians. They are unlike typical pharmacies, where patients can walk in and pick up prescriptions.

Technician Responsibilities in Prescription Processing

Within community and ambulatory care pharmacies, pharmacy technicians have a variety of responsibilities, including

- Communicating with patients
- Ensuring patient privacy
- Receiving prescriptions and registering patients
- Transferring prescriptions
- Entering prescriptions in a computer
- Handling restricted-use medications
- Resolving third-party payer issues
- Filling and labeling pharmaceutical products

- Compounding prescriptions
- Collecting payment and offering patient counseling
- Fulfilling miscellaneous responsibilities

Communicating with Patients

Pharmacy technicians spend a larger percentage of their time communicating with patients in community and ambulatory care settings than in any other practice setting, with the exception of mail-order settings. A technician is likely to be the first person to interact with a patient when he or she arrives, and the last before he or she leaves. Technicians also assist patients on the telephone with technical issues regarding their prescriptions. In many cases, patients will actually interact more directly with technicians and other support staff than with pharmacists.

✔When communicating with patients, it is important for staff to act professionally and in a caring manner at all times.

Patients are often at the pharmacy because they do not feel well, and this may affect how they interact with you. It is important to be patient and show concern for their needs. Also, remember to respect patients' privacy when discussing personal information in the presence of other patients and staff. Communication and professionalism are explained in greater detail in Chapter 8: Communication and Teamwork.

Rx for Success

Sometimes confrontations with patients are inevitable, but a calm approach can help to avoid them. If an interaction with a patient seems to be escalating toward confrontation, it is best for the technician to involve the pharmacist.

Ensuring Patient Privacy

In 1996, the **Health Insurance Portability and Accountability Act (HIPAA)** was passed. This important legislation included a "privacy rule" that was established to provide a national standard for protecting individuals' private health information. Essentially, this provides pharmacies with specific guidelines regarding how to handle private patient information. A technician's responsibility mostly involves using care when discussing private patient information and ensuring that any documents that contain private information be placed in the appropriate location for destruction (e.g., never with general refuse).

HIPAA also requires each pharmacy to have a written policy for handling private patient information. This policy must be given to new patients the first time they have a prescription filled, and a reasonable attempt must be made to record the patient's signature to verify their receipt of a copy of the policy.[3] A pharmacy can fulfill this requirement when the prescription is dropped off or when it is picked up. HIPAA and other relevant legislation are described in more detail in Chapter 2: Pharmacy Law.

Receiving Prescriptions and Registering Patients

When a patient is welcomed to the pharmacy, it is important to first identify him or her. If the patient has been to your pharmacy before, another piece of identifying information, such as date of birth, address, or phone number, should be obtained to confirm the patient's identity. If the patient is bringing a prescription to you for the first time, he or she needs to be registered by providing the following information:

- Correct spelling of name
- Address and phone number(s)
- Insurance information from patient's insurance card
- Date of birth
- Any drug allergies
- Other prescriptions or OTC medications the patient takes regularly
- Significant health conditions

Prescriptions may be received directly from the patient or from the prescriber by telephone, fax, or electronic transmission.

Receiving a prescription includes determining whether the prescription will be filled with generic or brand-name drugs. **Generic drugs** are less expensive alternatives to **brand name drugs** and can significantly drive down the cost of the drug to patients. The FDA regulates generic drugs so that they are equivalent in quality to corresponding brand name drugs. State regulations vary regarding the specifics of when a generic substitute may be used, so technicians should be familiar with their state's regulations. A general question that may be asked when the patient presents a prescription is, "Would you like us to fill your prescription with a less expensive generic alternative, if one is available?" Technicians may offer a generic drug to a patient only if the prescriber has indicated that substitution is acceptable. Some drugs are not available in generic form, thus should not be offered to the patient.

It is also important for customer service and workflow to ask the patient if he or she will be waiting for the prescription or if he or she will be coming back later. With this information, prescriptions can be processed in the order in which they are due, and when patients expect them to be ready.

Transferring Prescriptions

Prescriptions may be transferred between pharmacies subject to specific state regulations, which vary somewhat among states. Prescription information may be transferred by telephone or electronically between pharmacies within the same chain. A technician may be allowed to assist with prescription transfers made by telephone, but the pharmacist is responsible for the information transferred out and received. In many states, the transfer of a prescription from one pharmacy to another must be accomplished only pharmacist to pharmacist.

If a patient requests to have a prescription transferred from another pharmacy, it is important for the technician to obtain as much information about the prescription as possible, including at least the patient's name and date of birth, the name and telephone number of the other pharmacy, and the prescription number and/or name of the medication. If a patient brings in a prescription container from the other pharmacy, the label can be used to get the necessary information and to double-check the information received by telephone.

Entering Prescriptions in a Computer

There is a wide variety of prescription processing software on the market, so the specific steps for entering information into computers varies among systems. Some software now requires the prescription to be scanned into the system to make the information on the hard copy readily accessible (figure 3–1). Once the prescription has been scanned (if needed), the information on the prescription is entered into the appropriate fields. See Chapter 14: Processing Medication Orders and Prescriptions for more information.

Handling Restricted-Use Medications

There are certain medications that can be prescribed and dispensed only in a community or ambulatory care pharmacy under specific conditions due to special precautions regarding their use. The FDA requires a Risk Evaluation and Mitigation Strategy (REMS) when it determines that a strategy is necessary to ensure the benefits of using the drug outweigh the potential risks. A REMS may require registration and other specific action by the physician, pharmacist, and patient before the medication can be dispensed. It may also apply specifications as to how prescriptions may be written (i.e., limits on how many units may be dispensed or if refills are allowed, and requiring standard stickers or other documentation on the face of the prescription). Examples of drugs with REMS include: alosetron (Lotronex), clozapine (Clozaril, Fazaclo), isotretinoin (Accutane, Amnesteem, Claravis, Sotret), thalidomide (Thalomid), and dofetilide (Tikosyn).

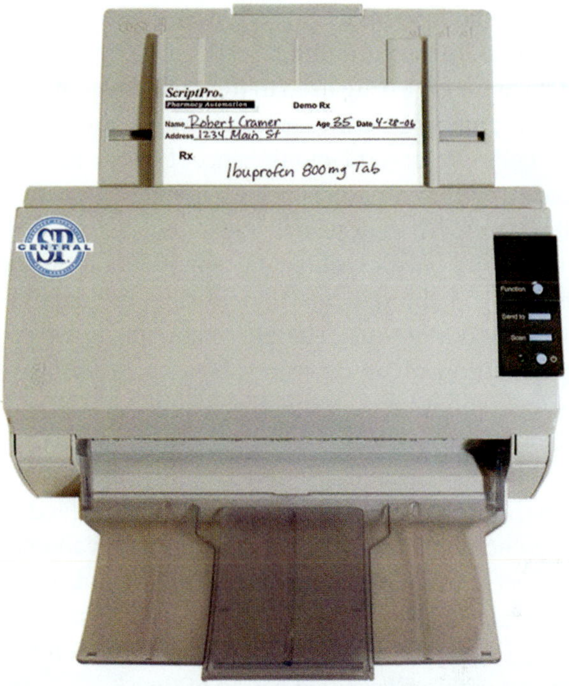

Figure 3–1. Prescription scanner; used to capture an image of the prescription for easy reference and retrieval. Photo courtesy of ScriptPro.

Alosetron is a drug used to treat severe diarrhea-predominant irritable bowel syndrome (IBS). Due to serious adverse reactions of the gastrointestinal tract—some necessitate a blood transfusion or surgery, and some even lead to death—alosetron's use is restricted by the Prescription Program for Lotronex (PPL). The program requires physician enrollment, including submission of the Patient-Physician Agreement Form. Prescriptions must be written by the physician and must include a PPL sticker on the face of the prescription. Refills may be authorized on the prescription.[4]

Clozapine is a drug used to treat patients with schizophrenia. This drug can cause a serious drop in white blood cells, so careful monitoring of these levels must be done regularly, based on the patient's condition and medical history. Pharmacies must register to dispense clozapine and only a specific day supply (1, 2, or 3 weeks depending on the patients' monitoring frequency) may be dispensed at a time. The pharmacy must also receive documentation of blood work showing a normal white blood cell count before each dispensing.[5]

Isotretinoin is a drug used for severe acne. Its use is restricted because it can cause serious birth defects. Doctors, patients, and pharmacies must register with the iPledge Program, which monitors the drug's use. Doctors and patients must meet specific requirements and answer questions with the iPledge Program each time the drug is dispensed. The quantity dispensed is limited and the prescription must be picked up within a specified period of time.[6]

Thalidomide is a drug that is used to treat multiple myeloma (a specific type of cancer) and erythema nodosum leprosum (a specific skin condition). The use of thalidomide is also restricted due to concerns about birth defects. Prescribers, patients, and pharmacies must register with the System for Thalidomide Education and Prescribing Safety (S.T.E.P.S.) program. The pharmacy must verify that the prescriber is registered with S.T.E.P.S. before dispensing the medication.[7]

Dofetilide is used to treat irregular heart rhythms. It can cause serious complications, particularly when therapy is first started, so patients must be hospitalized to initiate therapy. Prescribers and pharmacists must register with the Tikosyn in Pharmacy System (T.I.P.S.) program, and the pharmacy must verify the prescriber's registration with the program before dispensing an outpatient prescription.[8]

The FDA has designated other drugs that are required to be dispensed with **Medication Guides**. A Medication Guide is patient information approved by the FDA to help patients avoid serious adverse events, inform them about known serious side effects, and provide directions for use to promote adherence to the treatment. These are available for specific drugs or classes of drugs and must be dispensed with the prescription.[9] Common examples dispensed in community and ambulatory care pharmacies include non-steroidal anti-inflammatory drugs (NSAIDs) and antidepressants. Pharmacy technicians may be required to help maintain adequate supplies of these Medication Guides and to locate the appropriate guide when completing the prescription filling process.

REMS and Medication Guides are important to address patient safety issues. Additional programs and guides could be mandated by the FDA in the future, as new drugs are developed or new risks associated with drugs already on the market are discovered.

Resolving Third-Party Payer Issues

After a prescription is entered into the computer system, if the patient has prescription coverage by a third-party payer, a claim will be sent electronically to the payer. If the claim is accepted, the payer has agreed to pay the claim, and the appropriate copayment for the claim will be noted. The **copayment**, or copay, is the amount of the cost of the prescription that the patient is responsible for paying. Copays vary among plans, with some charging patients a percentage of the total cost of the prescription, and other plans charging a flat dollar amount per prescription. Three-tier copays are common: in this system, a low copay is charged for most generic drugs, a higher copay is charged for "preferred" brand name drugs, and a still higher copay is charged for "non-preferred" brand name drugs. A **formulary** is a list of drugs and their tiers that a specific third-party payer will cover.

Most claims are now handled by pharmacy benefits managers (PBMs), which are companies that contract with multiple third-party payers to process transactions and help establish and enforce their formularies.

If there is a problem with a claim, the pharmacy will receive a message that the claim has been rejected. Unfortunately, resolving third-party rejections has become a time-consuming part of prescription processing. Rejections may be resolved by simply verifying the information that was submitted, but often they require a telephone call to the third-party payer or PBM. Some of the most common rejections include missing/invalid patient ID number, refill too soon, plan limitations exceeded, and prior authorization required. See Chapter 20: Billing and Reimbursement for more information on resolving rejected claims.

Filling and Labeling Pharmaceutical Products

Today, most drug products are manufactured in their final dosage forms by manufacturers. The prescription filling process involves selecting the correct drug product, packaging the proper quantity in a suitable package, and then labeling the package. When the prescribed drug product is located and retrieved, care must be taken to select the correct drug, with the correct dose or strength, in the correct dosage form. Tablets, capsules, powder packets, and suppositories may need the specific number of units required by the prescription to be counted, and then packaged in a prescription container before labeling. Likewise, liquid medications may need to be poured from bulk bottles into smaller prescription bottles before labeling. Some manufacturers now package tablets and capsules in commonly dispensed quantities (e.g., 30, 60, or 90). Also, products such as topical preparations, inhalers, and nasal sprays are self-contained in sealed packages, which means they simply require applying the prescription label to the manufacturer's package. When a manufacturer's drug container is labeled, it is important to ensure that expiration date, lot number, and storage requirements are visible.

Safety First The process of filling and labeling is very important and must be accomplished with great care and accuracy. Any mistake presents a possible danger to the patient if the error is not detected before the patient receives the medication. Even if the error is identified, the process of correcting it takes additional time and obstructs work flow.

After completing the prescription filling and labeling process, the technician should re-check to make sure he or she has prepared the correct drug, with the correct dose or strength, in the correct dosage form. Each unique drug, strength, and package size is assigned a unique **National Drug Code (NDC) number** that is printed on the drug package.

Rx for Success

A product's NDC number can be used as a double check to make sure the correct drug product has been selected for filling.

Although tablets and capsules are still hand-counted and packaged in many pharmacy settings, technology is now available to assist in some or all of the filling and labeling functions. Counting devices use a scale to count units based on their weight (figure 3–2) or light beams to count units as they are poured through a machine (figure 3–3). Other machines store the most commonly used drugs in bulk quantities in "cells" that dispense the required number of units into a vial to be labeled. Some also place the label on the vial (figure 3–4). When a pharmacy utilizes technology as part of the dispensing process, technicians are required to fill, clean, and maintain the equipment so it performs correctly.

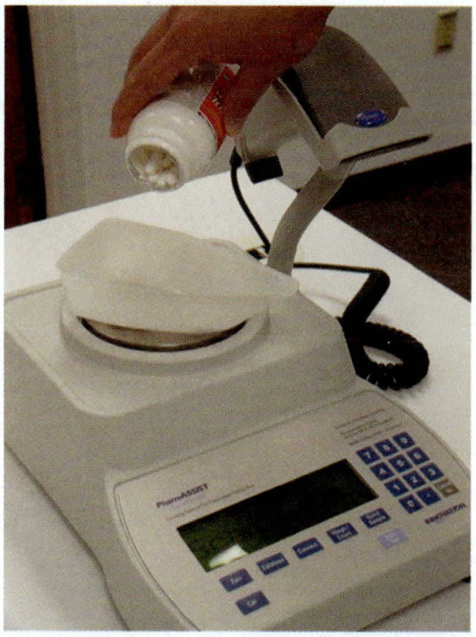

Figure 3–2. Scale counter. Photo courtesy of Innovation.

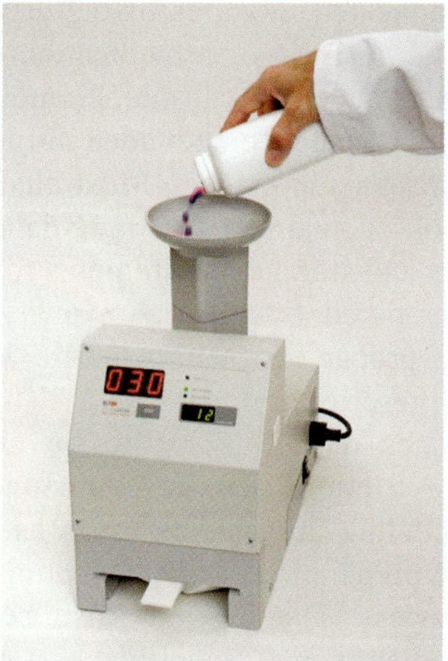

Figure 3–3. Counting device that utilizes light beams to quickly and accurately count tablets or capsules. Photo courtesy of Kirby Lester, LLC.

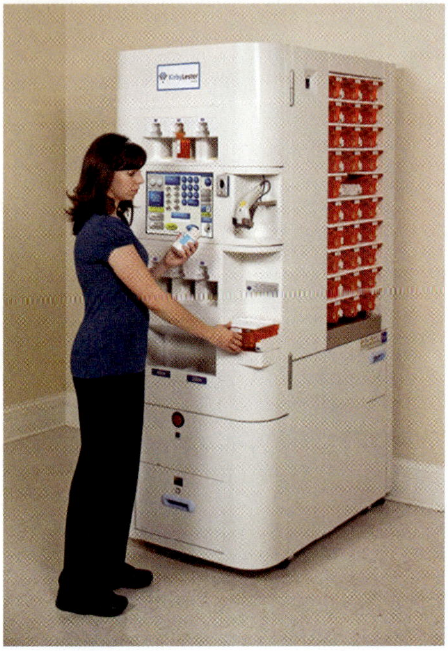

Figure 3-4. Robotic dispensing machine fills and labels prescriptions. Photo courtesy of Kirby Lester, LLC.

Compounding Prescriptions

Although most drug products are now manufactured by the pharmaceutical industry, there are still times when a special formulation must be prepared. Often these are simple mixtures of liquids or creams, but they may be more complicated mixtures of ingredients, such as preparing a liquid form of a medication that is available only as a tablet or capsule. Some states allow technicians to prepare compounded formulations under a pharmacist's supervision. Most pharmacies have a "recipe book" containing the ingredients, directions for preparing, and storage requirements for compounds commonly prepared by the pharmacy. A technician must receive proper instruction before attempting to compound a prescription.

Many states require a log to be maintained in which all prescriptions that are compounded are documented, including information (such as who was involved in the preparation) and verification of the compounding process. The log may also be required to include ingredient names, quantities, lot numbers, and expiration dates. Drug compounding is more fully described in Chapter 15: Nonsterile Compounding and Repackaging.

Collecting Payment and Patient Counseling

Technicians are usually involved in point-of-sale (POS) transactions, which involve checking out patients and collecting payment when prescription orders are complete. There are four important aspects to this task. First, the patient's name and some other identifying information (e.g., date of birth, address, phone number) must be verified to ensure that the correct medication is being given to the correct patient. Second, legal requirements must be met regarding patient counseling. State laws vary regarding whether new prescriptions and refills require patient counseling, and whether technicians are allowed to offer counseling. It is important to make sure all legal requirements are met. Also, patient counseling by the pharmacist is an important part of the dispensing process to ensure that the patient understands how to safely and effectively use his or her medication. Third, new patients must be given a copy of the pharmacy's patient privacy policy in compliance with HIPAA regulations. Finally, collecting patients' signatures is required by HIPAA when they receive the pharmacy privacy policy, by some states if they refuse patient counseling, and by some third-party payers when the patient takes possession of the prescription.

Safety First The patient's name and some other identifying information (e.g., date of birth, address, phone number) must be verified to ensure that the correct medication is being given to the correct patient.

Fulfilling Miscellaneous Responsibilities

In addition to duties related to prescription processing, technicians may perform other duties in the pharmacy. Other common responsibilities include managing inventory, managing pharmacy records, and helping patients locate OTC drugs, including the sale of products containing pseudoephedrine.

Managing inventory is an important part of pharmacy operations. The need to maintain adequate quantities of commonly used medications to meet patient needs must be balanced with the need to control operating expenses, i.e., avoiding tying up money in excessive inventory. Many community and ambulatory pharmacies' inventories are controlled by automatic inventory software systems that are incorporated into the prescription dispensing systems to reorder drugs as they are dispensed. Although these can be very efficient, human intervention is still necessary to ensure that quantities in the inventory system reflect the actual inventory in stock. Also, special orders often need to be entered manually. The topics of purchasing and managing inventory are more fully covered in Chapter 19: Purchasing and Inventory.

Pharmacy law requires accurate maintenance of pharmacy records. In addition to sequencing, sorting, and proper storage of prescription hard copies, other records that require regular maintenance include drug supplier invoices, particularly for controlled substances, insurance signature logs, patient counseling logs, and HIPAA signature logs. Inaccurate or incomplete maintenance of these records can result in disciplinary action or fines in the event of an audit by the state board of pharmacy, federal Drug Enforcement Administration (DEA), third-party payer, or other government agencies.

A technician's contact with patients will periodically involve responding to patients' inquiries about OTC medications. Care must be taken when responding to these inquiries. If a patient simply asks for the location of a specific product (e.g., aspirin) or type of product (e.g., pain relievers), a technician may help with these types of requests; however, if a patient has a question that requires clinical knowledge or judgment, such as which product to use for a specific condition, such inquiries must be referred to a pharmacist. If there is any question whether or not a technician is qualified to respond to an inquiry, the pharmacist should be consulted.

✔ If a patient has a question that requires clinical knowledge or judgment, such as which OTC product to use for a specific condition, the pharmacist should be consulted.

A specific area of concern is with the decongestant pseudoephedrine. Federal and state laws regulate the quantity of OTC medications containing pseudoephedrine that a person may purchase. These laws were passed because pseudoephedrine can be converted into illegal stimulants (i.e., methamphetamine, amphetamines). State laws vary somewhat, but generally patients are required to show valid photo identification, such as a driver's license, to purchase any of these products. Laws also limit the number of packages that an individual may buy per purchase and per month, based on the total amount of pseudoephedrine contained in each package. The pharmacy is required to keep these products behind the pharmacy counter and restrict sales based on these regulations. They are also required to keep records of who buys how much of which products. Technicians are allowed to process the transactions under these guidelines. See Chapter 2: Pharmacy Law for more information.

Practice Trends

As community and ambulatory pharmacy practice continues to evolve, pharmacies are finding new ways to serve their patients, while also generating revenue to offset the financial pressures from reduced third-party payer reimbursement. Newer practice trends include providing disease state management, health screenings, immunizations, dietary supplements, and specialty compounding. Providing one or more of these services may give a pharmacy or pharmacy chain a competitive advantage in the marketplace.

Disease State Management

As community and ambulatory care pharmacies have evolved from a focus on dispensing to a focus on clinical management of medication therapies, many pharmacists have developed specialties in disease state management. The ability of skilled technicians to assume many of the important dispensing functions that were previously performed by pharmacists has allowed pharmacists to participate in medication therapy management. Pharmacists collaborate with prescribers and other health care providers to monitor patients and make adjustments or changes to medications related to a specific disease. Disease state management is most common in the management of chronic conditions such as hypertension, hyperlipidemia, asthma, and anticoagulant therapy. Initially, third-party payers were reluctant to pay pharmacists for these services; however, as pharmacists have been able to demonstrate and document cost savings related to their services, more payers have been willing to cover at least some of the costs of these services. A pharmacist generally completes special training to become certified to provide disease state management. Technicians may also be involved in disease state management by helping collect and manage the data and records necessary for pharmacist monitoring.

Health Screenings

Another way for pharmacies to help patients monitor their health is to offer health screenings. This service is less involved than disease state management and can entail taking blood pressure measurements or checking blood glucose levels. Such services can be offered to patients as a free service or for a nominal fee. Pharmacies may also pay an agency to come in periodically to offer more complex screenings such as cholesterol panels or bone density scans. Providing health screenings is a way for a pharmacy to distinguish itself from its competitors by offering a unique and accessible service to its patients, while also increasing access to health care for many patients. Technicians may be trained to administer some screenings to collect data for the pharmacist to review with the patient.

Immunizations

Many pharmacies now provide immunizations for the prevention of various conditions. The influenza vaccine or the "flu shot" is probably the most common vaccine offered by pharmacies. Other examples may include shingles, pneumonia, and travel vaccines. In addition to being one of the most accessible members of the health care team, pharmacists have the opportunity to help identify patients who have certain risk factors that make them good candidates for specific vaccines. Most states now allow pharmacists with special training to administer vaccines themselves. Other pharmacies simply contract with an outside service to provide immunizations on the pharmacy's premises. Technicians may assist with immunizations by registering patients, ordering, storing and preparing vaccine doses, and keeping required records.

Dietary Supplements

With the decline in reimbursement from third-party payers for prescription drugs, many pharmacies have found an opportunity by specializing in dietary supplements, which generally include vitamins and minerals, amino acids, and herbs. Although supplements have become increasingly popular for patients to use to help or prevent various conditions, supplements remain loosely regulated and are often sold in health food stores and other non-pharmacy outlets where staff may have little or no medical training. Much of the information available to consumers about supplements is exaggerated or inaccurate, which can lead to overuse or misuse. Pharmacists have a unique opportunity to help their patients make reasonable decisions regarding supplement use. More and more medically credible resources are becoming available to help pharmacists make informed recommendations and provide important warnings. As with OTC drugs, pharmacy technicians should be familiar with the products that the pharmacy stocks and be able to help patients locate specific products they may request. It may also be appropriate to direct a patient to the pharmacist for more information or to answer questions about a product.

Specialty Compounding

As stated above, most pharmacies will prepare *simple* compounds, such as mixing two creams together or crushing tablets and suspending them in liquid, but many are no longer equipped to handle more complicated formulations with multiple ingredients or that require special equipment. These formulations may involve dosage forms in which a particular drug is not available, or for a drug that is no longer available in any form other than as a raw chemical. Some pharmacies meet this need by offering specialty compounding. This may involve making capsules, suppositories, transdermal gels, and topical preparations. Compounding supply companies provide the equipment and bulk chemicals used by compounding specialists, along with formulations and stability information for compounded products. In most states, technicians are allowed to assist in the compounding process under pharmacist supervision. For more information see Chapter 6: Specialty Pharmacy Practice and Chapter 15: Nonsterile Compounding and Repackaging.

Summary

In community and ambulatory care pharmacies, there continues to be a steady increase in the number of patients requiring prescriptions, the number of prescriptions required by each patient, the number of drugs available both as prescriptions and as OTC drugs, and the complexity of drugs and of drug therapies. This has increased the importance of the pharmacist's role as a manager of drug therapies, which in turn makes the role and responsibilities of the technician even more important. It is vital that technicians be conscientious in efficiently and accurately assisting in the prescription processing function, as well as treating patients in a professional manner at all times. It is likely that as these conditions continue to evolve, the technician's roles and responsibilities will continue to evolve as well.

Self-Assessment Questions

1. The practice of community and ambulatory care pharmacy has evolved from
   a. Preparing to dispensing to clinical
   b. Dispensing to preparing to clinical
   c. Preparing to clinical to dispensing
   d. Compounding to preparing to clinical
2. The term pharmaceutical care refers to
   a. The proper storage of pharmaceutical products
   b. The careful handling of private patient information
   c. The role of the pharmacist as a manager of drug therapy
   d. Patient counseling requirements for each prescription dispensed
3. Most community pharmacies are
   a. Independent
   b. Chain
   c. Mail-order
   d. Managed care
4. When communicating with patients, it is important to be all of the following, except
   a. Patient
   b. Caring
   c. Professional
   d. Quick
5. HIPAA regulates
   a. Guidelines for patient counseling
   b. Proper storage of drug products
   c. Rules for generic substitution
   d. Handling of private patient information
6. Which of the following questions may a technician answer for a patient?
   a. What can I take for a cold?
   b. Where can I find the aspirin?
   c. What is the best thing for pain?
   d. Can I take this drug if I have high blood pressure?
7. During a point-of-sale (POS) transaction, important technician functions include all of the following, except
   a. Verifying the patient's identity
   b. Meeting requirements for offering patient counseling by the pharmacist
   c. Collecting payment
   d. Answering a patient's questions about his or her prescription
8. In addition to the prescription filling process, a technician may be responsible for all of the following, except
   a. Managing inventory
   b. Managing pharmacy records
   c. Helping patients choose OTC drugs
   d. Preparing compounded drugs
9. With regard to the sale of OTC products containing pseudoephedrine:
   a. A pharmacy technician may process the transaction
   b. All products must be kept behind the pharmacy counter, but may be sold only by a pharmacist
   c. Patients are required to show photo identification, but are not limited to the number of packages they may purchase
   d. The pharmacy is not required to maintain a record of who buys how much of which products
10. Which of the following statements is true?
    a. Technicians play a critical role in the process of medication therapy management
    b. Technicians have less direct contact with patients in community and ambulatory care pharmacies than in other pharmacy practice settings
    c. Accuracy is not an important responsibility for a pharmacy technician during the prescription filling process because all prescriptions must be checked for accuracy by a pharmacist
    d. Technicians are not allowed to prepare compounded medications

Self-Assessment Answers

1. a. Pharmacists began their practice by preparing medications. As pharmaceutical companies began to manufacture more drugs, pharmacists shifted their focus to dispensing. As drug therapies became more complicated, pharmacists began to assume the clinical role of drug therapy managers.
2. c. The term "pharmaceutical care" describes a model that emphasizes the pharmacist's role as a drug therapy manager.
3. b. Originally, all community pharmacies were independent pharmacies, but due to financial pressures in the industry, the number of independent pharmacies has steadily declined and now most community pharmacies are chain pharmacies. Mail-order and managed care pharmacies aren't considered community pharmacies.
4. d. Patience, caring, and professionalism are important priorities at all times when taking care of patients in the pharmacy.
5. d. HIPAA regulates the handling of patients' private information in written, spoken, and electronic forms.
6. b. Technicians may direct patients to a particular product or type of product, but questions regarding clinical judgment should be referred to the pharmacist.
7. d. Questions about a patient's prescription require clinical knowledge and should be referred to the pharmacist.
8. c. Technicians may help a patient find OTC drugs, but should not give advice regarding which one to choose.
9. a. A technician may process a transaction for the sale of OTC products containing pseudoephedrine as long as they follow relevant federal and state laws. The number of packages purchased is limited by law. The pharmacy is required to record who buys these products.
10. a. An important part of medication therapy management is the proper handling and preparation of the actual drug product by technicians. Technicians have more communication with patients in community and ambulatory care pharmacy settings. Accuracy *is* an important responsibility for a pharmacy technician during the prescription filling process. Technicians may prepare compounded medications under pharmacist supervision.

References

1. Federal Food, Drug, and Cosmetic Act. U.S. Food and Drug Administration Web site. http://www.fda.gov/RegulatoryInformation/Legislation/FederalFoodDrugandCosmeticActFDCAct/default.htm. Accessed September 8, 2009.
2. Fink, J, Vivian, J. OBRA '90 at Sweet Sixteen: A Retrospective Review. *U.S. Pharmacist*. 2008;33(3)59–65.
3. Summary of the HIPAA Privacy Rule. U.S. Department of Health and Human Services Web site. http://www.hhs.gov/ocr/privacy/hipaa/understanding/summary/index.html. Accessed September 8, 2009.
4. Lotronex [package insert]. San Diego, CA: Prometheus Laboratories Inc.; 2008.
5. Clozaril [package insert]. East Hanover, NJ: Novartis Pharmaceuticals Corp.; 2008.
6. iPledge Program [online]. https://www.ipledgeprogram.com. Accessed April 14, 2009.
7. Thalomid [package insert]. Summit, NJ: Celgene Corporation; 2005.
8. Tikosyn [package insert]. New York, NY: Pfizer, Inc; 2003.
9. Medication Guides. U.S. Food and Drug Administration Web site. http://www.fda.gov/Drugs/DrugSafety/ucm085729.htm. Accessed April 14, 2008.

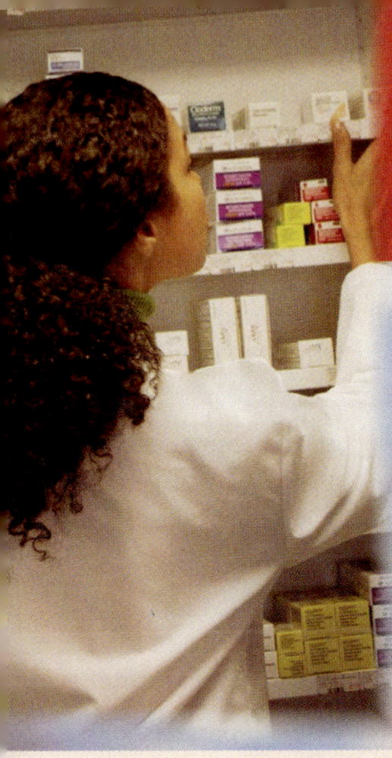

Chapter 4

Hospital Pharmacy Practice

Steven Lundquist

Learning Outcomes

After completing this chapter, you will be able to

- Describe the differences between centralized and decentralized pharmacies.
- List at least two types of services that are provided by hospital pharmacy departments.
- Explain how pharmacy policy and procedure manuals help technicians function efficiently in a large number of duties, responsibilities, and situations.
- List at least three different methods of drug distribution in which technicians play an active role.
- List the components of—and the role the technician has in—the medication management process.
- Describe the role accrediting and regulatory agencies play in a hospital pharmacy.
- List two types of technology that a pharmacy technician will work with in a hospital pharmacy.
- Describe quality control and quality improvement programs, including how they are used in hospital pharmacy practice.
- List at least three organizations that are involved with patient safety.
- Describe the financial impact that third-party payers have on hospitals.

Key Terms

automated medication dispensing device A drug storage device or cabinet that contains an inventory of medications that are electronically dispensed so they may be administered to patients in a controlled manner.

centralized pharmacy services Pharmacy services that are provided from one location (usually centrally located) in the hospital. Pharmacy personnel, resources, and functions primarily reside within this self-contained location.

clinical pharmacy services Services provided by a pharmacist focused on patient care. These services vary greatly by facility, but the goal is to ensure that each medication is appropriate, safe, and cost effective (based on the diagnosis of the patient).

closed formulary A predetermined, specific list of medications approved by the hospital's P&T committee (or equivalent) to be used for the patients it serves.

decentralized pharmacy services Pharmacy services that are provided on or near a patient care area. These services are often supported by a central pharmacy. A pharmacy satellite is an example of one form of a decentralized pharmacy service.

drug distribution services The system(s) used to distribute medications that begins when the medication is received by the pharmacy and ends when the medication is administered to the patient.

hospital formulary An approved list of medications that are routinely stocked in the hospital pharmacy to treat the types of patients the hospital typically serves.

investigational drug services Services provided to support clinical trials involving medications.

medication use evaluation (MUE) A performance improvement method that evaluates how medications are being utilized to treat patients in the hospital. The goal is to improve medication use and optimize patient therapy.

non-formulary drug A drug that is not included on the hospital's approved formulary list.

open formulary A system in which all medications are available for a prescriber to use on his or her patient.

pharmacy satellite A physical space located in or near a patient care area that can provide a variety of distributive and clinical services.

quality control A method to check and validate the steps throughout a process to ensure that the final product will be free of defects or medication errors.

quality improvement A process of systematic steps to achieve desired results with the goal of sustaining and improving medication use processes to reduce the number or variances of medication errors. Quality Improvement (QI) programs describe the desired performance and then identify gaps between the desired and actual performance. QI uses various tools to collect and measure data to identify root causes of variation, implements appropriate improvements to fix the root causes, then measures the impact these changes had in the system.

unit dose A single or individually packaged medication in a ready-to-administer form for the patient.

unit dose distribution system A system that provides all or most medications to patients in a unit dose ready-to-administer form.

Hospital pharmacy practice offers many interesting and challenging opportunities for pharmacy technicians. Many valuable services are provided by pharmacies in the hospital setting, including the traditional duties of drug procurement, storage, preparation, and administration, as well as the distribution of drugs and supplies to patients. Hospital pharmacy professionals also ensure that medications are used in a safe and effective manner, which involves clinical services, drug therapy monitoring, medication safety, patient education, and other related activities.

As in other settings, the scope of hospital pharmacy practice is ever changing and expanding to meet advances in technology, rising health care costs, and the increased requirements of regulatory and accrediting agencies. Technicians are an integral part of the pharmacy team that provides these services in the hospital setting. As the pharmacy profession continues to expand its realm of activities to include direct patient care, the responsibilities and opportunities for technicians are also expanding. This chapter provides a general overview of hospital pharmacy practice and describes the current roles and responsibilities of pharmacy technicians.

Historical Perspective

Pharmacy services have existed in hospital settings in one form or another for many years. In the past, the typical hospital pharmacy was primarily involved with traditional functions related to distributing drugs to patients. These services were primarily performed from a central pharmacy that was usually located away from patient care areas, such as in the basement of the hospital. Pharmacy services were often limited in scope, responsibility, and number of personnel. The focus was on medication products, including procurement, repackaging and labeling bulk supplies, and delivery to patient care areas.

At this time, it was common for bulk supplies of medications to be stored on nursing stations as floor stock. When a patient needed a medication, the nurse would take the medication from the floor stock and perform all necessary calculations and preparations before administering it to the patient. Nurses would also prepare all intravenous (IV) medications in the patient care area without the use of a laminar flow hood and often without proper quality control procedures. As a result, the potential for medication errors was very high.

The practice of hospital pharmacy has made tremendous advances over the past 40 years. In the mid-1960s, pharmacies began to assume more accountability for the entire medication use process in order to reduce the potential for medication errors. In fact, efforts to improve medication safety continue to be a major focus for hospital pharmacies today. As hospitals become more knowledgeable about the common causes of medication errors, there is a corresponding change in requirements by regulatory and accrediting agencies, which helps all hospitals continue to improve the safety and quality of care provided to patients.

Technology Topics

Automation and technology have also played a major role in changing the practice of hospital pharmacy. These technological changes have improved not only the efficiency of the drug distribution processes, but also medication safety.

In addition, the pharmacy profession has been moving from a primary focus on medication preparation and distribution to one that focuses on patient care by providing services that help patients realize safe and effective drug therapy outcomes.

The impact of changing reimbursement and the financial burdens placed on health care systems with rising costs and diminishing resources have required hospital pharmacies to adapt as well. These changes have resulted in greater efforts to provide the best quality care possible in an efficient and timely manner. The ultimate goal when treating patients is to achieve positive outcomes without causing harm—harm that could lead to additional days in the hospital and an increased use of limited health care resources.

Organizational Structure

Health care institutions are usually organized into several levels of management. Managers at the top of an organization are primarily involved in setting a direction and vision for the hospital. As you move down the organizational structure, the responsibilities become more defined and are targeted to meet specific goals of the hospital. Each level of management is designed to allow a distinct range of activities to be performed in an organized manner. Defining clear levels of responsibility and hierarchy ensures that the activities of employees are organized, efficient, and productive. Organizational structures also allow for appropriate lines of communication throughout the institution.

Typically, at the top of the hospital organization is the board of directors. Just below the board of directors is the chief executive officer (CEO), president, or hospital director. The CEO helps set a direction for the hospital by creating a vision and mission for the institution. The CEO reports to the hospital's board of directors and is responsible for ensuring that necessary budget, personnel, and operations are in place to help achieve the mission of the hospital. The medical staff and the second level of management report directly to the CEO.

Hospitals usually have a chief operating officer (COO) or vice president who represents a second level of management. The COO is responsible for the daily operations of the hospital. A chief financial officer (CFO) is also a second-level manager who is responsible for the financial management of the hospital. Another second level of management commonly seen today is the vice president of patient care services. This manager is usually responsible for departments that provide direct patient care, such as the pharmacy, nursing, and respiratory therapy departments. The number of additional levels of management is dependent on several factors, including the size and scope of services provided, the financial status of the facility, and the management philosophy of the CEO or equivalent manager. Individual departments are routinely grouped either by patient care (e.g., nursing, pharmacy, or radiology), ancillary services (e.g., materials management or environmental services), or support services (e.g., medical records or information systems).

Variations of organizational structures can be found depending upon a facility's size, needs, and goals. One such variation is the patient-focused care model. In this model, managers are given responsibility for all employees and activities provided to specific patient types (e.g., surgical, pediatric, or medical patients). The philosophy underlying this structure is that all health care workers function as a team, with everyone having a role in providing patient care, regardless of discipline or the tasks performed.

Pharmacy Department Structure

The director, or chief of pharmacy services, is at the top of the pharmacy department hierarchy. The director of pharmacy is responsible for all activities within the pharmacy, including, but not limited to, the budget and drug expenditures, medication management, regulatory compliance, and medication safety. The number and levels of management reporting to the director of pharmacy depend on the department's size and scope of services. For example, a hospital affiliated with a university may need one manager to coordinate pharmacy students and the residency program and another to coordinate staff development and all clinical pharmacy services. Pharmacy technicians may be assigned to management or lead responsibilities. In this capacity, the technician supervises the activities of other technicians. The lead technician will be responsible for management functions such as scheduling and performance evaluations. The structure of the pharmacy department is based on the types of pharmacy operations provided, such as centralized or decentralized pharmacy services.

Centralized Pharmacy Services

Centralized pharmacy services, as the name implies, handle pharmacy personnel, resources, and functions from a central location. A typical centralized pharmacy contains a sterile preparation area, known as a clean room, which is designed for the aseptic preparation of IV medications (e.g., antibiotic piggybacks, large-volume parenteral solutions with additives, total parenteral nutrition, and chemotherapeutic agents), a medication cart filling area, an outpatient prescription counter, and a storage area for medications and supplies. Central pharmacy services are beneficial when resources (i.e., personnel, equipment, and space) are limited. The advantage of centralized services is that fewer staff members are needed to control, store, inspect, prepare, and dispense medications for the entire institution. The disadvantages of offering only centralized pharmacy services are the lack of face-to-face interactions with patients and other health care providers and the increased time to deliver medications to patient care areas.

Many centralized pharmacies now have better access to patient care information through the use of computerized documentation. Although patient information is readily available in the pharmacy, the pharmacist may still need to go to the patient care floor when making therapeutic assessments regarding medication orders. Unless a hospital is completely electronic, there will be information written on the patient's chart that may be needed when drug therapy is reviewed. The pharmacist may also need to consult with the health care professionals treating the patient to obtain additional information, as well as interview or assess the patient for information regarding drug therapy decisions.

As mentioned above, it may take longer to deliver medications to all areas of the institution from a central location.

TECHNOLOGY TOPICS

Technology and automation, such as **automated medication dispensing devices** (e.g., Pyxis® MedStation™ and MedDispense™) can help hospitals improve the availability of medications for administration to patients. These are secured storage cabinets that allow medications to be kept in a patient care area (figure 4–1). Technicians have now expanded their scope of responsibility to include operating and maintaining these forms of automation, including checks to ensure adequate supplies of medications are in the devices.

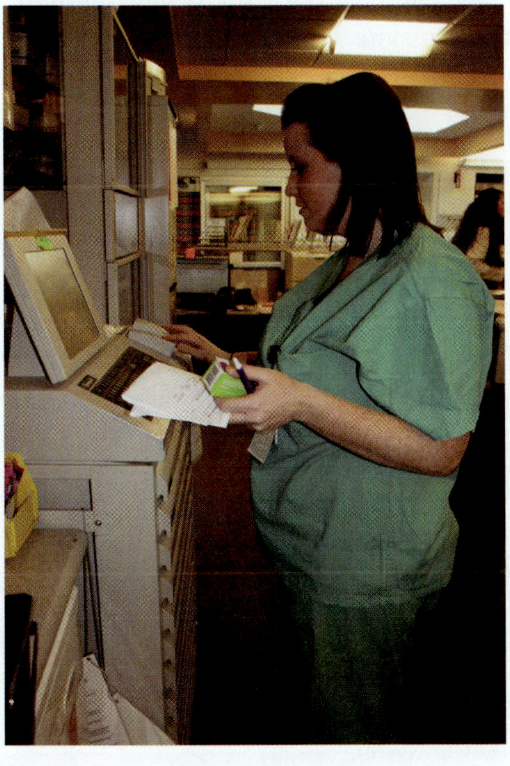

Figure 4–1. Pharmacy technician restocking an automated dispensing device in a patient care area.

Other technician responsibilities in a central pharmacy involve preparing IV medications (e.g., total parenteral nutrition and chemotherapeutic agents), filling patient medication carts, delivering narcotics, extemporaneous compounding (i.e., preparing products not available from a manufacturer), performing functions related to quality control and quality improvement, billing, and completing miscellaneous paperwork.

Decentralized Pharmacy Services

Decentralized pharmacy services do not replace centralized pharmacy services; rather, they are used in conjunction with a central pharmacy. **Decentralized pharmacy services** are provided from patient care areas. There are many types of decentralized pharmacy services, but one common form of a decentralized pharmacy (with opportunities for pharmacy technicians) is a pharmacy satellite. **Pharmacy satellites** have designated areas on a hospital floor or a patient care unit where drugs are stored, prepared, and dispensed for patients (figure 4–2). Pharmacy satellites may be staffed by one or more pharmacists and technicians. The proximity of a pharmacy satellite to the patients and other health care providers has several advantages. It allows the pharmacist more opportunities to interact with patients in order to obtain pertinent information, monitor and assess their response to drug therapy, provide patient education, and disseminate educational materials. The pharmacist also has more

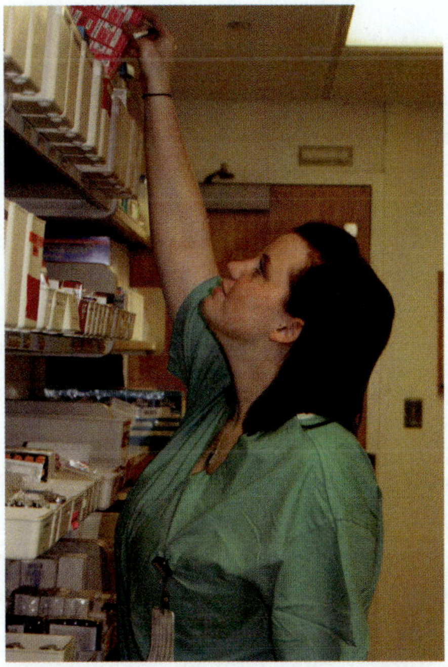

Figure 4–2. Pharmacy technician in a pharmacy satellite.

opportunities to discuss the plan of care, answer drug information questions, and make appropriate drug therapy recommendations while being face-to-face with other health care providers. Technicians have the advantage of being close to medication storage areas used by nurses. They can respond quickly to any problems with medication storage cabinets and prepare any needed medications in a timely manner. Technicians are an accessible, helpful source of non-clinical information to health care providers in decentralized pharmacy satellites.

The disadvantage of decentralized pharmacies is that they require additional resources, such as personnel to staff a decentralized satellite, equipment (e.g., laminar flow hoods, computers, and printers), references, and a second inventory of medications and supplies.

The technician's role in decentralized pharmacies varies from institution to institution. Technicians are given considerable responsibility in pharmacy satellites to free up the pharmacist to provide pharmaceutical care. Some responsibilities of satellite technicians are to maintain appropriate inventory (e.g., medications and supplies), including the disposal of expired medications; clean and maintain laminar flow hoods; and prepare all unit-dose and IV medication orders in a timely fashion. The experienced technician may answer specific non-clinical questions from nurses and make judgments regarding when to refer a question to the pharmacist. Technicians can be responsible for all aspects of running the pharmacy satellite under the supervision of a pharmacist.

Use of Clinical Practitioners

A pharmacy department may also have patient-focused care or **clinical pharmacy services** as part of its structure.[1] These services require clinical skills from a trained clinical pharmacist or practitioner. Clinical practitioners are involved in all aspects of drug therapy to ensure appropriate, safe, and cost-effective care. Patient-focused care is accomplished by ensuring all patient-specific problems requiring drug therapy are being treated, the medication selected is appropriate for the indication, the dose ordered is correct, and the dosage form and administration technique meet the patient's needs.

After the medication has been administered, clinical practitioners monitor the effects of the medication through laboratory results (e.g., serum drug levels, culture and sensitivity results, or serum creatinine levels) as well as patient-specific parameters (e.g., heart rate, temperature, or respiration rate). Clinical practitioners also play a significant role in the education of patients and other health care providers regarding the use of medications. They are able to spend more time with patients directly and in the patient care areas than centralized pharmacists.

Pharmacy technicians are being used to help pharmacists in these patient-focused models by collecting routine clinical data, tracking medication errors, and assisting in other clinical projects.[2–6]

Committee Participation

Committees are essential to effectively plan and implement the day-to-day working decisions in hospitals. There are two common types of committees: standing committees and ad hoc committees. Standing committees are permanent or on-going. They are often incorporated into official documents, such as policies and procedures. An example of a common standing committee is the Pharmacy and Therapeutics (P&T) Committee. This committee is multidisciplinary, with typical membership including, but not limited to, representatives of the medical staff, pharmacy, nursing, hospital administration, and dietary. The committee is required to meet on a routine basis to make decisions about the care of patients, with a focus on the safe and effective use of medications. The P&T committee will oversee and make decisions for the institution's formulary as an example of this responsibility. A **hospital formulary** is an approved list of medications to treat the types of patients the hospital typically serves.

Ad hoc committees are temporary and formed to address a specific purpose. An example of an ad hoc committee is a committee formed to address the implementation of a new computer system for the hospital. This type of initiative takes a great deal of work and coordination between departments. Once the new computer system is implemented, the ad hoc committee may no longer be needed.

Rx for Success

Pharmacy technicians are often asked to participate in a variety of hospital committees, based on their training and understanding of many hospital processes, especially as they relate to drug distribution systems.

Pharmacy Department Services

The services that a particular pharmacy department provides varies from hospital to hospital. This section describes a few examples of these services, including drug distribution services, clinical services, and investigational drug services. The policy and procedure manual is a great resource to identify the services provided by a hospital pharmacy department.

Policy and Procedure Manuals

Every hospital pharmacy is required by The Joint Commission to maintain a policy and procedure manual. Such a manual is critical for the successful operations of the department. Policy and procedure manuals contain descriptions of all of the functions and services that a pharmacy department provides, as well as written documents that describe the policies for operations and the procedures explaining how to execute them. They include detailed directions on how to perform a wide variety of functions to meet the needs of the hospital and its patients. These written procedures allow the functions in the pharmacy to be carried out in a consistent and standardized manner. They also serve as a way to communicate and educate new employees on how to do their jobs. Many policies and procedures in hospitals are multidisciplinary, so one policy can be used by all health care providers who are involved with carrying out a particular service or patient care activity.

Drug Distribution Services

Drug distribution services in hospitals involve all of the steps required to get a drug from the pharmacy to the patient. Exactly how this is done in each hospital varies significantly, depending on the physical layout of the hospital, available space, types of patient care services provided (e.g., oncology, pediatrics), and the types of automation and technology available. Regardless of the specific drug delivery systems used, the pharmacy is ultimately responsible for providing medications to patients. Fulfilling that responsibility requires that several sequential processes, such as procuring, storing, preparing, and delivering medications to patient care areas, are executed accurately and efficiently. Drug distribution services are essential to allow for the medication use process, which starts when a physician orders a medication and runs through the time the medication is administered to the patient. Medical staff, nursing, and pharmacy personnel must work together to ensure that the medication processes occur in a safe and timely manner. As an example, for a patient to receive one aspirin tablet, the following steps must occur:

1. The drug must be in the inventory, which means it was ordered from the wholesaler, received, inspected, stored, inventoried, and periodically reviewed to ensure that it did not expire.
2. The medication order must be written (or submitted electronically) by the physician and received by the pharmacy.
3. The medication order must be reviewed and verified by the pharmacist.
4. The medication order must be processed and added to the patient's medication profile so the drug can be dispensed and delivered to the nursing station or made available in a medication dispensing cabinet.
5. Once at the nursing station, the drug is administered to the patient and the dose is documented as given in the patient's medication administration record (MAR).
6. Once the medication is administered, physicians, nurses, and pharmacists monitor the patient to ensure that the patient is responding to therapy, and they also watch for the development of any adverse events that may occur.

In the past, compounding and repackaging medications was a major part of drug distribution services. The advent of **unit dose drug distribution systems,** however, has eliminated or minimized this time-consuming process for most of the solid dosage forms dispensed. A **unit dose** is an individually packaged medication that is ready to be dispensed and administered to the patient, including all necessary labeling requirements (i.e., drug name, strength, lot number, expiration date, etc.).

The distribution services mentioned up to this point focused primarily on new medication orders. Once the initial order has been processed and is on the patient's medication profile and MAR, the pharmacy needs to ensure that an adequate supply of maintenance medications is available to be administered by the nurse. Two primary methods are used in hospitals to dispense maintenance medications to patient care areas. The first involves the use of automation and the second is a manual process.

There are many forms of automation used to distribute medications to patient care areas. This section will focus on automated medication dispensing cabinets. Regardless of which form of automation is used, pharmacy technicians play a key role in maintaining an appropriate inventory of medications to be stocked in these devices. Inventory in these devices requires frequent adjustments to meet the current needs of the patients served. Having the proper inventory in these devices is important; it allows the nurse to obtain the right medication and the right dose (in the right form) so it can be administered to the right patient at the right time.

The second distribution system is a manual process that usually requires the use of medication carts or cassettes. In this system, each patient is assigned to a medication drawer, usually arranged by bed number. To fill each medication drawer, a report known as a fill-list is generated. This list is typically sorted by bed number to correspond with the labeling of the drawers. The fill-list will contain patient information (i.e., weight, height, allergies, etc.) to help the pharmacist when checking the carts. All medications scheduled to be given during the selected fill-list time will print, usually within a 24-hour period. The technician will fill each patient's drawer based on the fill-list. Once these cassettes are filled, the pharmacist will check the carts for accuracy. In some states, technicians are able to check other technicians for filling accuracy. Studies have shown that technicians are as accurate at checking medication carts as pharmacists.[7] Once the cassettes are filled and checked, the technician can deliver the cassettes to the patient care area to exchange them with cassettes from the previous time frame.

It is common for automated and manual systems to be used simultaneously. When both systems are used, it is a matter of logistics, resources, and philosophy as to when one system is used over the other.

Some drug distribution needs require unique procedures. An example is filling emergency crash carts. These carts or trays supply medications that are commonly used in emergency situations. Each cart or tray will have a defined list of medications and quantities to be filled and stored. Once these carts/trays are filled and checked by a pharmacist, they are locked and sealed. They can then be delivered to the designated patient care area. These emergency carts/trays are subject to unit inspections, as described later in this chapter.

Pharmacy technicians are often involved in the discharge medication process. Once the decision is made to discharge a patient from the hospital, a series of activities needs to occur, which includes writing prescriptions for medications. This is an important opportunity for the pharmacist to review the discharge medication orders for appropriateness and also to counsel patients on their medications. Some hospitals supply discharge medications directly to patients; pharmacy technicians play a key role in helping with this process.

Clinical Services

Pharmacists began providing patient-focused services, often referred to as clinical pharmacy services, in addition to product services sometime in the 1960s. Examples of such services include pharmacokinetic dosing, infectious disease consultations, drug information, and nutritional support services. The pharmacy profession realized that, in order to achieve optimal outcomes and improve patient satisfaction, it had to be accountable for all patient medication-related needs.

Clinical services were incorporated into a model known as pharmaceutical care. Pharmaceutical care is defined as "the responsible provision of drug therapy to achieve definite outcomes intended to improve a patient's quality of life."[8] In this model, the pharmacist is an advocate for the patient. Not only are all medication therapy decisions made for the patient's benefit, but the patient is involved in the decision-making process.

The pharmaceutical care model also allowed for new roles for the technician. Some institutions are now relying on the use of technicians to record laboratory results in the pharmacist's patient database.[2–6] As an example, pharmacy technicians might record the serum creatinine levels for patients who receive certain medications. The pharmacist uses these values to assess kidney function in order to make appropriate recommendations for dosing medications.

Rx for Success

Pharmacy technicians may obtain lab test results for the pharmacist, such as serum creatinine, bacterial cultures and sensitivities, serum drug levels, electrolytes (e.g., potassium and sodium), and other biological markers (e.g., blood cell counts).

Technicians can screen medication orders for nonformulary status or to identify if the medication is on the hospital's restricted list based on its high cost, high toxicity, or potential for over-prescribing. In such cases, the technicians then notify the pharmacist that there is a need to take action on these types of orders. Technicians can also review and collect missing information for a patient's database, such as allergies, height, and weight.

Investigational Drug Services

Investigational drug programs are another form of service seen in hospital pharmacies. **Investigational drug services** are provided by hospitals that participate in clinical trials involving medications. Clinical trials evaluate the efficacy and safety of medications. There are many types of drug studies. For example, a new drug that is not FDA-approved is required to go through a series of clinical trials classified into four phases. Each phase is treated as a separate clinical trial. These phases are designed to determine the efficacy, safety, or dosing requirements before they are approved to be marketed. Other studies involve medications already approved by the FDA that are being studied for efficacy and safety for a new indication or a new dose. Another way of classifying trials is by their purpose—for instance, prevention trials, diagnostic trials, or treatment trials.

Before a study is approved to be conducted in the hospital, a study protocol is developed, reviewed, and approved by the Institutional Review Board (IRB), which often includes pharmacy representation. The protocol is the operating manual for the clinical trial. In order to carry out a successful drug study, there are specific requirements and procedures that must be followed. These include proper storage, record keeping, inventory control, preparation, dispensing, and labeling of all investigational drugs. Technicians may be involved with these procedures under the supervision of the pharmacist. Clinical trials are often conducted at multiple sites and it is important that each site perform the trial in the same way. Following a protocol accurately is an important responsibility because the validity of the research results and the conclusions of the study depend on the accuracy of the dispensing records. As an example, when a patient is enrolled in a study, depending on the study protocol, the patient will be randomized to determine which study treatment the patient will receive (i.e., study drug or placebo). The randomization is commonly done in a double-blind fashion, which means that both the patient and the researchers are unaware of which treatment is being given to prevent bias. Once the patient is randomized to a treatment arm, it is important to follow all protocol procedures for labeling the medication to prevent the researcher or patient from being aware of which treatment is given. All these processes need to be documented accurately as part of the analysis upon completion of the study. The results and recordkeeping of an investigational study can be audited by the FDA to see if they correctly followed the study protocol. In addition, all investigational medications must be stored in a separate section of the pharmacy with limited access and comply with all federal and state requirements.

Medication Management

Medication management involves the entire medication use process, including

- selection and procurement of drugs
- storage
- prescribing
- preparation and dispensing
- administration
- monitoring the effects of the medication
- evaluation of the effectiveness of the entire system

All of these processes are so important to the safety and quality of care provided to patients that each of the steps is part of a Joint Commission standard. Following is a brief discussion of each of these components using different scenarios, including you as a patient, to demonstrate what can happen if these steps are not performed accurately and appropriately.

Selection and Procurement

Imagine that you are a patient just admitted to the hospital for a lung infection. Your diagnosis is community-acquired pneumonia, and your doctor orders intravenous levofloxacin, a common antibiotic used to treat this type of infection. However, the hospital does not have this medication in stock. It will take 1–2 days to order it from the wholesaler, place the medication into stock, prepare the medication, and deliver it to the patient care area so you can receive the medication. This is not an ideal situation because treatment is delayed, which could impact your recovery.

To prevent this scenario, hospitals implement policies and procedures that describe the appropriate selection and procurement of drugs so that, when the pharmacy receives a medication order from the prescriber, the pharmacy has the medication available to dispense and administer to the patient.

To guide the pharmacy regarding which drugs to order and keep in stock, the hospital's Pharmacy and

Therapeutics (P&T) Committee establishes a hospital formulary. Formulary medications are approved based on several criteria, such as

- indications for use
- effectiveness
- drug interactions
- potential for errors and abuse
- adverse effects
- cost

Hospitals typically operate with a **closed formulary**, which means that the list of available drugs is limited. For example, a hospital may have only a few drugs in a specific class of medications. This is in contrast to an **open formulary,** seen in a community pharmacy, in which most of the common drugs in a therapeutic class are available.

When the pharmacy receives a request by a physician to add a drug to the formulary, a drug monograph is used, containing the information listed above. The P&T Committee will use the information in the monograph to decide whether to add the drug to the formulary. If the formulary already includes other drugs with the same indications for use, the P&T Committee will compare the drugs and decide which drug is the best choice based on efficacy, safety, and cost. In some cases, drugs are removed from the formulary when better drugs become available or when purchasing trends show that a drug is no longer being used. The technician may support the P&T Committee in formulary decisions by providing comparative drug costs or drug usage trends.

Pharmacy technicians play a key role in the procurement of medications. In fact, many pharmacy departments have created a specific position for pharmacy technicians to ensure that the appropriate amounts of medications are ordered to maintain an appropriate inventory. The specific procurement process is based on the hospital's approved formulary and the department's policy and procedures (see Chapter 19: Purchasing and Inventory for more detailed information).

In the levofloxacin example above, the hospital may have a different medication on its formulary that would be appropriate for your treatment, and the pharmacist may suggest that the physician prescribe the formulary drug instead of levofloxacin. If the physician thinks that levofloxacin is the best choice for you, however, the hospital will implement procedures to allow for its temporary use as a **non-formulary drug.** The technician would refer to the specific policy and procedure for how to handle this non-formulary request.

Storage

Let's return to the example above in which levofloxacin is prescribed to treat your pneumonia. This time the medication is in stock and available to be dispensed and administered. However, the technician identifies that the medication is past its expiration or "beyond use" date. In fact, the medication expired more than one year ago. Again, this is not an ideal situation.

✔The hospital pharmacy is responsible for the appropriate inspection of all medication storage areas to ensure that the "beyond use" dates of medications have not expired.

The proper storage of medications is critical to the safe use of medications. Though everyone who handles medications should check expiration dates, inspections are primarily performed by pharmacy technicians. All medication storage areas in the hospital are assigned to be inspected at least monthly. These inspections are often referred to as unit inspections. When expired medications are found, they need to be returned or disposed of according to regulatory and legal requirements. Each medication has specific storage requirements from the manufacturer, such as temperature (e.g., room temperature, refrigerated, or frozen) and protection from light. Such special storage requirements for temperature and light ensure stability and potency of the drug product throughout its shelf life.

There are also specific storage and documentation requirements for controlled substances. As this is the most highly regulated class of drugs, the requirements are stringent and based on the abuse and diversion potential. The hospital needs to comply with all legal and regulatory requirements and safeguards. Technicians need to be trained and knowledgeable about these requirements.

Prescribing

Your physician just explained to you that you have pneumonia, and he will be starting you on levofloxacin to treat your infection. He walks out of your room and verbally tells the nurse to start the antibiotic right now. However, since he did not electronically enter or write the order immediately and there was a lot of noise outside of your room at that time, the nurse mishears the name of the medication and administers the wrong drug to you.

This scenario is an example of what can happen without proper policies and procedures for ordering and prescribing medications. Policies and procedures for prescribing medications are created to prevent medication errors and patient harm. Verbal orders are not recommended, but there are times when a verbal order is necessary, such as in the event of an emergency or if the prescriber is off-site and is without access to the patient's chart. If a verbal order has to be given, there are procedures for carrying out these orders to minimize errors. For example, an authorized professional within his or her scope of practice may accept a verbal order, but the order needs to be reduced to writing immediately and read back to the prescriber to clarify its accuracy. In such cases, the prescriber signs the transcription of the verbal order later to validate it. Every medication order should be clear and concise and contain the drug name, the dose, frequency, and route. It is especially helpful if the indication is on the order as well, to prevent misinterpretation that could lead to a medication error and patient harm.

Prescribers can either initiate an order verbally (as mentioned above), enter the order electronically (i.e., computerized physician order entry [CPOE]), or write the order. All three methods of medication orders require a pharmacist to review the order for appropriateness.

The pharmacist will review each medication order to determine if it is the most appropriate medication for the indication being treated, check for any potential allergies, screen for drug-drug interactions or therapeutic duplications, check correct dose and correct route, and identify any other contraindications. If the order is written, the order has to be manually entered into the pharmacy patient profile system. With electronic order entry, the pharmacist simply verifies the physician's order, although a product may still need to be selected. The pharmacy system usually has patient safety features like drug-drug or drug-allergy interaction alerts, and it is used to print medication labels. Usually, the pharmacy system interfaces with the electronic chart, so that, when medication orders are entered into the pharmacy profile system, the medication order information appears on the Medication Administration Record (MAR), which lets the nurse know when a medication needs to be administered. In some hospitals, the MAR and Patient Medication Profile systems are separate, stand-alone systems. When this is the case, there needs to be an additional verification and reconciliation to assure that the pharmacy patient profile (i.e., what the pharmacy dispenses) matches the nurses MAR (i.e., what the nurse will administer) to avoid any medication errors. Technicians are often involved in transcribing these orders into the patient medication profile. The pharmacist must still review the accuracy of the transcription and review the order for appropriateness before the medication is dispensed and administered to the patient.

Safety First If a medication order has missing information or is unclear, the technician must alert the pharmacist, who will get clarification of the order before the patient receives the medication.

There may be times when a pharmacist is unable to review and verify an order in the hospital, such as if the hospital pharmacy is not open 24 hours a day. In order to comply with the legal and regulatory requirements that a pharmacist must review all orders before the medication is administered, some hospitals outsource this function to remote sites. One example of a company that provides this type of service is R_xe-source℠. Once an order is written or entered, it is sent by fax or scanning technology to the offsite pharmacist. The pharmacist logs into the hospital pharmacy computer system and reviews the medication profile and necessary lab values, enters the medication into the patient's profile, and authorizes the order for administration.

Preparation and Dispensing

You are in the hospital with pneumonia, but, in this scenario, the physician writes the order for intravenous levofloxacin 500 mg, which, according to the hospital's policies and procedures, is in stock in the automated medication dispensing cabinet on the nursing unit and it has not expired. The nurse grabs a levofloxacin vial and prepares the medication on the floor. She accidentally takes a 750 mg vial instead of a 500 mg vial, however, and mixes the medication. She does not notice that the vial is 750 mg and does not ask another nurse to double check her work. She labels the intravenous bag as 500 mg and administers too much medication to you. Although this scenario may be unlikely, it illustrates what can go wrong without proper review, preparation, and dispensing procedures.

One medication safety strategy is to order medications directly from wholesalers in a unit-of-use dosage form, referred to as a unit dose. Unit dose packages contain a single dose that is ready to be administered to a patient, thus avoiding potential errors caused by having to package or prepare medications in the hospital. If a medication is not available in a unit dose form, the pharmacy should prepare the medication in a unit-ready-to-use form for the nurse or health care provider administering the medication. Understanding the unit dose system is essential because technicians spend a significant part of their time obtaining, preparing, and labeling medications in this form.

Safety First To prevent errors, the pharmacy should dispense patient-specific unit dose packages to nursing units instead of multidose or bulk packages whenever possible.

Unit dose drug distribution systems allow a limited number of doses (usually a 12- or 24-hour supply) in a single unit of use (the exact dose specified for the patient) to be dispensed in medication carts or via automated floor stock systems. The advantages of using a unit dose system include[9]

- reduction in the incidence of medication errors
- decrease in the total cost of medication-related activities
- more efficient use of pharmacy and nursing personnel, allowing for more direct patient-care involvement by pharmacists and nurses
- improved overall drug control and drug use monitoring
- more accurate patient billing for drugs
- greater pharmacist control over pharmacy workload patterns and staff scheduling
- reduction in the size of drug inventories located in patient-care areas
- greater adaptability to computerized and automated procedures
- reduction in the potential for drug waste

Most medications are commercially available in unit dose form, but pharmacy personnel still must package some medications as unit doses. Although many IV medications are also commercially available in unit dose form, some are not stable in solution and must be mixed by the pharmacy just prior to administration. The preparation of IV medications is a key role for pharmacy technicians in the hospital setting. Intravenous medications require the knowledge and skill of aseptic or sterile techniques (see Chapter 16: Aseptic Technique, Sterile Compounding, and IV Admixture Programs).

Patient-specific characteristics are often a reason to extemporaneously prepare medications in a unit dose form. Pediatric patients, for example, require very small doses that may not be available from the manufacturer in a unit dose form. Some doses required for pediatric patients (especially neonates) are so small that they cannot be measured accurately from commercially available products, so a special dilution may need to be made for an IV solution. An extemporaneous oral solution or suspension must be compounded for patients unable to swallow a tablet. In this case, the technician will crush tablets and follow a recipe for that particular solution or suspension.

Regardless of what type of medication is prepared, the final step before dispensing is to properly label the medication. The major requirements for proper labeling include

- patient's name
- patient's location in the hospital
- medication name
- dose
- route of administration
- expiration date
- any special directions or cautionary instructions for storage or administration

Many hospital pharmacy departments use bar-coding systems as part of their labeling systems.[10] Medication labels are bar coded so that the nurse can scan the patient's wrist band and then the medication label to confirm that the right drug is given to the right patient.

After the medication has been prepared and labeled, it is dispensed according to the hospital's drug distribution procedures.

Administration

Assume you have been lying in your hospital bed for more than 18 hours after the doctor told you that you have pneumonia. The nurse finally enters your room to administer your first dose of levofloxacin 500 mg intravenously, which was scheduled to be given immediately upon your admission. The nurse said she was sorry for being late with the medication, but the pharmacy was busy. This would not be considered timely administration of your medication.

Procedures are in place to ensure that medications are administered appropriately to patients, which includes providing them in a timely manner. The health care provider administering the medication should review each medication before giving it to the patient. He or she goes through a series of checks to ensure that the *right medication*, in the *right dose*, is given to the *right patient* at the *right time,* and by the *right route*. This is referred to as the 5 rights of medication administration. There should also be a visual inspection of the medication (especially intravenous or liquid medications) for any particulates or discoloration, and the label should be reviewed to ensure that the medication has not expired.

Monitoring

In this scenario, the nurse has administered levofloxacin 500 mg intravenously to treat your pneumonia. Later that day, you begin to develop hives and have difficulty breathing. The nurse is about to give you your second dose when you complain about your symptoms. The nurse does not administer the medication and alerts the ordering physician of your adverse effect to the drug, which is most likely an allergic reaction. She then begins treating your reaction. This is an example of monitoring the effects of medications.

Monitoring the effects of medications for both adverse effects and positive outcomes is an important component of the medication management process. Many pharmacy departments are active in monitoring the effects of medications by reviewing information in the medical record, laboratory results, the patient's clinical response, and the medication profile to identify any anti-allergic or antidote orders that can be used to counteract adverse effects or toxicity to medications.

Technicians are being asked to help in this process by gathering certain lab values for pharmacists. They are trained to alert pharmacists when certain STAT orders are received in the pharmacy, especially as they relate to anti-allergic or antidote-type drugs such as epinephrine or diphenhydramine, which are commonly used to treat allergic reactions.

Evaluation

The last step in the medication management process involves evaluating the effectiveness of the entire system. There are many techniques and sources of data used to evaluate the effectiveness of medication use, such as tracking and identifying trends in adverse drug events and medication errors and performing a **medication use evaluation (MUE)**. An MUE is commonly performed with medications that fall into one or more categories identified by the hospital, including

- high-use drugs
- high-cost drugs
- high-risk drugs

Data are collected to evaluate the appropriate use of these drugs, including appropriate indications, dose, route, and clinical response. Using levofloxacin as an example from the previous scenarios, this antibiotic would typically fall under the category of a high-use medication. The MUE criteria for this medication may be designed to capture indication for use, dose, route, duration of therapy, and side effects. After the MUE data are collected on a predefined number of patients, the results are tabulated and presented to the appropriate health care providers and committees. Depending on the results, appropriate recommendations and actions are taken. For example, if the data show many patients are receiving doses too high based on the indication and renal function, recommendations and actions may be provided that include education and training to health care providers on the appropriate dosing criteria for this medication. Another action may be to give the pharmacist authority to automatically change the dose based on approved criteria by the P&T committee. No matter what technique or data source is used to evaluate the process, the primary goal is to identify areas for improvement and implement strategies or needed changes in the process to improve the medication management system.

Accrediting and Regulatory Agencies

Every hospital pharmacy is dedicated to offering the best pharmacy services possible and is committed to providing safe and effective medication therapy to all of its patients. Nevertheless, standards of care between hospitals would vary greatly without accrediting and regulatory agencies. These agencies exist to ensure that each facility provides a safe and effective standard of care to patients. They are dedicated to helping hospitals provide the best care through meeting various standards or elements of care. These standards are a result of identifying the best practices available, either through research or practical experience. Standards are continuously changing to help hospitals improve the care they provide to patients.

Regulatory and accrediting agencies make site visits to inspect and verify that their published standards of care are being met. They meet with hospital administrators, health care providers, and hospital staff to determine how patients are being cared for in the institution. As part of this site visit, the evaluation team may review the hospital's guidelines and policy and procedure manuals. They also meet with hospital staff to observe and ask questions about patient care guidelines or procedures. Ensuring that a hospital continually maintains compliance with these standards requires a great deal of work and preparation. This preparation is frequently a multidisciplinary effort in which technicians often participate as key members of the health care team.

One of the most recognized accrediting agencies for hospitals is The Joint Commission (TJC; formerly known as the Joint Commission on the Accreditation of Healthcare Organizations, or JCAHO). The Joint Commission is an independent, not-for-profit organization that accredits and certifies more than 15,000 health care organizations and programs in the United States. It publishes guides and checklists on how to prepare for on-site inspections. Pharmacy technicians need to be familiar with and trained in these published requirements and standards. Most hospitals will provide on-the-job training and competencies based on these requirements. Hospitals may also create various committees around these standards that technicians often participate in.

The benefits of Joint Commission accreditation and certification include[11]

- strengthens community confidence in the quality and safety of care, treatment, and services
- provides a competitive edge in the marketplace
- improves risk management and risk reduction
- provides education on good practices to improve business operations
- provides professional advice and counsel, enhancing staff education
- enhances staff recruitment and development
- recognized by select insurers and other third parties
- may fulfill regulatory requirements in select states

Technology

Technology has had a significant impact on our everyday lives. We are able to obtain information and communicate faster and easier with the use of wireless telecommunications, cellular phones, pagers, fax machines, and computer networks. Technology has helped industries improve the quality of the goods they produce and the speed of production. These technological advances have certainly found their way into the health care system. Drug companies can now manufacture mass quantities of medications in ready-to-use, unit dose forms. The use of technology for patient care has made great advances in monitoring the effects of drug therapy. These technologies are becoming more integrated, including the capability of monitoring multiple patient parameters at the same time. Some of these integrated systems have built-in alarms to alert health care providers when a change in therapy is needed based on predefined patient parameters, such as heart rate or lab values.

The profession of pharmacy has integrated the use of technology and automation into nearly every function and service provided by the pharmacy department. Two important benefits of these technological advances include more accurate record keeping (e.g., inventory control) and a decreased need to prepare medications that are not available in a unit dose form, which results in reduced errors, waste, and costs.

Automation

Automation technologies have replaced many of the manual tasks within the pharmacy. Automation allows pharmacy technicians and pharmacists to devote more time and resources to patient-focused activities. A few examples in institutional practices are automated compounders (e.g., Baxa Micromix® and Automix® machines) used to prepare total parenteral nutrition solutions (figure 4–3), automated medication dispensing systems (figure 4–4), and the use of robotics (e.g., Cardinal's Pyxis Medstation®, OmniCell's SinglePointe™, and McKesson's ROBOT-Rx®), which can be used in the pharmacy and in patient care areas to allow health care providers to obtain medications at the point of use. These systems can track which medication was removed, who removed it, and to whom it was administered. This tracking system also notifies the pharmacy when a specific drug needs to be restocked and can help identify any potential diversion activity.

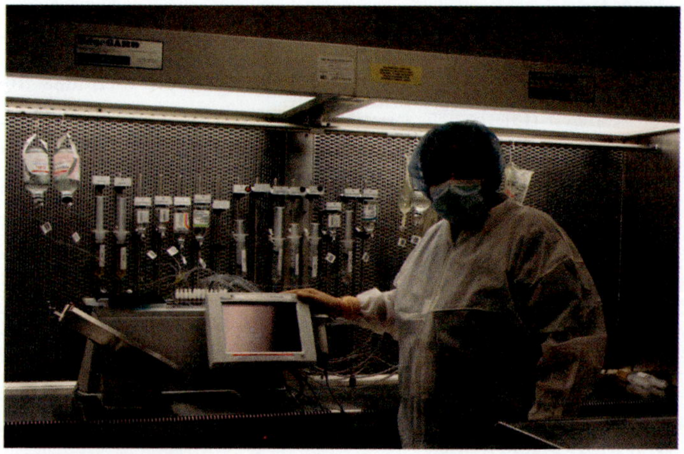

Figure 4–3. An automated TPN compounder.

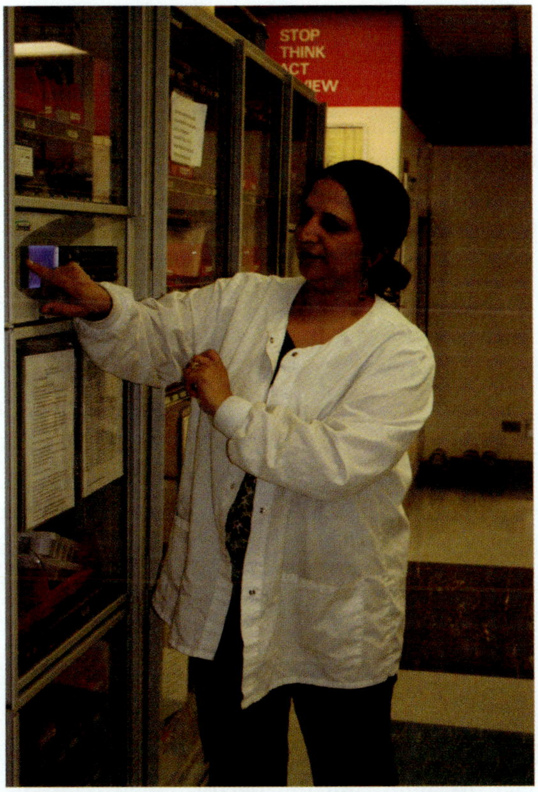

Figure 4-4. An automated dispensing cabinet (Omnicell) for narcotics.

Computer Systems

Computer systems and highly innovative software applications are used throughout the hospital for almost every imaginable process. A computer application that is becoming more common in hospitals is Computerized Physician (or Prescriber) Order Entry (CPOE; also referred to as Direct Physician Order Entry, or DPOE). These systems allow prescribers to enter medication orders directly into an institution's computer system, which prevents the need to transcribe, manipulate, or re-enter medication orders.

✔CPOE significantly reduces the number of steps in the medication use process and can reduce both interpretation and transcription errors and the time it takes to get medications to patients.

When a physician enters an electronic medication order, the pharmacist is able to review and verify the order much faster than with a manual system. A label will automatically print in the pharmacy to be filled, or the nurse can remove the drug from a unit-based medication cabinet if it is a drug that is stocked on the unit. This process is much more efficient and helps reduce preparation and delivery time to patient care areas.

There are a number of new and exciting technological applications related to data mining and surveillance of health care information. MedMined™ is one example of a program that detects opportunities to reduce infection rates based on specific best-practice recommendations. It provides real-time alerts to pharmacists regarding opportunities to improve the use of antimicrobials. An example is an alert that notifies the pharmacist if a patient has a positive culture result for a particular bacterial species and is not currently receiving an antibiotic. The pharmacist will also get an alert if the patient is on the wrong antibiotic or if a patient's renal function is changing, which may require a change in dose.

There are many new products on the market to help hospitals and pharmacies become more efficient while providing safe and effective care, but it is not within the scope of this chapter to describe each one. Although automation has replaced many tasks performed by technicians, it has also created new opportunities. Technicians are playing innovative roles relating to technology, such as data analysis of pharmacy-related patient care and financial information.[5]

Rx for Success

Technicians are often responsible for operating, stocking, and maintaining automation devices related to drug distribution.[12–14] The time saved on traditional product-focused tasks offers a variety of new opportunities for technicians, such as assisting pharmacists with patient-focused tasks and medication safety.

Quality Programs

Regardless of what service is provided by a hospital pharmacy, it must be provided in a manner that guarantees a high level of quality. Quality and the prevention of adverse events is an important topic, not only for pharmacy, but for any organization providing a product or service.[15] Medication safety continues to be in the public spotlight, and many hospitals have made quality improvement (sometimes referred to as performance improvement) a main initiative for their institutions. Many hospitals have performance or quality improvement departments that are dedicated to these programs. Quality improvement is also a key agenda for many regulatory and accrediting agencies, such as the Centers for Medicare and Medicaid Services (CMS) and The Joint Commission.

Quality itself is difficult to describe, because the term has a positive connotation but denotes nothing measurable. Quality may be identified when a product or service meets predetermined standards, such as accreditation or certification standards. Quality may also be defined by what customers perceive. The pharmacy's customers may be patients, nurses, other pharmacists, and even accrediting agencies. There are many tools, definitions, concepts, and systems that revolve around managing quality. The terms used to describe these tools and programs can be confusing because they are often used interchangeably (i.e., quality assurance, quality control, quality improvement, total quality management, etc.). This section will focus on quality control and quality improvement and provide examples of how pharmacy technicians can be involved in these quality programs. This section will also describe infection control which is a program to prevent infections in hospitalized patients and health care workers.

Quality Control

Quality control (QC) is a process of checks and balances (or procedures) that are followed during the manufacturing of a product or provision of a service to ensure that the end products or services meet or exceed specified standards (e.g., zero errors, zero problems). The start of any quality control program requires complete written procedures and training for all staff involved in that procedure. Checks and balances usually occur at critical points in the process. For example, a quality control system for the preparation of cefazolin 1 gram IVPB may begin with the technician pulling the cefazolin vial from stock and checking to make sure it is the right drug and strength and that it has not expired. Next, the technician will reconstitute the drug using a proper aseptic technique, calculate the correct volume, draw up the drug from the vial, inject it into the bag, and check for any particulate matter or leaks. The technician will then check the label for accurate and complete information (e.g., correct patient's name, drug, dose, route, time, and diluent). Once the preparation is complete, the pharmacists will check the final product to ensure that the label is correct, the correct medication and dose was used, and any other safety checks were done, as required by the department's policy and procedure for preparing IV medications. Both the technician and the pharmacist will initial the product, verifying that the medication is complete, accurate, and ready to be dispensed for the patient. Quality control is necessary to prevent defective products from reaching the patient and is critical when IV products are being prepared, as an error or defect in an IV medication can cause significant morbidity and even death.

A disadvantage of quality control is the time and resources it adds to the process. Although quality control identifies and prevents errors or defects from reaching the patient, the underlying cause of errors or defects are not always identified or corrected. As a result, the underlying problem still exists and defects will continue. Quality improvement, on the other hand, identifies the source of problems within a system. Once a problem is identified, appropriate actions are taken with the goal of improving the system to reduce the chances of future errors.

Quality Improvement

Quality improvement (QI) is a formal or systematic approach to analyzing the performance of a system or process.

There are numerous QI models used today, including Six Sigma, Zero Defects, Total Quality Management (TQM), and Continuous Quality Improvement (CQI).[16] There are also many tools used to identify problems, collect data, and analyze data. An example of a tool involving statistics is a run chart, which tracks patterns and trends over a period of time. The temperature of a medication refrigerator, for example, can be plotted each day on a run chart, allowing immediate action before medications are affected (if the temperature becomes too high or too low).

✔The ultimate goal is to improve the system or process, such as making a process more efficient or reducing the number of defects or errors. The focus of QI is to apply steps and techniques to analyze problems within a system, not within people. It requires that decisions be based on facts (data), not on hunches or opinion.

Quality improvement procedures can be prospective to identify system problems before they occur, such as a Failure Mode and Effects Analysis (FMEA), or retrospective after a problem has occurred, such as Root Cause Analysis (RCA). Both are systematic approaches with the goal of improving care to patients

Rx for Success

Technicians play key roles in many of the performance improvement activities of the hospital, such as participating on performance improvement teams to collect and analyze data. Technicians may also assist in database management for quality improvement services, such as adverse drug reaction (ADR) reports, medication error reports, and medication use evaluations.

Infection Control

Imagine you are a patient who is hospitalized for a specific condition, but during your stay you develop an unrelated infection that complicates your therapy and extends your admission by four days. During this time you receive many unplanned diagnostic and laboratory tests and medication therapy. What makes this situation most frustrating is the fact that the infection you developed was completely preventable and was a direct result of poor infection control procedures. Hospital-acquired, or nosocomial, infections have gained a great deal of attention in hospitals and communities. In fact, reducing the risk of health care-associated infections was added to The Joint Commission's National Patient Safety Goals program for 2008.

In order to prevent hospital-acquired infections, many policies and procedures are needed related to infection control. The most basic and widely communicated infection control procedure is hand washing.

Safety First Proper hand washing is one of the easiest and most effective ways to prevent the spread of infections in hospitals.

Other infection control strategies that apply to health care workers include covering coughs and sneezes; staying up-to-date with immunizations; using gloves, masks, and protective clothing; making tissues and hand cleaners available; and following hospital guidelines when dealing with blood and other contaminated items.[17] In the pharmacy, technicians play a key role in the control of infections, especially related to the sterile preparation of IV medications.

Pharmacy professionals often participate as members of the infection control committee of the hospital. This committee has several responsibilities, such as the surveillance of antibiotic utilization and bacteria susceptibility trends. One of the main causes of antimicrobial resistance is the overuse and misuse of drugs.[18] The committee develops organizational policies and procedures related to the prevention and control of infections.[19] A policy and procedure to prevent and control infections may include the creation of formulary restrictions on certain broad spectrum antibiotics that may have the potential of being over-prescribed. When the pharmacy receives an order for a restricted formulary medication, the technician can alert the pharmacist and follow the approved procedure for this restriction.

Medication Safety

Throughout this chapter and book, the topic of medication safety is repeatedly emphasized. Medication safety is at the heart of many decisions and processes, such as implementing new technology or automation, ordering drugs that are labeled clearly and ready to administer to patients without manipulation (i.e., unit dose), and applying performance improvement techniques. The number of organizations that are involved with quality and patient safety is growing, and includes

- The Institute for Safe Medication Practices (ISMP)
- American Society of Health-System Pharmacists (ASHP)
- Institute for Healthcare Improvement (IHI)
- The Joint Commission (TJC)
- Institute of Medicine (IOM)
- Agency for Healthcare Research and Quality (AHRQ)
- The Leapfrog Group
- National Quality Forum (NQF)
- Centers for Medicare and Medicaid Services (CMS)
- National Committee for Quality Assurance (NCQA)

These organizations offer a variety of medication safety initiatives, tools, and publications for hospitals to use. These resources offer many opportunities for pharmacy technicians to be trained and to participate in medication safety initiatives to ensure that no harm occurs to patients. Some of these medication safety resources are listed at the end of the chapter under Resources; also see Chapter 17: Medication Errors.

Financial Implications

The financial burden on health care systems continues to have enormous ramifications for patients and institutions. Health care costs have increased for many reasons, but many feel the major cause is the way in which health care services are paid. Health care is usually reimbursed by third-party payers, such as insurance companies and the government. An example of how this reimbursement arrangement has led to increased cost and consumption of health care resources is from past Medicare and Medicaid legislation that allowed institutions to receive full reimbursement for services determined to be necessary by the physician. This removed the incentive for institutions to control their costs and did not promote competition, which meant institutions were not stimulated to provide the best services at the lowest cost.

Today, institutions and payers are trying to reduce costs and improve the quality of care by developing alternative practice settings (e.g., home health care and mail-order prescription services), establishing reimbursement guidelines, and implementing changes to streamline patient care services. Insurance providers are finding new ways for employers to offer health care benefits that shift more responsibility of their health care to the patient. As an example, employees may be given a health care fund with a fixed amount of dollars for their health care needs, and the patient decides how and when to apply these resources. When the dollars in this fund are exhausted, the employee pays out-of-pocket up to a pre-defined amount, and once that deductible is met, the health care provider will again offer reimbursement.

Health maintenance organizations (HMOs) are a type of managed care organization. Employers may use an HMO to provide health benefits for their employees. The HMO centralizes the delivery of care to improve efficiency and reduce waste and cost. The reimbursement that HMOs receive from employers is capitated, which means HMOs receive a fixed amount of money for each employee enrolled in the plan, regardless of the amount or type of care the patient receives. HMOs, in turn, pay health care providers an agreed-upon reimbursement based on the number of patients and types of diagnosis and treatments provided. Thus, it is in the best interests of HMOs and the health care institutions, including hospitals with which they partner, to provide cost-effective care. This is why HMOs are also focused on preventive care and wellness.

In addition, annual hospital drug expenditures in 2008 increased by 2.1%, increased in 2009 by 3%, and are expected to increase 2% to 4% in 2010.[20] These increases are based on the net effect of changes in drug prices and expected changes in the utilization of medications. Although these projections represent a moderate increase in drug expenditures, they still represent an area of concern for hospitals. The hospital department continues to play a key role in ensuring that all drugs are used in a cost-effective manner.

Summary

Pharmacy technicians are essential to the functions and operations of a hospital pharmacy. There are many exciting roles for technicians as the profession of pharmacy continues to expand, not to mention the ever-changing environment based on new technology, regulatory requirements, and innovations in pharmacy practice. It is difficult to determine what the future holds for hospital pharmacy, but history has shown that, as the practice of pharmacy changes, technicians are called upon to expand their roles to make these changes happen. For example, a recent trend in hospitals is the increased number of critically ill and intensive care patients. In critical care settings, pharmacy technicians are already a valuable asset because they can accurately prepare emergency IV admixtures.

Automation and technology offer many opportunities for pharmacy technicians. These are areas in pharmacy that will continue to change and, because the role of technicians is already integral to automation, these will no doubt offer more opportunities for technicians. In addition, there continues to be a shortage in pharmacist manpower. This shortage will provide additional responsibilities for technicians to further help pharmacists with non-patient care functions, including pharmacy operations management.

The role of pharmacy technicians in the hospital setting has changed and will continue to change as health care systems change. The pharmacy technician will need to continue to be flexible, adaptable, and knowledgeable about new technologies and services. Thus, the technician is encouraged to attend educational sessions or in-services on new skills, automation, and technology. The technician should volunteer and participate in any available programs, such as quality improvement, data collection, and implementing new Joint Commission standards. Following these guidelines, the technician can stay one step ahead of change.

Self-Assessment Questions

1. Why was Medicare/Medicaid a possible cause for the rise in health care costs?
   a. Medicare/Medicaid overpaid for services provided to patients
   b. Medicare/Medicaid underpaid for services provided to patients
   c. Medicare/Medicaid, in the past, reimbursed for all services provided to the patient without any standards or justification for use of these resources
   d. Medicare/Medicaid have not been a contributing factor for the rise in health care costs
   e. Medicare/Medicaid only reimbursed for the best and most expensive treatments which forced hospitals to increase their costs
2. Which of the following forms of technology are primarily located in patient care areas that dispense medications to nurses for administration to their patients?
   a. Micromix®, Automix®
   b. Pyxis Medstation®, OmniCell SinglePointe™
   c. Medication cassette drawers
   d. Crash carts
   e. Medication Administration Record (MAR)
3. Which hospital committee is responsible for approving the formulary?
   a. Pharmacy and Therapeutics Committee
   b. Infection Control Committee
   c. Pharmacy-Nursing Committee
   d. Institutional Review Board (IRB)
   e. Medication Safety Committee
4. The formulary is an approved list of medications that is used to treat the types of patients the hospital serves. Which of the following criteria should not be used when deciding to include a medication in the hospital's formulary?
   a. Indications for use
   b. Effectiveness
   c. Potential for errors and abuse
   d. Costs
   e. The friendliness of the pharmaceutical representative
5. Although these can occur from either a centralized or decentralized pharmacy, which activity is more likely to occur in a decentralized pharmacy?
   a. Filling medication cassettes
   b. Conducting an investigational drug study inventory
   c. Preparing total parenteral nutrition solutions
   d. A pharmacist attending patient care rounds in the intensive care unit (ICU)
   e. Making an intravenous medication
6. Which of the following is an advantage of a decentralized pharmacy?
   a. Pharmacy services closer to the patient
   b. Fewer resources required
   c. Usually have more space than a centralized pharmacy to store medications
   d. Takes longer to deliver medications
   e. Difficult to have face-to-face interactions with other health care providers
7. The following functions can be performed by a technician under the supervision of a pharmacist, except which function?
   a. Prepare doses in a unit-dose form
   b. Perform pharmacokinetic calculations for a gentamicin dosing regimen
   c. Collect patient laboratory results for the pharmacist
   d. Screen questions in the satellite
   e. Prepare an intravenous medication for a patient
8. In which of the following activities is it appropriate for a technician to assist the pharmacist in order to free up time to provide pharmaceutical care to patients?
   a. Ordering laboratory results on a patient
   b. Making drug therapy recommendations to a physician to optimize the care to a patient
   c. Screening orders for non-formulary/restricted drugs
   d. Making a nutritional consult for a neonatal patient

Self-Assessment Questions

e. From the pharmacy satellite, the technician can answer most clinical questions from physicians or nurses

9. Which of the following best defines a unit-dose distribution system?
   a. All medications are stored on the nursing station in bulk quantities
   b. All medications are packaged in a single dose that is ready to be administered to a patient
   c. A unit dose system increases the number of errors compared with a system in which bulk supplies of medications are dispensed
   d. Very few manufactures provide medications in a unit dose form, making this system less desirable and more labor intensive
   e. Unit-dose medications usually lack the necessary labeling requirements (i.e., drug name, strength, lot number, expiration date), making them unsafe for distribution systems

10. Which of the following statements is true regarding unit-dose ready-to-use systems?
    a. Increases the potential for waste
    b. Increases the potential for errors
    c. Increases the time nurses spend preparing medications
    d. Increases the time pharmacy technicians spend preparing medications
    e. Decreases the potential for errors compared to preparing medications from bulk supplies

11. Which of following statements regarding ordering and prescribing is false?
    a. The hospital and pharmacy department have approved policies and procedures regarding how to order medications for patients
    b. The goal of every medication order is that the drug, directions, and indications are clear, concise, and misinterpretation that could lead to a medication error and patient harm is avoided
    c. Verbal orders are encouraged so that everyone can hear what the prescriber wants to order for their patient
    d. If a verbal order is necessary, it should only be accepted by an authorized professional within his or her scope of practice; the order needs to be reduced to writing immediately and read back to the prescriber to clarify the accuracy of the order
    e. Pharmacy technicians can screen medication orders for formulary status. If the technician identifies that a non-formulary drug has been ordered, he or she can notify the pharmacist to review and take appropriate action

12. Which of the following statements regarding organizational structures is false?
    a. A typical organizational structure will have the board of directors at the top of the hierarchy
    b. All health care institutions have the same organizational structure
    c. Organizational structures are important to maintain clear levels of responsibility and hierarchy
    d. Organizational structures allow for appropriate lines of communication throughout the institution
    e. Each level of management within an organizational structure is designed to allow a distinct range of activities to be performed in an organized manner

13. Which of the following statements regarding evaluation of the medication management process is false?
    a. The main reason for evaluating the medication management process is to identify which employee is not doing his or her job
    b. Various techniques and tools are used to assess the medication management process, such as medication use evaluations (MUEs)
    c. A typical evaluation of medication use will focus on appropriate indications, dose, route, and clinical response
    d. The main reason for evaluating the medication management process is to identify areas for improvement and then to implement strategies to improve the process
    e. Medications that are prescribed frequently are often targeted for a medication use evaluation

Self-Assessment Questions

14. Which of the following statements about quality improvement is false?
    a. Root Cause Analysis (RCA) is a procedure that is done proactively to improve the quality of care for a particular service before an adverse event occurs
    b. Quality improvement is an important part of meeting standards set by The Joint Commission
    c. Quality improvement concentrates on problems within a system rather than on individuals
    d. Failure Mode and Effects Analysis (FMEA) is a prospective process to identify problems within a system before they occur
    e. Pharmacy technicians are involved in many quality improvement activities and may be asked to participate on a multidisciplinary quality improvement team
15. All of the following are true about infection control except?
    a. Pharmacy professionals often participate as members of the Infection Control Committee of the hospital
    b. Infection control is an important patient safety goal of The Joint Commission
    c. Proper hand washing has never been proven to prevent the spread of infections in hospitals
    d. Staying up-to-date with immunizations is an infection control strategy
    e. In the pharmacy, technicians play a key role in the control of infections, especially related to the sterile preparation of IV medications
16. Which of the following statements is true regarding Computerized Physician Order Entry (CPOE)?
    a. Computers are frequently used with success by pharmacy departments; however, physicians using computers for medication order entry have increased errors and add several steps to the medication use process
    b. CPOE can decrease the number of steps in the process and reduce the potential for errors
    c. Physician order entry will eliminate the role of pharmacists in the review of appropriate medication therapy
    d. CPOE systems allow prescribers to enter medication orders directly into an institution's computer system, but the pharmacy still needs to transcribe and re-enter medication orders
    e. CPOE systems increase the time it takes for a pharmacy technician to create and affix a label to the medication ordered
17. For the following scenario, indicate which medication management process was not followed.
    You are in the hospital with pneumonia and the physician writes an order for oral levofloxacin 750 mg. The pharmacy technician went to pull the medication from the shelf and noticed the unit-dose supply for levofloxacin 750mg tablets is out-of-stock, but there is a bulk bottle with about 25 tablets available. The technician removes a few tablets from the bulk bottle, places them in a plastic baggie, handwrites "Levofloxacin 750 mg" on the outside of the baggie, and sends the medication to the patient care area.
    a. Monitoring
    b. Storage
    c. Ordering and prescribing
    d. Preparation and dispensing
    e. All steps in the Medication Management process were followed
18. For the following scenario, indicate which medication management process was not followed that nearly resulted in a potential adverse event for this patient.
    You are in the hospital with an upper respiratory tract infection and the physician writes an order for an antibiotic. You received this same antibiotic three years ago and developed a severe allergic reaction. The physician did not ask about your medication allergy history and the order is received in the pharmacy as a STAT medication. The pharmacist working in the satellite noticed that there were no allergies documented on your profile. The pharmacist goes to your room and conducts a medication history, learns about your allergy, and contacts

Self-Assessment Questions

the physician immediately to recommend an alternative medication.
a. Monitoring
b. Storage
c. Ordering and prescribing
d. Preparation and dispensing
e. None of the above

19. All of the following help to ensure the proper administration of medications to patients except
a. A visual inspection of all IV medications for any particulates or discoloration
b. Review of the medication label for accuracy prior to administration
c. A series of checks to ensure the right medication and the right dose is given to the right patient at the right time and by the right route before administering the medication to a patient
d. Written policies and procedures regarding the appropriate administration of medications to patients
e. Aseptic technique is not necessary for the routine use of IV medications, but is recommended in emergency situations

20. All of the following statements about monitoring drug therapy are correct except
a. Monitoring the effects of medication can identify any potential allergic reactions a patient may have after a medication has been administered
b. Technicians can assist monitoring the effects of medications by gathering certain lab values for the pharmacist
c. Monitoring the effects of drug therapy helps determine if patients are having the intended outcomes of their therapy
d. Monitoring the effects of medications are the sole responsibility of a nurse
e. The pharmacy technician can alert the pharmacist when certain STAT orders are received in the pharmacy, especially as they relate to anti-allergic or antidote-type drugs such as epinephrine or diphenhydramine, which are commonly used to treat allergic reactions

Self-Assessment Answers

1. c. Medicare and Medicaid have been identified as potential causes of rising health care costs by reimbursing for services determined to be necessary by physicians, removing the incentive to control costs.
2. b. Pyxis Medstation® and OmniCell's SinglePointe™ are examples of automated dispensing cabinets. This technology is primarily located in patient care areas.
3. a. The Pharmacy and Therapeutics Committee is the committee responsible for approving the hospital formulary.
4. e. the friendliness of a pharmaceutical representative (i.e., sales representative) should have no bearing on formulary decisions.
5. d. Because of the close proximity to patient care areas, a decentralized pharmacist is more likely to attend patient care rounds. Although it is possible for a centralized pharmacist to attend these types of rounds, it is more difficult.
6. a. A decentralized pharmacy based on its close proximity to patient care units allows pharmacy services to be closer to the patient.
7. b. Pharmacokinetic calculations involve clinical skills, which are the responsibility of a pharmacist to perform. A technician can collect

certain laboratory results that are used in these pharmacokinetic calculations.

8. c. Screening orders for non-formulary/restricted drugs is a common activity the technician can perform to assist the pharmacist in order to free up time for the provision of pharmaceutical care.
9. b. A unit-dose system involves preparing each dose in ready-to-use form. All other responses are false statements.
10. e. Unit dose ready-to-use systems decrease the potential for errors compared to preparing medications from bulk supplies. They also decrease the potential for waste and decrease the time to prepare medications for nurses.
11. c. Verbal orders are discouraged because they can be a source for misinterpretation and cause for errors.
12. b. Many organizational structures exist depending on the size, type of institution (e.g., teaching vs. community), and other factors.
13. a. Evaluating the medication management process is intended to assess and identify any potential system problems, not employee problems.
14. a. Root Cause Analysis is retrospective; it is performed after a problem is identified.
15. c. Proper hand washing is one of the simplest and most effective methods to prevent the spread of infections in hospitals.
16. b. Although computers cannot eliminate errors, they have reduced errors related to transcription and manipulation of orders. In addition, computer order entry reduces the number of steps in the medication use process.
17. d. This scenario illustrates a breakdown in the preparation and dispensing of the medication. Not only was the product not prepared in a unit dose package, the labeling would not meet standards set by regulatory and accrediting agencies.
18. c. When a medication is ordered and prescribed, it is important to obtain an accurate medication history to prevent adverse outcomes as described in this scenario. Pharmacists play an important role in ensuring medications are prescribed appropriately by checking each order for appropriateness, and reviewing for potential allergies, therapeutic duplications, drug-drug interactions, and other contraindications.
19. e. Aseptic technique is recommended for all routine preparation of IV medications. At times proper aseptic techniques may not be feasible during emergency situations.
20. d. Many health care providers are responsible for monitoring the effects of medication therapy. Pharmacy technicians may be asked to obtain certain laboratory values for pharmacists as part of the monitoring process of medication therapy.

Resources

ASHP. *Best Practices for Hospital and Health-System Pharmacy: Position and Guidance Documents of ASHP.* Bethesda, MD: American Society of Hospital Pharmacists; 2009.

Uselton JP, Kienle P, Murdaugh LB. *Assuring Continuous Compliance with Joint Commission Standards: A Pharmacy Guide*, 8th ed. Bethesda, MD: American Society of Health-System Pharmacists; 2010.

The American Society of Health-System Pharmacists: www.ashp.org.

The Institute for Safe Medication Practice (ISMP): www.ismp.org.

The Institute for Healthcare Improvement (IHI): www.ihi.org.

The Joint Commission: www.jointcommission.org.

References

1. American College of Clinical Pharmacy. The definition of Clinical Pharmacy. *Pharmacotherapy* 2008;28(6): 816–817.
2. Koch KE, Weeks A. Clinically oriented pharmacy technicians to augment clinical services. *Am J Hosp Pharm.* 1998;55:1375–1381.
3. Weber EW, Hepginger C, Koontz R, et al. Pharmacy technicians supporting clinical functions. *Am J Hosp Pharm.* 2005;62:2469–2472.
4. Schumock G, Walton S, Sarawate C, et al. Pharmaceutical services in rural hospitals in Illinois—2001. *Am J Hosp Pharm.* 2003;60:666–674.
5. Ervin KC, Skledar S, Hess MM, et al. Data analyst technician: An innovative role for the pharmacy technician. *Am J Health-System Pharm.* 2001;58:1815–1818.
6. Hudkins JE, Crane VS. Role of pharmacy technicians in hospital formulary maintenance. *J Pharm Technol.* 1988;4(Jul/Aug):144–156.
7. Ambrose AJ, Saya FG, Lovett LT, et al. Evaluating the accuracy of technicians and pharmacists in checking unit

dose medication cassettes. *Am J Health-System Pharm.* 2002;59:1183–1184.

8. Hepler CD, Strand LM. Opportunities and responsibilities in pharmaceutical care. *Am J Hosp Pharm.* 1990;47:533–543.
9. American Society of Health-System Pharmacists. Practice standards of ASHP 1995–1996. Bethesda, MD: ASHP, 1995; p.11.
10. Pedersen CA, Schneider PJ, Scheckelhoff DJ. ASHP national survey of pharmacy practice in hospital settings: Dispensing and administration—2005. *Am J Health-System Pharm.* 2006;63:327–345.
11. The Joint Commission Home Page. "Benefits of Joint Commission Certification." http://www.jointcommission.org/CertificationPrograms/cert_benefits.htm. Accessed 2009, June 23.
12. Fox BI, Poikonen J, Gumpper K, Sharing experience with information technology. *Am J Health-Syst Pharm.* 2008;65:1012–1014.
13. American Society of Health-System Pharmacists. ASHP Statement on the Pharmacist's Role in Informatics *Am J Health-Syst Pharm.* 2007;64:200–203.
14. Bross BA, Ness JE, Rudisill R. Benefits of forming pharmacy technician teams. *Am J Health-Syst Pharm.* 2004;61:1389–1391.
15. Bates DW, Laird N, Peterson LA, et al. Incidence of adverse drug events and potential adverse drug events. Implications for prevention. ADE Prevention Study Group. *JAMA*. 1995; 274: 29–34.
16. Walton M. The Deming management method. New York: Putnam Publishing Co; 1986.
17. Infection Control. http://www.nlm.nih.gov/medlineplus/infectioncontrol.htm. Accessed 2009, June 23.
18. Dent S. American Academy of Family Physicians. Deadly risks of antibiotic overuse warrant widespread education. http://www.aafp.org/fpr/20000300/01.html. Accessed 2009, June 23.
19. American Society of Health-System Pharmacists. ASHP Statement on the Pharmacist's role in infection control. *Am J Health-System Pharm.* 2008; 55: 1724–1726.
20. Hoffman, JM, Doloresco, FL, Vermeulen LC, et al. Projecting future drug expenditures—2010. *Am J Health-System Pharm.* 2010;67:919–28.

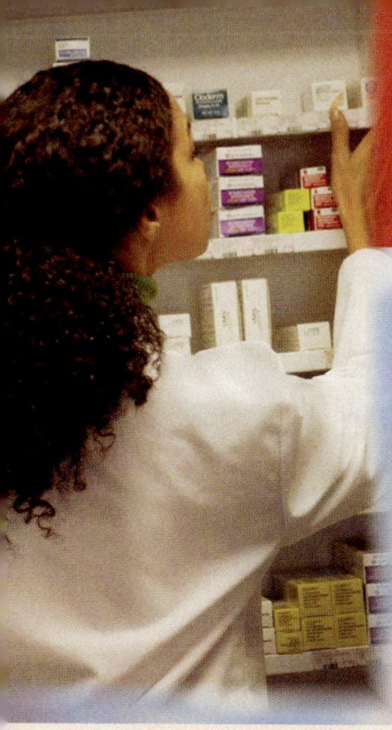

Chapter 5

Home Care Pharmacy Practice

Karen E. Bertch

Learning Outcomes

After completing this chapter, you will be able to

- Identify the historical reasons for establishing home care services and the growth of the home care industry.
- Cite the seven goals of home care therapy.
- Identify the members of the home care team and describe their primary roles in the home care process.
- Identify the most common diseases or conditions treated with home care services.
- Identify the top drug classes used in home infusion therapy. List one or two parameters for these drugs that affect how they are used in the home environment.
- Compare the advantages and disadvantages of the types of infusion systems available for use in a patient's home.
- List the labeling requirements for sterile products that are to be used in a patient's home.
- Outline the factors that are important to consider when determining expiration dates for sterile products used in the home care setting.

Key Terms

case manager Helps determine the location of the therapy. The case manager may work for the insurance company, the hospital, or the home care company. The case manager works to manage the cost of medical care for the patient and may be very influential in steering a patient toward home care.

elastomeric balloon system An intravenous administration system containing reservoirs that consist of multiple layers of elastomeric (i.e., stretchy, elastic-like) membranes within a hard or soft shell. When the device is filled with diluent and a drug, the elastomeric material expands like a balloon. When tubing is attached to the device and the patient's catheter, the elastic balloon forces the solution through the tubing and into the patient.

extravasation Leaking of intravenous solutions into areas outside of the vein, resulting in potentially severe tissue damage.

intake coordinator The person from the home care company who receives the patient referral. This person is responsible for getting the patient's contact information (address, phone number, etc.), diagnosis, requested home care therapy, pertinent medical data, and insurance information.

patient-controlled analgesia (PCA) A type of pain management in which the patient receives parenteral narcotics with a basal/continuous rate and/or has the capabilities to give fixed bolus doses to himself or herself using an electronic ambulatory infusion pump. The PCA pump allows one or both of the features to be in use at one time; the clinician may choose to use only the bolus option with lock-out periods or only the continuous rate to meet patient needs.

patient service representative Responsible for controlling the patient's inventory of supplies and screening for problems. This person's job is to contact the patient or caregiver weekly or on a routine basis, depending on the anticipated delivery schedule. Often, this individual helps coordinate pickup of supplies and equipment when the patient's therapy is completed.

peripherally inserted central catheter (PICC) An intravenous catheter that can be inserted at the hospital bedside or at home by specially trained nurses. They are inserted through a vein in the arm, threaded through other veins in the arm, and end up with the tip resting in the superior vena cava.

rate-restricted IV administration set systems An intravenous administration system used with proprietary fluid reservoirs that are designed specifically for use in the home care setting. The tubing used with these systems is designed to infuse the solution at a set rate. The only way to change the rate of infusion is to change the tubing.

smart pumps Infusion pumps equipped with IV medication error prevention software. These devices have specific drug libraries, dose calculators, programming limits, and remote communications capabilities.

universal precautions Treating all patients as if they were potentially infectious to prevent employees from exposure to human blood or other potentially infectious material. For example, wearing personal protective equipment (e.g., gloves, masks, gowns), hand washing, and proper handling and disposal of potentially infectious material.

Home health care is the provision of health care services in the patient's home, rather than an institutional setting or provider's office.[1] Home care pharmacy is part of home health care practice. The majority of pharmaceuticals in non-institutional settings are provided through the community pharmacy system. The role of home care pharmacy is to provide intravenous (IV) medications and high-technology services in the home. In the home care setting, the pharmacy technician can assist the pharmacist in the preparation of parenteral products as well as being involved with inventory maintenance and control, creating and maintaining patient supply inventory, and making deliveries to patients' homes. Much of the material covered in Chapter 16, Aseptic Technique, Sterile Compounding, and Intravenous Admixture Systems, complements this chapter. Technicians planning to practice in a home care setting should review both chapters thoroughly.

Historical Overview and Current Practices

Patients first began receiving infusion therapy in the home, rather than in an institutional setting, in the late 1970s. The driving force for sending patients home was twofold: keeping patients in the hospital to receive long-term intravenous antibiotic therapy or parenteral nutrition was becoming too expensive, and patients and their families considered it a hardship to "live" in the hospital for the duration of the patients' treatment. These long-term patients often required minimal intensive medical care other than the care associated with their infusion therapy. The search for alternatives to hospitalization led to the development of programs to treat long-term infusion patients at home, and the home infusion industry was born. In the past 25 years, home care, and in particular home infusion, has become one of the fastest growing segments of health care.[2] The alternate-site infusion therapy sector continues to expand. This is being driven by heightened emphasis on cost-effectiveness and cost containment, and the desire of patients to resume normal lifestyles and work activities while recovering from illness. This sector is currently estimated to represent approximately 9 to 11 billion dollars per year in U.S. health care expenditures serviced by 700 to 1,000 infusion pharmacies.[3]

Home infusion has grown rapidly for several reasons. First, a number of studies have shown that administration of long-term IV therapy in the home is safe and effective, as well as less expensive, which helped physicians and insurance companies overcome any fear or reluctance they may have had in sending their patients to home health care agencies. In addition, the explosion of technology has supported the movement of patients to the home care setting. New developments have brought infusion pumps that are portable, small, easily programmable for a wide range of therapies, and, in some cases, disposable. These new infusion pumps have made it easier to teach nonprofessionals, such as patients and their families, to administer complicated therapies at home. Although consumers have demanded home care—citing improved quality of life, ability to return to work, and greater independence—the strongest impetus for home health care came from the dramatic changes in our health care system. Escalating health care costs forced hospitals to decrease the length of time patients spent in the hospital. As a result, patients are discharged earlier in the course of treatment and often need additional care when they get home. The need for more intensive medical care and support in the home provided opportunities for the home health care industry to grow. Finally, treating patients at home has the advantage, in some cases, of helping them to avoid the development of new infections in the hospital, such as hospital-acquired pneumonia.

Home infusion services are provided by a number of organizations, including hospitals, community pharmacies, home health nursing companies, integrated health care systems, and independent home infusion companies. After the tremendous expansion of home health care organizations, we are now seeing a consolidation, with mergers of companies and shifting of dominance among the providers of home infusion services.

In addition, there appear to be more home infusion services that are providing therapies for niche markets, including national specialty pharmacies. These providers often focus care on patients requiring growth hormone and anti-hemophilic factor; however, in the past few years, their practice has expanded into the provision of biotechnology products and the treatments of rare, chronic diseases.[4]

Summary of Home Care Practice

Purpose and Goals of Home Infusion Therapy

The purpose of home care pharmacy practice is to provide high-technology therapy, which is usually available in an institutional setting, at home. The goals of home care services are summarized in table 5-1.

✔Overall, the major goal of home care pharmacy practice is to provide safe and effective infusion therapy in the home that is also cost-effective.

The Home Care Process

A patient may enter the home care process a number of ways. Usually a physician will recommend that a patient complete therapy at home. In some instances, the patient and the patient's family advocate home therapy, or the patient's insurance company may dictate where therapy will be provided. Sometimes an individual called a **case manager** will mediate the location of the therapy. The case manager may work for the insurance company, the hospital, or the home care company. The case manager works to manage the cost of medical care for the patient and may be very influential in steering a patient toward home care. The hospital may also initiate the process as it tries to control its costs by reducing patients' length of stay.

Once the decision has been made to send a patient home, a social worker or a discharge planner contacts the home care agency and initiates the process. In many hospitals, the discharge planner is a registered nurse with home care experience, who will begin preparing the patient for home therapy.

An **intake coordinator** at the home care company receives the patient referral. This person is responsible for retrieving the patient's contact information (address, phone number, etc.), diagnosis, requested home care therapy, pertinent medical data, and insurance information. Home care personnel must keep patient information confidential, especially in light of the regulations inherent to the Health Insurance Portability and Accountability Act (HIPAA). The intake coordinator is often a nurse but may also be a technician specially trained for the job.

When all the necessary data have been obtained, the home care team decides whether to accept or refuse the referral. This determination is based on the ability and willingness of the patient or the caregivers to perform the tasks required to administer therapy at home. Other factors used to decide if a referral is acceptable include the appropriateness and feasibility of the therapeutic plan and the assurance that home care therapy will not place too much of a financial burden on the patient or the home infusion company.

Once the patient is accepted, the home care team begins providing services, which include determining the necessary medical supplies (e.g., tubing, dressing, needles, and syringes), selecting an appropriate infusion device (e.g., gravity system, pump) depending on the patient's therapy, preparing the drug for the infusion device in a sterile environment, assembling the appropriate patient educational materials and home care paperwork, and negotiating charges with the insurer. When all materials and supplies are ready, a delivery is made to the patient's home. The pharmacy technician may be involved in gathering supplies, educational material, and paperwork and in arranging deliveries. The technician is always involved in preparing the drugs.

A registered nurse trained in home infusion makes the initial patient visit. Once the patient has been informed of his or her rights and responsibilities as a home care patient, the nurse begins to teach the patient about the

Table 5-1. Goals of Home Care

- Allow patients to leave the hospital earlier
- Allow patients to receive treatment without being hospitalized
- Allow patients to return to work or normal activities sooner
- Allow patients to recuperate in the comfort of the home environment
- Decrease health care costs
- Provide safe and effective treatment and care
- Decrease the risk of hospital-associated complications (e.g., infections)
- Achieve a smooth, non-stressful transition of treatment between the hospital and the patient's home

supplies and drugs and how to care for the catheter so the patient can eventually administer the medications. If a patient cannot administer the medications, a caregiver learns how to do it, or, on rare occasions, a nurse will administer the medications. Several nursing visits are often required to ensure that the patient can perform medication administration and other procedures properly.

The initial referral process usually takes 24 to 48 hours; occasionally, it must be performed in just a few hours. Empathy is essential in this process. Many times the idea of home infusion of medications overwhelms patients and their caregivers. What is routine for the home care professional is often very foreign to the patient. Therefore, crucial members of the team (home care nurse, pharmacist) must be available (usually by cell phone or pager) to the patient 24 hours a day, 7 days a week.

After the initial visit, the home care team develops a care plan for the patient. The care plan includes how the home care team will monitor the patient's therapy and watch for complications of therapy, as well as signs that the therapy is effective. Home care team members visit or contact the patients on a regular basis to assess their status, inventory their supplies, and make interventions when necessary. Generally, supplies and drugs are prepared and delivered weekly. Nevertheless, this schedule may vary, depending on the stability of the medications or solutions and the laboratory work that is being conducted on the patient. The home care team maintains records of the patient's home care course. These records become the patient's home care chart and include documentation of all communications concerning the patient, physician orders and prescriptions, records of drugs and supplies sent to the patient, and laboratory results. The goal of the home care process is for the patient to experience a successful course of therapy without any adverse events. Once home care therapy is completed, the patient is discharged from the home care service.

The Home Care Team and Specific Roles

The primary members of the home care team are actively involved in the care of the majority of home infusion patients. Secondary members are involved only when a particular patient requires their service. Examples of secondary members include registered dietitians, respiratory therapists, social workers, physical and occupational therapists, and certified nursing assistants (CNAs).

Physician

The physician is the leader of the team, and he or she is ultimately responsible for the care of the patient. The physician provides the direction of care. Any major changes in therapy require the physician's approval. To ensure that the physician remains in charge of the patient's care, the physician reviews and signs a Certificate of Medical Necessity and Plan of Treatment. Physician drug orders (prescriptions) are usually given to the pharmacist over the phone, as in the community pharmacy setting. Written and signed physician orders received via facsimile machine, however, are becoming more common. Rules and regulations regarding prescriptions may be specific to each state, especially for narcotics. The technician should be aware of the regulations of the state in which the home care pharmacy is located. In the home care environment, the physician does not see the patient daily or even weekly. The physician often relies on the nurse or pharmacist to evaluate and report the patient's clinical condition.

Nurse and Pharmacist

The infusion nurse and pharmacist are key members of the team. They work together to coordinate patient supplies, develop a plan of care, monitor and document the patient's status, communicate with the physician, coordinate physician orders, and make appropriate interventions. The nurse and pharmacist should not only be responsible for selecting the infusion devices, but also be proficient in programming and troubleshooting the devices. Both disciplines are intensely involved with assessing and educating home care patients and work jointly to perform the organization's clinical quality assurance activities, such as measuring and documenting catheter infections, re-hospitalizations, adverse events, and outcomes of the plan of care. Together, the nurse and pharmacist are responsible for communicating and coordinating all patient care activities.

Nurse

The nurse is the primary educator of the patient, responsible for teaching all aspects of home care therapy. When visiting the patient, the nurse assesses the patient's physical status, the patient's adherence to the treatment plan, the condition of the catheter, and any psychosocial issues the patient may be facing. Maintenance of intravenous catheters is the sole responsibility of the nurse. Home care infusion nurses are skilled in the placement of peripheral catheters, and many are skilled in the insertion of peripheral long-term catheters or the peripherally inserted central venous catheter (PICC), discussed later in this chapter. Nurses also schedule and perform all blood work that is ordered.

Pharmacist

The pharmacist is solely responsible for the proper acquisition, compounding, dispensing, and storage of drugs. The pharmacist is also an educator, responsible for instructing the patient and the nurse on the drugs being administered.

✔The pharmacist regularly assesses the home care patient with a focus on monitoring the laboratory data, the patient's symptoms, and the patient's compliance with drug therapy.

Important additional clinical pharmacy roles are pharmacokinetic dosing of vancomycin and aminoglycosides, providing nutritional support services, and having input in the selection of the most appropriate drug for the patient. The pharmacist is the drug information source for all other team members.

Pharmacy Technician

Pharmacy technicians support the pharmacist by performing the majority of the technical pharmacy functions. These functions consist of generating medication labels; compounding, preparing, and labeling medications; and maintaining the compounding room and drug storage areas. The technician is the coordinator of the IV room, working with the pharmacist to arrange the mixing schedule, ordering and maintaining drug and mixing supplies, and performing quality assurance on compounding activities. Pharmacy technicians are often responsible for managing the warehouse and inventory of non-drug supplies, keeping track of accounts receivable, picking and packaging supplies for shipment to patients, and arranging for delivery of supplies to patients. In smaller companies, the pharmacy technician may wear many of these hats. In larger companies, separate individuals (who may be pharmacy technicians) perform each of these functions. For example, some technicians may be experienced drivers who only make patient deliveries.

Reimbursement Specialist

Although not active in direct patient care, the reimbursement specialist is key to the economic viability of the company. The reimbursement department is the interface among the insurer, the home infusion company, and the patient. The primary responsibility of this department is to coordinate all the billing and collection for services provided. To fulfill this responsibility, reimbursement specialists brief staff regarding the services and drugs that are paid for by the insurers, negotiate the price of services with insurers, and brief the insurers regarding the status of the patient and the therapeutic plan. The timeliness of this function is crucial to the financial survival of the organization. The reimbursement specialist is also well-versed in public aid and government reimbursement programs, such as Medicaid and Medicare.

Patient Service Representative

Many companies employ a **patient service representative**. The representative is responsible for controlling the patient's inventory of supplies and screening for problems. This person's job is to contact the patient or caregiver weekly or on a routine basis, depending on the anticipated delivery schedule. Often, this individual helps coordinate the pickup of supplies and equipment when the patient's therapy is completed. Occasionally a pharmacy technician may be responsible for this job.

Patient and Caregiver

Not to be forgotten as team members are the patient and the caregivers. In home care, much of the burden falls on their shoulders. They must be involved in the decision making and the development of the care plan. The patient's right to be involved is clearly stated in the rights and responsibilities document that is presented on the initial visit. This document outlines how the patient and caregivers are included in the management of the patient at home.

Types of Home Care Therapies

Anti-Infectives

Anti-infectives account for the majority of pharmaceuticals used in home infusion therapy. The most common IV antibiotics and anti-infectives used in the home are listed in table 5-2 and are discussed below.[5,6] Relatively few infectious diseases require long-term infusion therapy. The most common infectious diseases seen in home care patients are listed in table 5-3.

Table 5–2. Common Antimicrobials Used in Home Care

Drug Class	Examples
Cephalosporins	Cefazolin (Ancef), cefepime (Maxipime), ceftriaxone (Rocephin)
Penicillins	Ampicillin/sulbactam (Unasyn), nafcillin, oxacillin, penicillin G, piperacillin/tazobactam (Zosyn)
Fluoroquinolones	Ciprofloxacin (Cipro), levofloxacin (Levaquin), moxifloxacin (Avelox)
Carbapenems	Ertapenem (Invanz), imipenem/cilastatin (Primaxin), meropenem (Merrem)
Other	Vancomycin, daptomycin (Cubicin), linezolid (Zyvox), quinupristin/dalfopristin (Synercid)
Antifungals	Amphotericin B, fluconazole (Diflucan), voriconazole (Vfend), anidulafungin (Eraxis), caspofungin (Cancidas), micafungin (Mycamine)
Antivirals	Foscarnet, acyclovir, ganciclovir

Antibiotics

The administration of antibiotic therapy is the leading home infusion service, comprising 40 to 70 percent of the current home infusion business.[5,7] Most available IV antibiotics can be used in the home environment. In general, antibiotics are chosen based on the organism(s) identified in the blood, bone, joint, and/or wound cultures and their susceptibilities to the various antibiotics, as well as individual patient characteristics.

Cephalosporins, such as ceftriaxone (Rocephin), cefazolin (Ancef), and cefepime (Maxipime), comprise most of the IV antibiotic courses administered in the home. Cephalosporins are very easy to use in home care because they have a low incidence of adverse reactions and require minimal monitoring.[6] Ceftriaxone is often prescribed because it can be given once daily, which decreases the costs of supplies and requires less work for the patient or caregiver. Most cephalosporins are stable for 10 days after admixture, so they are ideal for weekly deliveries. Moreover, many of the cephalosporins can be administered as IV push, a method of administration in which the drug is directly injected into the patient's catheter slowly over 2 to 5 minutes. This

Table 5–3. Common Infectious Diseases Treated in Home Care Patients

Infectious Disease	Definition	Common Anti-infectives Used for Treatment	Typical Duration of IV Therapy
Osteomyelitis	Infection that occurs when bacteria (e.g., *Staphylococcus aureus*) invades bone	Nafcillin, oxacillin, vancomycin, daptomycin	4–6 weeks
Cellulitis	Acute inflammatory infection of the skin that often extends deep into the subcutaneous tissue (tissue under the skin)	Nafcillin, oxacillin, cephalosporins, vancomycin	10–14 days
Septic arthritis	Infection of the tissue that lines the joints (synovium)	Vancomycin, cephalosporins, penicillins, carbapenems	Initially 2–3 weeks, may be as long as 6 weeks
Endocarditis	Infection of the heart valves or heart tissue	Vancomycin, penicillin plus gentamicin, daptomycin	4–6 weeks
AIDS-related infections	Fungal Infections	Amphotericin, other antifungals	1–2 months
	Viral Infections Cytomegalovirus (CMV)	Ganciclovir, foscarnet	2–3 weeks initially for induction treatment, followed by daily maintenance therapy for an indefinite period of time

is a convenience for the patient because of the short administration time.

Penicillins are also a common IV antibiotic used in the home.[6,7] Typical drugs used in this class are ampicillin/sulbactam (Unasyn), piperacillin/tazobactam (Zosyn), ticarcillin/clavulanate (Timentin), nafcillin or oxacillin, and penicillin G. Penicillins are more difficult to use in the home because they need to be given frequently (every 4 to 6 hours). These types of dosing regimens are difficult for some patients to adhere to because of the time they have to take out of their day for administration. Portable pumps, called ambulatory pumps, that can automatically give continuous or intermittent doses throughout the day are often used for penicillin therapy. Stability is another problem with this class. Ampicillin has short stability and must be mixed in the home prior to infusion. The availability of the ADD-Vantage® and Add-Ease® systems (see Chapter 16, Aseptic Technique, Sterile Compounding, and IV Admixture Programs) makes mixing in the home much easier and safer. Most of the other penicillins have just 7 days of stability. Pushing penicillins to their stability limit is a concern because they may break down as they expire, and the breakdown products are associated with an increased risk of allergic reactions. The most common adverse effect in this class is an allergic reaction, such as a rash. Penicillins are also very irritating to veins, frequently causing phlebitis (redness and inflammation of the vein). It is highly recommended that patients receiving penicillins at home have a central venous catheter, a catheter that is placed in a large central vein such as the subclavian vein.

Vancomycin is also a frequently prescribed drug in home care.[6,7] Vancomycin should be infused at a rate of no greater than 1 gram over 60 minutes to prevent Red Man Syndrome, which is an infusion-related reaction that causes a redness or flushing of the head and torso. This can be accomplished by using a pump or infusion control device, or by placing vancomycin in larger amounts of fluid (e.g., 150 to 250 mL). The pharmacist uses pharmacokinetics and the results of vancomycin blood levels to individualize patient dosing of vancomycin. Vancomycin is irritating to the veins and, in the home setting, is best given through a central catheter. If a peripheral catheter is used, vancomycin should be placed in larger amounts of IV solution (e.g., 250 to 500 mL of solution) to avoid vein irritation.

Additional antibiotics that are becoming more frequently used in the home care setting include azithromycin (Zithromax), doxycycline, and the fluoroquinolones, such as ciprofloxacin, levofloxacin (Levaquin), and moxifloxacin (Avelox). Azithromycin, doxycycline, and many of the newer fluoroquinolones can be given via IV once daily, thus making them convenient for patients receiving therapy at home.[8] The carbapenems, namely, imipenem/cilistatin (Primaxin), meropenem (Merrem), and ertapenem (Invanz), are being used more and more in the home care setting. However, because of their short stability, administration often requires the use of a bag and vial attachment system such as the Add-Ease® or Minibag® Plus systems.[9] Because of widespread cases of resistance to vancomycin, newer antibiotics such as daptomycin (Cubicin), linezolid (Zyvox), and quinupristin/dalfopristin (Synercid) are being more frequently prescribed in home infusion patients. Their use should be reserved for limited situations since resistance to these agents is somewhat limited at this point in time.[9] Limited stability information is available for these agents, which may pose some challenges in the home care setting and require that patients "home-mix" the medications themselves.

Antifungals

Antifungal agents may be used in the home care setting when a provider services a large transplant or immunocompromised patient population, such as those patients with acquired immunodeficiency syndrome (AIDS). Intravenous amphotericin B products are commonly prescribed for severe fungal infections. Many patients experience fever, chills, and shakes from amphotericin infusions. This reaction often requires premedication with oral acetaminophen and diphenydramine. Some patients have such severe reactions that IV meperidine and hydrocortisone are given. The home care infusion pharmacy usually supplies these premedications. Infusions of amphotericin should always be given with an infusion pump. Normal saline, commonly used to flush the catheter before and after the infusion of medication, is incompatible with amphotericin B—mixing the two results in a precipitate. Therefore, the pharmacy compounds dextrose 5 percent syringes for flushing the catheter when amphotericin is used in the home. Lipid-based amphotericin B (Amphotec) and liposomal amphotericin B (Ambisome) are being used more often, especially for patients who cannot tolerate plain amphotericin B or who have compromised renal function.[9]

Safety First To prevent errors, the technician should work closely with the pharmacist when preparing amphotericin B formulations. Dispensing the correct product is essential and dosing guidelines vary widely between the traditional and the lipid-based products.[9]

Intravenous azole antifungal agents such as fluconazole (Diflucan) and voriconazole (Vfend) are used in home infusion patients as an alternative to the amphotericin B products for some severe systemic fungal infections. A relatively new class of antifungal agents, the echinocandins, are being used more frequently in the home care setting. Anidulafungin (Eraxis), caspofungin (Cancidas), and micafungin (Mycamine) comprise this class of agents. Caspofungin is approved for use in pediatric patients;[10] thus its use in this patient population is growing in the home care setting. Caspofungin is not compatible with dextrose-containing solutions.

Antivirals

Ganciclovir is a commonly prescribed parenteral antiviral agent used in transplant patients or patients with human immunodeficiency virus (HIV) who have cytomegalovirus (CMV) infection. Special precautions must be taken when preparing and administering ganciclovir due to its cytotoxic nature. Ganciclovir almost always causes bone marrow toxicity in AIDS patients. Filgrastim (Neupogen) therapy is often added to offset bone marrow toxicity. An alternative to ganciclovir is foscarnet. Patients must receive hydration fluids while receiving foscarnet because it may have effects on the kidneys. To help prevent kidney damage, foscarnet is compounded in 500 to 1,000 mL of fluid and infused with a pump, or 500 to 1,000 mL of normal saline is given prior to each infusion. Intravenous acyclovir is sometimes administered to immunocompromised patients in the home and is usually given every eight hours. Because it can cause phlebitis, patients receiving this agent must have adequate intravenous access.[9]

Other

Pentamidine is occasionally given in immunocompromised patients as prophylaxis for a particular type of pneumonia. The route of administration for this agent for prophylactic use is inhalation, via a special nebulizer, Respigard®, every 4 weeks.[9,11] Patients may receive the nebulized treatments at home or in an ambulatory infusion suite.

Parenteral Nutrition

Total parenteral nutrition (TPN) is intravenous nutrition that provides a patient with all of the fluid and essential nutrients he or she needs when oral nutrition is difficult or impossible. Patients with Crohn disease (inflammatory disease of the small and large intestines) and bowel loss or dysfunction are the major recipients of parenteral nutrition. Malnutrition associated with cancer and AIDS is another indication for parenteral nutrition. Patients who absorb some nutrients from the food they eat, but not enough to completely sustain them, may require supplementation with parenteral nutrition. These patients require smaller volumes of parenteral nutrition and may not need daily infusions.

Parenteral nutrition may be infused continuously over 24 hours, or, typically in the home infusion patient, it is given cyclically. The cycles can range from 12 hours to 20 hours, whereby the patient will not infuse the nutrition solution during some hours of the day. Allowing the patient to be off of the parenteral nutrition solution for some time during the day gives him or her the opportunity to have a more active lifestyle and may cause less long-term adverse effects versus a continuous infusion. Patients receiving parenteral nutrition often require other IV medications. Many of these medications are not compatible with parenteral nutrition, which creates a difficult situation to manage in the home, especially if the patient is receiving the parenteral nutrition continuously. The patient must learn to stop and start the parenteral nutrition and adequately flush the catheter to administer other medications. One alternative is for these patients to have a central catheter with at least two separate lumens, which are tunnels within the catheter. The parenteral nutrition is infused in one lumen, while other medications are administered in the other lumen. Another alternative (as noted earlier) is for the parenteral nutrition to be cycled to infuse over 12 to 14 hours at night, instead of continuously over 24 hours. Medications could be administered while the parenteral nutrition solution is not infusing.

Typical ingredients in a parenteral nutrition solution include dextrose, amino acids, electrolytes (e.g., potassium, sodium, calcium, etc.), trace minerals, and multivitamins. Lipids are another important component and can be infused separately from the parenteral nutrition solution in their own bag or bottle, or directly admixed with the other ingredients. Commonly, parenteral nutrition 3-in-1 solutions (containing lipids), also referred to as total nutrient admixtures (TNAs), are used in home infusion patients for convenience. They are stable for a shorter time period than bags without lipids, but extended stability may be achieved by using a dual-chamber bag in which the lipids are housed separately above the dextrose and amino acids. The patient "activates" the bag just before infusing it. Pre-mixed parenteral nutrition formulations (e.g., Clinimix®) are also available and may have some use in the home care setting. These formulations contain a standard amount of dextrose and amino acids, and, in some cases, electrolytes. The patient's nutrient requirements and volume of TPN formula will need to be considered prior to using a pre-mixed parenteral formulation. The home infusion pharmacy staff may need to include additional ingredients (e.g., lipids or other electrolytes) prior to sending these formulations to a patient.

✔A number of ingredients in parenteral nutrition are stable for only 24 hours. These drugs are called patient additives and must be injected into the bag prior to infusion by the patient or caregiver.

Examples of drugs that the patient must add are insulin, heparin, vitamins, and H_2-receptor antagonists (e.g., famotidine, ranitidine). Drugs a patient needs to add should be supplied in vials rather than in ampules whenever possible, for patient convenience. It is also advisable to limit the medications a patient must add to a parenteral nutrition bag to those that are absolutely necessary. This limitation is not only for sterility reasons but also for the sake of compliance and patient stress. The more medications that are added, the greater the complexity of the solution and the greater the chance for incompatibility or contamination.

Patients receiving parenteral nutrition require intensive monitoring, which usually includes weekly laboratory tests (chemistry and complete blood count [CBC]), blood glucose, fluid status, and patient weights. Monitoring progress toward the therapeutic goals of increasing the patient's weight and improving his or her nutritional status, as well as screening for complications such as liver toxicity and bone breakdown, is a continual process. Before a week's supply of solution is mixed, the pharmacist must review these parameters, as well as others. If these values are abnormal, the pharmacist must make recommendations to the physician, followed by appropriate changes in the parenteral nutrition formula (e.g., electrolyte content; volume; or amount of glucose, lipid, or protein in the solution). The pharmacist may do this in consultation with a dietician. To avoid making parenteral nutrition bags that cannot be used, the technician should coordinate mixing of a patient's parenteral nutrition to follow scheduled laboratory blood draws and pharmacist and nursing assessments and visits. Changes to parenteral nutrition formulas are common, especially in the first few months of therapy. Patients on long-term parenteral nutrition tend to stabilize after several months and require less monitoring.

Rx for Success

The pharmacy technician can play an instrumental role in collecting the laboratory and patient data, then recording it on patient flow sheets so that the pharmacist has this information readily available for monitoring the patient.

Enteral Nutrition Therapy

Some home infusion pharmacies may also provide enteral nutrition therapy. Enteral nutrition is the administration of specialized formulas that are high in required nutrients through the stomach or part of the small intestine (jejunum) to meet a patient's nutritional needs. Patients who can eat will drink the enteral formula. Patients who cannot eat (e.g., those who are comatose) but have a working stomach or small intestine receive the formula through tubes placed either through their nose down into their stomach (nasogastric tube [NG tube]) or surgically to their stomach (gastrostomy tube [G tube]) or jejunum (jejunostomy [J tube]). Home infusion companies become involved when enteral nutrition is being administered continuously via a feeding tube, with or without a pump. When this technology is used, the expertise of the home health care team is often required. Patients who can drink their enteral formulas can usually get their therapy much cheaper through a community pharmacy and do not require home care services. Monitoring patients receiving enteral nutrition includes following their nutritional status and detecting drug-nutrient interactions.

Chemotherapy

Most chemotherapy is given in a clinic setting, but a number of chemotherapy agents may be given in the home environment. Chemotherapy regimens given in the home are those requiring prolonged infusion, usually greater than 24 hours. The agents that tend to be used in this manner are 5-fluorouracil, cyclophosphamide, doxorubicin (Adriamycin), oxaliplatin (Eloxatin), vincristine, vinblastine, and paclitaxel (Taxol).

One of the most common agents administered in the home care environment is 5-fluorouracil. Continuous infusions of 5-fluorouracil are used in treatment protocols for stomach, intestine, colon, and liver cancers. A central line is highly recommended for patients receiving chemotherapy at home to avoid the risk of **extravasation,** which is when the solution leaks into the areas outside of the vein, resulting in potentially severe tissue damage. Side effects of chemotherapy such as bone marrow toxicity (low platelets [thrombocytopenia], low white blood cells [neutropenia], and low red blood cells [anemia]) and stomatitis (sores in the mouth), are frequent with this class of drugs. Many patients require the addition of colony-stimulating factor therapy such as filgrastim (Neupogen) or sargramostim (Leukine) to counteract the chemotherapy-induced drop in white blood cells. Other supportive therapies, such as IV fluids and anti-nausea medications (e.g., prochlorperazine [Compazine], metoclopramide [Reglan], or ondansetron [Zofran]), are often administered to patients receiving chemotherapy.

Some oncology clinics and offices have home infusion pharmacies mix chemotherapy for their patients. The chemotherapy is usually compounded for IV push or short IV infusion in the clinic or office. When the home infusion company assumes this role, the home care team does not routinely monitor these patients.

Biological Response Modifiers

The biological response modifiers include filgrastim (Neupogen), a long-acting colony-stimulating factor called pegfilgrastim (Neulasta), erythropoietin (Epogen, Procrit), a long-acting erythropoietin called darbepoetin alfa (Aranesp), interferons, and growth hormone. These agents are considered *high-technology or biotech drugs* because they are produced through genetic engineering. They are fairly easy to administer by subcutaneous and IV routes in the home. These drugs are often administered to patients because of adverse effects associated with chemotherapy or depletion of red blood cells in patients with chronic kidney disease who receive dialysis.

Filgrastim is used for treatment of chemotherapy- and AIDS-induced neutropenia (low white cell count). Erythropoietin is used to treat anemia. Interferons have roles in the treatment of multiple sclerosis, chronic hepatitis, cancer, and certain rare diseases. Growth hormone is used in children under 14 years old who are short in stature because of a deficiency in the hormone. All of these agents are proteins that should not be shaken and that require refrigeration to ensure stability.

Pain Management

Patients with chronic pain and pain associated with terminal illnesses often receive pain management therapy at home. Many home infusion pharmacies will care for hospice and/or palliative care patients with severe pain who are at the end stages of their lives. Intravenous medications are used when oral, rectal, or transdermal alternatives are not effective. Ninety percent of home care narcotic orders are for morphine.[6] When morphine is not acceptable, other drugs used for pain control include hydromorphone (Dilaudid), fentanyl, or fentanyl with bupivacaine, an anesthetic. Usually one bag or cassette with enough narcotic to last the patient a week is dispensed at a time, with a back-up bag being available in case the connected bag runs out in the middle of the night. The morphine solution is usually provided in concentrations of 5 to 50 mg per mL.

In the home environment, narcotics can be given intravenously, subcutaneously, intrathecally, or epidurally. When the patient has an IV catheter, pain management is given via this route. The subcutaneous route is often used in patients without IV access. Intrathecal (injection into the fluid surrounding the brain and spinal cord) and epidural (upon or external to the membranes surrounding the brain and spinal cord) routes are saved for those patients who cannot achieve adequate pain control with IV therapy. Infusion of narcotics is accomplished using **patient-controlled analgesia (PCA)** pumps (see Chapter 16 for a complete description). Patients receiving PCA therapy may receive a continuous basal infusion with or without patient-activated bolus doses.

✔Attainment of adequate pain control, such that the patient has a decent quality of life, is the goal of the home care team. Team members assess the patient's pain on a continual basis.

Cardiovascular Agents

Patients with congestive heart failure (CHF) may receive continuous infusions of parenteral inotropic agents at home. Inotropic drugs help increase the force of contractions of the heart muscle. Specific agents that may be used include dobutamine, dopamine, inamrinone (Inocor), and milrinone. Because dopamine and inamrinone have a more serious side effect profile than dobutamine and milrinone, they are used less often in the home care setting.[9] These therapies are often used as an interim approach to improve the patient's signs and symptoms of CHF, as they await a heart transplant. Patients receiving these therapies must be monitored very closely, including weight fluctuations and fluid status.

Other Therapies

Numerous other therapies are becoming more common in the home health care setting. In some cases, patients with pulmonary arterial hypertension, women with premature labor, patients with the genetic disorder alpha-1 antitrypsin deficiency, and patients with simple dehydration are being treated at home with drugs that were previously infused in institutional settings. Other specific medications that the technician should become familiar with because they may be used in the home care setting are intravenous immunoglobulin (IVIG), anticoagulants, intravenous corticosteroids, deferoxamine, and blood factor replacement products. Additional parenteral medications that the technician may see used in the home health care setting include the following:[12–14]

- Alemtuzumab (Campath), a monoclonal antibody for chronic lymphocytic leukemia
- Anakinra (Kineret), an interleukin-1 inhibitor for rheumatoid arthritis
- Infliximab (Remicade), a monoclonal antibody used in rheumatoid arthritis and Crohn disease
- Nesiritide (Natrecor), a natriuretic hormone for congestive heart failure
- Pantoprazole (Protonix IV), a proton pump inhibitor for gastroesophageal reflux disease
- Treprostinil sodium (Remodulin), a direct pulmonary and systemic arterial vasodilator
- Zoledronic acid (Zometa), a bisphosphonate for malignant hypercalcemia

Administration of Medications in the Home Care Patient

High-Technology Systems

The home infusion therapy industry's needs for technology to improve the patient's quality of life and save money have resulted in a number of products that allow medications to be delivered to patients at home.

✔In most cases, the device chosen by the home care provider dictates the type of bag the medication or solution will be dispensed in and, to a greater extent, the type of supplies the technician will have to assemble for the patient (e.g., tubing, needles).

Technicians should become familiar with the infusion products and supplies the home infusion company uses to care for its patients.

Five types of infusion systems are available for patients to use at home: (1) minibag infusion via gravity system, (2) syringe infusion via syringe device, (3) syringe infusion via IV push method, (4) rate-restricted IV administration set systems, and (5) ambulatory electronic infusion pumps. Home care providers, such as nurses, case managers, pharmacists, and pharmacy technicians with the help of other health care professionals, select the most appropriate infusion device on the basis of several factors, the most important being the patient's needs (see table 5–4). In addition, cost and reimbursement are important factors that home care providers consider when selecting a system.[15,16] A range of issues to consider when selecting an infusion system are listed in table 5–5. All these factors have an impact on the cost-effectiveness and appropriate selection of infusion devices.

Minibag Infusion via Gravity System. The minibag infusion via gravity system is one of the most cost-effective methods to deliver medications. In fact, it is the standard IV administration set used for hospitalized patients in the United States. Nevertheless, this system may be more expensive in the home care setting than in the

Table 5–4. Patient Needs Assessment for Selecting Infusion Systems

■ Age	■ Diagnosis
■ Clinical condition	■ Manual dexterity
■ Ambulatory status	■ Working status
■ Number of therapies	■ Training ability for self-administration
■ Language interpreters	■ Caregiver presence in the home
■ Nursing support requirements	
■ Travel time from home infusion provider	

Adapted from: Saladow J. Ambulatory systems for i.v. antibiotic therapy: making sense of the options. Infusion. 1995;April:17–29.

Table 5-5. Issues Associated with Infusion System Selection

■ Product design	■ Storage space needed in patient's home
■ Product reliability	■ Manufacturer and/or distributor support
■ Product compatibility and stability	■ Ease of product disposal
■ Ease of staff training	■ Inventory costs
■ Nursing interaction time	■ Product efficacy
■ Pharmacy filling time	■ Product availability
■ Ability of device to minimize complications	■ Downtime and repair cost
■ Ability of device to minimize waste	■ Ease of patient/caregiver training
■ Storage space needed at provider's facility	■ Pharmacy handling time

Adapted from: Saladow J. Ambulatory systems for i.v. antibiotic therapy: making sense of the options. Infusion. 1995;April:17–29.

institutional setting because of the cost associated with nurses teaching patients and caregivers and troubleshooting problems.[15] Other limitations of the system are the expectation that patients or caregivers will manually connect the bag to the infusion tubing and set and maintain the infusion rate, the increased risk for touch contamination, and the problems the cumbersome IV pole (on which the bag hangs) causes patients who are ambulatory or trying to work.

The Add-Vantage®, Add-Ease®, and Minibag® Plus systems are special types of minibags used for drugs with short stability. They are also referred to as bag and vial attachment systems. The term "binary connector" is also commonly used for Add-Ease®, which is a separate connector, not part of a specialized bag. With these systems, the patient or caregiver activates the vial just before administration so that the drug mixes with the diluent in the minibag. This is more expensive than the minibag system mentioned above because of the specially designed minibags these systems use and the special drug vials used with the Add-Vantage® system. All of these systems have the same limitations as the traditional minibag system. See Chapter 16 for a more detailed description of special types of minibags.

Syringe Infusion System. The syringe infusion system is very cost-effective. Syringes are easier to prepare and store than the containers used with other systems. The limitation of the syringe systems is the small volume of fluid that can be stored in one syringe, resulting in the preparation of concentrated dilutions. The potential for increased time spent educating patients and caregivers, for malfunctions of the electrical devices used to push the solution from the syringe, and for restrictions on ambulatory or working patients are other concerns associated with syringe infusion systems.[15] Syringe infusion systems include the Baxa MicroFuse® Syringe Infuser; Baxa MicroFuse® Extended Rate Infuser; Baxa MicroFuse® Rapid Rate Syringe Infuser; Baxter Auto Syringe® AS50 Infusion Pump; Baxter InfusO.R. Syringe Pump; B. Braun Medical Perfusor® Basic; Excelsior ESP Syringe Pump; Smiths Medical Medfusion Syringe Pumps, models 2010i, 3010a, and 3500; and Graseby® syringe pumps, various models.[17,18] These devices are commonly used to administer IV antibiotics to home care patients. The Excelsior ESP syringe pump is ideal for home use because of its simplicity, which aids in simple education for patients and/or caregivers in terms of its use. The Repro-Med Systems, Inc., Freedom60® Syringe Infusion System is unique in that it uses a mechanical rather than an electronic syringe driver along with a series of proprietary infusion sets that control the medication rate. It does not require batteries to operate. One model, the Freedom60-FM® Flow Monitor Syringe Pump, is available with a flow monitor alert system that provides an audible tone if flow stops or an infusion has ended.[19,20]

Part 1

Syringe Infusion via IV Push. Administration of medications via the IV push method using a syringe and slowly giving the drug over several minutes directly into the patient's IV catheter is common in the home care setting. Its popularity is due to the cost savings associated with using a syringe, labor savings in the preparation of the product, and convenience and ease of administration for the patient. Many of the IV cephalosporin antibiotics can be given via the IV push route.

Rate-Restricted IV Administration Systems. **Rate-restricted IV administration set systems** are used with proprietary fluid reservoirs that are designed specifically for use in the home care setting. The tubing used with these systems is designed to infuse the solution at a set rate. The only way to change the rate of infusion is to change the tubing. Three general types of proprietary fluid reservoirs can be used in this system: (1) the elastomeric balloon system, (2) the mechanical system, and (3) the controlled pressure system.

Elastomeric Balloons. Elastomeric balloon systems are used to deliver antibiotics and chemotherapy agents to patients outside the hospital setting. These reservoirs consist of multiple layers of elastomeric (i.e., stretchy, elastic-like) membranes within a hard or soft shell. When the device is filled with diluent and drug, the elastomeric material expands like a balloon. When tubing is attached to the device and the patient's catheter, the elastic balloon forces the solution through the tubing and into the patient. The tubing controls the rate of the infusion, which can range from 0.5 to 200 mL/hour.[15] These devices do not have alarms or safety features, so they may not be suitable for medications that require a critical infusion rate (e.g., dobutamine) or that cause tissue damage if extravasation occurs.[16] The advantages of elastomeric balloons are that they are small and lightweight, thus convenient for use in ambulatory or working patients, and they are easy to use, which makes patient training simple.

Examples of elastomeric balloon systems include Baxter's Intermate® Elastomeric Infusion System, Cardinal Health, Inc. ReadyMed®, and I-Flow Homepump Eclipse®.[17,21] Baxter Healthcare's Infusor™ System and I-Flow's Homepump® C-Series Continuous Infusion System are designed specifically for administering chemotherapy and other long-term continuous infusions.[17] Acacia Medflo®MultiRate is used for continuous infusion of non-narcotic pain medications at home during the post-operative period, directly to the operative site,[22] as is the Curlin Medical, Inc. Accufuser® device. This device is also equipped with a bolus button, for patients to give themselves additional doses of pain medication as needed.[23] Elastomeric balloon reservoirs can be filled by syringes manually, via an automated filling pump, or by using a pump designed specifically for filling the elastomeric system.

Safety First It is extremely important to prime the tubing to remove any air before providing an elastomeric balloon device for a patient. If air gets into the patients' bloodstream, it could cause an air embolus, which could be fatal.

Manipulation of these devices may take the pharmacy technician more time than other systems because of the need to add diluent and drug. Automated filling pumps can reduce the preparation time.

Mechanical Systems. Several mechanical systems that rely on positive pressure similar to elastomeric balloons have been developed. The Paragon® Ambulatory Infusion System holds 100 mL of fluid and its spring mechanism is designed for more accurate delivery and slower infusion rates. It was designed to give longer-term continuous infusions, such as chemotherapy. It can also be used for pain management and includes the ability for a patient to receive a basal or continuous infusion along with patient-controlled bolus capability. The Paragon® device can also be used with a Select-a-Flow variable rate controller. This controller offers the ability to titrate medications. Models are available with multiple rate ranges.[24] These devices are manually filled by a syringe or a pharmacy-automated filling pump.

Other mechanical systems include I-Flow's ON-Q® PainBuster® post-op pain relief system. This system automatically and continuously delivers a local anesthetic, to relieve post-operative pain, through an antimicrobial (SilvaGard®) catheter, which may destroy or inhibit the growth of microorganisms on the catheter. It comes with a Fixed Flow Rate that delivers medication at a continuous infusion rate. A Select-a-Flow™ variable rate controller or ONDEMAND™ device can be used with this system also, whereby the patient can activate a bolus dose of anesthetic when needed. The ON-Q C-bloc continuous nerve block system is a continuous peripheral nerve block system that slowly infuses a local anesthetic for effective pain relief.[25] These systems would most likely be filled with medication in a hospital pharmacy or outpatient pharmacy, but once the patient is sent home, the home infusion pharmacy may need to provide supplies related to the patient's care and monitor the patient's pain status. If a patient happens to stay on these systems for longer than 5 days, the home infusion pharmacy may then fill one of the devices with medication and send it to the patient.

Controlled Pressure Systems. A unique rate-restricted IV administration system is the Eureka infusion pump by Universal Medical Technologies, Inc. The delivery rate of the IV solution is determined by the selection of the IV administration set, which is designed to deliver solution at a controlled flow rate. The pumping mechanism on this device is a controlled positive pressure displacement. It maintains a constant pressure on an IV solution container to evacuate all of its solution. It is an electronic plus elastomeric hybrid. The Eureka infusion pump will accommodate standard solution containers plus the reconstituted drug solution.[17] The Eureka-IP (intermittent) infusion pump model can be utilized to deliver antibiotics and chemotherapy intravenously, while the Eureka-LF (low flow) infusion pump model delivers medication solutions intravenously or subcutaneously. It is intended for 24- or 48-hour medication administration.[26,27]

Curlin Medical manufactures a disposable non-electronic device using springs that create a positive pressure to deliver medication at a low or high flow based on the integrated tubing set. The beeLINE® features a large-volume polypropylene syringe reservoir and patented drive mechanism. This system is ideal for administration of chemotherapy, antibiotics, and pain medications.

Rate-restricted IV administration systems offer significant advantages in the delivery of antibiotics and other medications to home care patients. Unfortunately, many of them still require the addition of diluent to the reservoirs. When more are available with prefilled diluents, these systems will be more convenient, reduce pharmacy admixture time, increase flexibility of use, and be more cost-effective.

Ambulatory Electronic Infusion Pumps. Ambulatory electronic infusion pumps integrate infusion and computer technologies. Some are designed to administer a single therapy, such as parenteral nutrition, while others can accommodate multiple types of therapies used in the home.[15,16] Today, more than 30 ambulatory electronic infusion devices are available.

Ambulatory electronic infusion pumps are small and lightweight, and they can be worn by the patient during infusions. They offer a wide range of infusion rate settings and volumes that are controlled by the electronic components of the individual device. Moreover, these pumps can infuse out of standard IV containers or proprietary reservoirs. Selection of an ambulatory device depends on patient-, therapy-, and infusion service-related factors. Table 5–6 reviews these factors. The device selected for a patient receiving home infusion therapy may ultimately determine how the patient views his or her home care experience.[28,29]

Ambulatory infusion devices are typically divided into two broad categories: therapy-specific and multiple-therapy devices.[30] Therapy-specific devices are designed to provide single therapies, such as pain management or total parenteral nutrition (TPN). Operation of these devices is fairly straightforward and can be done by clinicians or patients. Common therapy-specific devices include the Automed® 3400-C and Automed® 3400 PCA by Curlin Medical, some of the Smiths Medical CADD® infusion pumps, and WalkMed Infusion WalkMed® pumps. The CADD® pumps are some of the most widely used ambulatory infusion devices in the United States. Most of these devices are therapy-specific and relatively simple to program.[17,29] The CADD-Legacy® PCA and CADD-Legacy® Plus are designed specifically for pain medications and for continuous and intermittent infusions, respectively. These devices use proprietary 50-mL or 100-mL cassettes with attached tubing that contain the diluent or drug. These devices are manually filled using a luer-lock syringe. Other IV containers can be used with these two devices by attaching a bypass spike adaptor with tubing. Filling the cassettes or containers requires the technician to remove air from them because the pumps do not contain air-eliminating filters.

The growth of the product offerings in ambulatory electronic infusion devices took hold in the mid-1990s with the introduction and acceptance of multiple-therapy devices. Multiple-therapy devices allow providers to carry a single device that may be used for patients with different therapies. Inventory can be consolidated, capital equipment costs can be overcome more quickly, and clinical staff training is simplified. These devices can infuse continuously or intermittently and may be

Table 5–6. Factors Influencing Selection of Ambulatory Infusion Device[28,29]

Patient-Related	Therapy-Related	Infusion Service-Related
■ Age	■ Number of drugs	■ Distance from home care office
■ IV access	■ Drug stability and compatibility	■ Reimbursement issues
■ Ambulatory status	■ Duration of infusion	■ Nursing support requirements
■ Level or presence of caregiver assistance	■ Dosing schedule or pattern	
■ Environment	■ Volume of infusate	
■ Language interpreters	■ Patient-controlled dose needs	
	■ Accuracy of small volume delivery	
	■ Life of battery	

used to infuse TPN solutions, antibiotics, antineoplastic agents, and pain medications. Most are single-channel, allowing infusion of only one medication at a time. Others are multiple-channel, capable of infusing up to several different drugs at different rates.[28,30,31] In addition, newer devices offer telemedicine capabilities whereby information can be transmitted over standard telephone lines via the use of modems from the patient's home to the health care provider's office. Providers can change infusion rates, correct alarm conditions, track patient compliance, and view or print infusion status reports without making a home visit.

New ambulatory infusion devices continue to be developed. Disposable devices that infuse large volumes of fluid using disposable batteries are on the horizon. In addition, infusion pump safety, including reduction in medication errors, has been put in the spotlight by consumer groups and federal agencies as device use has become more widespread. **Smart pumps** started to be used in the home care setting in the 2000s.[31] Home infusion providers must keep up with the latest infusion device technology so they can provide the high quality of care that patients and third-party payers expect. Pharmacy technicians must become familiar with the different ambulatory infusion devices available. This knowledge will help technicians choose the appropriate supplies (e.g., container to prepare medication in, tubing if attachment of it is required, filters, etc.) when preparing products and sending the supplies to patients who need to use the devices.

TECHNOLOGY TOPICS

"Smart pumps" are equipped with IV medication error prevention software. These devices have specific drug libraries, dose calculators, programming limits, and remote communication capabilities.

Compounding in the Home Care Setting

Pharmacy technicians, under the supervision of pharmacists, are responsible for the correct preparation of sterile products. Chapter 16 on Aseptic Technique will cover the process of sterile compounding and specific equipment needed. In this chapter, the general guidelines and principles will be introduced relative to the home care environment.

Guidelines for Sterile Compounding

Most infusion providers look to voluntary practice standards for guidance on quality assurance. Two professional organizations have provided guidance to help pharmacy personnel ensure that pharmacy-prepared IV admixtures are of high quality: the American Society of Health-System Pharmacists (ASHP) and the United States Pharmacopeial Convention (USP). ASHP publishes guidelines on quality assurance for pharmacy-prepared sterile products.[32] The United States Pharmacopeial (USP) Convention issued an informational chapter (Chapter 797) on "Sterile drug products for home use."[33,34] This chapter was recently revised and renamed "Pharmaceutical compounding—sterile preparations." The revised USP chapter focuses on the practices of personnel who compound sterile formulations for patients' use rather than the site in which sterile formulations are used.[35] USP Chapter <797> is part of an educational/advisory section of the USP standards, which are required and enforceable. USP itself does not have the authority to enforce these standards, but they are potentially enforceable by the Food and Drug Administration (FDA) as well as by state boards of pharmacy. In the ASHP guidelines, sterile products are grouped into three levels of risk to the patient. The risk categories depend on how much time elapses between when the drug is compounded and when it is administered—in other words, the expiration dating—as well as the use of non-sterile ingredients. These levels increase from least (level 1) to greatest (level 3) potential risk, and they have different quality assurance recommendations for product integrity and patient safety.[8,33,36]

The rationale behind the risk-level approach in the ASHP guidelines is that the greater the chance of contamination or the greater the risk of microbial growth in the product, the more careful providers should be to safeguard the sterility of the IV admixture. For example, a parenteral nutrition solution prepared by gravity transfer from manufacturers' bottles or bags, refrigerated for 7 days or fewer before administration, and given to a patient over a period not exceeding 24 hours is a relatively low-risk product. The highest risk of contamination would entail batch preparation of parenteral nutrition solutions with investigational L-glutamine prepared from non-sterile powdered glutamine in an open reservoir.

✔Most products prepared for use by home care patients fall into risk level 2 (medium risk) because they are stored for more than 7 days.

In USP Chapter <797>, maintenance of sterility is required when compounding with sterile ingredients (low- and medium-risk levels), and achievement of sterility when compounding with non-sterile ingredients (high-risk levels)[33,35]

Methods to assess aseptic technique and environmental monitoring programs are two ways of identifying potential sources of contamination. Once a source is identified, steps can be taken to improve the environment. Pharmacy technicians can play a major role in preserving clean environments by maintaining them properly. Pharmacy technicians should become familiar with USP Chapter <797> and the ASHP Guidelines as well as review sections pertinent to the home care setting. Chapter 16 reviews the principles relating to sterile compounding and maintaining clean environments.

Devices Used for Sterile Compounding

Laminar Airflow Workbench. A laminar airflow workbench (LAFW) is considered the working area where compounded sterile products are prepared while subjected to laminar airflow. The area can include a workbench, workstation, or hood. There are two types of LAFW, horizontal airflow benches and vertical airflow benches. These devices differ based on how air is blown across the workspace toward the operator. It is recommended that these devices be recertified at least every six months or when moved or renovated.[33,35]

Biological Safety Cabinets. A biological safety cabinet (BSC) is a vertical flow hood specially designed for the safe preparation of cytotoxic and other hazardous drugs. There are five different types of BSCs, differing based on the amount of air re-circulated and exhausted through a high-efficiency particulate air (HEPA) filter, and whether the exhaust air is blown into the workspace room or to the outside of the building.[33]

Barrier Isolators. Barrier isolators, also known as glove boxes or compounding aseptic isolators (CAI) are being used more and more to prepare compounded sterile preparations. They are a cost-effective alternative to LAFWs. The operator uses a pair of gloves that are integrated into a clear view screen within the device. They are designed to maintain an aseptic compounding environment throughout the compounding and material transfer processes.[35] The major difference with these devices over LAFWs is that the work area in a barrier isolator is physically separated from the surrounding environment.

Automated Compounding Devices. Automated compounding devices are based on peristaltic pump principles similar to those of infusion pumps. Peristaltic pumps control rate by squeezing tubing. Newer devices integrate gravimetric pumping principles, using the specific gravity of the solution component to determine the flow rate. Patient-specific parenteral nutrition formulations and the benefits of providing 24-hour, single-container TPN and hydration bags have driven the need for automated compounding devices. The need is especially prevalent in home care practice because the patient usually gets a 1- to 2-week supply of TPN or fluids. Automated compounding devices are also used to prepare complex multicomponent sterile products, such as nutrition formulations and multiliter hydration solutions with electrolytes, as well as batch preparations of other solutions.

The advantages of the automated compounding devices are increased efficiency and accuracy, automatic calculations (software-driven systems), potential reduction in labor, reduction in materials, and demonstrated cost-effectiveness.[37,38] The disadvantages of a completely automated system are the potential for equipment malfunction and power outages. Automated compounding devices are available with proprietary tubing that attaches to the device. Proprietary or other manufacturers' containers are then connected to the tubing. The device operator must remove air from the filled container before sending it to the patient. Removing air avoids setting off device alarms and eliminates other problems.

Special considerations are needed when using automated compounding devices. Home infusion pharmacies use a compounding sequence or manufacturing practice that minimizes the potential for gross (large) or subtle (slight) incompatibilities, especially when mixing total nutrient admixtures (TNAs).

✔It is essential that technicians recognize the importance of these sequences and practices because technicians often play a major role in, or are completely responsible for, following the sequence.

The order of mixing of components as well as their final concentrations is important for TPN solution stability.

Facility/Pharmacy Name, Address, Telephone Number(7)	
Rx: 1234567(1)	Date: 2/11/04(1)
Patient: Jane A. Doe(2) 110 S. Elm St. Anywhere, MD(2)	Physician: J.R. Smith(1) No refills(1) Bag: # 1 of 5(8)
Nafcillin 24 gm/250ml SWFI(4) Cadd Prizm Pump to infuse Nafcillin 2 GM(4) IV every 4 hours via intermittent infusion for 10 days. Change bag every 48 hours. Keep bag refrigerated and warm to room temperature prior to infusion.(3)	
Pump settings(3): Res Vol = 250ml; Dose = 20ml(4); Dose Infusion Tim = 1 hour Cycle = 4 hours; KVO = 0.2ml/hour ***Bag will last 48 hours ****	
Use before 12N 2/24/04(5) Prepared by: AP(6)	Checked by: TK(6)

KEY: Required Labeling

1 - Prescription number, date, and prescribing physician—These are typically required by state boards of pharmacy. Used by dispensing pharmacist to verify original order.

2 - Patient name and address—The patient's name should be printed as part of the label.

3 - Directions to the patient for use of the medication—These should be easy to understand. They should include rate and frequency of administration. Any special handling or storage requirements should be stated.

4 - Name and volume of the admixture solution—The amount of admixture solution per dose should be stated. In the case of a container housing more than one dose, the volume listed should be equivalent to the total volume in the container.

5 - Beyond-use date—The date is usually the actual beyond-use date established for the product.

6 - Initials of persons who prepare and check IV admixture—State boards of pharmacy often require that this information appear on the label. In addition, this information is helpful when questions arise about product preparation.

7 - Name, address, and telephone number of the compounding facility/pharmacy—This information provides an easy mechanism for the patient to contact the dispensing pharmacy when questions arise.

8 - Optional labeling—The bottle or bag sequence number can help to track the doses ordered and/or doses administered.

Adapted from: Kuban PJ. Labeling sterile preparations. In: Compounding sterile preparations, 2nd ed. Bethesda, MD: ASHP; 2005:102.

Figure 5–1. Sample home care label.

Many manufacturers of automated compounding devices have predetermined additive sequences available for use by operators of these devices.[39] Because many pharmacies are using automated compounding devices, ASHP has developed guidelines to outline the key issues that should be considered to incorporate this type of technology into pharmacy operations safely and cost-effectively.[40] The development of dual-chamber bags in which the lipid is in the upper portion of the bag while the other TPN components are in the lower portion also may improve the safety of TNA formulations. These bags extend stability (up to 30 days), which is convenient for the home care patient because deliveries may only be made every 7 to 10 days. The patient or caregiver activates the bag by removing a white strip and gray bar just prior to infusing. These bags can be filled using an automated compounding device. To ensure stability throughout the administration period, the patient adds some medications, such as multivitamins and insulin, just prior to infusion.

Automated Filling Devices. These devices are used to automate routine filling procedures for syringes, minibags, large volume bags, and/or elastomeric devices. They ensure accuracy for IV admixture and batch production, and they reduce touch contamination. Use of these devices may save the technician time.

Labeling and Expiration Dating of Compounded Products

Labeling in home care practice is similar to labeling in institutions. Nevertheless, home care practice has some unique requirements. The product is considered an outpatient prescription, so it must meet state board of pharmacy requirements. The label should be written so that lay people (people who are not medically trained, such as patients and caregivers) can interpret and understand the directions.

The information required by law for a home care product label includes the patient's name, prescription number, prescribing physician, and date (see figure 5–1). The patient's address is optional; however, an address may simplify delivery procedures. Directions for use should state the rate and frequency of administration and any special handling or storage requirements. The name and amount of drug contained in one dose and the appropriate volume for that amount are listed. Then, the name and volume of the admixture solution equivalent to one dose of drug is indicated. The actual expiration date established for the product is noted. The individual(s) who prepared and checked the admixture must initial the label. Finally, auxiliary labeling should include federal transfer labeling, and, as an option, specific precautionary labels or storage instruction labels may be applied to the product. The bottle or bag sequence may be listed as well to help track the number of doses ordered or the total number of doses administered.[34]

Expiration dating has important implications in home care practice because it may dictate whether the pharmacy can prepare batches, reduce waste, and decrease the frequency of deliveries to the patient.

✔Expiration dates for admixtures are based on stability and sterility data.[34,35] Each compounded sterile product must be labeled and must indicate its storage requirements and beyond-use date (BUD).

New guidelines for BUD incorporating the concept of microbiological limits or loads came about with the adoption of USP Chapter <797>.[32] Most home care pharmacists have references that list expiration dates for products or their components. The most common reference is *Trissel's Handbook on Injectable Drugs,* but many pharmacists keep files containing published research articles on stability. *Extended Stability for Parenteral Drugs* is a reference that contains stability information on the most commonly used medications in alternate site infusion practice. Technicians need to be aware of expiration dates on products they use to make sterile admixtures. When a product expiration date is a particular month, it can be used through the last day of that month.

A product can quickly change or deteriorate as a result of changes in pH, temperature, and drug structure that may cause solubility problems; drug adsorption to and absorption within, or volatility leading to leaching out of product containers; and chemical degradation due to hydrolysis, oxidation, reduction, or exposure to light. The method of delivery—either the system or technique—and the environment of drug administration can also affect stability.[34,35] In home care practice, the pharmacist must assign a maximum expiration date that is still within appropriate stability limits. A common problem is the use of drugs with limited stability at room temperature. For drugs to be given via an ambulatory infusion device, at least 24-hour stability at room temperature or warmer is required.[28] For drugs that have limited room temperature stability, the patient or caregiver must be taught how to prepare the drug immediately before administration. Although a product may be stable for an extended period, its sterility and potential for bacterial growth must also be considered in assigning an expiration date. Sterile products not intended for prompt use should be stored at no higher than 4°C (25°F) to inhibit microbial growth, unless room temperature storage is warranted.[35] This temperature is generally provided by refrigerating the products.

Packaging and Transport of Compounded Products

Temperature control during transportation of sterile products to a patient's home is critical. Appropriate packaging must be used to keep the temperature near the midpoint of the product's specified range.[35]

✔Technicians should be familiar with the storage requirements for specific drugs and the pharmacy's procedures for packaging to ensure the integrity of the products.

Most admixtures are placed in a zip-loc bag to prevent a problem if leakage occurs. Hazardous substances should be double bagged to protect the shipper, patient, and caregiver if leakage occurs. These individuals should be trained to deal with a spill in case it occurs. Certain product containers, such as pre-filled syringes, should be packaged in hard plastic or cardboard tubes or within bubble packs to prevent movement during transit. Refrigerated items should be transported in coolers, and post-delivery temperature checks should be made to ensure that an adequate temperature was maintained. Delivery personnel should be familiar with the shipping requirements for each package.

Supplies for the Home Care Patient

Pharmacy technicians should become familiar with the supplies used by home care patients so the technicians can communicate about supply issues with the patient and other health care professionals. Familiarity entails being aware of the various venous access devices (catheters that reside in the patient's vein through which medication or solution flows) as well as specific supplies that the patient or caregiver uses to set up an infusion, such as tubing and needles.

Venous Access Devices

Peripheral access (infusing drugs through a needle placed in an arm vein) is one of the most common ways patients receive infusions in the hospital, but it does not always work well in the home care environment. Peripheral access is better for short courses of therapy than for long courses of therapy. Peripheral veins often collapse or rupture, so a new vein must be used, and, in some cases, no usable peripheral veins are available. To avoid this scenario, other types of venous access devices are used for patients who need long-term access. A number of extended venous access devices that can be used for weeks to months even years have been developed for patients who require repeated venipuncture (blood draws) or who have suboptimal peripheral venous access due to advanced age, obesity, or previous irritating drug therapy. These devices are classified as tunneled central venous catheters, subcutaneous vascular access ports, or **peripherally inserted central venous catheters (PICC).**[28] A general understanding of the venous access devices commonly used is important for technicians. This knowledge helps technicians select patient supplies more accurately and efficiently.

Two commonly used tunneled central venous catheters are Broviac and Hickman catheters. These catheters were introduced in the 1970s and are made of barium-impregnated silicone rubber (Silastic®). They facilitate long-term vascular access with minimal complications. These catheters are surgically inserted into a central venous site, such as the subclavian vein, and passed through the vein until the tip of the catheter stops at the entrance of the heart's right atrium. After insertion, the catheter is tunneled subcutaneously for a short distance to establish a barrier between the skin exit site and vascular entrance site. An external dressing or bandage is applied to the site. Available tunneled models are distinguished by the catheter material (silicone or polyurethane), number of lumens (single, double, or triple), catheter diameter (from French size 3 = pediatric up to 12.5 or 13 = double or triple lumen), lumen diameter (0.2 to 2 mm), and type of catheter tip.[28,41,42] A lumen is a tunnel within the catheter. Some catheters contain two or three separate tunnels running parallel along their entire length, with access ports or openings to specific tunnels so incompatible solutions can be administered at the same time, through different lumens. To prevent the formation of blood clots when the catheter is not in use, a heparin solution of 100 units/mL is "locked" into each lumen at least daily. Another type of tunneled catheter, the Groshong® catheter, is unique in that it has a pressure-sensitive, distal-tip slit valve (a valve at the end of the catheter with a slit in the rubber). Infusing or withdrawing fluid causes pressure that opens the valve. When the valve is closed, blood cannot flow back into the catheter. This eliminates the need for heparin locking and also decreases the risk of air embolism. These catheters are flushed with 5 to 10 mL of saline after each use and weekly when the catheter is not in use. Infections are the most common complications of tunneled venous access devices. Other complications include catheter occlusion (clogging), dislodgement (moving out of the vein), incorrect catheter positioning, and venous thrombosis (blood clots).

Subcutaneous vascular access ports (e.g., Port-a-Cath® and Infusaport®) consist of a small-volume reservoir with a self-sealing septum that is connected to a central venous catheter. This system is placed subcutaneously (under the skin) by a surgeon, usually in the chest wall, and is hardly noticeable. A dressing or bandage is unnecessary. The device is accessed by inserting a specially designed, noncoring needle, called a Huber needle, through the skin and port septum.[28] Single- and double-lumen devices are available. These devices are suitable for intermittent or prolonged continuous infusions. Between infusions, the port is flushed and locked with heparin 100 units/mL, 5 mL at monthly intervals. Complications are similar to those of tunneled catheters and include infections, occlusion, and thromboses. Needle dislodgement from the septum may occur, as may pocket (the opening under the skin where the device resides) infections.

The use of PICCs has continued to increase because of their unique features. PICCs can be inserted at the hospital bedside or at home by specially trained nurses. They are inserted through a vein in the arm, threaded through other veins in the arm, and end up with the tip resting in the superior vena cava.[28,42] PICCs can remain in place for weeks to months. An X-ray is used to confirm placement before infusing solutions that are very hypertonic (solutions that have a greater osmotic pressure than normal body fluid, and that may cause irritation to veins), such as TPN. PICC lines, also known as *long-arm* or *long-line* catheters, are made of silicone or flexible polyurethane and are available in single- and multi-lumen designs. They require daily flushing with heparin and routine dressing changes. Complications include phlebitis at the insertion site or along the vein, infection, cellulitis, occlusion, catheter tip migration, and thrombosis.[28,42,43]

Peripheral catheters are available in a number of gauges and lengths, commonly from 18- to 24-gauge and ¾ to 1 inch in length. These catheters are desirable for short-term therapies. Most home care providers' protocols call for changing peripheral catheters every 72 hours.

Midline catheters (e.g., Landmark®) are peripheral catheters but have the advantage of being 6 inches long and able to remain in place on average 7 to 10 days or even up to months. For this reason, they are appropriate for longer-term therapy, such as the treatment of endocarditis with IV antibiotics. Midline catheters are usually placed in one of the large veins of the upper arm, basilic or cephalic veins. Because they are in a large vein, they are ideal for infusing caustic drugs, which should not be infused in other peripheral catheters.

Other Supplies

Patients receiving home infusion therapy require a number of other supplies. Many home care providers have standard supplies that are sent to most patients, whether they have a peripheral or a central venous catheter. In general, these supplies include alcohol pads, injection caps (caps that go onto the end of the catheters), non-sterile gloves, a sharps container, medical waste bags, and tubing. A sharps container is a hard plastic or thick cardboard container used to dispose of any needles or sharp objects, which is essential to avoid needlestick injuries to patients and health care professionals. Additional supplies depend on the type of venous access and therapy, the physician, or the account specifications. For drugs or fluids requiring filtration, an appropriate filter should be included. If a patient has a peripheral line, an IV start kit will be needed, whereas a central venous catheter (CVC) kit is required for midline or central lines. These kits are self-contained packets of supplies required to insert IV lines or change the dressing at the line insertion site. Several catheters should be available in the home for patients with peripheral lines so that the nurse has one when the catheter is scheduled to be changed. The only centrally placed catheters that are inserted in the home are PICC lines. Other central venous access devices are placed in the hospital, outpatient clinic, or surgical setting.

For patients requiring an ambulatory infusion device, the appropriate tubing should be sent. Thus, keeping a record of which device a patient is using is important. Batteries are required for devices that are battery-operated. Patients receiving their therapy via minibag or using a non-ambulatory infusion device may need an IV pole. IV poles are available in portable, collapsible designs or the standard, rugged type seen in hospitals. Pitch-It, by SCI, a line of disposable IV poles designed specifically for home infusion therapy patients, is also available.

Heparin is supplied in different concentrations depending on the type of venous access device. Generally, heparin 10 units/mL is used for peripheral catheters, while 100 units/mL is used for central venous catheters. The concentration of heparin used may also differ in neonatal, pediatric, and adult patients. Many home infusion companies or institutions have specific protocols that are followed for heparin flushes. Technicians should be familiar with these protocols so the appropriate flushing materials accompany the patient's supply order. If flush materials are sent in vial form, or if drugs will need to be drawn from vials, the appropriate syringe(s) and needles should be included.

Safety First Heparin is available in a number of different concentrations (10 unit/mL, 100 unit/mL, 1000 unit/mL). To prevent errors, read the label carefully and double check that the correct concentration and volume of the drug is selected.

Patients using a needleless system should receive the proper materials, including injection caps, vial adaptors, syringes, and syringe cannulas. Interlink®, CLAVE®, and Smartsite™ are some of the needleless system products currently available.[43] Home care personnel should determine the appropriate amounts of supplies needed based on anticipated delivery frequency and send supplies accordingly. In many cases, patients are taught to take inventory of their supplies and review the inventory with the appropriate personnel—which may be a responsibility of the pharmacy technician—each time a delivery is anticipated. This minimizes oversupply or undersupply and helps to reduce costs.

Rx for Success

Timely delivery of drugs and supplies is important to avoid any interruptions in therapy.

Infection Control and Safe Disposal

All patients in the home care setting should be treated as if they were potentially infectious. Thus, home care personnel must follow **universal precautions**. Nurses should wear sterile gloves when manipulating catheters to maintain their integrity and non-sterile gloves when drawing blood to protect themselves. Delivery personnel should also wear non-sterile gloves or rugged work gloves when picking up medical waste and unused supplies to prevent needlestick injuries or contact with contaminated spills.

Patients or their caregivers are taught to use appropriate sterile techniques when preparing their medications or fluids and when manipulating the catheter. Occasionally, a break in technique may occur that could lead to a catheter infection or sepsis (an infection in the blood stream). In some cases, these infections can be treated with IV antibiotics, but many cases require removal of the catheter.

Collection and Disposal of Medical Waste. Most state boards of pharmacy prohibit reuse of repackaged or compounded items, including sterile products. Thus, products returned from the home environment are not recycled for use by another patient. Supplies returned by patients to the home infusion company should be dealt with according to the company's disposal policies and procedures.

In the 1980s, improper disposal of medical waste was a nationwide issue. Since then, disposal methods and waste recycling have become much more regulated. All home care patients and their caregivers should be taught to dispose of hazardous and nonhazardous waste properly.[35] With the move to the use of more needleless systems, the need for sharps containers has been reduced. Nevertheless, needles and other sharp materials should be placed in a hard plastic or cardboard sharps container to prevent injury. An isolated area in the home should be identified for the storage of medical waste. A schedule for waste removal should be developed and agreed upon by the patient and the home care provider. If patients notice that their sharps container will be full before their next scheduled delivery, they should contact their home care provider as soon as possible. Some home infusion companies offer patients the use of a mail-back medical disposal process whereby medical waste is sent in commercially available containers via the U.S. Postal Service to regulated collectors.

Summary

Home infusion pharmacy offers a unique and challenging opportunity for pharmacy technicians. The role of the home care pharmacy technician involves substantial responsibility, and the technician's role in the maintenance of the mixing room, inventory control, and product preparation continues to expand. Home care technicians have an opportunity to learn skills not found in other types of practice sites, such as dealing with specialized technologies, infusion supplies, and venous access systems. Often, there is an opportunity for patient contact as well. In some home infusion pharmacies, a "clinical" technician, sometimes referred to as a clinical service representative, triages for the pharmacist. This technician asks the patient a scripted set of questions designed to uncover side effects or complications of the patient's medications. If a potential problem is found, the technician then hands the phone call over to the pharmacist to handle. This is an expanding role for pharmacy technicians and provides the technician with the opportunity to have more one-on-one interaction with the patient. Home infusion pharmacy is a growing field that depends on skilled pharmacy technicians to help the team provide pharmaceutical care to its patients.

Self-Assessment Questions

Case 1

Tom is 54 years old with a 10-year history of diabetes. Tom stepped on a tack while working in the garage. He did not notice the tack in his shoe until he took off his shoes and socks that evening. The tack had cut his right foot behind the big toe and caused it to bleed. He cleaned the wound. Three weeks later, Tom began experiencing severe pain and tenderness in his right foot. He went to his doctor, who noted a swollen and red right foot with a 2-cm-wide and 4-cm-deep ulcer behind the big toe. The patient was hospitalized for surgery to drain the wound. Cultures of bone were obtained during surgery. A diagnosis of osteomyelitis of the right foot with *Staphylococcus aureus* was made.

Tom supports a family of six. Three of his children are in college. Because of recent layoffs at his place of employment, he is concerned about his illness causing him to lose time at work. He is also concerned about the financial drain this illness will cause his family because his HMO requires him to pay 20 percent of all health care expenditures.

1. Tom's diagnosis is often treated in the home health care environment.
   a. True
   b. False

2. Which of the following would be home care goals for this patient?
   a. Allow the patient to stay in the hospital longer to make sure he can handle his care at home.
   b. Allow the patient to return to work sooner.
   c. Keep health care costs associated with his therapy the same.
   d. Complete the course of therapy quicker at home than in the hospital.

Tom's physician started nafcillin 2 gms IV every 6 hours to treat his infection and gave orders to arrange home care services for him. Tom is very nervous about going home. He is not sure he will be able to do what the nurses have been doing for him in the hospital. Although he knows going home will be less costly, he is still concerned about how much this is going to cost.

3. Which of the following hospital employees coordinates Tom's transfer into the home care system?
   a. pharmacy technician
   b. reimbursement specialist
   c. discharge planner
   d. intake coordinator

4. The most appropriate team member with whom Tom should discuss the cost of therapy is the
   a. pharmacy technician
   b. reimbursement specialist
   c. home care nurse
   d. home care pharmacist

5. The pharmacist and nurse decide to use an ambulatory pump to administer Tom's nafcillin so he can return to work. The pump is chosen because
   a. the company will make more money.
   b. the ambulatory pump will automatically infuse the drug every 6 hours, allowing the patient more time to work.
   c. nafcillin is more stable in ambulatory pumps.
   d. the patient or his caregiver will need to make multiple manipulations to the pump.

6. Which team member would be the most appropriate to teach Tom how to use the system chosen to administer his medication?
   a. home care nurse
   b. physician
   c. pharmacy technician
   d. delivery personnel

Tom is ready to be discharged to home from the hospital. Besides the prescription, orders are written for a PICC catheter to be inserted at home and for a CBC and erythrocyte sedimentation rate to be done weekly.

7. Which home care team member is ultimately responsible for giving the above orders and for the care of the patient?
   a. home care nurse
   b. home care pharmacist
   c. physician
   d. discharge planner

Self-Assessment Questions

8. Which team member will insert the PICC catheter?
   a. nurse
   b. physician
   c. pharmacist
   d. pharmacy technician

9. The pharmacy technician is assisting the pharmacist in creating a laboratory tracking sheet for Tom while he is on nafcillin. The pharmacist requests that the routine laboratory collection dates be listed on the tracking sheet for the patient's entire length of therapy. The technician notes that Tom's diagnosis is osteomyelitis. Based on this, how long will his therapy last and how far out will the technician list the laboratory values to monitor on the tracking sheet?
   a. five days
   b. four to six weeks
   c. one week
   d. three months

10. The pharmacy technician is entering the orders for Tom into the computer system at the technician's home infusion company. He or she comes to the CBC and erythrocyte sedimentation rate orders and recognizes that
    a. the nurse will need to schedule blood draws.
    b. the pharmacist will not need to set up a monitoring plan because the patient's therapy does not require these labs for monitoring.
    c. the patient will need to obtain blood draw supplies from a retail pharmacy before the nurse comes to draw labs in the home.
    d. blood draws can only be performed in the hospital setting.

Tom has now received 5 weeks of therapy without complications. At the weekly patient rounds, the nurse reports Tom's right foot looks great. There is no more swelling or redness, and the ulcer has completely healed.

11. The patient service representative tells the pharmacy technician that the patient needs seven more cassettes of nafcillin. She is a little concerned because Tom has not been feeling "quite right" the last few days. He thinks he may have prickly heat because he has red bumps all over his chest. What should the technician do?
    a. Tell the pharmacist about the patient service representative's concerns and wait to make the nafcillin until the pharmacist has evaluated the situation.
    b. Mix 7 days' worth of nafcillin, because a rash is a common reaction to nafcillin.
    c. Arrange to return the nafcillin to the drug supplier because it appears to be a faulty product.
    d. Call Tom and tell him to take some oral diphenhydramine (Benadryl) for any itching he may have.

Case 2

Ken is 35 years old and was diagnosed with AIDS two years ago. He was recently started on ganciclovir for CMV retinitis. Over the past six months, Ken has lost 60 pounds, and now he feels very weak. Ken and his physician have decided to treat his malnutrition with parenteral nutrition.

12. Parenteral nutrition is used to treat malnutrition associated with AIDS.
    a. True
    b. False

13. Parenteral nutrition is a very complicated therapy and needs to be administered in an institutional setting. Ken will have to be admitted to a hospital or long-term care facility.
    a. True
    b. False

14. Ken would like to continue his job as an accountant and wishes to start his parenteral nutrition at home. His physician and insurance case manager approve this plan because home care therapy for parenteral nutrition
    a. allows patients to transition from continuous therapy to cyclic therapy much quicker than in the hospital.
    b. allows patients to return to work or normal activities sooner.

Self-Assessment Questions

c. will not change health care costs versus those in the hospital setting.
d. administration will be safer at home than in the hospital.

15. The pharmacist recommends the following formula for Ken:

Dextrose 50%	1,000 mL
Amino acids 10%	1,000 mL
Lipids 20%	500 mL
Multiple electrolyte vial	40 mL
Sodium phosphate	30 mMol
Trace metals	5 mL
Multivitamins	10 mL

The technician is preparing to compound Ken's parenteral nutrition solutions. Which of the following will the technician *not* add to the solution?

a. Lipids 20%	500 mL
b. Trace metals	5 mL
c. Sodium phosphate	30 mMol
d. Multivitamins	10 mL

16. The pharmacist tells you that the electrolytes on Ken's most recent labs are all normal, but his liver enzymes are elevated. The pharmacist reviews potential reasons as to why Ken's liver enzymes are abnormal. The pharmacist tells the technician to
    a. go ahead and mix his TPN because his electrolytes are normal.
    b. hold the mix of TPN because the elevated liver enzymes may be TPN-induced and result in a change in formula.
    c. go ahead and mix his TPN because the elevated liver enzymes are due to the ganciclovir.
    d. go ahead and mix his TPN because the elevated liver enzymes are due to the multivitamins and the pharmacist will get an order to hold them.
17. Which of the following is an advantage of using minibags as a delivery system?
    a. Manually connecting the bag to the infusion system and setting the infusion rate is an easy process for patients to grasp.
    b. There is a decreased risk for touch contamination.
    c. They require less nursing interaction than other delivery systems when teaching patients how to use them.
    d. It is one of the most cost-effective methods to deliver medications.
18. Which of the following is true regarding delivering medications via syringe infusion?
    a. Syringes are difficult to batch fill, thus making it harder for a pharmacy to prepare them in advance.
    b. Syringes take up more storage space than other delivery systems.
    c. Drugs stored in syringes are stable longer than in minibags.
    d. Administration of medications by syringe via IV push offers convenience and ease of administration for patients.
19. Which of the following groups was *initially* responsible for establishing three levels of risk to patients who are receiving a sterile product, labeling them risk level 1, 2, and 3?
    a. American Society of Health-System Pharmacists
    b. Food and Drug Administration
    c. United States Pharmacopeial Convention
    d. National Institutes of Health
20. A pharmacy technician is preparing a 1-week supply of TPN for a patient at home using an automated compounding device. Investigational L-glutamine is being added at the end of the mixing process. Which risk level of compounding describes this situation?
    a. risk level 1
    b. risk level 2
    c. risk level 3
    d. no risk level
21. Required labeling information for a product going to a home care patient includes which of the following?
    a. patient name, address, prescribing physician
    b. prescription number, date, prescribing physician
    c. precautionary labels, patient name, date of dispensing

Self-Assessment Questions

d. bag sequence, patient address, federal transfer label

22. Selecting an appropriate expiration date for sterile products used in home care practice is important because it determines all of the following except
    a. whether the product can be prepared in batches.
    b. how much of the product will be wasted.
    c. the frequency of deliveries to the patient.
    d. whether the product is considered hazardous.
23. Which of the following statements is true regarding expiration dating for sterile products used in the home care setting?
    a. At least 24-hour stability at room temperature is required for drugs to be given via an ambulatory infusion device.
    b. Changes in pH and drug structure do not affect extended stability for sterile products.
    c. Sterile products not intended for prompt use should be stored at no more than 25°C to inhibit microbial growth.
    d. Physical degradation due to hydrolysis, oxidation, and reduction do not need to be considered when determining expiration dating.
24. Tunneled central venous catheter models are distinguished from each other by which of the following features?
    a. surgery versus bedside placement
    b. likelihood that it will become occluded
    c. flushing protocol
    d. number of lumens
25. Which of the following is true about peripherally inserted central venous catheters (PICCs)?
    a. They are also called midlines.
    b. They do not require flushing with heparin.
    c. They may be inserted in the hospital or at home.
    d. Their complication rate is less than any other catheter.

Self-Assessment Answers

1. a. Osteomyelitis is one of the most common diseases seen in the home care environment, primarily because it requires long-term IV antibiotic therapy.
2. b. By allowing the patient to be treated in his home with IV antibiotics, he will be able to return to work sooner than if he continued therapy in the hospital. A goal of home care is to allow the patient to leave the hospital earlier, not stay longer. Health care costs in the home are less than in the hospital. The patient's total course of therapy for the treatment of osteomyelitis is the same whether he is managed at home or in the hospital.
3. c. The discharge planner or a social worker coordinates the discharge of a patient to home care from the hospital.
4. b. The reimbursement specialist is the most knowledgeable about the cost of home care therapy and insurance coverage.
5. b. Ambulatory infusion pumps can be used to automatically infuse doses throughout the day. They are ideal for patients who may have a problem adhering to an infusion schedule that requires frequent dosing. In addition, ambulatory infusion pumps are convenient for patients who may require ambulation during their therapy.
6. a. The nurse is the primary educator of the patient in the home.
7. c. The physician is the leader of the team and is ultimately responsible for the care of the patient. The physician provides the direction of care. The physician is the primary individual who gives orders that alter the therapeutic plan. Nevertheless, in some cases, a home care nurse practitioner or home care pharmacist may write orders based on protocols approved by the physician.
8. a. The home care nurse has primary responsibility for IV catheters. Many home care nurses are trained in the insertion and maintenance of PICC catheters.

9. b. Osteomyelitis is usually treated for four to six weeks.
10. a. The nurse is responsible for scheduling and drawing blood for laboratory tests on the patient. The pharmacist is responsible for evaluating laboratory results as part of the patient assessment and monitoring function. The lab orders the technician comes across are typically drawn in home care patients on IV antibiotics. The home care company is usually the source for all the patient's medical supplies, and many of the supplies for blood draws would not be stocked by a retail pharmacy. The labs can be drawn from the patient either in the home care setting or at the hospital.
11. a. A rash developing well into therapy with nafcillin is a common occurrence in the home care environment. Nevertheless, it is best to find out how the rest of the home care team wants to deal with the rash before mixing or returning the nafcillin. That way the nafcillin will not be wasted. A pharmacy technician should not provide advice to the patient regarding a drug reaction.
12. a. Parenteral nutrition may be used to treat malnutrition associated with AIDS. AIDS patients, because of chronic diarrhea, often cannot absorb enough nutrients from the food they eat to sustain adequate nutrition.
13. b. This may have been the thought 35 years ago; however, long-term infusion therapy such as parenteral nutrition has been shown to be safe, effective, and less costly in the home care environment.
14. b. A major goal of home care therapy is to allow patients to return to work or normal activities sooner. The speed of transition of the patient on parenteral nutrition from continuous to cyclic therapy is not dependent on the setting in which the patient is receiving therapy. A goal of home care therapy is to decrease health care costs compared to the hospital setting. There are no data to indicate that administration of parenteral nutrition is safer in the home care setting.
15. d. Multivitamins are the only component of Ken's formula that have limited stability (24 hours) and must be added by the patient in the home prior to infusion. The remaining ingredients—lipids, electrolytes, sodium phosphate, and trace metals—are stable in solution for nine days.
16. b. Because elevated liver enzymes are a long-term complication of parenteral nutrition, the TPN order may be changed to avoid further complications. It is best to wait until a decision has been made regarding the composition of the TPN, rather than to mix the wrong TPN and waste material, time, and money.
17. d. From an acquisition standpoint, minibags are considered one of the most cost-effective methods to deliver medications. It is the standard IV administration set used for hospitalized patients in the United States. Their limitations in home care practice include the need for an IV pole; patient or caregiver needs to manually set and maintain the infusion rate; patient or caregiver needs to connect the set and the bag in the home, increasing the risk of touch contamination; and the need for more nursing interaction with the patient than other systems. Use of minibags for drugs that are given frequently can pose a problem for patients who are ambulatory or working because of the cumbersome IV pole.
18. d. There is a revived interest in the delivery of medications via syringe infusion because of attempts to reduce cost. Administration of medications via the IV push method using a syringe is becoming more popular in the home care setting because of convenience and ease of administration for the patient. As drug containers, syringes are the least expensive. In addition, syringes are easy to batch fill and require less storage space.
19. a. The American Society of Health-System Pharmacists (ASHP) was the first group to categorize risk levels. These categories depend on how much time elapses between when the drug is compounded and when it is administered (i.e., expiration dating). These levels increase from least (level 1) to greatest (level 3) potential risk and have different quality assurance recommendations for product integrity and patient safety. The USP Chapter <797> also uses three levels of risk; however, the risk levels are labeled low-, medium-, and high-risk.

20. c. The rationale behind the risk-level approach is that the greater the chance of contamination or the greater the risk of microbial growth in the product, the more careful providers should be to safeguard the sterility of the IV admixture. The product being prepared by the pharmacy technician falls into risk level 3 because of the preparation of investigational L-glutamine from a powder (a non-sterile component) in an open reservoir. Indeed, the TPN solutions are being prepared using an automated compounder, which alone renders them risk level 2. Because of the L-glutamine, however, risk level 2 is superseded by risk level 3.

21. b. Required labeling includes prescription number, date, and prescribing physician. This is usually required by state boards of pharmacy and is useful to the dispensing pharmacy to verify an original order. The patient's name is mandatory but the address is optional; however, an address may simplify delivery procedures. Directions for use should be simple and easy to understand. The name and amount of drug contained in one dose and the appropriate volume for that amount is listed. Then, the name and volume of admixture solution equivalent to one dose of the drug is indicated. The actual expiration date established for the product is noted. The individual who prepared and checked the admixture must initial the label. Finally, auxiliary labeling should include federal transfer labeling, and, as an option, specific precautionary labels or storage instruction labels can be applied to the product. The bottle or bag sequence may be listed as well to help track the specific number of doses ordered or the total number of doses administered.

22. d. Expiration dating has important implications in home care practice because it may mean the ability to do batch preparation in the pharmacy, a reduction in waste, and less frequent deliveries to the patient.

23. a. Expiration dates for admixtures must be based on stability and sterility considerations. Physical and chemical breakdowns are possible. Changes in pH, temperature, and drug structure may cause solubility problems. Chemical degradation due to hydrolysis, oxidation, reduction, or photolysis can quickly cause a product to deteriorate. Home care practice demands that the pharmacist assign a maximum expiration date that is still within appropriate stability limits. A common problem is the use of drugs with limited room temperature stability. For drugs to be given via an ambulatory infusion device, at least 24-hour stability at room temperature or warmer is required. For drugs that have limited room temperature stability, the patient or caregiver may be taught how to prepare the drug immediately before administration. Although a product may be stable for an extended period, its sterility must also be a factor in assigning an expiration date. The potential for bacterial growth must be considered. Sterile products not intended for prompt use should be stored at no more than 4°C to inhibit microbial growth, unless room temperature storage is warranted.

24. d. Available tunneled central venous catheter models are distinguished by the catheter material (silicone or polyurethane), number of lumens (single, double, or triple), catheter diameter (from French size 3 = pediatric up to 12.5 or 13.0 = double or triple lumen), lumen diameter (0.2 to 2.0 mm), and type of catheter tip.

25. c. The use of PICCs is continuing to increase because of their unique features. PICCs can be inserted at the bedside or at home by specially trained nurses. These lines may remain in place for weeks or months. PICC lines, also known as long-arm or long-line catheters, are made of silicone (Silastic®) or flexible polyurethane and are available in single- and multi-lumen designs. They require daily flushing with heparin and routine dressing changes. Complications include phlebitis at the insertion site or along the vein, infection, cellulitis, occlusion, catheter tip migration, and thrombosis.

Resources

ASHP Guidelines: Minimum standard for home care pharmacies. Available at: www.ashp.org/DocLibrary/BestPractices/SettingsGdlMinHC.aspx.

ASHP Guidelines on the pharmacist's role in home care. *Am J Health-Syst Pharm.* 2000;57:1252–7.

ASHP Compounding Resources Center. Contains information and resources on compounding standards and practices. Available at www.ashp.org/Import/PRACTICEANDPOLICY/PracticeResourceCenters/CompoundingResourceCenter.aspx.

References

1. Anon. Home health care. *Ann Int Med.* 1986;105:454–460.
2. American Society of Hospital Pharmacists. Increase in market for home infusion products and services predicted. *Am J Hosp Pharm.* 1990;47:958.
3. National Home Infusion Association. Infusion FAQs. What is the size of the U.S. alternate-site infusion therapy market? National Home Infusion Association Web site (copyright 2009). Available at: http://www.nhia.org/faqs.cfm#spltyIVmeds. Accessed March 21, 2010.
4. American Society of Health-System Pharmacists. National specialty pharmacies focus on rare, chronic diseases. *Am J Health-Syst Pharm.* 2004;61:133,138,140.
5. Kliethermes MA. Adverse drug reactions in home care: report of five-year data collection. Paper presented at: HomeCare 95 Meeting of ASHP; August, 1995; Boston, MA.
6. Tice AD, Rehm SJ, Dalovisio JR, et al. Practice guidelines for outpatient parenteral antimicrobial therapy. *Clin Infect Dis.* 2004;38;1651–1672.
7. The University of Wisconsin Board of Regents and CME Enterprise. Home antimicrobial infusion therapy: issues in planning, treatment, and patient care. cmeInsight™ 2008;1–12.
8. Tice AD, Nolet BR. Update on outpatient parenteral antimicrobial therapy. *Home Health Care Consultant.* 2001;8(12):22–29.
9. Yocom SJ. Introduction to home infusion therapies: anti-infectives, chemotherapy, pain management, and miscellaneous therapies. In: Monk-Tutor MR, ed. NHIA Home Infusion Pharmacy Certificate Program. Alexandria, VA: NHIA;2005:9–18.
10. Cancidas (caspofungin acetate) for injection, for intravenous use [package insert]. Whitehouse Station, NJ: Merck & Co, Inc.; July 2009.
11. Yeong KT, Chan M, Chan C. The safety of IV pentamidine administered in an ambulatory setting. *Chest.* 1996;110:136–140.
12. Nowobilski-Vasilios A. New drugs and biologicals. *Infusion.* 2002;July/August:32–42.
13. Counce J. Home infusion & specialty pharmacy: a marriage whose time has come? *Infusion.* 2005;January/February:16–20.
14. Flores K. Ambulatory infusion suites: appropriate therapies. *Infusion.* 2005;March/April;22–23,26–32.
15. Saladow J. Ambulatory systems for i.v. antibiotic therapy: making sense of the options. *Infusion.* 1995;April:17–29.
16. Kwan JW. High-technology i.v. infusion devices. *Am J Hosp Pharm.* 1991;48(suppl. 1):S36–51.
17. Saladow J. Infusion device technologies: consolidation and change. *Infusion.* June 2000;9–42.
18. Smiths Medical Web site. Available at: http://www.smiths-medical.com/catalog/syringe-pump/medfusion-3500-syringe-pump/medfusion-3500.html. Accessed March 21, 2010.
19. Repro-Med Systems, Inc Web site. Available at: http://www.rmsmedicalproducts.com/Freedom60info.htm. Accessed March 21, 2010.
20. Saladow J. Ambulatory infusion pump technologies. New developments and how they might affect alternate site care. *Infusion.* 2007; July/August:17–22.
21. Skryabina EA, Dunn TS. Disposable infusion pumps. *Am J Health-Syst Pharm.* 2006;63:1260–1268.
22. Acacia Web site. Pain management. Available at: http://www.acaciainc.com/pain-management.php?PHPSESSID=8322add86044c4d77aff733e60bd2993. Accessed March 21, 2010.
23. Moog, Inc. Web site. Available at: http://www.moog.com/products/medical-pump-systems/post-operative-pain-management-systems/accufuser/. Accessed March 21, 2010.
24. I-Flow Corporation Web site. Available at: http://www.iflo.com/prod_paragon.php. Accessed March 21, 2010.
25. I-Flow Corporation Web site. Available at: http://www.iflo.com/products.php. Accessed March 21, 2010.
26. Universal Medical Technologies Inc Web site. Available at: http://www.umtinc.com/index.html. Accessed March 21, 2010.
27. Counce J. Infusion pump. Several market factors contribute to increased sales. *Infusion.* 2006;July/August:10–18.
28. Finley RS. Drug-delivery systems: infusion and access devices. *Highlights on Antineoplastic Drugs.* 1995;13:15–20,23–29.
29. Bowles C, McKinnon BT. Selecting infusion devices. *Am J Hosp Pharm.* 1993; 50:228–230.
30. Saladow J. Ambulatory electronic infusion systems. Making sense of the options. *Infusion* 1995;July:9–21.
31. Saladow J, Prosser B. Improving the continuity of care: new infusion pump technologies. *Home Infusion Continuum.* 2007:1(1):1, 8–11.
32. American Society of Health-System Pharmacists. ASHP guidelines on quality assurance for pharmacy-prepared sterile products. *Am J Health-Syst Pharm.* 2000; 57:1150–1169.
33. Thoma LA. Sterile product design, preparation, and management. In: Monk-Tutor, ed. NHIA Home Infusion Pharmacy Certificate Program. Alexandria, VA: NHIA; 2004;9–16,18–20,33,42–45,48.
34. Sterile drug products for home use. In: United States Pharmacopeia, 24th rev./national formulary. 19th ed. Rockville, MD: United States Pharmacopeial Convention; 1999:2130–2143.
35. The United States Pharmacopeial Convention. <797> Pharmaceutical compounding—sterile preparations. Revision bulletin. 2007:1–61.

36. Kaplan LK. How clean is clean enough? *Infusion.* 1995;August:11–18.
37. Dickson LB, Somani SM, Herrmann G, Abramowitz PW. Automated compounder for adding ingredients to parenteral nutrient base solutions. *Am J Hosp Pharm.* 1993; 50:678–682.
38. Seidel AM, Woller TW, Somani S, Abramowitz PW. Effect of computer software on time required to prepare parenteral nutrient solutions. *Am J Hosp Pharm.* 1991;48:270–275.
39. Driscoll DF. Total nutrient admixtures: theory and practice. *Nutr Clin Pract.* 1995; 10:114–119.
40. American Society of Health-System Pharmacists. ASHP guidelines on the safe use of automated compounding devices for the preparation of parenteral nutrition admixtures. *Am J Health-Syst Pharm.* 2000;57:1342–1348.
41. Viall CD. Your complete guide to central venous catheters. *Nursing 90.* 1990;20:34–41.
42. Masoorii S, Angeles T. PICC lines: the latest home care challenge. *RN.* 1990;44–51.
43. Moureau N. Vascular access with a focus on safety. *Infusion.* 1991;October:16–35.

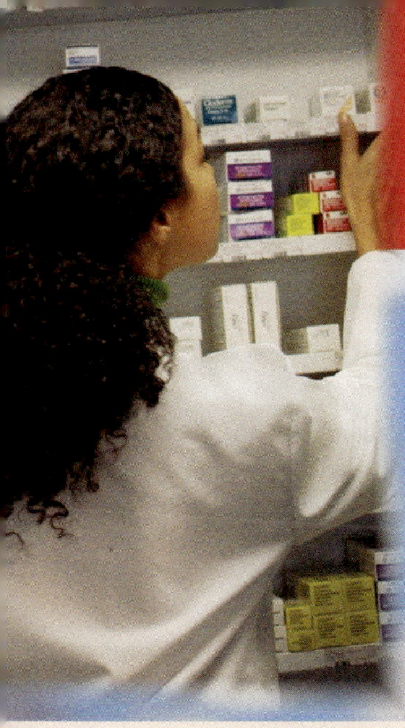

Chapter 6

Specialty Pharmacy Practice

Kara D. Weatherman

Learning Outcomes

After completing this chapter, you will be able to

- Describe the historic development of nuclear pharmacy practice.
- Explain the basic concepts of radioactivity and nuclear medicine as they relate to nuclear pharmacy practice.
- Explain the role of nuclear medicine and nuclear pharmacy in patient diagnosis and treatment.
- Describe the various aspects of nuclear pharmacy practice.
- Identify the common areas for technician involvement in the practice of nuclear pharmacy.
- Explain the role of pharmacy technicians in compounding specialties such as veterinary pharmacy practice.

Key Terms

activity units (mCi) Radiopharmaceuticals are described by activity units, which relate to the number of atoms that give off a radioactive emission per unit of time. The most common activity unit used in the United States is the Curie (Ci). In a nuclear pharmacy, the amount of radioactivity is small, so the millicurie (mCi) unit is mainly used.

assay Describes the activity per unit of volume, measured as mCi/mL.

gamma photon Type of radioactive emission. Gamma photons are electromagnetic waves (like x-rays) that have the ability to travel far enough to leave the patient's body and be detected by nuclear medicine imaging equipment.

half-life The amount of time required for one-half of the amount of radioactivity to decay.

hazardous material Any material that poses a risk to people, animals, property, or the environment.

ligand Chemical substance that will behave in a certain way when injected into the body. For nuclear medicine imaging, a small amount of radioactivity is attached to the ligand, and the ligand "carries" the radioactivity with it as it moves around the body.

naturally occurring radioactive material (NORM) Radioactivity that is present naturally in the environment.

nonrestricted areas Areas of a nuclear pharmacy where radioactive materials are prohibited.

nuclear pharmacy A specialty area of pharmacy practice involving the compounding and dispensing of radiopharmaceuticals for diagnostic imaging and therapy.

positron emission tomography (PET) An advanced nuclear imaging technique that involves the use of short-lived radioactive materials to produce three-dimensional, colored images of those materials functioning in the body.

radioactive decay The process of providing stability to an unstable nucleus by removing excess energy. Radiopharmaceutical products essentially become inactive when they have undergone decay.

radioactivity The emission of radiation that is released from an unstable nucleus.

radiopharmaceuticals Prescription drugs that contain a radioactive component that are used for diagnostic imaging and therapy.

restricted areas Areas of a nuclear pharmacy where radioactive materials are used and stored.

The pharmacy profession has always provided multiple practice opportunities for practitioners, both pharmacists and technicians alike. The profession has evolved, as practitioners of the past recognized that the multifaceted training and skill set that form the backbone of the pharmacy profession could be applied to a variety of unique practice settings. With the formation of the Board of Pharmaceutical Specialties (BPS) in 1976, a mechanism was put into place that allowed these practitioners to unify and establish standards that recognize the significance of these nontraditional practice settings.

The role of the pharmacy technician has expanded into these new areas, providing a broader number of choices for professional development and advancement. This chapter focuses on two specialties: nuclear pharmacy (the first specialty area recognized by the BPS) and veterinary pharmacy (a unique compounding practice site). The intent of this chapter is to give a pharmacy technician a brief overview of these two areas of practice and increase awareness of these (and other) specialty areas of practice. It does not attempt to provide every detail that would be needed to work in these settings. Although specialty areas of practice are not as common as traditional pharmacy employment opportunities (and may be more challenging to identify and pursue), they provide yet another choice for technicians who are interested in broadening their experience and expertise as pharmacy practitioners.

Nuclear Pharmacy

Nuclear pharmacy is an area of pharmacy practice that involves the preparation and dispensing of radioactive pharmaceutical products, or **radiopharmaceuticals**, for use in the diagnosis and treatment of disease. Nuclear pharmacy works closely with nuclear medicine departments in hospitals and clinic settings to provide these agents in a safe, effective, and timely manner for use in their patient population. The use of radioactivity in the products that are compounded and dispensed from nuclear pharmacies adds a significant layer of complexity to the process; as a result,

✔ The practice of nuclear pharmacy involves considerable regulatory oversight to ensure the safety of both patients and practitioners who are involved in the preparation and dispensing process.

Basic Concepts

Radioactivity involves the transfer of excess energy into a radioactive emission. Within an atom, the nucleus contains protons (positive [+] charge) and neutrons (neutral charge). Surrounding the nucleus are electrons (negative [-] charge). Some atoms contain an imbalance in the ratios between the protons and neutrons within the nucleus, which makes them unstable. In order to return to a more stable state, the atom must release some of the excess energy. In some atoms, this excess energy is given off as a radioactive emission.

Radioactive material has a distinct characteristic called a half-life. The **half-life** of a radioactive material is the amount of time that it takes for one-half of the material to give up its excess energy in the form of a radioactive emission.

Radioactive materials can occur naturally or be created using various techniques. **Naturally occurring radioactive material (NORM)** is the radioactive form of a naturally occurring element. Radon gas, which is a concern to many homeowners, is a radioactive emission that occurs due to the elemental composition of the earth. The sun- and energy-creating events that occur throughout the universe create cosmic radiation, a naturally occurring radiation source that is enhanced when traveling by air or residing at high altitudes. Even the human body contains small amounts of radioactive carbon and potassium. Naturally occurring radiation is always present in small amounts, and it is impossible to completely remove radioactivity from daily life. Naturally occurring radioactive material is not particularly useful for medical imaging because most such elements have a very long half-life.

Most medical applications use radioactive materials that are created in a nuclear reactor or an accelerator. People are generally familiar with the concept of a nuclear reactor, which can be used to generate power. Medical isotopes are produced using the same technology, but on a significantly smaller scale. In a reactor, a large atom (usually uranium) is split in a process called fission. Some of the byproducts generated are radioactive and can be collected and purified to be used in medical applications. In an accelerator, a stable atom is bombarded with a positively or negatively charged particle which creates an imbalance in the atom. These agents have shorter half-lives and are more useful for performing nuclear medicine imaging.

Nuclear medicine plays an important role in the diagnosis and treatment of disease. Although detailed information about this radiologic practice specialty is beyond the scope of this book, in broad terms, diagnostic nuclear medicine studies involve attaching a small amount of radioactive material to a compound (called a **ligand**) that is known to behave a certain way when it is introduced into the body. Once administered, the ligand moves through the patient's body, following a physiologic process that occurs within that patient (e.g., elimination of waste through the kidney, remodeling of bone structure, and blood flow to the heart muscle). As the ligand moves through the body, the radioactive material gives off a radioactive emission called a **gamma photon,** which passes out of the patient's body and into a detector located near the patient. The radioactive emissions are detected and mapped to identify how the tracer moves through the patient's body. From these data, physicians can gain information about how the particular organ is working, as well as the physiologic process that should be occurring. As an example, in renal imaging, the organ of interest would be the kidney, while the physiologic process of concern would be excretion of waste products. The agents used for renal imaging are taken up by the kidney just like typical waste products in the blood would be. The agent is removed from the kidney in the urine and moves to the bladder. By watching the movement of the radioactive emissions as the agent moves through the kidney, it is possible to determine if there is adequate blood flow to the kidneys, if the kidneys are functioning properly, and if urine is able to pass out of the kidney and into the bladder. Examples of common renal images are found in figure 6-1.

The functional information provided by nuclear medicine studies is used to augment the anatomic information that is obtained by traditional imaging modalities such as x-ray, computed tomography (CT), or magnetic resonance imaging (MRI). Although these modalities provide excellent information about what the organ in question looks like, they can provide only limited information about how well the organ is working.

Nuclear medicine is also used as a form of treatment for certain diseases by taking advantage of the destructive effects of certain types of radioactive emissions to provide localized treatment of disease. The most common example of this is the use of a radioactive form of iodide for the treatment of thyroid diseases such as overactive thyroid or thyroid cancer. The thyroid gland typically takes iodide from the bloodstream to make thyroid hormones that play an important role in maintaining basic functions of the body. When a radioactive form

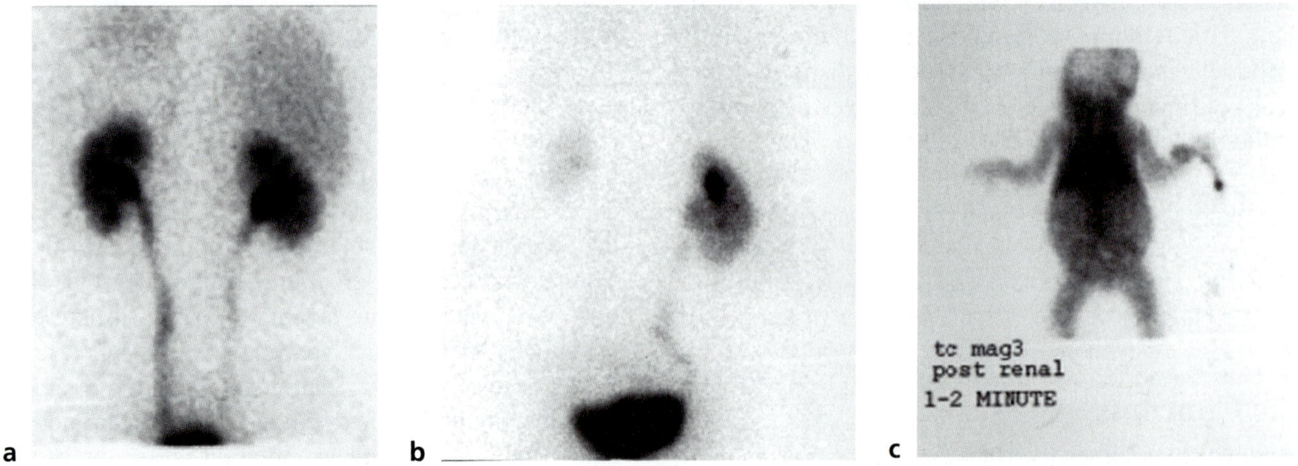

Figure 6–1. Nuclear Imaging of the kidney (a) An example of normal renal function—good uptake in kidney with radioactivity moving to bladder. (b) Renal scan showing good function of left kidney, with extremely poor function of right kidney due to blockage of blood flow. (c) Complete absence of renal function (no kidneys seen) in 3-day-old child with polycystic kidney disease.

Table 6–1. Common Nuclear Medicine Procedures

Procedure	Purpose
Bone imaging	Evaluation of metastatic cancer that has spread to bone Evaluation of small fractures Evaluation of trauma
Cardiac imaging	Evaluation of myocardial perfusion (blood flow to cardiac muscle) Evaluation of cardiac ejection fraction (amount of blood pumped per heartbeat)
GI imaging	Evaluation of rate of gastric emptying Evaluation of presence and extent of gastric reflux
Liver/spleen/biliary imaging	Evaluation of liver function Evaluation of bile formation and excretion
Renal imaging	Evaluation of renal (kidney) function (GFR, ERPF) Evaluation of post-renal transplant function Evaluation of vesicourethral reflux (reflux of urine from bladder to kidney)
Thyroid imaging/therapy	Evaluation of hyperthyroidism (type and severity) Evaluation of thyroid nodules Effectiveness of treatment of hyperthyroidism and thyroid carcinoma

of the iodide molecule is administered, the thyroid gland takes up the radioactive iodide molecule just like it takes up the normal iodine molecule. Once in the gland, the radioactive emissions from the molecule cause damage to the thyroid tissue. In patients with an overactive thyroid, this is enough to return function back to normal levels. In thyroid cancer, the dose is substantially higher. The goal is to completely damage all thyroid tissue, which treats the cancer and prevents disease recurrence. There are more than 100 different nuclear medicine imaging procedures available today (table 6-1), with approximately 16 million imaging and therapy procedures performed annually in the United States alone, the majority being related to cardiac and oncology applications. These procedures can be performed on any patient population, including pediatric patients.[1]

Historical Perspective

The development of the specialty of nuclear pharmacy is primarily credited to Dr. John Christian, a professor at the Purdue University School of Pharmacy, and Captain William H. Briner of the National Institutes of Health (NIH). As early as 1948, Christian recognized the potential relationship between pharmacy and the use of radioactivity.[2] Throughout his career in academia, Christian continued to focus on the role that pharmacy could play in the medical use of radioactivity by establishing a series of training courses at Purdue University that are still in existence today. Captain Briner established the first radiopharmacy at the NIH in 1958, and he is widely recognized in the nuclear pharmacy community as the "Father of Radiopharmacy."[2]

In the 1970s, several leaders in the yet unrecognized field of nuclear pharmacy began to focus on creating formalized educational programs within several schools of pharmacy, recognizing that pharmacists with specialty training would be best prepared to provide the services needed to support the nuclear medicine community. In 1978, thanks to the work of several pioneers in the field, nuclear pharmacy was recognized by the American Pharmaceutical Association (APhA) as the first specialty area of pharmacy practice.[2] Development of a board certification specialty examination (BCNP) followed, with the first exam administered in 1982.[3] Currently, there are more than 500 nuclear pharmacists who have earned board certification.[4]

Nuclear pharmacy practice today takes many different forms. Early practitioners of nuclear pharmacy were hospital pharmacists who took an interest in the agents used in the nuclear medicine department of their institution. Hospitals that used radiopharmaceuticals were primarily academic medical centers that used their own "in-house" radiopharmacies to dispense radiopharmaceuticals to patients treated in their particular institutions.[5]

In the late 1970s and early 1980s, several centralized nuclear pharmacy companies were established that placed nuclear pharmacy "labs" at various locations throughout the United States. This type of nuclear pharmacy provided unit dose service to hospitals, clinics, and physicians' offices within a localized geographic area. Unit doses are individual doses, generally dispensed in a syringe, that contain the correct amount of radioactivity for the actual time of administration to the patient.

Currently, there are three major chain nuclear pharmacies with more than 200 locations, and more than 100 independently owned nuclear pharmacies throughout the United States.[6] The majority of pharmacist and technician employment opportunities are found in the centralized nuclear pharmacy practice setting.[7] There are still several hospital-based pharmacies that employ nuclear pharmacists and nuclear pharmacy technicians; however, these are mostly limited to very large hospital systems or academic medical centers.

Rx for Success

While PTCB training does not cover the scope of nuclear pharmacy practice at this time, many states and some nuclear pharmacy providers require PTCB certification in order for nuclear pharmacists and technicians to work in the pharmacy.

Some nuclear pharmacists choose to practice in specialized facilities that focus on the production and dispensing of a slightly different type of radiopharmaceutical agent for performing **positron emission tomography (PET)** imaging. PET is a type of nuclear imaging study that uses very short-lived radioactive materials.[8] PET imaging has become more popular in recent years and, as a result, has led to increased numbers of dedicated facilities that specialize in this area.

Nuclear Pharmacy Operations

Stepping inside a nuclear pharmacy is a distinctly different experience than in most other types of pharmacies. In addition, nuclear pharmacy involves some unique workflow patterns that are followed on a daily basis. The pharmacy technician is an integral part of almost every aspect of nuclear pharmacy practice and an essential member of the nuclear pharmacy team. It is important to realize that the role of the pharmacy technician varies from pharmacy to pharmacy, in part based on the pharmacy regulations set forth by each state's board of pharmacy.

Rx for Success

Nuclear pharmacy technicians generally receive most of their training "on-the-job." Having no experience in nuclear pharmacy is expected when hiring new pharmacy technicians in this area of practice.

Nuclear pharmacy is a 24-hour-a-day operation. Even though not every nuclear pharmacy is physically open all hours of the day, several nuclear medicine studies are considered emergent, and radiopharmaceuticals must be made available at any time of the day. As such, most nuclear pharmacists also have an "on-call" component to their job, during which they must be available at any time of the day or night to provide appropriate services to the end user.

The most critical component of the preparation and dispensing of radiopharmaceuticals is the presence of the radioactive material in the final preparation. The concept of radioactive decay fundamentally drives all of the processes and procedures in nuclear pharmacy operations. When a radioactive material gives off a radioactive emission, it eventually becomes nonradioactive, or stable. Because every isotope has a distinct half-life, we can predict approximately how long a product will give off enough emissions to allow imaging to take place. **Radioactive decay** means that the radiopharmaceutical products essentially become inactive, which creates significant logistical issues when preparing and dispensing products.

Unique aspects of nuclear pharmacy operations include

- Location of nuclear pharmacies
- Workflow and staffing
- Restricted and nonrestricted areas
- Preparation and dispensing

Location of Nuclear Pharmacies

The location of nuclear pharmacies is unique—centralized nuclear pharmacies are not located on every street corner in every city, as you might see with traditional community pharmacies. Nuclear pharmacies are generally found in larger metropolitan areas and other locations where there are several hospitals in a fairly close geographic area. Generally, because of the challenge of working with radioactivity, most pharmacies can only deliver final materials to hospitals within a two- or three-hour travel distance from the pharmacy.

The outward appearance of a nuclear pharmacy also differs from what most people expect in a pharmacy. Nuclear pharmacies are often located in strip malls, medical office complexes, and, occasionally, as freestanding buildings. In fact, there may be few outward signs that a pharmacy is located in the building. Movement into and out of nuclear pharmacies is fairly restricted due to the strict regulations involving control of radioactive materials, so it is unlikely that an individual would be able to just walk into a nuclear pharmacy off the street. Because nuclear pharmacies must deliver their products to the end users, nuclear pharmacies are often located in areas where there is ample room for a fleet of delivery vehicles to be maintained. Due to the emergent need and time sensitivity associated with radiopharmaceuticals, most nuclear pharmacies have quick access to major transportation routes (interstates, highways, etc).

Workflow and Staffing

Because nuclear pharmacies are either open or available 24 hours a day, 7 days a week, 365 days a year, there are generally several dedicated shifts. The most important and productive time in a nuclear pharmacy is the early/opening shift, also known as the "night shift." Because radiopharmaceuticals must be compounded on a daily basis due to the radioactive component of the products, the nuclear pharmacy must prepare, dispense, and deliver agents to their customers *before* the first patient is seen in the nuclear medicine department. Most nuclear medicine departments begin seeing patients as early as 7 A.M., so a majority of the work done in the nuclear pharmacy is performed during the early morning shift. In pharmacies that are not open 24 hours, the early shift consists of at least one pharmacist and one technician who both begin work between midnight and 2 A.M. In larger nuclear pharmacies, there may be more than one technician who works the early shift. A majority of the doses dispensed from the pharmacy will be en route to the hospitals or clinics before 6 A.M. each day.

Customers will have "add-on" doses that will be needed throughout the day, so nuclear pharmacies also have typical day shifts, generally beginning as early as 6 A.M. to meet these needs throughout the day. Again, depending on the size of the pharmacy, there may be one or two pharmacists and pharmacy technicians working at any given time in the pharmacy. The day-time shift consists of filling add-on doses called in by customers, performing daily regulatory tasks, taking prescription orders for materials needed the next day, and setting up the pharmacy to get ready for the preparation of the next day's doses.

Generally, if a pharmacy is not open 24 hours, the end of the workday occurs between 4 and 5 P.M. each day. Once the last pharmacist leaves the pharmacy, the pharmacist who is on-call begins coverage. Some pharmacies implement a rotating shift so that all pharmacists and technicians work every shift, whereas other pharmacies have dedicated staff working the opening shift to maintain continuity. The staffing and scheduling of a nuclear pharmacy is specific to each nuclear pharmacy and is usually established based on customer demand, workload levels, and input from the pharmacy staff.

Restricted and Nonrestricted Areas

Commercial nuclear pharmacies are often referred to as "labs" because of the way they are set up. Every nuclear pharmacy has two distinct areas: the restricted (radioactive) and nonrestricted (nonradioactive) areas. The **nonrestricted areas** are the general areas of the pharmacy where the staff and visitors can be assured of having no contact with radioactive materials. Examples of these areas include the kitchen and eating areas, office areas for the pharmacy manager and other staff members, bathrooms, and the general reception area. These areas are designed so there is no reason for radioactive materials to be brought into them, either intentionally or unintentionally. The nonrestricted areas are monitored on a regular basis to ensure there has been no inadvertent introduction of radioactive materials.

The **restricted area** is the area of the pharmacy where all radioactive materials are stored, handled, and dispensed. Because the radioactive materials are being manipulated, there is a risk that individuals might come into contact with radioactivity. Each radiopharmacy has its own specific layout to meet the daily preparation, dispensing, and storage needs of the facility, but all restricted areas of radiopharmacies contain the following:

- Order entry area—All radiopharmaceutical doses are dispensed pursuant to an order from a nuclear medicine physician. A nuclear medicine technologist working at a hospital usually calls orders into the pharmacy each afternoon and at various times throughout the day. Depending on state regulations, telephone orders can be taken by pharmacists and, in some cases, pharmacy technicians. Telephone orders are entered into the pharmacy computer system, which allows for prescription labels to be generated that will accompany the patient's dose to the hospital.
- Compounding area—Because most radiopharmaceuticals are administered via the intravenous (IV) route, to

ensure compliance with sterile product compounding guidelines, the agents are compounded in a laminar flow hood. These hoods are located in a fairly segregated area in the pharmacy, away from major traffic areas, yet fairly close to the areas where radioactive materials are stored for easy access. Pharmacists are primarily responsible for the compounding of radiopharmaceuticals in most nuclear pharmacies.

- Dispensing area—The dispensing of unit doses is done in a laminar flow hood found in close proximity to the compounding area, within the same segregated area of the pharmacy. Pharmacy technicians are primarily responsible for taking the batch of prepared radiopharmaceutical (prepared in the compounding area) and withdrawing a designated amount of the material from the source vial into one or more patient doses.
- Blood labeling area—One common procedure performed in most nuclear pharmacies is the isolation and radiolabeling of white blood cells that have been withdrawn from a patient in the hospital nuclear medicine department to assist in the detection of the body's infection sites. The blood labeling area is usually segregated from the rest of the radiopharmacy due to the biohazard risk of handling blood products, but it still must be contained in the restricted area due to the use of radioactive materials. It is also located in a segregated area away from traffic to comply with sterile product compounding guidelines. In many pharmacies, both pharmacists and pharmacy technicians are responsible for the isolation and radiolabeling process.
- Packaging and transport area—Because all doses dispensed must be delivered to the end user at a facility outside of the radiopharmacy, a large area of the pharmacy is dedicated to the safe packaging and transport of these doses. Driver/courier staff members in the pharmacy are responsible for ensuring that the dose containers are not contaminated with external radioactive material, placing the correct doses in appropriate shipping containers, completing inventory before shipping, and following the appropriate regulatory requirements for shipping radioactive materials. Technicians are sometimes involved in these activities once they have completed the dose drawing process to expedite the packaging and transport process.
- Radioactive material storage area—In the restricted area, there will always be significant amounts of radioactive materials that are not in use, and these are generally stored in a designated area within the pharmacy. This area is designed to prevent the unintended release of radioactive materials into the work area, as well as to provide increased protection to the pharmacy staff.
- Radioactive waste areas—One of the major benefits of a centralized nuclear pharmacy for the customer is the fact that waste materials (e.g., used syringes) can be returned to the pharmacy. Because these materials will still be radioactive for some period of time, all radioactive waste must be stored until the radioactivity decay is below a certain level. Because most nuclear medicine departments have limited space for holding this waste, the ability to ship it back to the nuclear pharmacy for storage and disposal is a major benefit of using a centralized radiopharmacy service. Once the radioactive waste (which is also biohazardous because it was most likely injected into a patient's blood stream and may have some blood contamination) has reached appropriate levels of radioactivity, it is sent to a medical waste facility for disposal. This is a highly regulated area of the pharmacy; very often, pharmacy technicians are responsible for maintaining appropriate recordkeeping and waste disposal.

There is no mandated size for a commercial radiopharmacy's restricted area; it generally depends on how many doses are dispensed from the facility and how much equipment and staff are needed to perform the daily tasks.

One interesting change that will occur in most commercial nuclear pharmacies relates to the recent release of the United States Pharmacopeia (USP) Chapter "<797> Sterile Product Compounding." The USP is an official public standards-setting authority for medications, food ingredients, and dietary supplements. In response to increasing concern about the quality of sterile products (e.g., IVs and eye drops), this group released updated standards for preparation, dispensing, and release of sterile products, which became official in June of 2008. Because the primary dosage form for radiopharmaceuticals is an IV injection, the preparation and dispensing of radiopharmaceuticals falls under the scope of this document. Radiopharmaceuticals are specifically addressed, along with detailed requirements for equipment, training, appropriate attire when compounding and dispensing, and cleaning of the work and surrounding areas. Many commercial nuclear pharmacies are making significant changes to their compounding facilities to become compliant with these new recommendations.[9] The general scope of USP <797> is described in other chapters of this textbook, but should be reviewed for nuclear pharmacy-specific requirements when employment is begun in a commercial nuclear pharmacy setting.

Preparation

In nuclear pharmacies, a significant amount of preparation must take place before the first product is made each day. The same general procedure for the preparation of radiopharmaceuticals is followed by most nuclear pharmacy operations, with minor deviations depending on pharmacy-specific needs.

Prescription Processing. As stated above, most prescriptions for radiopharmaceutical agents will be called in to the pharmacy the evening before they are needed. A majority of patients who are treated in nuclear medicine departments are seen on an outpatient basis and are scheduled well in advance. Most hospital facilities have add-on doses that are ordered during the nighttime hours or put on the schedule as a "STAT" (at once, immediately) procedure, but these are only a few doses each day, generally.

When a prescription for a radiopharmaceutical is taken, there are some differences when compared to traditional prescription orders. First, radiopharmaceuticals are not dispensed based on the milligram (mg) amount of the product, but instead on the amount of radioactivity that will be administered to the patient. Therefore, assays are used rather than traditional concentration values (e.g., mg/mL). An **assay** in nuclear pharmacy describes the number of **activity units (mCi)** per mL and is expressed as mCi/mL. Just like concentration values for non-radiopharmaceuticals, the assay of radiopharmaceutical products is extremely important when radioactive doses are prepared and dispensed. A challenge in the nuclear pharmacy environment is the fact that the assay of the products is constantly changing due to the continual loss of activity from radioactive decay. This is one of the most difficult concepts for new practitioners (pharmacists and technicians) in a nuclear pharmacy practice.

When a prescription order for a radiopharmaceutical is placed, the following information must be obtained:

1. agent to be administered
2. amount of radioactivity (mCi) to be dispensed to the patient
3. time of administration to the patient
4. patient name

✔ When radiopharmaceuticals are dispensed, the activity for the dose must be accurate *at the time the material is to be injected into the patient.*

For example, a dose to be administered to a patient at 10 A.M. might be prepared and dispensed at 3 A.M., so it is necessary to dispense enough material at 3 A.M. to account for radioactive decay, resulting in the correct dose when it is needed at 10 A.M. This is very different from pharmaceuticals in other pharmacy practice settings, in which the concentration of a compounded product does not change with time, and the amount dispensed is the same regardless of when it will be given to the patient.

When prescription orders are called in to the pharmacy, they are entered into the computer system. A prescription label is generated that contains all pertinent information that will be needed when the dose is dispensed and all board of pharmacy labeling requirements. Prescriptions are reviewed for accuracy by a pharmacist, segregated by product, and placed near the compounding and dispensing area for easy access during the morning dispensing period.

Production and Acquisition of Radioactive Material. Fundamentally, the job of a radiopharmacist when preparing radioactive pharmaceuticals is to attach radioactivity to a ligand. The radioactivity, because of the inherent nature of radioactive materials, must be produced or ordered on a fairly frequent basis. The ligands are supplied in commercially prepared radiopharmaceutical "kit" formulations, and they are supplied by a variety of manufacturers. There are more than 40 different radiopharmaceutical "kits" on the market today. Figure 6-2

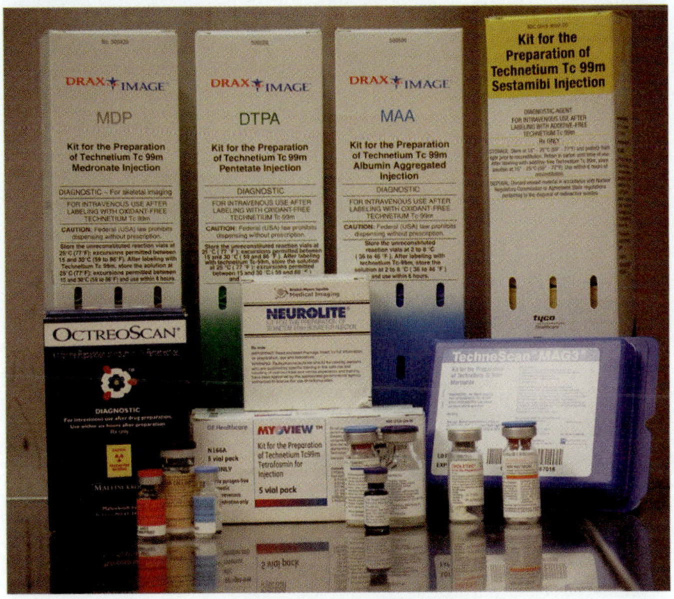

Figure 6–2. Radiopharmaceutical kits

shows several commonly used kits employed in practice today. The radiopharmaceutical kits are not radioactive, so they can be ordered in larger quantities and stored for use when needed. The radiopharmacist acquires radioactivity from the desired source; introduces the radioactivity into the pre-formulated kit product, which contains the ligand; allows the radiolabeling reaction to occur (in which the radioactive atoms bind to the ligand); verifies the quality of the radiolabeling reaction; and supervises the dispensing of doses for each patient.

On-site production and acquisition of radioactive material is done for the majority of the radioactivity used in a nuclear pharmacy on a daily basis. The success of radiopharmacy is due mostly to the advent of the radionuclide generator system in the late 1950s/early 1960s. This compact system is designed to allow continual production of the radioisotope Tc-99m, which is used in most of the radiopharmaceutical products administered today. Examples of the two commercially available generator systems are shown in figure 6-3. Most commercial nuclear pharmacies have several radionuclide generators available at any given time to assure that a sufficient amount of material is available to meet the daily needs of the pharmacy.

To prepare a radiopharmaceutical, a specified amount of the Tc-99m radioactive material is added to a commercially available radiopharmaceutical kit. In most cases, all of the components needed to attach the radioactive material to the ligand are provided in the kit vial. The radiopharmacist withdraws the desired amount of radioactivity that will be added to the kit from the generator system. For most preparations, the radioactivity is added directly to the kit, and all of the chemical reactions necessary to form the radioactivity-ligand bond occur without further manipulations. Some products may require the addition of other materials, such as acids, bases, or stabilizing agents; others require either a boiling step to drive the reaction to completion or an extended labeling time (up to 30 minutes) to ensure that the radioactivity is attached firmly to the ligand.

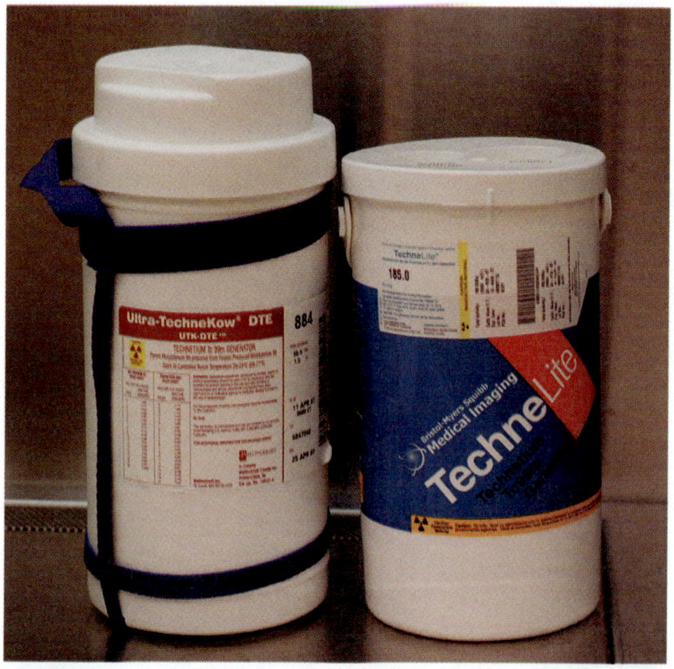

Figure 6-3. Radionuclide generators provide a continuous source of radioactivity, which is used in the compounding of most radiopharmaceuticals.

After every product prepared is compounded, it undergoes quality control testing before any patient dose is released from the pharmacy. Because the chemical reaction involved in the radiolabeling takes place within the container, there is no way to ensure that the reaction went to completion unless the product is tested. Testing ensures that the desired product was formed and there are no impurities that may adversely impact the quality of the imaging study.

Common quality control tests performed in a nuclear pharmacy are quick (generally less than 1 minute to complete) and easy to perform. Generally, quality control testing is performed while the pharmacy technician dispenses the final doses. If the quality control test reveals a problem, all of the doses from that kit are pulled, a new product is compounded, and all of the original doses are re-dispensed using the new product. Fortunately, the incidence of kit failure is extremely rare, so it is acceptable to begin dispensing doses while the quality control testing is being completed. In extremely busy nuclear pharmacies, the pharmacist may compound more than 100 kits each morning, so performing quality control on every kit before starting the dispensing process is not feasible. Nevertheless, no doses should leave the pharmacy before all quality control checks are completed and reviewed by the pharmacist. Generally, quality control testing is a task assigned to a pharmacy technician or a very advanced member of the delivery staff.

Dispensing

Radiopharmaceuticals are most often dispensed as a unit dose, meaning one dose for one patient in one administration vessel. Because most radiopharmaceutical agents are administered by IV injection, radiopharmaceuticals are usually dispensed in a 3- or 5-mL syringe. The preparation of these unit doses is the primary responsibility of the pharmacy technician. For each kit that is prepared, there may be only a single dose removed or several doses, depending on the orders needed for the day. After the kit is prepared by the pharmacist, the product and the dose to be withdrawn from that product are given to the pharmacy technician who will draw up the designated volume listed on the prescription label. This is done using radiation safety tools that are described below. It is important that the pharmacy technician utilizes the same basic sterile techniques that would be used for any IV preparation when dispensing unit dose radiopharmaceuticals. Next, the dose must be verified to ensure that the appropriate amount of material is dispensed. After the desired volume of material is drawn up, the syringe is placed in a dose calibrator, which is a standard piece of equipment in a nuclear pharmacy that determines the amount of radioactivity present in the syringe. Because radioactivity is random, the amount of activity is not constant, but varies slightly from the average activity amount. Because this is a characteristic of radioactivity that can't be controlled, when radioactive materials are dispensed, some small variance (usually 10 or 20%) from the prescribed dose is allowed.

Once the dose is verified to be within the desired range, it is placed in an appropriate container made of lead or another shielding material to prevent loss of material during shipping. The shielding material also minimizes radiation exposure to the delivery staff, who may need to travel long distances with the radioactive material in the delivery vehicle, as well as to members of the public who may come in contact with the shipment during the delivery process. The doses are then given to the delivery staff who place each dose in the appropriate transport container for each hospital, perform mandated shipping tests to ensure that the containers are free from radioactive contamination, and place the containers in delivery vehicles to be taken to the nuclear medicine departments at various hospitals within the pharmacy's delivery area.

The number of doses dispensed from radiopharmacies varies greatly, but, generally, smaller nuclear pharmacies may dispense between 100 and 300 doses per day, and medium-sized pharmacies dispense between 300 and 800 doses per day. Some very large pharmacies that service highly populated areas of the country may dispense as many as 1,500 doses per day.

Unique Aspects of Nuclear Pharmacy

Many aspects of nuclear pharmacy practice are similar to those of traditional pharmacy practice. Nuclear pharmacies are licensed as pharmacies with the state board of pharmacy and follow all of the regulatory requirements set forth in state pharmacy regulations. However, there are several areas that are specific to nuclear pharmacy practice that translate to different job responsibilities and an enhanced level of regulatory compliance that must be examined when considering nuclear pharmacy as a career. These include handling radioactive materials and using specialized instrumentation.

Handling Radioactive Materials

Without question, radioactive material is considered hazardous by international, federal, state, and local regulatory agencies. A **hazardous material** (sometimes called a dangerous good) is any material that poses a risk to people, animals, property, or the environment. The hazardous material classification means that all aspects involving radioactivity are regulated extensively. In the nuclear pharmacy, in addition to state and federal regulations that dictate how the pharmacy is operated, there are countless other regulatory requirements that must be met at every stage in the acquisition, preparation, dispensing, and transport of radioactive materials.

Safety First There are several tools and processes that the staff of a nuclear pharmacy are required to use to make sure that their exposure to radioactivity is as low as possible.

The primary source of regulatory compliance involves the Nuclear Regulatory Commission (NRC), which has oversight for all activities related to radioactive materials. Most of the nuclear pharmacy regulations are listed in Part 10 of the Code of Federal Regulations (10 CFR). An additional source of regulatory oversight for nuclear pharmacy operations is provided by the Department of Transportation (DOT), which covers the shipping and receiving of radioactive materials. This regulatory compliance is essential, because all products must be transported to and from nuclear pharmacies, which increases the chances that members of the public could come in contact with dangerous amounts of radioactivity. Most of the regulatory areas of oversight are in place to ensure the safety of the public, who may be exposed intentionally or unintentionally to sources of radioactive materials.

From the standpoint of the nuclear pharmacy employee, some of the most important regulatory guidance is found in 10 CFR, part 20, entitled Standards for Protection from Radiation.[10] It is critically important that employees who handle radioactive materials as part of their daily duties be allowed to work in an environment in which they can ensure their personal safety. Handling radioactive materials while preparing, dispensing, and transporting radiopharmaceuticals requires that practitioners be exposed to some amount of radioactivity.

Safety First Women can safely work in nuclear pharmacy, even if they are pregnant or nursing. Additional monitoring and safety precautions are used to assure that the fetus of pregnant women have little to no exposure to radioactivity.

One of the major tenets of nuclear pharmacy practice is the concept of ALARA—the practice of keeping exposure to radioactivity As Low As Reasonably Achievable.

✔ There are three major factors that influence the amount of exposure that is received by nuclear pharmacy staff and that nuclear pharmacy practitioners use to maintain ALARA: time, distance, and shielding.

Obviously, *time* is one of the easiest factors to control; the more time spent handling radioactive materials, the more exposure occurs. Generally, nuclear pharmacy staff members are encouraged to use time wisely. Procedures and dispensing functions should be planned out ahead of time to provide organization to the workflow and minimize the amount of contact time with the radioactive material.

Distance is a unique aspect of practice that should be considered in the techniques of any person who practices in a nuclear pharmacy. By increasing the distance from the source, radiation exposure can be decreased. This is carried out in nuclear pharmacy practice by utilizing tongs and other remote handling devices whenever radioactive materials must be handled. This aspect of practice can easily be incorporated into compounding and dispensing techniques.

The most substantial factor used to decrease radiation exposure to the radiation worker is *shielding.* A large amount of shielding materials are present in various areas of nuclear pharmacies. Figure 6-4 shows examples of some of the shielding materials that are used in most nuclear pharmacies. To be effective, shielding material is made of very dense materials such as lead and tungsten. The dense shielding serves to prevent the penetration of radioactive emissions from the source to the person handling the radioactive materials; i.e., it is a barrier between the user and the radioactivity. Shielding materials surround any area where radioactive materials are stored in the pharmacy and are used in the compounding and dispensing process as well to minimize exposure to the pharmacist and the pharmacy technician.

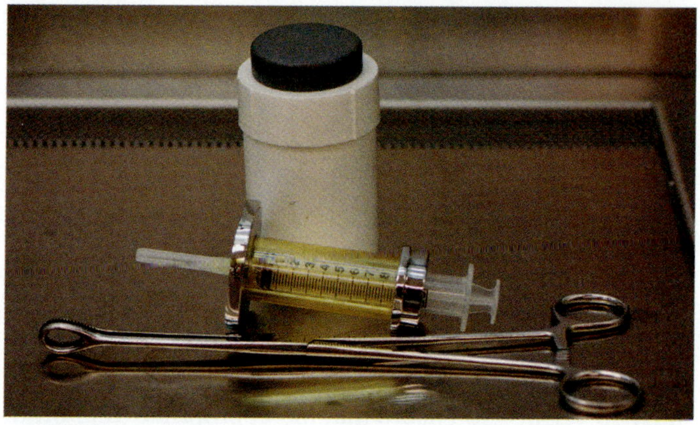

Figure 6-4. Radiation safety tools. Shown are examples of the most common radiation safety tools used during the preparation and dispensing of radiopharmaceuticals. In the back is a vial shield, designed to hold the bulk radiopharmaceutical kit from which all single doses are withdrawn. In the middle, a syringe properly placed in a syringe shield. The leaded glass protects the user from excessive radiation exposure, while still allowing visualization of the syringe markings. In front, a pair of tongs, used to move the syringe containing radioactive material when removed from the syringe shield. The increased distance between the unshielded syringe and the user's fingers helps to keep the exposure to the fingers as low as possible.

In the compounding and dispensing hoods, all radiopharmaceutical kits are shielded by a lead or tungsten vial shield, and every dose should be drawn up using a syringe shield, which is a specially designed hand-held shield made of leaded glass. The syringe is placed inside the shield to provide radiation protection while allowing visualization of the markings on the syringe. An example of dose drawing using these shielding tools is shown in figure 6-5. As with the use of tongs to increase distance, the incorporation of shielding materials during the compounding and dispensing processes has a significant impact on the safety of the pharmacist and technician, making them an integral part of nuclear pharmacy practice.

Although it is not possible to completely eliminate radiation exposure when working in a nuclear pharmacy, there are mechanisms for monitoring the amount of radiation exposure received and the total dose of radiation

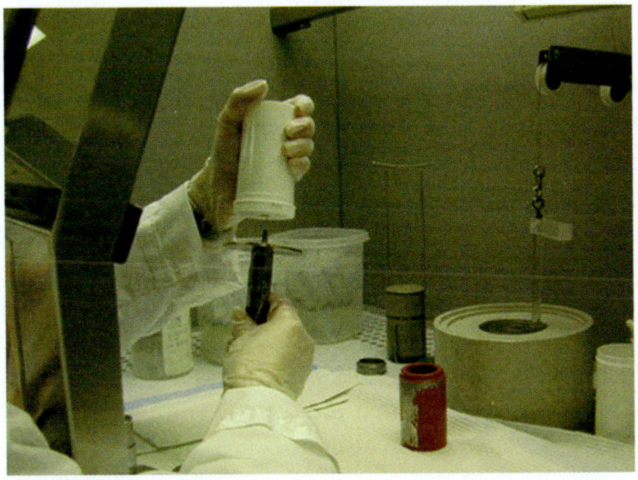

Figure 6–5. Dose drawing with shielding. The above photo shows the proper technique and shielding tools used when radiopharmaceutical unit doses are drawn. Note the white shielding container which houses the prepared radiopharmaceutical kit held in the left hand. In the right hand, a syringe is shielded using a device called a syringe shield made of leaded glass, which provides protection to the hand while allowing the user the ability to see the markings on the syringe for accurate dose dispensing.

that is deposited. Any person working in a nuclear pharmacy must wear a film badge to estimate the dose received by the whole body and ring badges on the fingers to determine the dose to the fingers and hands, the areas most likely to receive the highest exposure to radioactivity. The film badges are worn at the collar to give a general estimate of the dose to the torso of the worker, and the ring badges are worn on the fingers that receive the highest radiation dose to most closely reflect the total radiation dose to the hands. Examples of common monitoring tools are shown in figure 6-6.

The film and ring badges are worn for a preset period of time; then they are returned to the manufacturer for developing and reporting of the radiation dose received during the monitoring period. Each worker's radiation dose reports are maintained in the pharmacy and must be made available to the employee and regulatory inspectors to ensure that appropriate radiation safety measures are being followed. The NRC has set limits for the maximum permissible dose that can be received for each part of the body each year.

Part 1

Safety First A key part of nuclear pharmacy practice is continuous monitoring of the amount of radiation that each employee receives during working hours.

Using Specialized Instrumentation

It is impossible to see, hear, taste, smell, or touch radioactivity. As a result, it is difficult to monitor for the presence of radioactive material, either intentional or unintentional. Specialized instruments are necessary to determine how much radioactive material is present in a given location, identify the location of radioactive materials that may have been spilled to assist in clean up, and ensure that the amount of radioactive material in a patient dose matches the amount that was ordered for the patient. These instruments can be used to detect, identify, and quantify radioactive materials present in the pharmacy. There are several instruments that have been designed to take advantage of the methods by which radioactivity

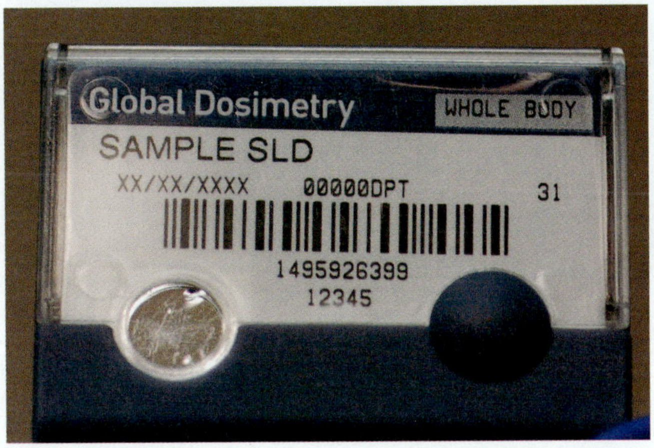

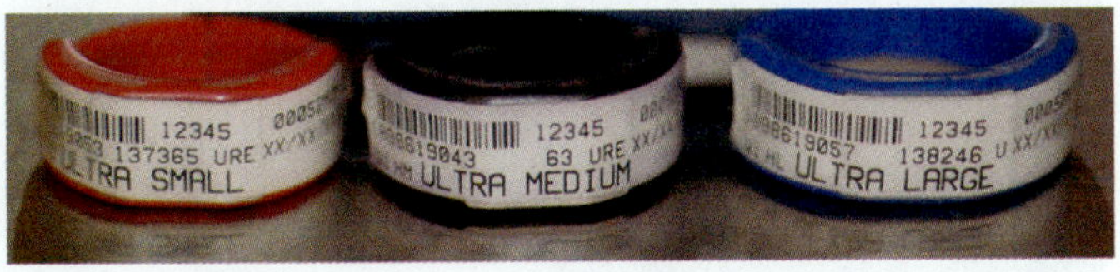

Figure 6–6. Radiation dosimetry. The film badge (left) is worn on the collar to provide an estimate of whole body exposure. The ring badges (above) are generally worn by pharmacists and technicians on both hands. Ring badges come in various sizes to assure correct fit and comfort.

interacts with matter to allow us to quantify the amount of radioactive material being used in radiopharmaceutical preparation and dispensing.

A Geiger Mueller (GM) survey meter is a portable radiation detector that can be used to identify the presence of radioactive material and quantify the amount present at a particular location. Because the device is portable, it is possible to use this piece of equipment at various places within the pharmacy. Ideally, a survey meter is used to monitor a work area upon completion of a task utilizing radioactive materials. It is important to locate and clean up any uncontrolled radioactive material in the work area to prevent the unintentional spread of radioactive materials and the unwanted contamination of people and places in the pharmacy. An example of a GM survey meter used to perform surveys is shown in figure 6-7.

The dose calibrator is the most widely used piece of equipment and the most essential for the preparation and dispensing of radiopharmaceutical doses that will be administered to patients undergoing nuclear medicine studies. The regulations for the medical use of radioactivity stipulate that every patient dose must be assayed in a dose calibrator prior to administration to the patient. Every radiopharmaceutical kit prepared in the pharmacy uses a dose calibrator to verify the total amount of radioactivity that is added to the kit during the preparation process. Every patient dose undergoes a final check in the dose calibrator to ensure that the dose dispensed matches the dose ordered for the patient at the time of administration. Because doses are prepared and dispensed significantly earlier than the time they are administered to patients, they will have significantly more radioactivity at the time of dispensing than when the dose is administered to the patient. Today's dose calibrators are capable of identifying the level of radioactivity at the time of dispensing and can perform the required calculations to determine how much radioactivity will be present at the time of patient administration. This allows the person dispensing the dose to verify that the final dose meets the requirement of being within 10% of the prescribed dose at the time of administration to the patient. Figure 6-8 shows an example of a radionuclide dose calibrator.

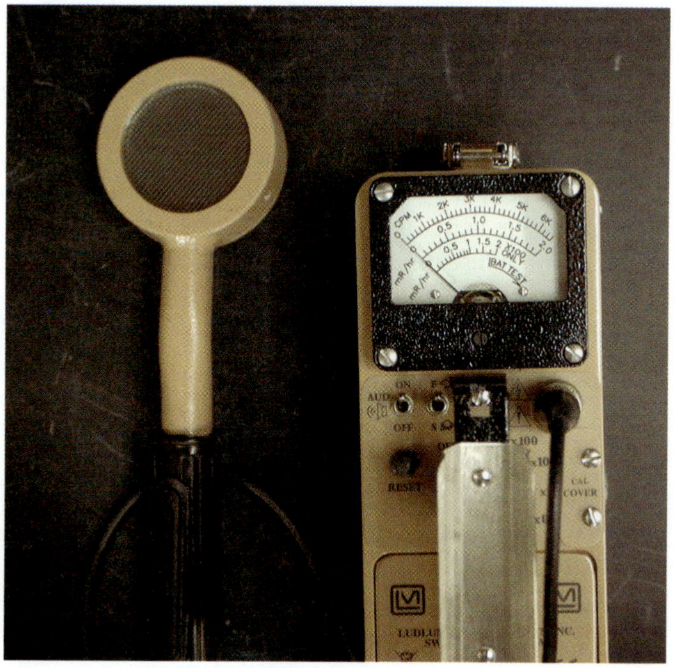

Figure 6–7. Geiger Mueller survey meter. The probe (left) is slowly moved over areas of the pharmacy to detect the presence of radioactivity. If present, the needle on the scale of the unit (right) will move, allowing an approximation of the amount of radioactivity present. In addition, the unit emits audible "chirps" to notify the user that radioactivity has been detected.

TECHNOLOGY TOPICS

Newer models of dose calibrators allow the user to specify the time the dose will be injected, and the machine will determine how much radioactivity will be present at that time.

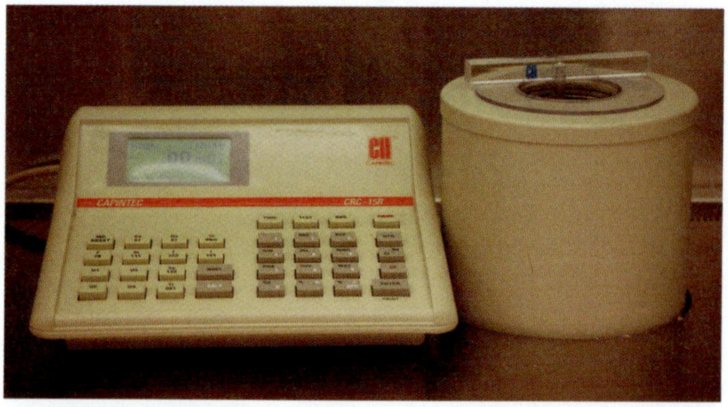

Figure 6–8. Radionuclide dose calibrator used for determining the amount of radioactivity in each dose dispensed from the pharmacy. The syringe is placed in the well (right) and the activity is read on the display (left).

Another unique piece of equipment found in nuclear pharmacies is a scintillation detector. This instrument is used to quantify small amounts of radioactivity. It is used to count samples and quantify the amount of radioactivity present at given locations in the pharmacy. It can also identify what type of radioactive material is present in the sample. This type of detector is also used when quality control is performed on the prepared radiopharmaceutical kit formulations to ensure purity of the final product before dispensing. An example of a scintillation detector is shown in figure 6-9.

The use of instrumentation in the nuclear pharmacy setting requires that each piece of equipment be capable of accurately detecting or quantifying the amount of radioactive material present. Each piece of equipment must be tested to ensure that it is working properly. Some instrumentation tests are conducted daily, whereas others are done on a quarterly or yearly basis. A common component of a nuclear pharmacy technician's daily responsibilities involves performing and documenting the quality control verification of the instruments used in a nuclear pharmacy. This is essential to ensure the accurate dispensing of patient doses and to maintain appropriate radiation safety for the workers in the pharmacy by identifying any unwanted contamination before radiation exposure occurs.

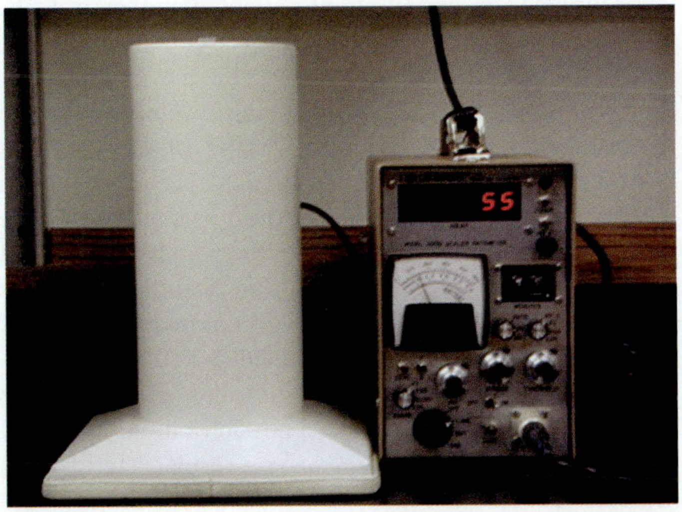

Figure 6–9. Typical scintillation detector consisting of a well (on left) in which samples are placed for analysis and the electronic detector (right) which analyzes and displays data. Data are provided in "counts," which relate to the number of atoms in the sample that gave off a radioactive emission.

Future Directions of Nuclear Pharmacy

Currently, the nuclear pharmacy technician is an integral part of the preparation and dispensing of radiopharmaceutical agents used in the diagnosis and treatment of disease. In the future, as the role of the nuclear pharmacist changes and develops, so too will the role of the nuclear pharmacy technician. Currently, pharmacists are responsible for all aspects of the preparation and dispensing of radiopharmaceuticals used for *therapeutic* purposes due to the risk involved for both the pharmacist and the patient if errors are made in these doses.

In considering future developments in the area of nuclear pharmacy, it can be assumed that the majority of products that will be brought to market will be focused on the therapeutic side of the nuclear medicine spectrum because we already have diagnostic agents available for most of the organs and organ systems in the body. Also, the Joint Commission, which accredits and certifies healthcare entities, including the hospitals and clinics that are serviced by nuclear pharmacies, requires more emphasis on maintaining certain quality standards and providing clinical pharmacy services to benefit the patient. This mandate may increase the direct role of nuclear pharmacists in the provision of pharmaceutical care for patients who receive radiopharmaceuticals for diagnosis and treatment. More of the pharmacist's time will be dedicated to these tasks, requiring that the nuclear pharmacy technician establish a greater role in the preparation of diagnostic radiopharmaceuticals. Regardless of how the job descriptions change in the future, the nuclear pharmacy technician will play an essential role in the provision of nuclear pharmacy services, which provide high-quality radiopharmaceutical products that play an important part in the diagnosis and treatment of disease.

Other Compounding Specialties

Many areas of pharmacy include a compounding function that is associated with daily preparation and dispensing of pharmaceuticals for patient care. In some cases, the use of compounding becomes an essential part of the process because of the lack of commercially available products with the appropriate mixture of multiple ingredients, the appropriate amount of medication for the specific patient, or the appropriate dosage form for the specific patient. To review, compounding involves the practice of creating prescriptions to meet the specific needs of an individual patient upon receipt of a valid prescription. Manufacturing, on the other hand, generally involves the preparation of large batches of material (without a specific prescription) with the intent of delivering to large numbers of patients. In such situations, the ability to compound products to meet the needs of a special population becomes an integral part of providing excellent pharmaceutical care.

Compounding patient-specific pharmaceuticals provides a number of benefits, including patient-specific dosing, delivery of specialized dosage forms, dosing of products for specialized populations, and the ability to address stability issues that may limit the ability to provide commercially available products. For more information on the practice of compounding, see Chapter 15, Nonsterile Compounding and Repackaging.

Custom compounding of specific dosages may occur in several areas of practice, including pediatrics, women's health, fertility, pain management, ophthalmology, and veterinary pharmacy practice.

The focus of the following section is on veterinary pharmacy practice, an area that is becoming more popular because of the increasing need to provide treatment to the animal population (i.e., household pets, farm animals, and animals used as a food source) and develop prescription products for use in animals.

Veterinary Pharmacy Practice

The provision of pharmaceuticals for animals is an area of pharmacy practice that has led to the development of a small number of dedicated veterinary pharmacies, as well as increased potential for traditional pharmacists and pharmacy technicians to become involved in the preparation and dispensing of pharmaceuticals for this specialized patient population.

Historical Perspective

Veterinary medicine in some form has been in existence for as long as human medicine. There is evidence that early cultures such as the Greeks and Egyptians described diseases of common animals. The first veterinary school of medicine was founded in France in 1761, and the first formalized school in the United States was founded in 1852 in Philadelphia.[11] Currently, there are more than 45,000 veterinarians practicing in the United States. Veterinarians are involved in the care of household domestic pets; large animals such as horses, cows, and pigs; and zoo animals. Veterinarians also play an important role in the regulatory aspects of using animals for food and preventing the spread of diseases that can impact both animal and human health.[11]

Veterinary medicine is also a federally regulated specialty. The Center for Veterinary Medicine (CVM) of the U.S. Food and Drug Administration (FDA) regulates the manufacture and distribution of food additives and drugs that are given to animals. In addition, the Food, Drug and Cosmetic Act includes a subsection specific to veterinary medicine. As with drugs used for humans, medications to be given to animals can be over-the-counter (OTC) or prescription. Pharmaceuticals for animal use are restricted to prescription status if the FDA determines that it is not possible to provide adequate directions for the use of the medication by a layperson, and that the medical use must be supervised by a licensed veterinarian. Prescription veterinary products are labeled with the statement "Caution: Federal law restricts this drug to use by or on the order of a licensed veterinarian."[12]

The use of medications (OTC and prescription) provides an added concern when being used on animals that will serve as a food source for consumption by humans or other animals. In addition to safety and efficacy of the medication, other issues, such as withdrawal time before slaughter, become relevant because residual medication in the animal could potentially be passed on to the consumer and result in unnecessary exposure to the drug substance.

Veterinarians have the authority to dispense prescription medications from their site of practice as long as an appropriate veterinarian-client-patient relationship exists. The American Veterinary Medical Association (AVMA) has published guidelines that cover the use and distribution of prescription drugs.[13] Generally, veterinarians are encouraged to utilize animal-specific pharmaceuticals for treatment of the animal population. The FDA "Green Book" is a listing of all animal drug products that have been approved for safety and effectiveness. Published annually and updated monthly, this document is available electronically and currently lists more than 30 pages of FDA-approved agents designated as veterinary medicines.[14] In addition, veterinarians are authorized to utilize drugs approved for human use if no such animal-approved pharmaceutical product exists. As a result, veterinarians may use a written prescription to authorize the dispensing of a legend drug for use in animals for the treatment of disease. If the veterinarian chooses a "human" drug and writes a prescription for that drug, it can be filled at any licensed pharmacy pursuant to the state board of pharmacy regulations for that practice site. It is important to emphasize, however, that all of this is possible only if the veterinarian has documentation of the veterinarian-client-patient relationship, and that appropriate records are maintained regarding the use of the medication on the animal. In veterinary practice, the veterinarian-client-patient relationship generally requires that the veterinarian has sufficient knowledge of the animal and should have recently seen the animal, be acquainted with the care of the animal, and be available in the event of adverse reactions or failed treatment regimens.[12, 13]

Unique Aspects of Veterinary Pharmacy

The practice of compounding medications for use in animals has decreased in recent years, as more and more drug products have become available for use in animals. Nevertheless, in some cases, materials may need to be specifically compounded to meet the specific need of the animal. Compounding is intended to be a patient-driven process, and both veterinarians and pharmacists are allowed to provide this service on an as-needed basis. As with compounding for the human patient population, compounding in the animal population has the potential for causing harm to both animals and members of the public if these agents are used without having appropriate safety and effectiveness data, or if they are compounded in the absence of sound manufacturing practices. In 2003, the FDA released a compliance policy guide that was designed to assist practitioners in understanding the role that compounding plays in veterinary medicine practice.[15]

As in any other pharmacy that provides compounding services, the role of the technician varies. In some situations, technicians are responsible for the actual compounding activities. For technicians who would like to work in this environment, the most difficult issue is finding a location that specializes in providing pharmacy services for an animal population. The American College of Veterinary Pharmacists provides information about member pharmacies that compound veterinary-specific medications.[16] Most of these pharmacies are designated "compounding pharmacies" and compound for both human and animal patients. The Society of Veterinary Hospital Pharmacists is an organization consisting of pharmacists who work exclusively at hospitals dedicated to the care of animals, mostly in academic teaching hospitals within colleges or universities that have veterinary medicine schools. This organization has published a position statement on compounding practices in the animal population.[17]

Most of the compounding duties in these environments involve the incorporation of common medication into dosage forms that fit the specific needs of a particular animal, such as the creation of liquid dosage forms from oral tablets, flavored medications that increase palatability (often beef- or chicken-flavored), and adjustment of commercially available dosage forms to meet the dose requirement for an animal outside the normal dosage range. It is not uncommon to see standard "recipes" in the compounding area of the pharmacy that are commonly compounded for local veterinarian needs.

The use of medications in the animal population is very unique, as the bioavailability, biodistribution, and kinetics of drugs can differ greatly as compared to that for the human population.[11] Interestingly, these same factors can vary greatly between animal species as well due to differences in metabolism, gastric transit, absorption, and pH.[18] Although it seems unlikely that a large-sized animal may require a smaller dose than a traditional house pet, it is possible due to the intrinsic physiologic differences. In addition, a fairly innocuous drug used in the canine population (aspirin, for example) can be lethal to felines, because they have a deficiency in the normal metabolic pathway for this drug.

✔ Practitioners in a veterinary pharmacy should become somewhat familiar with some of these differences and be aware of the sometimes significant differences in prescribing patterns between species.

Several pharmacy references are available that are dedicated to veterinary medicine, and these should be consulted when one is working in this practice area.[19–21]

Summary

The pharmacy profession has multiple areas of practice in which pharmacy technicians can play an important role in the provision of pharmaceutical care. This chapter describes two less common areas of pharmacy practice: nuclear pharmacy and veterinary pharmacy—these are areas of practice that utilize the pharmacy technician in a variety of roles. Again, the scope of this text is an introduction to these areas of practice and is not intended to provide all of the information specific for each area of practice. For pharmacy technicians who are looking for a unique area of practice to utilize their skills, both of these areas require expertise in compounding and dispensing pharmaceuticals, and introduce a different variety of daily duties that provide an interesting and challenging twist to the pharmacy technician's career.

Self-Assessment Questions

1. Radioactivity occurs when there is instability due to an imbalance in the ratio between the components of an atom (protons and neutrons).
   a. True
   b. False
2. The half-life is the amount of time required for a radioactive isotope to decay (or decrease) by
   a. 10%
   b. 20%
   c. 25%
   d. 50%
3. Which of the following is an imaging specialty that provides FUNCTIONAL information about an organ or organ system?
   a. CT scanning
   b. MRI imaging
   c. Nuclear imaging
   d. Ultrasound
4. Nuclear pharmacy was the first recognized specialty area of pharmacy practice.
   a. True
   b. False
5. Which of the following is FALSE about nuclear pharmacy practice?
   a. Radioactive pharmaceuticals decay with time
   b. Extensive shielding and personnel protection is required when dispensing
   c. Nuclear pharmacies operate with limited patient contact
   d. Nuclear pharmacies do not need to comply with state pharmacy regulations
6. Which of the following is NOT part of the UNRESTRICTED area of the pharmacy?
   a. Compounding area
   b. Kitchen
   c. Office area
   d. Restrooms
7. Which of the following is NOT part of the pharmacy technician's duties when working in a nuclear pharmacy setting?
   a. Dispensing DIAGNOSTIC radiopharmaceuticals
   b. Dispensing THERAPEUTIC radiopharmaceuticals
   c. Performing daily instrumentation checks
   d. Performing quality control testing on prepared products
8. Traditional pharmacy settings will never have occasion to dispense pharmaceuticals for the animal population.
   a. True
   b. False
9. It is legal to compound a prescription for an animal and then sell the compounded pharmaceutical to other animal owners without a prescription for that product because it is intended for animal use.
   a. True
   b. False
10. An additional challenge for practitioners in veterinary practice is introduced because a prescription drug may behave differently in an animal patient than it does in a human patient.
    a. True
    b. False

Self-Assessment Answers

1. a. True. An unstable atom will try to reach a more stable state. A radioactive emission is a mechanism by which the unstable atom gives off excess energy and corrects the imbalance.
2. d. The half-life of an isotope is the time needed for 50% (or one-half) of a radioactive material to decay.
3. c. Nuclear imaging. Nuclear imaging enables visualization of a physiologic process within the body, allowing for the determination of the *function* of the organ or organ system being evaluated. The other procedures provide far greater details regarding the anatomic features of the organ *structure*.
4. a. True. Nuclear pharmacy was recognized as the first area of specialty pharmacy practice in 1978.
5. d. Nuclear pharmacies must comply with state pharmacy regulations. A nuclear pharmacy is licensed as a pharmacy by the state board of pharmacy, just like any other pharmacy. All rules and regulations that are applied to traditional practice settings apply to nuclear pharmacies.
6. a. All of these areas are considered the "unrestricted" areas of the pharmacy except "a"—the compounding area, which is restricted. This is the area where radiopharmaceuticals are compounded and dispensed, so there are substantial amounts of radioactivity present in this area.
7. b. Dispensing THERAPEUTIC radiopharmaceuticals. Due to the significantly greater risk of therapeutic radiopharmaceuticals to both the patient and the person involved in preparation and dispensing, only pharmacists dispense therapeutic radiopharmaceuticals.
8. b. False. If an animal requires treatment with a pharmaceutical that is used in humans, a veterinarian may write for that agent using a standard prescription, which will need to be filled in the same manner as if the drug were being prescribed for a human patient.
9. b. False. Compounding is designed to provide a product to a single user (or limited number of users) only when a valid prescription is written for each specific animal. In addition, a compounded product that is prepared using a prescription drug component must always be dispensed following a prescription order.
10. a. True. Biodistribution in animals differs from that in humans, and there are often differences in biodistribution among species. To verify the validity of dose, administration route, and dosing interval in a prescription written for an animal, it is important to recognize the intrinsic differences in how the agent will behave between species.

Resources

Most nuclear pharmacies do not extensively advertise technician positions. If nuclear pharmacy is an area of practice that interests you, it is best to contact the pharmacy directly to inquire about possible positions. The following Web sites contain lists and contact information for nuclear pharmacies around the country and may be helpful in your search

1. Purdue University Division of Nuclear Pharmacy
   - http://nuclear.pharmacy.purdue.edu
   - click on "Nuclear Pharmacies in the US" for a map and contact information
2. University of Arkansas Nuclear Pharmacy Web site
   - http://nuclearpharmacy.uams.edu
   - click on "Nuclear pharmacies" link

References

1. Society of Nuclear Medicine. What is nuclear medicine? [online educational brochure]. Reston, VA: 2009. Available at http://interactive.snm.org/docs/whatisnucmed.pdf. Accessed June 14, 2009.
2. Shaw SM, Ice RD. Nuclear pharmacy, part I: emergence of the specialty of nuclear pharmacy. *J Nucl Med Technol*. 2000; 28:8–11.
3. Grussing PL, Allen DR, Callahan RJ, et al. Development of pharmacy's first specialty certification examination: nuclear pharmacy. *Am J Pharm Ed*. 1983; 47:11–16.
4. Board of Pharmaceutical Specialties. *2008 Annual Report — For Skills that Pay. . . .* Washington DC; 2009.
5. Ponto JA, Hung, JC. Nuclear pharmacy, part II: nuclear pharmacy practice today. *J Nucl Med Technol.* 2000;28: 76–81.
6. United Pharmacy Partners, Inc. Pharmacy locations. Suwanee, GA: 2008. Available at http://www.uppi.org/businesses/businesseslist.php. Accessed February 2010.
7. Callahan RJ. The role of commercial nuclear pharmacy in the future practice of nuclear medicine. *Semin Nucl Med.* 1996; 26:85–90.

8. Callahan RJ, Dragotakes SC. The role of the practice of nuclear pharmacy in positron emission tomography. *Clin Pos Imag.* 1999; 2:211–216.
9. United States Pharmacopeia. USP <797> Sterile product compounding. 32nd revision and the National Formulary, 27th edition. Washington, DC: 2009.
10. Nuclear Regulatory Commission. Code of Federal Regulations, Part 10. Washington, DC. 2008. Available at http://www.nrc.gov/reading-rm/doc-collections/cfr/. Accessed February 2010.
11. Wick JY, Zanni GR. Patients large and small: role of the pharmacist in veterinary medicine. *J Am Pharm Assoc.* 2004; 44(3):319–323.
12. US Food and Drug Administration. Center for Veterinary Medicine. Rockville, MD. 2010. Available at http://www.fda.gov/AnimalVeterinary/default.htm. Accessed February 2009.
13. American Veterinary Medical Association. *Guidelines for Veterinary Prescription Drugs*. November, 2006. Available at http://www.avma.org/issues/policy/prescription_drugs.asp. Accessed February 2010.
14. US Food and Drug Administration. The Green Book On-line. Center for Veterinary Medicine, Rockville, MD 2008. Available at http://www.accessdata.fda.gov/scripts/animaldrugsatfda/. Accessed February 2010.
15. US Food and Drug Administration. Compounding of Drugs for Use in Animals (CPG 7125.40). Office of Regulatory Affairs, 200. Available at http://www.fda.gov/ICECI/ComplianceManuals/CompliancePolicyGuidanceManual/ucm074656.htm. Accessed February 2010.
16. American College of Veterinary Pharmacists. Member directory. 2010. Available at http://www.vetmeds.org/aboutus/member_websites.asp. Accessed February 2010
17. Society of Veterinary Hospital Pharmacists. *Position Statement on Compounding of Drugs for Use in Animals*. 2007. Available at http://www.svhp.org/CompoundingStatement.pdf. Accessed February 2010.
18. Ahmed I, Kasraian K. Pharmaceutical challenges in veterinary product development. *Adv Drug Deliv Rev.* 2002; 54:871–82.
19. American Academy of Veterinary Pharmacology & Therapeutics. *USP Veterinary Drug Information monographs.* Available at http://www.aavpt.org/USPmonographs.shtml. Accessed February 2010.
20. Kahn CM, Line S, eds. Merck Veterinary Manual 9th ed., Whitehouse Station, NJ. 2008. Available at http://www.merckvetmanual.com/mvm/index.jsp, Accessed February 2010.
21. Plumb, D. *Plumb's Veterinary Drug Handbook 6th ed.* Hoboken NJ: Wiley Blackwell; 2008.

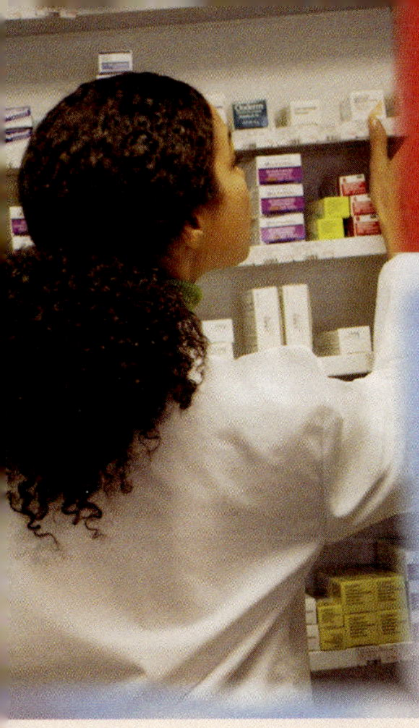

Chapter 7

Drug Information Resources

Bonnie S. Bachenheimer

Learning Outcomes

After completing this chapter, you will be able to

- Classify a drug information request.
- Explain how to obtain appropriate background information for a drug information request.
- Distinguish between questions that may be answered by a technician and those that should be answered only by a pharmacist.
- Given a specific pharmacy-related question, identify the best resource to use to find the answer.
- Describe how to find answers to drug information questions at the workplace.

Key Terms

drug information request A question regarding a medication.

drug monograph Written information about a drug or class of drugs that contains product details, indications for use, safety information, dosing, administration, and other useful information about the drug(s).

material safety data sheets Information sheets provided by manufacturers for chemicals or drugs that may be hazardous in the workplace. They provide information about the specific hazards of the chemicals or drugs used at the worksite, guidelines for their safe use, and recommendations to treat an exposure or clean up a spill.

Medline A searchable database containing over 16 million references to journal articles and abstracts published in approximately 5,200 biomedical journals.

MedlinePlus An online database sponsored by the government that contains health information for the public on over 500 health conditions

package insert A manufacturer's product information sheet that provides general drug information, such as how it works, indications, adverse effects, drug interactions, dosage forms, stability, and dosing information.

primary references Original research articles published in scientific journals.

PubMed A Web-based searching system, sponsored by the National Library of Medicine, which can be used to access Medline journal citations.

requestor The person requesting the information. A requestor could be a nurse, doctor, other health care professional, or a patient.

secondary references Indexing systems such as Medline, which provide a list of journal articles on the topic that is being searched.

tertiary references General references that present documented information in a condensed and compact format, such as textbooks or manuals.

The provision of drug therapy has become increasingly complex and the number of new drugs approved for use has significantly increased during the past decade. The result is that pharmacy technicians are frequently challenged with drug information questions throughout the workday and must become more knowledgeable about the handling, availability, and uses of medications. A basic knowledge of the drug information resources available will help prepare technicians and leave them better equipped to assist pharmacists with certain drug information requests.

Pharmacy reference books and electronic media, including the Internet, that are available in all practice settings often hold the answers to typical, day-to-day practice-related questions. These resources can also be used as study aids for the technician certification examination and to expand a technician's general knowledge about medications. Therefore, it is essential that technicians understand the basics about frequently used, reputable pharmacy references.

The purpose of this chapter is to classify the various types of drug information requests, explain which types of questions are appropriate for pharmacy technicians to answer, and describe where technicians can find answers to drug information requests. With time and practice, technicians will be able to find the information that they need quickly and efficiently; in doing so, they will become even more valuable members of the health-care team.

The Drug Information Request

A **drug information request** is simply a question regarding a medication. The person requesting the information, the **requestor**, can be a nurse, doctor, other health-care professional, or patient. The request might be asked over the telephone, in person, or via fax or email. The request may be simple, requiring little time to research and answered quickly, such as "what is the generic name of Lipitor?" Other requests may be complicated, requiring a significant amount of research before they can be answered. An example of a complicated request is "what is the safety of fluoxetine (Prozac) in pregnancy?"

✔ Before responding to a drug information request, technicians must clearly differentiate questions that fall within their scope of practice from those that may be answered only by a pharmacist.

In general, if a question requires specific knowledge about a medication and/or professional judgment, it should be answered by a pharmacist.

An example is a patient wanting to know whether he or she is experiencing a side effect from a medication. The pharmacist needs to research whether the medication could cause the side effect, obtain patient-specific information, and use his or her professional judgment to determine whether the side effect could be due to the medication or something else going on with the patient. In some cases, the distinction between the two types of questions may not be apparent. If there is any doubt about the nature of the question, the technician should defer the question to the pharmacist.

✔ When approached with a drug information request over the telephone or in person, technicians should identify themselves as pharmacy technicians, so that the person asking the question will know the type of information that may be appropriately conveyed.

Keep in mind that consumers may not understand which questions a pharmacy technician can answer and which should be referred to the pharmacist. It is important to identify the person initiating the request and, when the request comes over the telephone, to obtain the necessary contact information (phone, pager, fax, etc.) in case the person needs to be called back. The search for and response to drug information requests will differ depending on who requests the information. Knowing information about the requestor, including his or her training and knowledge of the subject, will impact the final response and how it is given. For example, if a pharmacist is asked how the drug ondansetron (Zofran) works, he or she would respond differently if the request was from a patient compared to a physician. When answering questions from patients, medical terminology is avoided and the response is put into language that patients can understand. The answer would be more in-depth to a physician and written information might also be provided.

Obtaining information about the purpose of the request will help to determine the needs of the requestor and whether it involves clinical judgment, requiring the expertise of a pharmacist. It will also make the search for information more efficient. It is important to find out if the information is for general knowledge or if it pertains to a specific patient. If the question involves a specific patient, the pharmacist will need to obtain background information in order to respond to the question. For example, if a physician asks what the dose of gabapentin (Neurontin) is, the pharmacist would need to know if it was for a specific patient and, if so, what the indication is, the patient's age, kidney function, other medications, allergies, etc.

The urgency of the request and the extent of the information needed should also be determined so that an appropriate amount of time is allotted to answer the request. Often, part of the question can be answered initially (if needed urgently), with the remainder of the answer provided later, allowing time for research in order to give a more thorough response. For example, a physician calls and wants to know if the pharmacy stocks a new drug that has recently been FDA approved. Upon further questioning, she has a patient in her office who might benefit from the drug and she needs to know if the drug is available. She would also like some written information about the drug. This is an urgent request, and the initial answer is no, the drug is not stocked in the pharmacy and does not appear to be available at the wholesaler yet. Because the drug is not even available yet, the request is no longer urgent. The technician can call the wholesaler and/or the manufacturer to find out when the drug will be available and the pharmacist can gather information about the new drug and follow up with the physician at a later time.

Classifying the Request

After information is gathered about the request and the requestor, it is helpful to identify the type of question that is being asked, that is, to classify the request. Classifying the type of request helps to narrow the search and make

Table 7–1. Classifications of Drug Information Questions

Question Classification	Examples
General Drug Information	What is the brand name of warfarin? Do Naprosyn and Aleve contain the same active ingredient? Who manufactures Enbrel? Is Prilosec available as a generic? Is it a prescription or over-the-counter (OTC) product?
Availability and Cost	What dosage forms of Imitrex are available in your pharmacy? Is Zoloft available as a liquid? If so, what size and concentration is available? What are the prices of Adalat CC and Procardia XL? How long is the shortage of albumin expected to last?
Storage and Stability	Should Lovenox be stored in the refrigerator? How long is a flu shot stable after it is drawn up in a syringe?
Calculations	How many milliliters are in an ounce?
Preparation	How should ampicillin be reconstituted?
Pharmacy Law	In what controlled substance schedule is zolpidem (Ambien)? Can Tiazac be substituted for Cardizem CD (is it AB rated)? How many times can a prescription be transferred from one store to another?
Miscellaneous	Where can I find the phone number for Sanofi Aventis? When will the patent for Lipitor expire? Where can I get more Lovenox teaching kits? Where can I find the Vaccine Information Sheet for the influenza vaccine?

the search process more efficient. Many of the questions that technicians encounter fall into the categories outlined in table 7–1. The table also lists examples of questions within these categories.

As explained above, it is critical that technicians differentiate questions that fall within their scope of practice from those that may be answered only by a pharmacist.

✔ Technicians should not interpret a patient-specific question or provide information that requires professional judgment.

Sometimes a simply stated question can actually represent a complex patient-specific situation. For example, the pharmacist may need to learn more about the patient's specific problems and apply clinical judgment in order to answer the question appropriately and completely. Many times, the person requesting the information is indirectly asking for a pharmacist's point of view or interpretation of a situation, which requires an in-depth analysis and recommendation from the pharmacist. For a technician, attempting to interpret or answer such a question could result in miscommunication and the delivery of inaccurate information, both of which could be potentially harmful to the patient. If there is any doubt about the nature of the question, the technician should defer the question to the pharmacist.

Safety First Don't attempt to answer a question when there is any doubt about its nature.

Table 7–2 provides examples of questions that require a pharmacist's interpretation and should not be answered

Table 7–2. Drug Information Questions Appropriate for Pharmacists

Question Classification	Examples	Rationale
Identification and Availability	What is paracetamol and what is its U.S. equivalent?	Although it is appropriate for a technician to obtain technical information about availability (e.g., anticipated length/reasons for a shortage), questions that require clinical knowledge, such as therapeutic alternatives, must be answered by a pharmacist
Allergies	Which narcotic is safe to use in a patient with a codeine allergy?	For allergy questions, the pharmacist must obtain more patient-specific information, such as a description of the allergy and the condition being treated. Clinical judgment is required.
Dosing and Administration	What is the usual dose of propranolol? How long should ciprofloxacin be given for a urinary tract infection? What is the best way to give gentamicin IV?	Answers to dosing and administration questions depend on many factors, especially the indication for use and patient-specific information (e.g., age, weight, and kidney and liver function).
Compatibility	Is Primaxin compatible with dopamine?	More information is needed (e.g., doses, concentrations, fluids, and type of IV lines), and a pharmacist must interpret information found in a reference and apply it to the situation.
Drug Interactions	Is it OK to take aspirin with warfarin?	Drug interaction questions are complex and require patient-specific information and interpretation by a pharmacist in order to apply the significance of a potential interaction to a specific patient.
Side Effects	What are the side effects of Lexapro? Can Celebrex cause renal failure?	Package inserts and textbooks provide lists of side effects that are often difficult to interpret and convey. Also, a pharmacist must interpret whether the request is being made because an adverse event is suspected with one or more medications.
Pregnancy and Lactation	Is albuterol safe to use in pregnancy? Can I get a flu shot if I am breastfeeding?	Pregnancy and lactation questions are complicated because more information is needed about the patient, the stage of pregnancy, and/or age of the infant. A pharmacist must interpret the findings and apply them to the specific situation.
Therapeutic Use	Has clonidine been used to treat opiate withdrawal?	The use of drugs for non-FDA-approved uses often requires evaluation and interpretation of the literature and clinical judgment.

by pharmacy technicians, as well as the rationale for why it is necessary for a pharmacist to answer the question.

Conducting the Search: Choosing the Right References

There are a number of drug information resources available. The key to answering questions quickly and accurately is to know where the necessary information is likely to be found. Not all references contain every possible answer to every drug information question. At times, it may be difficult to find a reference that contains the information that you are seeking. Pharmacists usually search for information until they exhaust all possible resources. Often, they use multiple resources to verify the information that is found, such as in determining the dose of a medication in a pediatric patient. As part of a systematic search strategy, a pharmacist is taught to first consult tertiary references, then secondary references, and, finally, primary references.[1]

Tertiary references are general references that present documented information in a condensed and compact format. They may include textbooks; compendia (e.g., American Hospital Formulary Service Drug Information (AHFS DI), and Drug Facts & Comparisons); computerized systems, such as Micromedex® Clinical Information System; review articles; or information found on the Internet. Tertiary references are the most common references used because they are easy to use, convenient, readily accessible, concise, and compact. Disadvantages of tertiary references are that information may not be up to date, they may contain errors, and the level of detail on a specific topic may not be deep enough due to space restrictions.

Secondary references include indexing systems such as Medline (further explained later in the chapter), which provide a list of journal articles on the topic that is being searched. Secondary references are used when new or very up-to-date information is required, or when no information can be located in tertiary references.

Primary references are original research articles published in scientific journals, such as the *American Journal of Health-System Pharmacists (AJHP)* or the *Journal of the American Pharmacists Association (JAPhA)*.

Other resources that can be used include pharmaceutical manufacturers and specialized drug and poison information centers.

If the information cannot be found in a tertiary reference, then the technician should consult a pharmacist, who may advise an alternative search strategy or consult a secondary reference. If time permits, the technician should consult as many resources as possible and compare information from several different sources.

Common References

There are numerous resources that are extremely useful for pharmacy professionals. This section highlights common, reputable drug information resources. A brief discussion of the resource, its features, and questions that the reference will help answer are provided. The following discussion may not apply equally to the various practice settings and does not include all the information resources that are available. Technicians should familiarize themselves with the references in their practice settings to determine which resources best fit their needs.

General Drug Information

General drug information references are found in virtually every type of pharmacy setting and are used frequently by pharmacists and technicians. There are many general information references available in a variety of formats, including textbooks, PDAs, CD-ROMs, and online versions. Following are descriptions of the most common general references that are used by pharmacy professionals.

> **TECHNOLOGY TOPICS**
>
> Drug information databases are now integrated with many computer systems and automated dispensing cabinets, offering drug information directly at the point of care.

Facts and Comparisons. *Facts & Comparisons®*, a part of Wolters Kluwers Health, is one of the most widely used drug information references by pharmacy professionals. It is easy to use, updated regularly, and available in print and electronic (Internet, PDA, or CD-ROM) formats. It is a comprehensive, general drug information reference that provides complete **drug monographs**. The print version is organized by therapeutic or pharmacologic class (e.g., antihistamines or topicals) and includes tables that allow for quick comparisons of drugs within the same class.

Tables compare pharmacokinetic parameters (e.g., onset, duration, and metabolism), adverse effects, drug interactions, dosing, and multiple ingredient preparations (e.g., lists the individual ingredients of the cough and cold preparations and analgesic combinations).

Information that can be found in this reference includes the following: general drug information (e.g., pharmacology, drug interactions, dosing and administration, adverse effects, warnings, and precautions); product availability (e.g., dosage forms, brand and generic names, and manufacturers); active ingredients and strengths of multiple-ingredient products; controlled substance schedules; designation as over-the-counter (OTC) or prescription; whether products are sugar-free, alcohol-free, and/or dye-free; drug company contact information; color-coded pictures that can assist with tablet/product identification; and investigational and orphan drug information. Patient information in English and Spanish (MedFacts) and Medication Guides are also available, depending on the subscription.

Drug Information Handbook. Lexi-Comp publishes numerous handbooks for health-care professionals that provide drug and disease state information specific to health-care professionals (e.g., pharmacists, nurses, physicians, and dentists). *The Drug Information Handbook* and the *Pediatric Dosage Handbook* contain general drug information monographs. They are quick, convenient, and easy to use. They are alphabetically organized in dictionary format according to generic name. The monographs are comprehensive and include pharmacology, dosing, drug interaction and safety, as well as available doses and strengths. The *Pediatric Dosage Handbook* contains additional dosage information by age group (neonatal, pediatric, and adult) and extemporaneous compounding recipes.

Other Lexi-Comp handbooks include the *Drug Information Handbook for Oncology, Geriatric Dosage Handbook,* and the *Drug Information Handbook for Psychiatry*. All of the Handbooks contain extensive appendices with helpful charts, abbreviations, measurements, and conversions. The handbooks are also available in a variety of electronic formats and packages for PDA and Web-based applications. Lexi-Comp Online can be purchased with the electronic handbooks, as well as a drug interaction database (Lexi-Interact) (figure 7–1), a natural products database (Lexi-Natural), and an extensive patient drug information database (Lexi-PALs). Lexi-PALS contains Patient Advisory Leaflets that can be used for patient counseling and are available in 18 languages. Lexi-Comp Online has partnered with the American Hospital Formulary Service (AHFS) to provide more in-depth drug information.

American Hospital Formulary Service Drug Information. The American Hospital Formulary Service Drug Information (AHFS DI), published by the American Society of Health-System Pharmacists (ASHP), is a detailed, comprehensive, general drug information reference. This textbook provides complete drug monographs that are organized by therapeutic class, including detailed information about the use of a drug, its side effects, dosing considerations, etc. Its coverage is not limited to FDA-approved uses of medications. It is especially useful for injectable products with respect to preparation and administration instructions. AHFS DI is widely used by health-system pharmacists because it provides in-depth, unbiased, evaluative reviews of medications. This resource is extensively reviewed by editors and contains information from various reputable sources. Subscriptions include online updates. As mentioned above, AHFS DI is also available in an online version with Lexi-Comp Online.

Clinical Pharmacology. *Clinical Pharmacology* (published by Gold Standard) is an electronic drug information database that is widely used in retail chain pharmacies, pharmacy schools, and hospitals. It contains complete monographs for prescription and OTC drugs, dietary supplements, and investigational drugs. Drug information includes indications (FDA approved and off-label uses), pharmacology, pharmacokinetics, dosing and administration, drug interactions, warnings and precautions, pregnancy and lactation information, adverse effects, and available strengths with photos (figure 7–2). It has a drug identifier as well as patient information sheets in English and Spanish.

Micromedex® Healthcare Series. *Micromedex® Healthcare Series* (published by Thomson Reuters) is a comprehensive reference system that is accessed electronically via Internet, CD-ROM, and PDA (figure 7–3). Depending on the subscription, it contains comprehensive drug information (DRUGDEX®), poison information (POISONDEX®); Material Safety Data Sheets; foreign drug information; tablet and capsule identification; disease and trauma information; herbal information; stability, compatibility, and pregnancy information; patient information; and more. Drug information for patients (CareNotes®) is available in both English and Spanish.

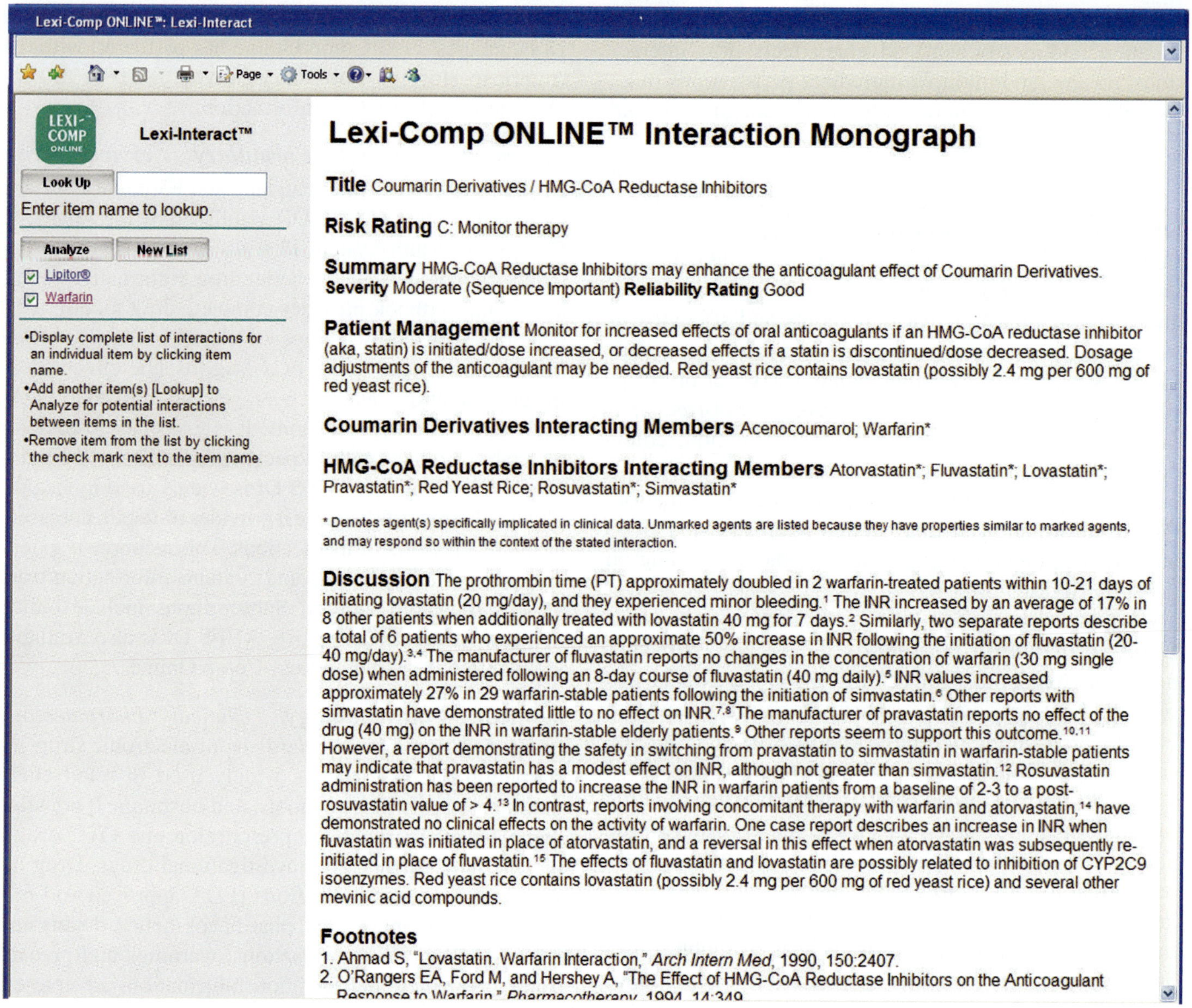

Figure 7–1. A screenshot from Lexi-Interact™ showing a drug interaction monograph of atorvastatin (Lipitor) and warfarin. Reprinted with permission. Copyright © 1978-2010 Lexi-Comp Inc. All Rights Reserved.

> **Rx for Success**
>
> Online drug information databases also have news sections that offer a great way to keep up-to-date with new drug approvals and safety information.

United States Pharmacopeia Drug Information. *United States Pharmacopeia Drug Information* (USPDI) (published by Thomson, Micromedex) is a three-volume set that provides medication information for health-care professionals (Volume I) and patients (Volume II). The third volume (*Approved Drug Products and Legal Requirements*) provides information on laws affecting pharmacy practice.

Volume I (*Drug Information for the Healthcare Professional*) provides comprehensive, general drug information. The drug monographs are arranged alphabetically, but similar medications are described in a single section. The monographs provide a description of how medications work, their indications and other uses, adverse effects, potential drug interactions, admixture information, storage requirements, auxiliary label recommendations, etc.

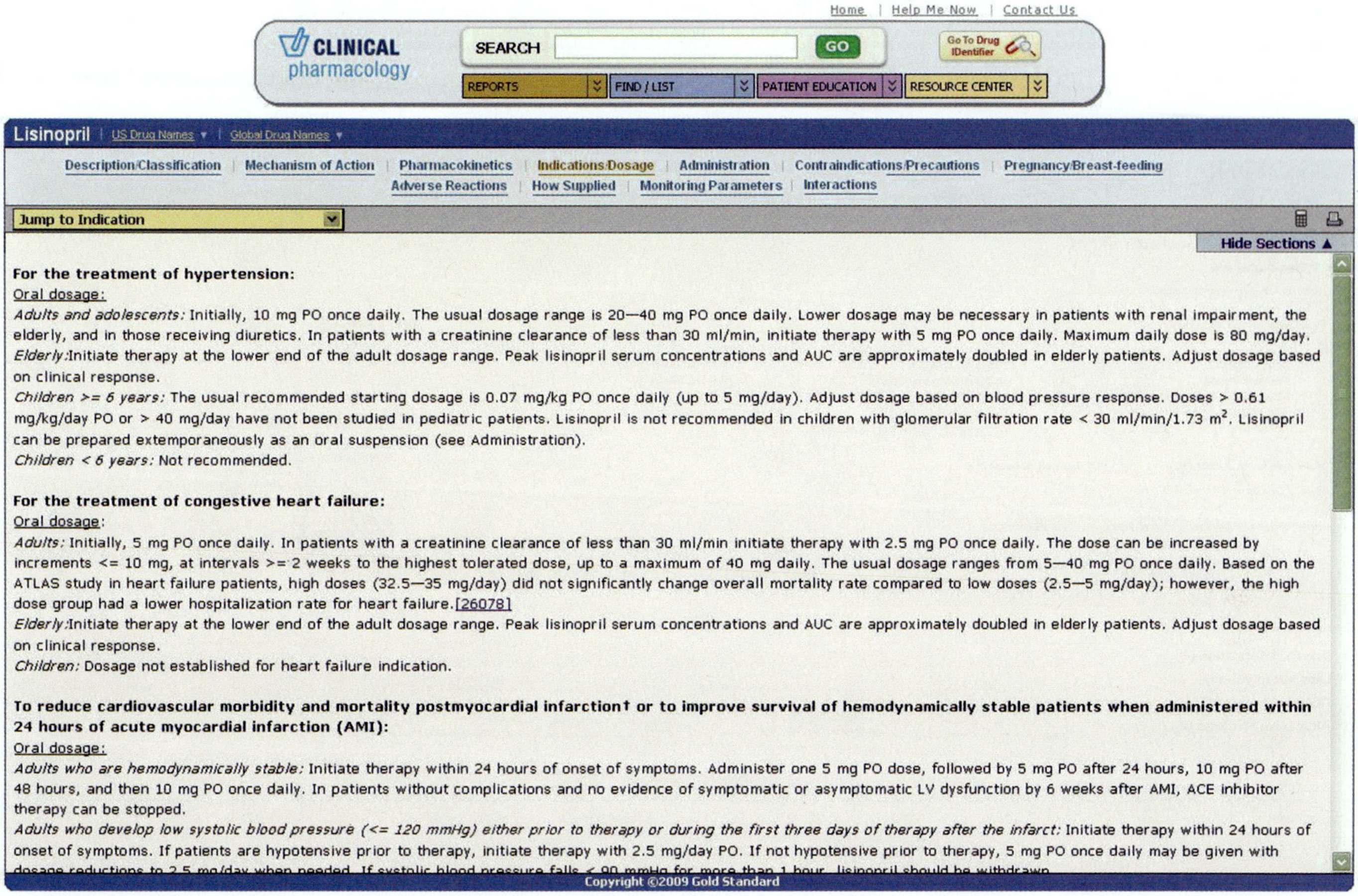

Figure 7–2. A screenshot from the Clinical Pharmacology Web site showing indications and dosing for the drug lisinopril. Reprinted with permission. *Clinical Pharmacology*, http://clinicalpharmacology.com. Gold Standard/Elsevier, Publishers, Tampa, FL, 2009.

Volume II (*Advice for the Patient*) provides a more general discussion of the medications in language that patients will understand. This volume answers questions that patients may ask, such as how to take the medication, special considerations about taking the medication during pregnancy and while breastfeeding; and common adverse effects that may occur when taking the medicine.

Volume III (*Approved Drug Products and Legal Requirements*) contains the FDA's published list of approved drug products: *Approved Drug Products with Therapeutic Equivalence Evaluations* (also known as the Orange Book). This section provides information related to bioequivalence of products, or whether generic drugs can be substituted. USP DI Volume III helps to identify a drug's chemical properties, determine if a drug has been discontinued, or select an appropriate generic substitute for a brand name drug. It also includes information about federal requirements regarding product quality, packaging, storage, and labeling.

The Physicians' Desk Reference. *The Physicians' Desk Reference* (PDR) (published by Thomson Medical Economics) contains manufacturer's **package inserts**. A package insert is a manufacturer's product information sheet that provides general drug information, such as how it works, indications, adverse effects, drug interactions, dosage forms, stability, dosing information, etc. The PDR is organized according to the manufacturer's products (as opposed to therapeutic class). The PDR contains other useful information, such as colored photographs of tablets, capsules, or packaging that may be used for product identification. Package inserts list active and inactive ingredients, preparation, administration, stability, and storage instructions, and availability. The PDR also lists manufacturer phone numbers and addresses and Drug and Poison Information Centers.

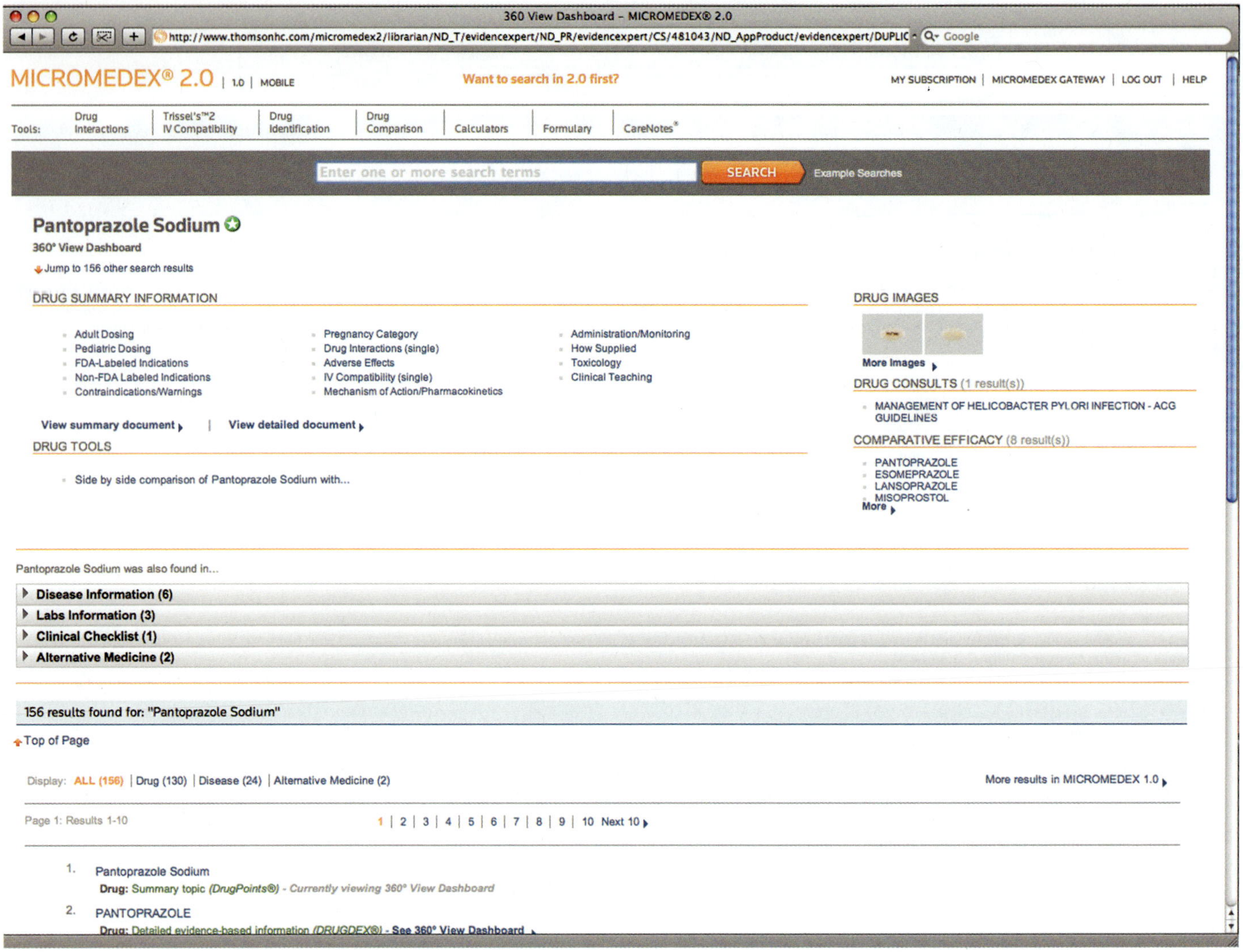

Figure 7–3. A screenshot of the Micromedex Healthcare Series database after searching for the drug pantoprazole.

The *PDR* is not comprehensive and only contains information on select brand name drugs. The information is written by the manufacturer and approved by the FDA. It only contains information about FDA-approved uses of the drug. It does not provide comparative information of that drug with similar medications. Therefore, the *PDR* may not be as useful as other resources in comparing products. Information about generic medications is typically not included.

Specialty References

Specialty references include those related to availability and cost, compatibility and stability, compounding, herbal medications, and dietary supplements.

Availability and Cost.

Red Book. *Red Book* (published by Medical Economics) contains product information and prices for prescription drugs, over-the-counter products, and medical supplies. It contains NDC numbers for all products, available packaging, and therapeutic equivalence ratings (according to the FDA's Orange Book). Red Book includes a comprehensive listing of manufacturers, wholesalers, and third party administrator directories. There are sections with other useful practical information, such as lists of sugar, lactose, galactose, and alcohol-free products; sulfite-containing products; medications that shouldn't be crushed; and color photographs of many prescription and over-the-counter products.

Compatibility and Stability. When addressing questions regarding injectable drugs, careful attention must be paid to the concentrations of all drugs, the admixture solutions, infusion rates and routes, and dosing frequency. It must not be assumed that medications listed as compatible under specific conditions will also be compatible at higher concentrations or in different solutions. Technicians should ask the pharmacist to help them learn how to interpret the tables provided in these references, and should always consult with the pharmacist before applying information learned or before providing another health-care professional with this information. Commonly used references for these types of questions are described below. They are available in both print and electronic versions.

Trissel's Handbook on Injectable Drugs. *Trissel's Handbook on Injectable Drugs,* published by American Society of Health-System Pharmacists (ASHP), is a textbook that is often used in hospital and home health-care pharmacies. It focuses solely on injectable medications. Information provided by this reference includes data on the solubility, compatibility, and stability of many different medications. Specifically, it is useful to determine when two medications may be safely mixed together in an IV bag, in a syringe, or at a Y-site on an administration set. This reference also addresses special handling requirements of certain agents (e.g., glass vs. plastic container, light restrictions, filters, refrigeration requirements, and expiration).

King Guide to Parenteral Admixtures. *King Guide to Parenteral Admixtures,* published by King Guide Publications, Inc., is another reference that is useful for compatibility and stability of injectable medications. It lists medications and their compatibility with common infusion solutions and, when available, compatibility of medications mixed together in a syringe, by Y-site, or in other types of sets. A section discusses reconstitution stability under different conditions, and precautions to be taken in the preparation and administration. There is also information regarding total parenteral nutrition solutions and total nutrient admixtures.

Extended Stability of Parenteral Drugs. *Extended Stability of Parenteral Drugs,* published by American Society of Health-System Pharmacists (ASHP), contains stability data of injectable drugs that extend beyond 24 hours. The reference is intended for use by alternate site infusion practices, such as home infusion. It includes information to help assign appropriate extended expiration dates, select the best container or administration system for individual drugs, and identify the best storage conditions.

Compounding.

USP Pharmacist's Pharmacopeia. The *USP Pharmacist's Pharmacopeia,* published by U.S. Pharmacopeia, is a reference that includes the official standards and procedures to ensure the strength, quality, and purity of sterile and nonsterile compounded preparations. The individual drug monographs contain information on compounding, packaging, labeling, and storage of pharmaceuticals. The reference also includes information on veterinary compounding and food ingredients, colorings, preservatives, and flavorings. It is a useful resource for pharmacy compounding because it provides information on legal requirements and laws that apply to compounding practices, as well as articles on the basics of compounding.

Trissel's Stability of Compounded Formulations. *Trissel's Stability of Compounded Formulations,* published by the American Pharmacists Association (APhA), summarizes formulation and stability studies that are published for compounded formulations. Its drug monographs provide guidance for preparing the products as well as expiration dating, proper storage, and repackaging. Each monograph contains three sections: Properties, General Stability Considerations, and Stability Reports. Compatibility with other drug products, if available, is also listed.

Herbal Medications and Dietary Supplements.

Natural Medicines Comprehensive Database. *Natural Medicines Comprehensive Database,* published by Therapeutic Research Faculty, is a commonly used reference for natural medicines, including herbal and dietary supplements. Individual monographs list the name of the product, its common and scientific names, uses, safety, effectiveness, dosage and interactions with drugs, foods, labs, or diseases/conditions. It is available in both print and electronic forms.

Miscellaneous Resources

Other useful resources of drug information include material safety data sheets, manufacturers, drug information, and poison control centers.

Material Safety Data Sheets. **Material Safety Data Sheets** (MSDS) are information sheets provided by manufacturers for chemicals or drugs that may be hazardous in the workplace. The primary purpose of the MSDS is to provide information about the specific hazards of the chemicals or drugs used at the worksite (i.e., to describe acute and chronic health effects), to provide guidelines for their safe use, and to provide recommendations to treat an exposure or clean up a spill. Materials commonly encountered in pharmacies that require MSDS information at the workplace site include chemotherapy agents (e.g., doxorubicin and methotrexate), hormonal agents (e.g., diethylstilbestrol), volatile or explosive agents (e.g., isopropyl alcohol and ethyl alcohol), and chemicals stocked for compounding purposes (even innocuous things like olive oil and simple syrup).

Material Safety Data Sheets contain information that may be used to answer the following questions:

- What precautions must be taken when preparing and dispensing doxorubicin?
- Where should isopropyl alcohol be stored?
- How should an employee exposed to doxorubicin be immediately treated?
- How should a chemotherapy spill be cleaned?

Manufacturers. Pharmaceutical manufacturers are valuable resources for drug information. Most large pharmaceutical companies have Medical Information Departments that have access to published and unpublished information about their products on file. Customer Service Departments of pharmaceutical companies are particularly helpful with product problems and availability questions (e.g., drug shortages, discontinuations, and availability of new drugs or dosage forms).

Drug Information and Poison Control Centers

Formal Drug Information Centers are another source of drug information. The centers throughout the country vary in the types of services they provide, but most centers provide drug information for health-care professionals, assist with formulary management, and train pharmacy students, residents, and pharmacists. Some centers provide drug information for consumers as well.

Poison Control Centers are available throughout the country to help with poison exposures 24 hours a day, 7 days a week. Contacting your local poison center is easy, since the American Association of Poison Control Centers (AAPCC) has a nationwide number. In case of poisoning or if over-exposure occurs, the Poison Control Center should be called at 1–800–222–1222. Callers will be automatically routed to their local Poison Control Center. Local Poison Control Centers have valuable resources and training materials for poison prevention activities. Pharmacists and pharmacy technicians play an important role in educating the public about poison prevention.

The PDR and RedBook list Drug Information Centers and Poison Control Centers in the United States.

Rx for Success

Contact your state Poison Control Center to see how you can become a poison prevention educator in your community.

The Internet

The Internet can be a very useful source for drug information when it is used appropriately. Pharmaceutical manufacturers often have reputable sites because they should only have FDA-approved content on them. Government sites are usually reputable because experts have reviewed the information and there is no conflict of interest (i.e., they aren't selling anything). Pharmacy and medical organizations often have their information reviewed by experts in the particular field and are therefore considered reputable. Commercial or personal sites can contain erroneous and/or misleading information, especially if a product is being sold.

✔ Information found on the Internet should always be evaluated for believability, the validity of the source, accuracy, supporting evidence, and timeliness.

The availability of the Internet has improved the efficiency of searching for drug information. Many pharmacy settings that are not affiliated with major medical center libraries now have the means to perform literature searches, purchase articles on-line, and view governmental publications, often at no additional cost. Most pharmacy settings today have access to the Internet, and most hospital settings have high-speed Internet connections, which speeds the process even more.

Most of the publishers of the references that have been identified in this chapter have developed Internet versions of their resources. Internet versions are advantageous because the end-user no longer has to update hard copy references, and they can be accessed with a username and password from any computer with Internet access. Table 7–3 lists useful Web sites that can be accessed for drug information, including a brief description of what each site contains.

Table 7-3. Useful Web Sites for Obtaining Drug Information

Web site	Address	Description
Food and Drug Administration:	www.fda.gov	Home page for the FDA; contains numerous useful links for both consumers and health-care professionals
FDA Center for Drug Evaluation and Research (CDER)	www.fda.gov/cder	Contains links for consumers and health-care professionals regarding drug information, such as new drug approvals, drug shortages, safety information, and generic drug bioequivalence (Orange Book)
Drugs@FDA	www.accessdata.fda.gov/scripts/cder/drugsatfda/index.cfm	Contains information about FDA-approved drugs. Users can find package labeling information, generic drug products for brand name products, patient information (including Medication Guides), and the approval history of drugs
Centers for Disease Control and Prevention (CDC)	www.cdc.gov	Home page for the CDC; contains information about diseases, health topics, vaccines, traveler's health, bioterrorism, etc.
CDC Vaccine Information Statements	www.cdc.gov/vaccines/pubs/vis/default.htm	Link to Vaccine Information Statements that explain the benefits and risks of vaccines
National Institutes for Health (NIH)	www.nih.gov	Home page for the NIH; contains information about health topics, clinical trials, and the various divisions of the NIH
National Library of Medicine: Medline/PubMed and MedlinePlus	www.nlm.nih.gov	Home page for the U.S. National Library of Medicine. Links to Medline Plus (health information for consumers) and Medline/PubMed (references and abstracts from biomedical journals)
American Society of Health-System Pharmacists (ASHP)	www.ashp.org	Home page for ASHP; contains news related to health-system pharmacy and many helpful links for pharmacy professionals
ASHP Drug Shortages Resource Center	www.ashp.org/shortage	Up-to-date information on current drug shortages, including which products are affected and why, the anticipated time to resolution, and alternatives.
ASHP Consumer Drug Information	www.safemedication.com	Reputable Web site for patient medication information
American Pharmacists Association (APhA)	www.pharmacist.com	Home page for APhA; contains news related to pharmacy and many helpful links for pharmacy professionals
Institute for Safe Medication Practices (ISMP)	www.ismp.org	Homepage for the ISMP; contains medication error alerts, a section for reporting, products available for purchase, and medication error prevention strategies
Virtual Library Pharmacy	www.pharmacy.org	Contains links to pharmacy associations, pharmaceutical manufacturers, governmental sites, hospitals, journals and books, and more

Safety First The Institute for Safe Medication Practice (ISMP) publishes a medication safety alert newsletter for acute care, community, and ambulatory care settings. There are many tips in these newsletters that can be incorporated into your worksite to make it safer for your patients.

Conducting a Search Using MedlinePlus

The National Library of Medicine (NLM) is the largest medical library in the world. It maintains **MedlinePlus**, a database that contains health information for both health professionals and consumers on over 800 health conditions.[2] The MedlinePlus Web site (www.medlineplus.gov) also features a medical encyclopedia and dictionary, health and drug information in multiple languages, drug information on prescription and over-the-counter products, health information from the media, and links to clinical trials. The information is government sponsored and updated daily.

Use of the MedlinePlus Web site to find information on diseases or consumer drug information is simple, using the following steps:

1. To search for a specific disease or medical condition, go to http://medlineplus.gov
2. Click on "Health Topics."
3. Diseases and conditions can be searched by the first letter of the topic, broad group (body location or system, disorders and conditions, diagnosis and therapy, demographics, or health and wellness), or frequently requested topics.
4. Clicking on the "Drugs & Supplements" tab will enable you to search for consumer drug information. There are also links to the FDA (recalls, warnings, and safety information), clinical trials listings, and Medline/PubMed. Click on the first letter of the brand or generic name of the drug or product to access drug information. The source of the drug information on this site comes from AHFS Consumer Medication Information, a product of the American Society of Health-System Pharmacists (ASHP) and FDA-approved package labeling.
5. Click on the first letter of an herb or dietary supplement to access detailed information. The source of this information is from Natural Standard®, which is an international research group that collects and evaluates evidence on natural products.

On the MedlinePlus home page, a topic can also be searched by typing in a key word in the "Search" window.

Conducting a Search Using Medline/PubMed

Although MedlinePlus has links to recently published health professions articles, the best way to research the science literature is to perform a Medline search. **Medline** is a database containing over 18 million article references published in approximately 5,400 biomedical journals.[3] **PubMed** is a free Web-based searching system, sponsored by the National Library of Medicine, which can be used to access specific Medline journal citations. PubMed also contains links to full-text articles and related articles.

Searching in PubMed is relatively simple, and there is an online help section to explain its features and assist with performing more complicated searches. Enter your search terms into the query box and then either hit the "enter" key on your keyboard or click "Go." You can type multiple terms into the search box, and PubMed will automatically combine similar terms. For example, if you type in "vitamin C common cold," PubMed will automatically combine "vitamin C" and "common cold." You can also use the terms *and, or*, and *not* to combine sets and narrow your search. For example, if you type "vitamin C AND common cold," you will access all of the citations that have "vitamin C" and "common cold" as subjects in the articles. This strategy is most commonly used to access citations that are pertinent to your topic. If you type in "vitamin C OR common cold," you will get all citations with either "vitamin C" or "common cold" as the subjects in articles (and many more citations). If you type "vitamin C NOT common cold," it will eliminate any citations that have "common cold" as the subjects in articles about vitamin C (and much fewer citations). The term NOT is the least used when doing searches, since it may eliminate citations that may be useful. To help to narrow down your search, you can apply limits, such as English language, human subjects, age, publication year(s), etc. You can also search by the author's name or the name of the journal if you are looking for a specific article.

Following is a sample search. Your quest is to search for articles on the value of pharmacy technician certification.

1. Go to www.nlm.nih.gov. Click on "PubMed" on the list of databases and resources to get to the PubMed Web site.
2. In the search window, type "pharmacy technicians *and* certification."

3. Either hit the "enter" key on your keyboard, or click "Search."
4. The results of your search contain all of those articles that contain both pharmacy technicians and certification as subjects in the articles.
5. To view more details of one of the citations, click on the blue hypertext title (to the right of the number of the citation).
6. If you would like to save multiple citations, select the citations you want by clicking the checkboxes to the left of the citations you want to save.

Just above and below the citations, there is a display option, which is set to "Summary," but can be changed to display abstracts and other details. After you have selected the citations you wish to save, select "Abstract" from the display menu and then click "Apply."

The citations you selected will show up with the abstracts (assuming there was an abstract available). Using your browser's print function, you can print out the citations with the abstracts.

As illustrated with this example, PubMed is useful for searching for practice-related issues, such as the value and/or role of pharmacy technicians, in addition to clinically focused questions. A PubMed search can be useful prior to expanding a service or evaluating an existing pharmacy service. Fortunately, many publishers have full-text articles available for purchase, enabling practice sites that are miles from a medical and/or pharmacy library to obtain pertinent articles at the click of a button.

Table 7–4 summarizes common types of drug information requests and the references likely to contain such information.

Table 7–4. Common Drug Information Requests and Reference Sources

Type of Information Needed	References Likely to Have the Information
Product Availability dosage form, product strength, brand and generic name, manufacturer, indication	Facts & Comparisons, Drug Information Handbook, Internet, PDR, Micromedex, Clinical Pharmacology, RedBook (not indication), USPDI, Pharmaceutical Manufacturer
Product Identification dosage form, product strength, brand and generic name, manufacturer, colored photographs of tablets/capsules	Facts & Comparisons, PDR, Clinical Pharmacology, USPDI, Micromedex
Drug Uses FDA-approved indications, other uses of the agent	AHFS, Clinical Pharmacology, Facts & Comparisons, Drug Information Handbook, PDR (FDA-approved indications only), Micromedex, USPDI
Drug Monographs general drug information, pharmacology, indications and uses, drug interactions, admixture information, doses, adverse effects, drug interactions	AHFS, Clinical Pharmacology, Facts & Comparisons, Drug Information Handbook, Micromedex, PDR, USPDI
Injectable Drug Compatibility/Stability Information drug diluent and solution, compatibilities, drug compatibility, conditions for handling and storing products (i.e., glass vs. plastic container, protection from light, filters, refrigeration, expiration, etc.)	AHFS, King's Guide, Trissel's Handbook on Injectable Drugs, Package inserts, PDR, Micromedex
Preparation	AHFS, King's Guide, Trissel's Handbook on Injectable Drugs, Micromedex, Package inserts, PDR
Calculations	Drug Information Handbook, Micromedex
Hazardous Chemicals and Drugs specifies hazards of the chemicals or drugs used at the worksite, guidelines for their safe use, recommendations to treat or clean up an exposure	Material Safety Data Sheets, Micromedex
Pharmacy Law Generic substitution (bioequivalence), Federal regulations regarding handling and dispensing	USPDI Volume III, Orange Book
Patient Information	Clinical Pharmacology, Facts & Comparisons, Internet, Lexi-Comp, MedlinePlus, Micromedex, Patient package inserts, Medication Guides, USPDI Volume I

Responding to the Drug Information Request

After the search for information is complete, all of the information gathered must be organized and evaluated before one responds to the drug information request. A verbal and/or written reply that restates the question and outlines the response should be made. Recommendations should be supported by references, if applicable. For example, if a pharmacist asks if a certain product is interchangeable, it may be necessary to provide proof that it is AB rated.

✔ One of the most important steps in answering a drug information question is follow-up. For example, questioning the requestor about whether the information was useful and/or if it was answered will ensure that the response was complete.

Asking if you can be of further assistance is also good practice.

Summary

Pharmacy technicians are frequently asked drug information questions by consumers, pharmacists, and other health-care professionals. Using a systematic approach when faced with a drug information question will aid in understanding the nature of the request, obtaining pertinent background information, and successfully answering the question. There are numerous resources available to assist with answering drug information requests. Becoming familiar with common resources will make the search process more efficient. It is critical for pharmacy technicians to be able to differentiate between basic drug information questions that can be answered by technicians and questions in which clinical judgment is required and, therefore, should only be answered by a pharmacist.

Self-Assessment Questions

1. When a drug information call is received, the technician should identify himself or herself as a pharmacy technician, obtain the name and contact information of the requestor, determine whether the requestor is a consumer or health-care professional, and elicit the general question, but if the question involves professional judgment, it should be deferred to the pharmacist.
   a. True
   b. False
2. A pharmacist needs to identify an over-the-counter, sugar free, non-alcohol-containing cough formula containing guaifenesin and dextromethorphan. How would this question be classified?
   a. Availability
   b. Storage and Stability
   c. Pharmacy Law
   d. Calculation
3. Drug information questions relating to side effects and drug interactions of medications are best answered by a pharmacist.
   a. True
   b. False
4. Pharmacists should answer any question that is related to a medication shortage.
   a. True
   b. False
5. An example of a tertiary reference is the following:
   a. MedlinePlus
   b. Medline
   c. The American Journal of Health-System Pharmacists
   d. American Hospital Formulary Service Drug Information (AHFS DI)
6. Which reference would have information to determine the strengths that fluvastatin (Lescol) is available as?
   a. Facts & Comparisons
   b. MSDS
   c. Trissel's Handbook on Injectable Drugs
   d. PubMed
7. Which reference would provide information to answer the following questions:
   "How is injectable amiodarone (Cordarone) prepared (with what solution)?
   How long is it stable?"
   a. Red Book
   b. MSDS
   c. Trissel's Handbook on Injectable Drugs
   d. Orange Book
8. Which reference would provide information on drugs or chemicals that may be hazardous in the workplace?
   a. PDR
   b. MSDS
   c. Facts & Comparisons
   d. Trissel's Handbook on Injectable Drugs
9. Conducting a search using MedlinePlus would help you find what kind of information?
   a. Drug stability and compatibility
   b. Cost
   c. General health information
   d. Manufacturer's phone numbers
10. A doctor calls and states he needs to know the identification of a white tablet with imprint code "M C2." Which reference would provide information to answer this question?
    a. Micromedex
    b. Trissel's Handbook on Injectable Drugs
    c. United States Pharmacopeia Drug Information (USP DI)
    d. AHFS
11. A patient asks if you have a medication that she heard about on the radio. Where can you find out if a drug has been FDA approved?
    a. Internet
    b. Facts & Comparisons
    c. PDR
    d. MedlinePlus
12. Which reference would help answer the question: "Does Prinivil have a generic equivalent?"
    a. Orange Book
    b. MSDS

Self-Assessment Questions

c. PubMed
d. PDR

13. Which reference will help answer the question: "What is the controlled substance schedule for Ambien?"
    a. Facts & Comparisons
    b. Trissel's Handbook of Injectable Drugs
    c. Red Book
    d. MSDS
14. Which reference would be used to find the answer to the question, "How many milliliters are in a teaspoon?":
    a. Drug Information Handbook Appendix
    b. PDR
    c. MSDS
    d. Facts & Comparisons
15. What is the best place to find the latest information on bioterrorism and the smallpox vaccine?
    a. Facts & Comparisons
    b. PDR
    c. MedlinePlus
    d. Red Book

Self-Assessment Answers

1. a. When approached with a drug information request, technicians should identify themselves as pharmacy technicians so that the person asking the question will know whom they are speaking with. It is important to know who the person initiating the request is and to get contact information (phone, fax, pager, etc.) in case the person needs to be called back. Knowing information about the requestor, his or her training, and knowledge of the subject will impact what and how the final response will be given. If there is any doubt about the nature of the question, the technician should defer the question to the pharmacist.
2. a. This drug information question is related to product availability. Pharmacy technicians may be asked by their pharmacist to help identify specific types of products or formulations to purchase.
3. a. Drug interaction and side effect questions are complex. They involve patient-specific information, interpretation of printed drug information, and clinical judgment. Therefore, a pharmacist should always answer them.
4. b. Although it is best for the pharmacist to approve alternative agents in the event of a medication shortage, the technician can find out more information about the shortage—for example, the reason for the shortage, if other dose forms are available, and how long the shortage is anticipated to last. Resources to assist in shortage information include the drug manufacturer, the FDA (www.fda.gov/cder), and ASHP's drug shortage Web site (www.ashp.org/shortage).
5. d. The American Hospital Formulary Service Drug Information (AHFS DI) is a general drug information textbook that is considered a tertiary reference. MedlinePlus and Medline are online databases that are considered secondary references. The American Journal of Health-System Pharmacists (AJHP) is a scientific journal, which contains original articles, and is therefore considered a primary reference.
6. a. Facts & Comparisons is the only reference listed that would provide the available dosage strengths of an oral drug such as fluvastatin.
7. c. Trissels' Handbook on Injectable Drugs provides information on the preparation of injectable products.

8. b. Material Safety Data Sheets (MSDS) provide information about the hazards of certain medications. They specify hazards of the chemicals or drugs used at the worksite, and provide guidelines for their safe use and recommendations to treat an exposure or clean up a spill.
9. c. MedlinePlus is a government-sponsored database that contains information on over 500 health conditions and general drug information on prescription, over-the-counter, herbs, and dietary supplements. It does not contain information on drug stability, and compatibility, cost or manufacturer's phone numbers.
10. a. Micromedex has a tablet identification database in which you can search by the imprint on the tablet.
11. a. Although the Internet versions of Facts & Comparisons and the PDR are more up-to-date than print versions, there may be a significant lag time until new drugs are included in the database. The Internet is the best place to find information that is "hot-off-the-press." New drug approvals can be found on the FDA's Web site.
12. a. The FDA's Orange Book contains generically equivalent products and lists the bioequivalence rating. The PDR does not contain information on generic drugs.
13. a. Controlled substance schedules can be found quickly in Facts & Comparisons.
14. a. Calculations such as this one can be found in the appendices in the Drug Information Handbook.
15. c. The National Library of Medicine's MedlinePlus contains information on numerous health topics and drug information in lay terms. Clicking on "Health Topics," then "B," and then "Biodefense and Bioterrorism" or "S" and then "Smallpox" will bring up the latest news and useful links to search for more specific information.

Resources

You can find a list of the top 200 selling drugs at http://www.drugs.com/top200.html.

Links to additional Web content, including ASHP Technical Assistance Bulletins and Practice Guidelines can be found at www.ashp.org/techmanual.

References

1. Kier KL, Malone PM. Drug Information Resources. In: Malone PM, Wilkinson Mosdell K, Kier KL, Stanovich JE, eds. *Drug information, a guide for pharmacists*, 2nd ed. New York, NY: McGraw-Hill; 2001:53-94.
2. United States National Library of Medicine. National Institutes of Health. MedlinePlus® Trusted Health Information for You. Available at http://medlineplus.gov. Acessed June 24, 2010.
3. United States National Library of Medicine. National Institutes of Health. Fact Sheet Medline®. Available at http://www.nlm.nih.gov/pubs/factsheets/medline.html. Accessed June 24, 2010.

Part Two

Foundation Knowledge and Skills

This section highlights the important foundation knowledge and skills that are necessary to understand the basics of medication use. A chapter on Communication and Teamwork is also included in this section since it is so important for all pharmacy settings.

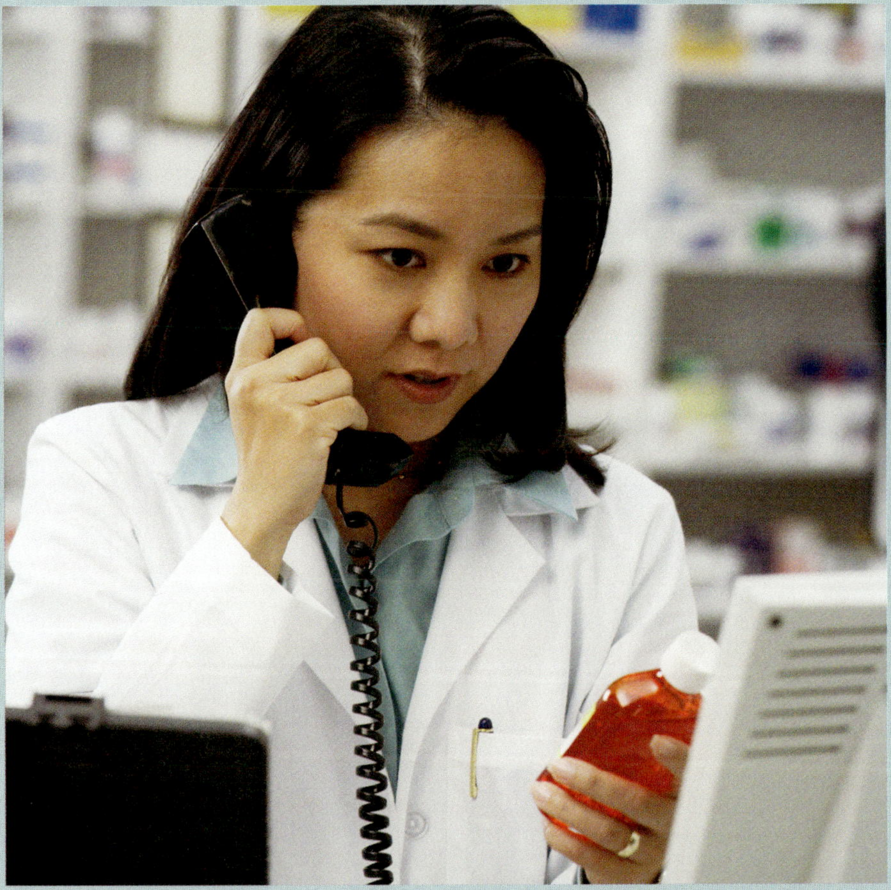

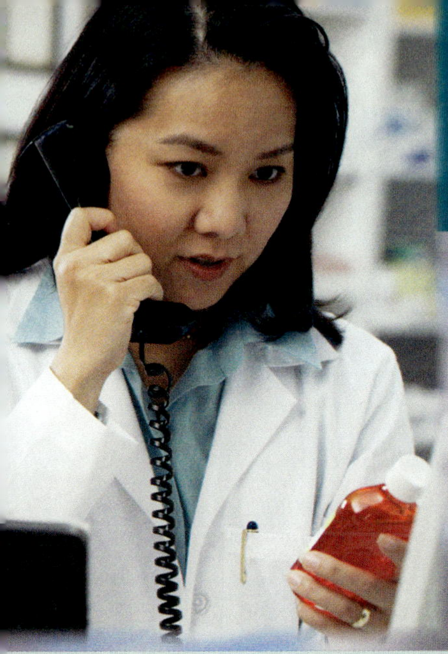

Chapter 8

Communication and Teamwork

Miriam A. Mobley Smith

Learning Outcomes

After completing this chapter, you will be able to

- Describe the purpose of various types of communications that occur within pharmacy practice settings, including the role of the pharmacy technician.
- List the basic elements of verbal and nonverbal communications.
- Given a specific patient encounter scenario, compare and contrast effective and ineffective communication skills.
- Describe how to vary communication techniques to improve success when working with special patient populations.
- Identify the types of health care professionals with whom a pharmacy technician may communicate, as well as effective strategies for those communications.
- Describe the types of behaviors that should be demonstrated by pharmacy technicians to promote effective working relationships with other health care team members.

Key Terms

body language Body movements or mannerisms that can be interpreted as conveying one's feelings or psychological state of mind.

closed-ended questions Questions that can be answered by a simple "yes" or "no."

communication The transfer of information, knowledge, facts, wishes, or emotions from one source to another.

empathy A sharing of or identification with another's feelings or state of mind without actually going through the same experience; the ability to view feelings from the patient's perspective, communicating acceptance or understanding.

health literacy The ability to read, understand, and act upon health care information to make appropriate decisions and follow instructions for treatment.

message Information, a point of view, or an idea that is being communicated.

nonverbal communication The exchange of messages by using means other than speaking to convey attitudes, beliefs, and emotions.

open-ended questions Questions that require a response other than a simple "yes" or "no"—designed to obtain as much information from an individual as possible.

patient-centered care The responsible provision of drug therapy for the purpose of achieving outcomes that improve a patient's quality of life; focuses on the patient's role and responsibility in his or her medication-taking and health-related behaviors.

receiver The recipient of a message.

response The reaction of a receiver upon receiving a message.

sender The individual who conveys a message to a receiver.

While performing their daily job responsibilities, pharmacy technicians must interact and communicate with many individuals. To facilitate successful communication, effective relationships must be established with patients, consumers, pharmacists, fellow technicians, and other health care professionals. Thus, it is important for pharmacy technicians to develop effective communication skills in order to help strengthen professional relationships and to ensure appropriate information exchange. These skills will help the pharmacy technician better assist the pharmacist in providing patient-centered care and managing pharmacy operations.

The purpose of this chapter is to help the pharmacy technician develop effective communication skills to enhance his or her value as a member of the pharmacy patient care team.

The Role of the Pharmacy Technician on the Patient Care Team

As pharmacists have expanded their roles in the provision of patient-centered care, the roles of pharmacy technicians have concurrently evolved. A pharmacy technician is defined as "[an] individual working in a pharmacy who, under the supervision of a licensed pharmacist, assists in pharmacy activities that do not require the professional judgment of a pharmacist."[1] As integral members of the pharmacy care team, pharmacy technicians work together with pharmacists to help ensure optimal and safe use of medications by patients and to help promote successful health outcomes.[2] This is accomplished through a synergistic application of knowledge, skills, abilities, and responsibilities. As described in Chapter 1, pharmacy technicians help the pharmacist with prescription preparation and distribution, with maintaining medication inventories, and with managing and administering pharmacy operations, and they also serve in other vital capacities within various pharmacy practice settings. These roles and responsibilities are not limited to interactions with pharmacists and other pharmacy technicians but also include other health care professionals and patients/caregivers as recipients of the health care–related services provided.

Whether pharmacy technicians are engaged in traditional roles or in more contemporary ones, the use of effective communication skills can play a major role in furthering successful versus unsuccessful encounters and greatly affect their related outcomes.

The Importance of Effective Communication Skills

Effective **communication** skills are essential if pharmacy technicians are to sustain successful interactions within the scope of their responsibilities. Strong communication skills help avoid misunderstandings and interpersonal conflicts and play a major role in ensuring patient safety. Miscommunications could also result in problems related to inventory control, financial and legal liability, licensure maintenance, breakdowns in organizational relationships, and potential loss of employment, so it is imperative that the value of effective communication by all members of the pharmacy patient care team be realized.

Safety First Effective communication strategies can help to prevent medication errors and improve the quality of patient care.

Effective Communication Skills

Communication occurs when one individual conveys information to another individual or group of individuals. The goal of effective communication is to ensure that the recipient party hears the same message, both in content and intent, as the deliverer, and that the intended result of that message is achieved. However, because there may be situations when the best communication efforts don't yield the intended result, it is important to develop strategies for identifying when this occurs.

The other important aspect of communication is listening. If the recipient of the message does not give the individual who is conveying information his or her full attention, he or she may misunderstand the message or fail to hear it in its entirety. Even under the best of circumstances, many things can go wrong with the communication process, in part because each individual processes information in his or her own unique way. The information is received and, in combination with the circumstances surrounding the reasons for the encounter, the recipient of the message draws his or her own conclusions. Consider the following scenario:

> A patient arrives at the pharmacy counter with a new prescription. After handing the prescription to the pharmacy technician, the patient is informed that the prescription will not be ready for at least an hour. The patient responds, "That's ridiculous! It can't take that long to take a few pills from a container and put them in a bottle. I want my prescription filled right now, or I'm taking it to another pharmacy where people know what they are doing!"

How should the pharmacy technician respond to this patient? How has the technician delivered the message about the prescription waiting time? How has the patient received the message given? What other factors need to be considered in this encounter? Specific information has been shared, but there is probably much information that has *not* been communicated that could play a significant role in the outcome of this encounter. In fact, each individual's views in these types of circumstances are based on different information. To improve communication, these different perspectives will be further explored.

The Patient's Perspective A patient is an individual who is receiving medical or health treatment. Regardless of the pharmacy practice setting, patients come into contact with pharmacists and pharmacy technicians in association with seeking or receiving health care–related services or information. Patients do not want to be viewed as objects, but rather as individuals who need the services that are being provided. A patient's underlying feelings and concerns about health conditions can produce behaviors that are challenging to deal with. Examples of health-related personal issues that patients may experience are listed in box 8–1.

Regardless of outward behaviors, patients need to feel that care and understanding is being extended to them. Even in circumstances when the correct words are spoken, unintentional confrontations can occur when underlying issues are present. This may be especially true when patients are facing acute illness, hospitalization, or other potentially debilitating circumstances. Viewing patients as objects instead of individuals with legitimate needs can get in the way of delivering patient-centered care (described below) by causing providers to mentally assign negative value to them (e.g., as unworthy, irrelevant, or unimportant).[3–4] It is important to show an active interest in the patient's concerns, to be attentive to emotional signals, to listen well, to exhibit sensitivity, to anticipate needs, and to meet expectations.[5] In addition, professional behavior should be exhibited by the health care professional at all times. Anything less will prevent high-quality care from being given.

In the scenario above, what was the patient's view of the circumstances? The patient had given the technician a new prescription. The medication could have been prescribed for an acute or new chronic health problem that is causing major stress for the patient. In addition, the patient could have been influenced by past experiences encountered at a pharmacy. Collectively, these feelings may have produced an unwelcome emotional response that was then directed at the pharmacy technician. In the patient's view, the length of time to fill the prescription was potentially connected to the level of competence of the pharmacist and pharmacy services being provided. The patient lacks more specific information about the circumstances necessitating the waiting time for the prescription. Was there more specific information that the pharmacy technician could

Box 8–1. Patient Perspective: Examples of Health-Related Personal Issues

Anger	Compromised coping skills	Grief	Loss of power
Anxiety	Denial	Health care insurance	Mental changes
Concern about body changes	Fear	Isolation	Social support availability
Concern about possible death	Financial worries	Loss	Spirituality

have shared to address the situation? Were there additional questions the pharmacy technician could have asked the patient to help clarify the patient's concerns? If so, how could these things have been accomplished to improve communication and increase the likelihood that the patient would allow the prescription to be filled—and return in the future for additional medications?

The Pharmacist's Perspective. Pharmacists are involved in providing **patient-centered care**, previously referred to as "pharmaceutical care." As defined, it is the "responsible provision of drug therapy for the purpose of achieving definite outcomes that improve a patient's quality of life."[6] Patient-centered care focuses on the patient's role and responsibility in his or her medication-taking and health-related behaviors. The pharmacist is responsible for ensuring that the patient will not be harmed by any given medication and for verifying that the patient understands how the medication should be used in order to prevent harm and achieve therapeutic goals. To achieve these goals, an important requirement is that the pharmacist must be able to develop the needed relationships with the patient and other health care professionals to provide the specified care.

It is important for patients to feel that health professionals care for them and are willing to address their needs. Pharmacists can accomplish this by communicating with patients in a manner that expresses and demonstrates a caring attitude in the degree, the method, and the expertise of the response. Of course, pharmacists cannot make patients take medication properly, but they can create supportive conditions under which patients can be encouraged to be successful.

But pharmacists are human beings just as patients are, and pharmacists do not want to be viewed as objects any more than the patients do. Pharmacists can struggle with their own personal lives. Pharmacy practice settings can be very stressful, and not all patient-related encounters are friendly or enjoyable. However, health care providers are expected to manage personal feelings while recognizing and considering the feelings of their patients. High-quality service is provided when better understanding of patient needs and feelings are achieved. When the goals of communication are clear, they help shape the responses—and, ultimately, the outcomes—of the encounters. The pharmacist does not carry these responsibilities alone. All members of the pharmacy team are accountable to the patient.

The Pharmacy Technician's Perspective. Pharmacy technicians also play an important role in the patient's safe use of medications and positive medication-related outcomes. This encounter may be in person, by telephone, or by another communication means. The first impression that the individual will have of the pharmacy and its staff and services may be the one provided by the technician. Thus, the importance of professionalism—appropriate appearance, behavior, knowledge, and responses—in a technician cannot be overemphasized. For example, if the pharmacy technician greets the patient by his or her first name instead of more formally without being asked to do so, this may be viewed by the patient as disrespectful. If the technician is engaging in a personal mobile phone call that causes an inappropriate wait for the patient, this could be viewed as unprofessional or disrespectful. Furthermore, inattention to personal hygiene, the wearing of inappropriate apparel (e.g., low-cut blouses or torn pants), the lack of a visible professional identification badge, and use of foul language, a loud voice, or belittling tones can undermine the relationships between patients and pharmacy personnel.

✔Often, the pharmacy technician is the first person the patient (and, in some cases, other health care providers) encounter in the pharmacy setting.

Rx for Success

Professional behavior should be exhibited by the pharmacy technician at all times to ensure the provision of high-quality patient care.

Returning to our scenario: the pharmacy technician had information impacting the wait time of which the patient was unaware (e.g., the number of prescriptions awaiting processing, the number of telephone calls being received, personnel availability issues, employee personal problems, and so forth). Raising the patient's awareness of these situations may not be easy, practical, or appropriate. Emotionally charged circumstances can be stressful and challenging and may feel somewhat threatening. Just like the pharmacist, the pharmacy technician may not have control over the circumstances facing the patient, but the technician's response to those circumstances is very much under his or her control. Remember that when the goals of the communications are clear, they help shape the responses—and, ultimately, the outcomes—of the encounters. The priority should be the well-being of the patient.

Using the previous scenario, how could the pharmacy technician have answered the patient to address the stated concern?

> A patient arrives at the pharmacy counter with a new prescription. After handing the prescription to the pharmacy technician, the patient is informed that the prescription will not be ready for at least an hour. The patient responds, "That's ridiculous! It can't take that long to take a few pills from a container and put them in a bottle. I want my prescription filled right now, or I'm taking it to another pharmacy where people know what they are doing!"
>
> "I can appreciate your concern about the waiting time. It may seem somewhat excessive. There have been several patients who arrived before you with complicated medication needs requiring discussions with their health care providers. Our goal is to ensure that every patient receives individualized care from our pharmacists, so it may take a little longer to complete a prescription than you may be used to. But please be assured that we value you as our patient and want to ensure that your medication and health care needs are met as safely and efficiently as possible. Maintaining our patients' good health is our first concern!"

Later in the chapter, we will revisit this scenario again and use specific concepts of effective communication to address the patient's concerns.

The Basic Elements of Communication

Interpersonal communication involves a complex array of processes focused on transmitting, receiving, and processing (or interpreting) information. This section will address the areas of verbal, nonverbal, and written interpersonal communication.

Verbal Communication. Verbal communication is the most common form of interpersonal communication. It involves a spoken message delivered from a sender to a recipient.

> ✔One of the most important things to remember about verbal communication is that "once it has been said, it can't be taken back."

For successful encounters, this key fact should never be forgotten and should always guide the communication. There are four main aspects of verbal communication: the sender, the message, the receiver, and the response.[7] A model representing these aspects is shown in figure 8–1.

Sender. To begin the communication, the **sender** conveys a message to the recipient. The initial sender of the message can be the pharmacist, pharmacy technician, another health care provider, or the patient. The message can be conveyed verbally (by talking), nonverbally (without talking), or both verbally and nonverbally.

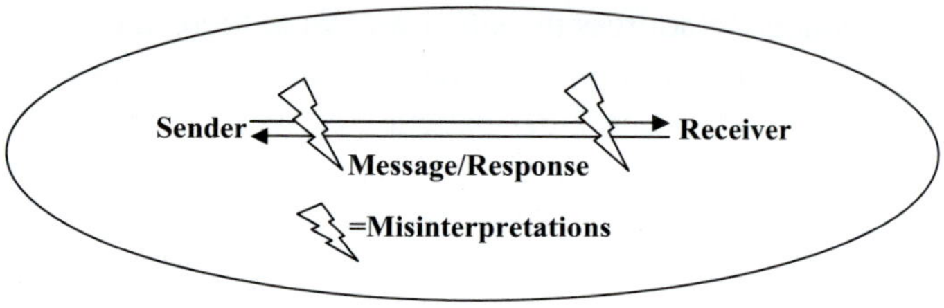

Figure 8–1. The Four Aspects of the Communication Model. *Source:* Adapted from Reference 7.

Message. The **message** is the information being conveyed from the sender to the recipient. Some messages are carefully considered before their delivery, whereas others are delivered more impulsively, sometimes as one of the results of an emotional situation. Messages can also be conveyed as sending "mixed signals" or with their real meaning hidden, confusing, or otherwise less than obvious. The vocal tone in which a message is delivered can also play a significant role in how the message is received. In many circumstances, nonverbal messages may also contribute to the wrong message being received by the recipient.

For example, a pharmacy technician in a hospital may call the nursing unit and say, *"Hello, Nurse Smith. This is Lois, the pharmacy technician. We* have *sent the STAT IV* [intravenous] *solution for Mr. Jones in room 271. Haven't you gone to the tube station to get it yet?"* A variation of the message could be the following: *"Hello, Nurse Smith. This is Lois, the pharmacy technician. We've sent the STAT IV solution for Mr. Jones in room 271. I'm just calling to make sure you've received the IV on time and to see whether there's anything else we need to send you for the patient."* Clearly, the second message is more patient-centered, and more likely to get a partnership-like response from the nurse.

Receiver. The **receiver** is the recipient of the message. This being the case, the recipient must interpret the message and decide what its meaning is. The recipient must not only understand what has been said, but also decide whether anything important has been omitted or conveyed with incorrect emphasis. Sometimes the perception of the receiver can be clouded by a personal opinion concerning the message's sender. The individual may focus on some facts that confirm/reinforce his or her prior perceptions and may disregard or misinterpret facts that change/challenge them. It is important to ensure that the recipient understands the message being verbalized, and to confirm that it is understood as the sender intended it to be. In that way, the conclusion that is reached by the recipient about the message is more likely to be consistent with the intent of the message being sent. Unfortunately, however, individuals process information and interpret it in their own unique ways, something that can lead to misinterpretation and conflict.

In the first message above, there was an implied tone of annoyance in the question. In addition, the nurse may have perceived that the message carried blame and the implication that something the nurse failed to do resulted in the lack of the product's receipt. This approach was more likely to foster disagreement, denial, and lack of cooperation. In the second message, the technician's approach was one of assisting and supporting, and voiced a concern aimed at ensuring that all the current needs had been met. The concern was extended on behalf of not only the patient but the nurse as well.

Response. After the recipient of the message interprets its meaning, the **response** or reaction to the message will indicate whether an understanding was mutual. The recipient will convey this response verbally, nonverbally, or through a combination of both. This is a point at which misunderstandings can be realized and clarifications offered, if needed, to help ensure that the intended message was the one that was received.

In the first message above, a typical response may have been: *"Don't you think I would have looked at the tube station first? You must think I have time to keep looking for something that should have been here already. People in the pharmacy are inconsiderate . . ."* The second message may have produced an entirely different response, such as: *"I really appreciate your double-checking to make sure I received the IV. Yes, I've got it, and I'll be able to administer it on time. Thank you for caring enough to check."* The second response reflects the type of response desired when communicating such a message.

Nonverbal Communication

Nonverbal communication is the exchange of messages by means other than speaking. This may include—but is not limited to—appearance and behavior, body language, physical distance, and physical contact. Nonverbal communication is usually interpreted to convey attitudes and emotions, and it can enhance (by adding clarity) or disrupt (by contradicting) verbal communication efforts. Awareness of nonverbal communication can help technicians communicate effectively.

Professional Appearance and Behavior. A pharmacy technician should maintain a professional appearance and behave professionally at all times. As a representative of the pharmacy team, the technician who maintains a professional appearance and behaves professionally helps form positive impressions of the pharmacy operations and services and inspires patient confidence. A professional appearance includes a visible identification badge, good grooming, cleanliness, and socially appropriate clothing. Professional behavior includes displaying a high level of respect to patients, coworkers, and other health care professionals. Jokes or political comments able to be overheard by patients should be avoided. Religious and ethnic comments, even when seemingly innocent, can cause many problems and are never acceptable. Telephone use should be restricted to conducting the business of the pharmacy except during designated breaks. Personal mobile phone calls and texting, except for emergency purposes, should be discouraged, for they can distract the technician from gathering accurate information from patients and can contribute to errors in the medication filling process by decreasing concentration.

Body Language. **Body language**, or bodily mannerisms that can be interpreted as unconsciously conveying one's feelings or psychological state of mind, can have a profound impact on how a message is received by the recipient. Facial expressions should correspond to the message being delivered. Pleasant smiles convey positive thoughts or feelings. Expressions representing concern should look different than those depicting humor or amusement. An expression conveying deep thought should accompany a discussion based on problem solving. Inappropriate expressions, such as lack of eye contact, eye rolling, and grimacing, can undermine effective communication, give the wrong impression about the intent of the message, or convey a lack of true interest in the patient.

To foster open communication and trust, the technician should use body postures that convey attention and interest, such as by standing with raised shoulders and head erect, slightly leaning toward the patient and with the arms at the sides, or slightly gesturing in a positive manner. Avoid body postures that may represent a lack of interest in or patience with the patient, such as arms crossed on the chest, hands on the hips, or a back turned to the patient during conversation.

Physical Distance. Physical distance, or the space between two individuals during an activity being carried out between them, may contribute to the success or failure of communication. The technician should determine an appropriate distance to maintain from the patient based on the nature of the encounter. Acceptable distances have been described as 1.5 to 4 feet for personal discussion and 4 to 12 feet for impersonal business.[7] The levels of privacy needed to be observed can help guide these distances. When gathering patient-related information that would be considered confidential, closer distances should be observed to protect privacy. When conveying concern for a patient's circumstances or situation, the distance of separation may reflect a higher level of closeness. When a conversation is ending, the distance between the patient and technician may increase, signaling closure. In addition, observation of the patient's body language is generally a clue as to whether the correct boundaries have been observed. Physical distance as it pertains to cultural differences will be addressed in a later section of the chapter.

Physical Contact. Physical contact, a situation in which two individuals actually touch, may help to convey caring or understanding. Some patients may appreciate this type of personal expression; others may not. The patient's comfort with being touched may arise from his or her personal beliefs, cultural norms, or traditions. As with the determination of appropriate physical distance, an observation of the patient's body language can help to guide a decision as to whether touching is appropriate, and, if so, when to do so. In addition, the technician can ask the patient if he or she desires to be touched. Physical contact as it pertains to cultural differences will be addressed in a later section of the chapter.

Written Communication

Written communication involves the transcribing of information onto paper or another medium for transmission, such as e-mail. Common written communications in pharmacies may include notes/memos, e-mails, shift reports, faxes, reports or documentation forms, entries in want books (inventory control), and prescriptions. As with verbal communication, once a message has been written and delivered to a recipient, it cannot be taken back, so it is very important that the correct message be conveyed to the recipient to elicit the intended response. Every effort must be made to prevent inaccuracies, errors, inappropriate content, and unprofessional attitudes or remarks. Care should be taken to compose clearly written information, spell words correctly, and avoid the use of slang or confusing terminology. In addition, written communications should be composed using a friendly tone, with brevity appropriate to their purpose, at a level for their intended audience, and including salutations/titles as needed.

In contemporary pharmacy practice settings, written communication may be required of the pharmacy technician in various roles and responsibilities. Written communication can be used when the pharmacy technician helps the pharmacist serve patients, engages in activities related to medication distribution and inventory control, and participates in pharmacy practice management and administration. Incorrect written communication in any of the above areas can result in undesirable consequences that can directly affect patient health and well-being, product availability, and overall pharmacy operations and finances.

The Patient Encounter

Pharmacy technicians can encounter patients in many of the pharmacy practice settings in which they are employed. The nature of the patient encounters will be determined by the type of practice environment, the designated role and responsibilities of the technician, the policies and procedures of the practice setting, and the method of interaction used.

Type of Environment. Different levels of pharmacy technician communications can occur in various practice settings. In all settings, technicians will communicate with their coworkers and supervisors. In community and ambulatory care pharmacy settings, common patient-related communications will occur when a new prescription or refill is requested, when patient profile information is gathered, and when a medication is being picked up. Communication also occurs when the technician answers the telephone and responds to questions about pricing, insurance, and product location.

In hospital pharmacy and other institutional care settings, most of the communications occur with other health care professionals rather than with patients. However, effective communication skills between pharmacy technicians and other health care professionals are essential for high-quality patient care and harmonious work environments. As the scope of technician responsibilities grows, the reasons and opportunities for direct patient communication may also increase. Patient and health care professional communications in other types of practice settings are based on the level of available or necessary direct contact.

Purpose of the Encounter. In proper communications, the purpose of the encounter needs to be understood by each individual involved in the communication exchange to establish essential relationships and provide for the exchange of necessary information. For example, when a technician asks a patient a question, such as when completing a patient profile, the purpose is to gather information to initiate a specific action or clarify an issue. In this case, an action would include recording a patient's allergy in the profile, which might facilitate a patient counseling session by the pharmacist. In a community or mail-order pharmacy setting, a technician may ask the patient for verification of medication insurance coverage or payment for the medications. In a hospital setting, a pharmacy technician may enter a patient's room to check on the status of an IV fluid or to return unused/expired medications to the pharmacy. If the goal of the communication is to solve a problem, the importance or urgency of the issue must be assessed, and the proper questions asked when gathering information to help ensure that the desired outcome is achieved.

Method of the Encounter. The method of the encounter determines the role that verbal and nonverbal communication factors play in its success. Common methods include face-to-face encounters, telephone encounters, and Internet and other electronic means of communication.

Face-to-Face Encounters. In a face-to-face encounter, both verbal and nonverbal communications are important. How individuals relate to each other during this type of encounter will depend on what was spoken and how, what body movements were used during the conversation, and the environment in which it took place. All conscious and unconscious actions have the potential to impact the intent of the communication and either prevent or cause misunderstandings, so great care should be taken to remain aware of personal behavior.

Telephone Encounters. In telephone encounters, nonverbal communication does not play as significant a role as in verbal communication. Clearly, what was spoken and how it was spoken (e.g., in an enthusiastic, abrupt, or negative tone) can affect how the message is perceived by its recipient. A pleasant tone, for example, helps convey courtesy and caring. A loud or abrupt tone may convey annoyance, impatience, or disrespect, all of which may prompt hostility during the encounter. A pleasant attitude and a smile, even though unseen by an individual on the other side of the telephone, can be very apparent.

At the beginning of a telephone conversation, pharmacy technicians should identify themselves by stating name and title and the name of the pharmacy or pharmacy department. It is also very important to speak clearly and not too rapidly, pronouncing words completely and avoiding the use of slang or potentially confusing terminology.

Internet and Other Electronic Communication Methods. The use of the Internet and fax for communications has greatly expanded in pharmacy practice settings. Evolving uses are for electronic transmittal of prescriptions, medication refill requests, drug information requests and retrieval, product ordering, and other potential time-saving uses. Neither verbal nor nonverbal communication factors play a significant role in these types of encounters, but the principles of effective written communication should be followed.

Internet "etiquette" also dictates that e-mail and business-related messages not be composed of all uppercase letters, to prevent the perception of "shouting" or "scolding." In addition, when sending a message to a patient or other business-related client, use the business e-mail address or official Web site address so that the recipient knows that the message is legitimate. Never ask patients to provide information over the Internet that could lead to "identity theft" unless it is transmitted through the use of a security-encrypted Web site. When faxing documents, be sure to include a cover sheet to ensure that all information reaches the appropriate person, and follow the Health Insurance Portability and Accountability Act (HIPAA) requirements to maintain the privacy of patient protected health information (PHI). For important documents, use a method of verification of information receipt.

Gathering and Delivering Information. When the intent of the communication effort is to gather information (i.e., by asking a question) or to deliver information (i.e., to answer a question), several key elements must be considered to bring about success.

Approach. When asking a question, a pharmacy technician makes a decision about the best way to approach and conduct a conversation with a patient. He or she makes a behavior choice to use passive, assertive, or aggressive behavior when making the request. Underlying this choice is the desire to avoid conflict and accomplish the goal. Passive behavior, in which an individual does not take an active role or lets others make decisions, is often used to avoid involvement; it can also be used to evade responsibility for something. This behavior is not an effective problem-solving technique and can actually lead to harmful results (e.g., not correcting a patient's medication adherence problem to avoid conflict). Assertive behavior, in which an individual displays a confident attitude and expression of ideas as well as opinions, is used to directly address an issue, resolve conflict, and actively participate in the conversation to produce a positive outcome. The element of mutual respect is usually present.[8] Aggressive behavior, in which an individual displays an overbearing or intimidating attitude, can result in conflict and create a combative atmosphere and a perception of disrespect. This approach usually results in an angry and disruptive encounter.[8] An assertive approach to communication and problem solving is superior to an aggressive one, because it promotes and builds the relationships needed for successful patient care and productive work environments.[8–9]

Asking the Question. In order for the pharmacy technician to receive an accurate and complete answer from the patient, the correct question needs to be asked in a manner likely to gather the most comprehensive level of needed information. This may require determination of the type of question to ask. Two common types of questions are "closed-ended" and "open-ended" questions.

Closed-ended questions are questions that can be answered with a simple "yes" or "no." An example of a closed-ended question is, *"Are you allergic to any medications?"* **Open-ended questions** are questions that require a more elaborate response. An example of an open-ended question is, *"What medications are you allergic to?"*

✔Open-ended questions should be used to gather more in-depth answers.

They can help verify or clarify understanding of information by requesting patients to elaborate on the concepts being discussed. A follow-up question may be needed to further elicit important information. If the patient indicates the presence of a medication allergy, an important follow-up question to ask would be, *"Can you describe what happens when you take the medication?"* The question, *"What else are you allergic to?"* would be asked until the patient verifies that no more allergies are present.

Listening. After asking the question, the technician must listen carefully to the answer and observe any nonverbal communication being displayed. Listening helps the technician better understand the patient's perceptions, sense the patient's emotions, and hear what the patient is saying. It is important to remember that when an individual is talking, he or she is not also listening. Listening improves not only what is heard, but what will be said in response. By paying attention, with only necessary interruptions to clarify, the patient can feel the satisfaction of being heard and understood. Otherwise, if the technician verbalizes a response that reflects an alternate point of view, the patient may believe that he or she may not have been heard, which can prevent the continuation of constructive dialogue. To understand the needs of others, an individual must listen to what is being said by the other individual in its entirety. Listening also helps determine whether the question was fully understood. Avoid the appearance of "faking" interest. If you are not in a position to help the patient, arrange for someone to help who is better able to do so. It is also essential to not assign a personal value judgment to what is being communicated, for to do so can affect your ability to appropriately address the situation or concern. While listening, also be careful not to craft a mental response before listening to the patient's complete concern. This will help you keep from developing counterarguments to what has been said, which may foster a breakdown in communication when they are verbalized.

Responding. Strong patient-provider relationships can be built when responses to questions or concerns are addressed in an empathetic manner. **Empathy**, in which an individual is able to identify with and understand another individual's feelings or difficulties, helps establish a caring and trusting relationship.[8] These types of responses help convey to patients that they have truly been heard and that their feelings are understood and respected. Other effective response types involve restating or paraphrasing the patient's expressed feelings to ensure complete understanding. These manners of responses help promote open conversation with the patient, particularly when there are potentially emotional issues present.[8]

Returning to our scenario again, examples of responses follow:

> A patient arrives at the pharmacy counter with a new prescription. After handing the prescription to the pharmacy technician, the patient is informed that the prescription will not be ready for at least an hour. The patient responds, "That's ridiculous! It can't take that long to take a few pills from a container and put them in a bottle. I want my prescription filled right

now, or I'm taking it to another pharmacy where people know what they are doing!"

An *empathetic response* to the situation could be: *"You seem to be concerned about our ability to provide you with the correct medication in a timely manner."*

A *restating or paraphrasing response* could be: *"I understand that you feel that it shouldn't take that long to fill your prescription."*

Each of the above responses allows the technician to gather more information from the patient in order to get a better understanding of the problem, to open the lines of communication, and to help the patient feel that the technician is listening to his or her expressed concerns. These responses are not given until the patient has finished stating the original concern or issue to be addressed. Counterarguments, meant to contradict or oppose something that an individual has said, should not be mentally rehearsed as responses, because they prevent the use of empathetic or paraphrasing techniques. A counterargument to the above scenario might be: *"We know what we're doing at this pharmacy. It always takes at least an hour to get your medicine. What do you think this is, McDonald's?"*

There are four types of responses that should be avoided because they can be perceived negatively by the patient and produce an undesirable outcome:

A *judgmental response* to the situation above could be viewed as devaluing the patient's concern, as in: *"You seem to be the only one concerned about our ability to provide you with the correct medication quickly. All our other patients really love us and don't seem to care about the wait."*

An *advice-giving response* to the situation could be viewed as evidence that the technician thinks that the patient doesn't understand, or hasn't thought through the comments; it might consist of the following statement: *"You need to talk to the other patients who are waiting here. They will tell you that we know more about medicine and the prescription-filling process than you do."*

A *quizzing response* to the situation could be viewed as evidence that the technician thinks that the patient is confused or wrong; for example: *"Think back to when you have picked up medication at other pharmacies. I don't believe that you have gotten it as quickly as we are going to give it to you."*

A *placating response* to the situation above could be viewed as condescending, for example: *"Oh, you shouldn't worry so much about the length of time. Just shop around for a while until it is ready, and try not to get yourself so worked up."*

There are times when, despite all best efforts, unmanageable conflict occurs. Personal limits on the extent of involvement should be set and the issue referred to appropriate supervisory personnel.

Verification of Understanding. It is important that an effort is made to verify the patient's understanding prior to the end of the conversation. In this way, actions can be summarized, agreements reached, or reasonable alternatives suggested.

Honesty and Ethics. When addressing a patient's question or concern, nothing can destroy confidence or trust in a health care provider or practice setting faster than discovering dishonest and fraudulent answers or practices. Examples of situations in which communications with patients are difficult include incidents of suspected medication-related errors. A health care professional should always put the health of the patient ahead of personal concerns. Suspected errors should be brought to the pharmacist's attention immediately so that full disclosure and proper management of the patient's health needs can be undertaken. Cover-ups and related negligent actions have no place in a patient-centered care facility because they can lead to patient harm, legal action against the pharmacy and against pharmacy personnel, and loss of employment.

Confidentiality. Confidentiality and privacy are not only patient rights, but also legal issues. The Health Insurance Portability and Accountability Act (HIPAA) is a federal law that prohibits the disclosure of protected health information (PHI) to anyone without the patient's permission or outside of the process of providing patient care.

✔ When gathering information for inclusion in a patient's profile, every effort should be made to conduct this conversation in a manner that ensures as much privacy as possible.

In addition, patients may ask for certain products that could be considered embarrassing. A patient has a right to expect that the pharmacy technician will exhibit the highest level of discretion in these situations and obey all laws regarding privacy requirements. In situations when a message must be left for a patient on a telephone answering machine, caution must be used by the technician to allow the information to be given without violating the patient's confidentiality. For a more in-depth discussion of these concepts, please refer to Chapter 2: Pharmacy Law.

Medication Information and Counseling. As described in Chapter 7: Drug Information Resources, numerous questions are posed to pharmacy technicians in every practice setting, and technicians must honor the boundaries of their scope of practice responsibilities. For example, when patients have questions about the dosages, effects, and administration of medications or the choice of medications to treat specific health concerns, those questions should be directed to the pharmacist. A pharmacy technician should ask a patient whether medication counseling is desired by using an open-ended question, such as, "*What questions do you have for the pharmacist about your medication?*"—but they should not provide the actual counseling. This is true for both over-the-counter (OTC) and complementary and alternative medication (CAM). Pharmacy technicians must be guided by their prevailing state laws, pharmacy practice acts, and organizational policies/procedures as to their roles and responsibilities in the areas of medication information and counseling.

Communication Strategies for Special Patient Populations

Certain situations warrant modification of typical communication strategies to help ensure effective communication.

Angry or Hostile Patients. Patients are often coping with a number of personal issues related to their health concerns. Some patients are better able to cope with these challenges than others. Even with angry or hostile individuals, it is important to show understanding and caring to help ensure effective communication. Communicating with individuals who are angry requires the technician to recognize what may have provoked the conflict, as well as how to address or resolve it. As previously discussed, the technician must actively listen to the patient and observe body language to better understand the individual's feelings and perceptions. Then, the technician should express an understanding of the problem in a meaningful way, seeking clarification of issues when needed. If possible, the technician should attempt to address or solve the problem, if it is in his or her ability to do so. Issues that are beyond the ability of the technician to address should be directed to the pharmacist or other supervisory personnel for resolution. During conflict resolution, it is important that professional attitudes and self-control be exhibited at all times.

Patients with Terminal Health Conditions. Patients who are facing terminal illness and death need supportive care and unique understanding. Some health care professionals may find it difficult to communicate with patients in this situation without first resolving their own feelings about death and dying. It is important to ask open-ended questions to inquire about the patient's state of being, to be understanding of his or her feelings, and to respect whatever strategies are being used to cope with their circumstances. Family caregivers may be responsible for patients who are unable to fully care for themselves.[10] In this role, caregivers may not only be responsible for administering medications, but also provide physical and emotional support for the patient. These individuals can experience many of the same emotions as the patient, so it is important that expressions of support, care, and understanding be extended to them as well.

Patients with Mental Illness. Communicating with patients with mental health illnesses can be challenging for health care professionals. It is important to ask open-ended questions to determine their level of understanding of health-related issues. In addition, mistaken belief, labeling, and stereotyping are unacceptable and greatly hinder communication efforts. Genuine interest and concern should be exhibited through the use of patient-centered communication strategies.

Older Adult Patients. Older adults are the fastest-growing population group and account for the highest percentage of medication use (both prescription and over-the-counter).[10] The aging process can present challenges for older adults when it comes to their communication abilities. These challenges can include changes in memory, attention span, perceptions, vision, hearing, speech, and mobility.

Strategies for improving communication in this population include using open-ended questions, information reinforcement materials, materials written in larger type, proper vocal tone and body positioning (avoid shouting), brighter environmental lighting, slower speech, and patience.[7–8] It is also important, as it is with patients with mental illness, to avoid mistaken beliefs, labeling, and stereotyping, all of which hinder communication efforts.

Another consideration when communicating with older adults is their increased use of patient caregivers who care for them and assist in the management of their medications and health conditions. Although the use of caregivers may prevent direct communication with the actual patient, it is important that the same level of care and understanding be extended to these individuals as well. They should also be encouraged to ask questions or to facilitate the patient's ability to ask questions when necessary.

Patients with Low Health Literacy. Current information shows that as much as half the U.S. population lacks the adequate general literacy (i.e., the ability to read and write at a capable level) to effectively carry out their necessary medical treatments and preventive health care plans.[11] Individuals with poor general literacy skills have associated poor **health literacy** skills.[11–12] Health literacy, or the ability of an individual to read, understand and act upon health care information, is an important predictor of health care outcomes. It affects how an individual understands wellness and illness, participates in disease prevention, decides health-related treatments, takes medications, and follows self-care instructions.[12] Poor health literacy is more prevalent in the poor, minority, older adult, and recent U.S. immigrant populations. The consequences of poor communication in individuals with low health literacy include poor health outcomes (e.g., errors, hospitalization, poor quality of life, and even death).

Rx for Success

Technicians who are able to identify patients with these types of special needs and can effectively communicate these concerns with the pharmacist and other health care professionals are invaluable for patient care.

Problems with health literacy are not confined to individuals with low general literacy (i.e., reading and comprehension difficulties). Some patients may possess strong literacy skills but may not be able to accomplish their health care plans because of their high level of complexity. This is another reason why it is important to identify patients with general and health literacy problems.

There are various strategies that can be used by technicians in the pharmacy to identify individuals who lack general and health literacy skills.[12] These "red flags" include patients who

- Decline when asked to read or fill out a form, explaining that they have "forgotten their glasses" or "have a headache"
- Always bring family members or friends to fill out paperwork on their behalf
- Rarely look at prescription labels when discussing medication but only want to look at the medication itself
- Ask the questions contained in the patient information handouts
- Exhibit problems with medication adherence

When pharmacy technicians encounter individuals who have low general and health literacy skills, special strategies can be implemented to improve communication efforts:[11]

- Speak slowly (but not loudly) and spend additional time with the patient.
- Use plain, nonmedical, nontechnical language.
- Use visual images to improve a patient's recall of information.
- Limit the amount of information given to the patient at one time.
- Use open-ended questions to verify understanding of information provided.
- Ask patient to repeat (or demonstrate) what has been explained to him or her. Then repeat the information to ensure that what was heard was the intended response and is accurate.
- Make patients feel comfortable asking questions.
- Additional health literacy resources can be accessed on the following Web sites:
  www.healthliteracy.com and www.npsf.org/pchc/index.php (The Partnership for Clear Health Communication)

Cultural Sensitivity

In many pharmacy practice settings, pharmacy technicians will come in contact with patients from many cultural and ethnic backgrounds. Sensitivity to the cultural differences in these patient populations is necessary to help ensure effective communication. To help prevent health-related disparities and provide multicultural patient care, all health care professionals should seek to become more culturally competent, and be able to adapt the care provided for the patient in a manner that is consistent with the patient's cultural, traditional, and societal needs and beliefs.[13–14] It is also important, as discussed in previous sections, to avoid mistaken beliefs, labeling, and stereotyping, all of which greatly hinder communication efforts.

In communicating with patients represented by different cultures, it is important to assess their ability to understand and communicate in English (or whatever language is being used). Open-ended questions are a useful tool for accomplishing this. It is also a mistake to assume that just because a person speaks another language, he or she has an adequate level of general literacy in that language. For example, it cannot be assumed that when a prescription label is printed in Spanish for a Spanish-speaking patient, the individual can read the label in a functional way. Professional interpreters should be used when available. When using an interpreter, the technician should look at the patient while speaking, not at the interpreter.

Particular attention should be given to verbal and nonverbal behavioral cues, which may be different within certain ethnic populations.[7] Direct eye contact may be valued in some cultures but may be a sign of disrespect in others, particularly when exhibited by younger individuals. Some cultures may show minimal emotion when discussing health-related issues and are likely to be less responsive to touch by the health care professional. Differences in acceptable personal space also exist among different cultures. As previously discussed, an observation of the patient's responses during specific situations can help the technician determine the best method of response. Asking a patient about his or her preferences is also a good way to identify how services can be provided to address his or her needs. However, at no time should general assumptions be made about patient behaviors and beliefs based on a cultural or ethnic identification.

Communicating with Other Health Care Professionals

Pharmacy technicians will interact with various other health care professionals in the practice settings in which they are employed—for example, doctors, nurses, and administrators, as well as other health professionals. In the pharmacy, technicians will work together with pharmacists, supervisors, and other technicians. Technicians will also interact with representatives from pharmaceutical manufacturers, with wholesalers, and with other individuals who are involved in the management of the pharmacy operations. In every case, technicians must use effective communication skills to promote a functional work environment.

As in patient-related encounters, communication with other health care providers can occur in person, on the telephone, and by electronic means. The principles of gathering and delivering information, explained above, will enhance communication with all other professionals. On the other hand, poor communication can lead to frustration and lack of respect between professionals and can compromise patient care if important information is misunderstood, ineffectively conveyed, or omitted. The pharmacy technician must abide by role responsibility boundaries and make the best use of effective communication strategies at all times.

Teamwork

Teamwork is when individuals work together, in collaboration or cooperation, to accomplish a common goal. The working relationship between team members is important to the success of the team's efforts. The essential elements that need to exist among the team are trust, understanding, respect, and friendship.[15] These features help individual team members feel good about themselves, their team members, and their own roles on the team. All members of the team are interested in satisfying their basic human needs, which include security, economic well-being, a sense of belonging, recognition, and control over one's own life. When these elements are present, the team has a high chance of success. When these elements are missing, team members can become angry, depressed, hostile, frustrated, and offended. There may be egos that are threatened. In addition, reality can be clouded by perceptions, leading to misunderstandings, negative impressions, and the assigning of blame.

Pharmacy technicians, as members of the health care team, have a responsibility to promote the principles of teamwork and further the advancement of the team's success. This can be accomplished by adopting the following behaviors:[16]

- Cultivating trust and confidence among team members
- Recognizing the contributions of all team members
- Working with other team members to solve problems and develop ideas
- Minimizing politics by respecting professional boundaries
- Helping align the team around the objectives and priorities the members have in common
- Establishing respect and appreciation among team members
- Holding oneself and other team members to the same high standards
- Putting the team's goals ahead of personal interests and goals

It is also the responsibility of team members to identify and disclose unprofessional behaviors among team members that could jeopardize the team and the services it provides. In pharmacy settings, these situations (e.g., medication errors, drug diversion, substance abuse impairment, patient discrimination or harassment, theft) could result in negative effects on services, operations, and patient health. The pharmacy technician should play an active role in the detection and prevention of these issues by bringing irregularities to the attention of the pharmacist or appropriate supervisory personnel.

Whether a technician is a member of a small team in a community pharmacy or a large team in an integrated health care setting, adhering to the above principles will help improve team performance and overall organizational success.

Summary

As members of the pharmacy team, technicians have an important role in ensuring that patients receive the highest level of service and care. Good communication skills are required to help achieve this goal. To this end, effective communication must also occur in the pharmacy workplace between technicians, coworkers, and other health care professionals. The process of effective communication requires a continuous effort as well as commitment by all individuals to improving overall relationships and providing successful collaborative care.

Self-Assessment Questions

1. Questions that can be answered with a "yes" or "no" are classified as
   a. open-ended
   b. closed-ended
   c. aggressive
   d. assertive
2. For which of the following may pharmacy technicians instruct a patient in a community pharmacy setting?
   a. the selection of a liquid cough and cold reliever for flu symptoms
   b. the location of a liquid cough and cold reliever for upper respiratory symptoms
   c. the brand of aspirin that should be taken with warfarin
   d. which prescription blood pressure medication should be substituted due to cost

Questions 3 and 4 pertain to the following scenario:

A pharmacy technician discovers a medication error while preparing the next set of doses for a patient. Unfortunately, a day's worth of medication therapy has already been sent by the pharmacy and administered to the patient. After retrieving the original medication order, the technician discovers which pharmacist made the original error. This pharmacist has been known in the past to disrespect, "put down," and devalue pharmacy technicians in the department. The technician shares the uncovered problem with a fellow technician to seek advice on how to deal with this situation.

3. The problem described above and its resolution should be
   a. the concern of the pharmacist.
   b. the concern of the technician and the pharmacist.
   c. ignored because it has already happened.
   d. covered up to prevent a possible lawsuit.
4. The technician coworker recommends that the pharmacist who made the error be confronted by the technician, in front of the pharmacy supervisor, to put him in his place and make a point that pharmacists are not perfect. This type of behavior could be classified as
   a. passive
   b. assertive
   c. aggressive
   d. justified
5. It should be expected that the pharmacy technician would not take an active role in detecting and communicating, to the appropriate individual, which of the following situations?
   a. drug diversion
   b. patient medication nonadherence
   c. patient discrimination or harassment
   d. the determination of a medication dosage change
6. Making the statement, "Don't worry, I'm sure that you can take all of these HIV medications and live a long time," is an example of what type of a response?
   a. quizzing
   b. empathetic
   c. placating
   d. judging
7. Printing a medication vial label in a patient's native language
   a. will ensure that the directions will be easily read and understood.
   b. can help prevent medication errors if the patient is literate.
   c. adequately addresses concerns about health literacy issues.
   d. eliminates the need for verbal medication counseling.
8. Compassion, not returned hostility, should be extended to a patient who may exhibit anger toward the pharmacy technician during an encounter in the pharmacy, because the patient
   a. may be experiencing difficulty in coping with uncontrolled chronic illness.
   b. really doesn't like the technician and needs to be shamed.

Self-Assessment Questions

   c. will get the technician fired if all patients are not treated nicely.
   d. will not be able to detect a "faked" caring attitude.

9. Which of the following strategies can be used to improve teamwork?
   a. place the sole responsibility of accountability on the team leader
   b. revisit discussions and decisions again and again after finalized
   c. admit weaknesses and mistakes
   d. hesitate to offer help outside of own areas of responsibility

10. Strategies to improve communications when assisting older adults can include which of the following?
    a. shouting the information so they can hear it
    b. using larger font on prescription labels so they can see the information
    c. using medical and technical language so they can understand the directions
    d. eliminating medication counseling if the patient has a caregiver

Self-Assessment Answers

1. b.
2. b. Counseling patients on the selection of an appropriate over-the-counter or prescription product is the responsibility of the pharmacist. After the initial product determination, the technician may direct the patient to the location of the product in the pharmacy.
3. b. Pharmacy technicians are members of the pharmacy patient care team and are also accountable to promote positive patient outcomes. Even though, ultimately, a clinical judgment will be needed to determine the best therapeutic course of action to address the error, it is the responsibility of the technician to report the error to the pharmacist or pharmacy supervisor.
4. c. The technician coworker was seeking to "win"—to "get even" with the pharmacist for past offensive behavior. This behavior would not be patient-centered and would only be used to promote self-interest.
5. d. Each of the other listed situations are classified as either "unprofessional behavior" by employees or undesirable actions by patients that could have a negative effect on the provided pharmacy services, pharmacy operations, or patient health. As such, it is the responsibility of the pharmacy technician to play a role in the detection and prevention of these situations.
6. c. This response, although it may seem helpful on the surface, may be perceived by the patient as a suggestion that he or she should not actually be upset by the circumstances of illness. It does not acknowledge or respect the patient's feelings.
7. b. It cannot be assumed that a patient who speaks another language will possess the necessary level of general literacy in that language to read and fully understand the label instructions. If a patient is literate in the target language, this can help him or her understand the printed directions on the label, but even this does not eliminate the need to use other methods of counseling and verification of understanding.
8. a. Underlying feelings and concerns about health conditions may produce behaviors in patients that may be challenging to deal with.
9. c. Admitting weaknesses and mistakes gives team members a chance to help in the growth and development of others and helps increase overall trust among its members.
10. b. Using a larger font on the prescription label can help improve readability for an older adult with visual impairment if he or she is sufficiently literate.

References

1. White paper on pharmacy technicians 2002: needed changes can no longer wait. *Am J Health-Syst Pharm.* 2003;60:37–51.
2. Muenzen PM, Corrigan MM, Mobley Smith MA, Rodrigue PG. Updating the pharmacy technician certification examination: a practice analysis study. *Am J Health-Syst Pharm.* 2005;62:2524–2526.
3. The Arbinger Institute. *Leadership and Self-Deception: Getting Out of the Box.* San Francisco, CA: Berrett Koehler Publishers; 2002.
4. The Arbinger Institute. *The Anatomy of Peace: Resolving the Heart of Conflict.* San Francisco, CA: Berrett-Koehler Publishers; 2006.
5. Goleman D. *Working with Emotional Intelligence.* London, England: Bloomsbury Publishing; 1998.
6. Hepler CD, Strand LM. Opportunities and responsibilities in pharmaceutical care. *Am J Pharm Educ.* 1989; 53(suppl):7S-15S.
7. Rantucci MJ. *Pharmacists Talking with Patients: A Guide to Patient Counseling.* Baltimore, MD: Lippincott Williams & Wilkins; 2007.
8. Beardsley RS, Kimberlin CL, Tindall WN. *Communication Skills in Pharmacy Practice: A Practical Guide for Students and Practitioners.* Baltimore, MD: Lippincott Williams & Wilkins; 2008.
9. Stone D, Patton B, Heen S. *Difficult Conversations: How to Discuss What Matters Most.* New York, NY: Penguin Books; 2000.
10. IOM. *Retooling for an Aging America: Building the Health Care Workforce.* Washington, DC: The National Academies Press; 2008.
11. Weiss BD. *Health Literacy: A Manual for Clinicians.* Chicago, IL: American Medical Association; 2003.
12. Osborne H. *Health Literacy from A to Z: Practical Ways to Communicate Your Health Message.* Sudbury, MA: Jones and Bartlett Publishers; 2005.
13. McDonagh MS. Cross-cultural communication and pharmaceutical care. *Drug Topics.* 2000;144(18):95–102.
14. Brown CM, Nichols-English G. Dealing with patient diversity in pharmacy practice. *Drug Topics.* 1999;143(17):61–68.
15. Fisher R, Ury W. *Getting to Yes: Negotiating Agreement without Giving In.* New York, NY: Penguin Group; 1991.
16. Lencioni P. *The Five Dysfunctions of a Team.* San Francisco, CA: Jossey-Bass; 2002.

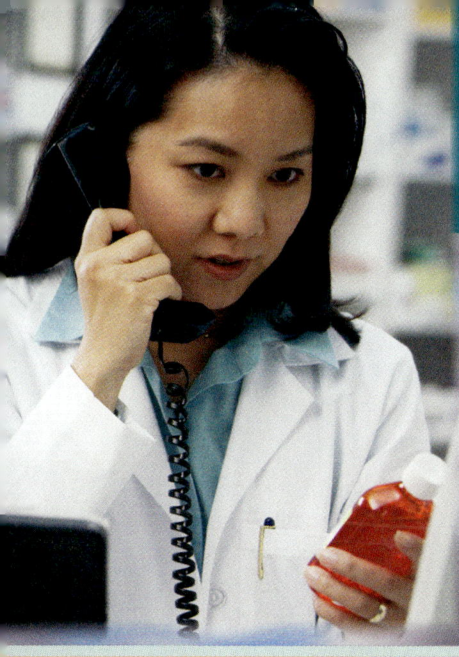

Chapter 9

The Human Body: Structure and Function

Alice J. A. Gardner, Bertram A. Nicholas Jr.

Learning Outcomes

After completing this chapter, you will be able to

- Identify the major structures of each of the body systems presented.
- Describe the major functions of each of the body systems presented.
- Describe common diseases and disorders that can develop when something goes wrong in a body system.
- Recognize the role of drug therapy in the common diseases and disorders of the body systems.

Key Terms

anatomy The study of body structure.

antigen A substance that is capable of causing the production of an antibody.

autoimmunity A misdirected immune response that happens when the body attacks itself.

diastole When the heart muscle is relaxed and the chambers are filling with blood; the pressure is at the lowest point in a normal heart.

digestion The process whereby ingested food is broken up into smaller molecules by chemical or mechanical means.

endocrine The internal secretion of substances into the systemic circulation (bloodstream).

endocrine glands Glands that have no ducts; their secretions are absorbed directly into the blood.

gonads Reproductive organs; testes in the male, and ovaries in the female. Gonads function to produce reproductive cells and sex hormones.

hormone A chemical substance produced in the body that controls and regulates the activity of certain cells or organs. Usually, it is a chemical made by a gland for export to another part of the body; it is not active at its site of synthesis.

pathophysiology Unhealthy function in an individual body system or an organ due to a disease.

pH The hydrogen ion concentration in a solution/fluid. The lower the pH, the more acidic the solution and the greater the hydrogen ion concentration; a pH of 7.4 is considered to be normal for blood.

perception The mental process of becoming aware of or recognizing an object or idea.

peristalsis Waves of involuntary muscular contractions in the digestive tract. In the stomach, this motion mixes food with gastric juices, turning it into a thin liquid called chyme.

physiology The study of how living organisms function normally, including such processes as nutrition, movement, and reproduction.

receptors A structure on the surface of a cell (or inside a cell) that selectively receives and binds a specific substance.

secrete To form and give off.

sphygmomanometer An instrument for measuring blood pressure. Sphygmomanometers are available as a mercury column, a gauge with a dial face, and an electronic device with a digital display. A sphygmomanometer consists of a measuring unit attached to a cuff that is wrapped around the upper arm and inflated to constrict the arteries.

systole When the heart muscle is contracting and ejecting blood from the chambers of the heart; the pressure is at the highest point in a normal heart.

tolerance A state of unresponsiveness to a specific antigen or group of antigens to which a person is normally responsive. Immune tolerance is achieved under conditions that suppress the immune reaction and is not just the absence of an immune response.

This chapter provides an overview of the structure and function of the human body. By organizing the information by body system, we can become familiar with the major parts of each system (i.e., the structure) and what they do (i.e., the function), as well as what can go wrong (which results in diseases and disorders). You'll find that the organization of this chapter is similar to that of Chapter 10: Drug Classifications and Pharmacological Actions, wherein detailed information about the drugs used to treat common diseases and disorders is explained.

Overview of the Human Body

In the human body the simplest functioning unit is the cell, which is the basic unit of life. There are many different types of cells in the body, and when cells with the same function or origin are organized in groups, the formation of tissue results. In turn, combinations of tissues form organs, such as the heart, lungs, brain, and skin. Organs within the body are then connected into highly organized body systems that work together within the body.

Each body system is linked to function as a single working unit to ensure that all body functions are in balance, which is referred to as homeostasis.

Anatomy is the study of body structure; the study of the collective functions and processes of the body systems is known as **physiology**. It is important to remember that none of these body systems work alone; in order to maintain a stable internal environment, the proper functioning of each system requires and depends upon the proper functioning of one or more of the other body systems. When the normal physiological function of a body system becomes abnormal and a disease state occurs, this is known as **pathophysiology.**

The Nervous System

Overview of Structure and Function

The anatomy (structure) of the nervous system consists of the brain, spinal cord, and a system of nerve cells (neurons) that connect to organs and tissues throughout the body (see figure 9–1). There are two major parts to the nervous system: the central nervous system and the peripheral nervous system. The central nervous system consists of the brain and the spinal cord, whereas the peripheral nervous system consists of a network of nerves that exit from the spinal cord and extend throughout the entire body.

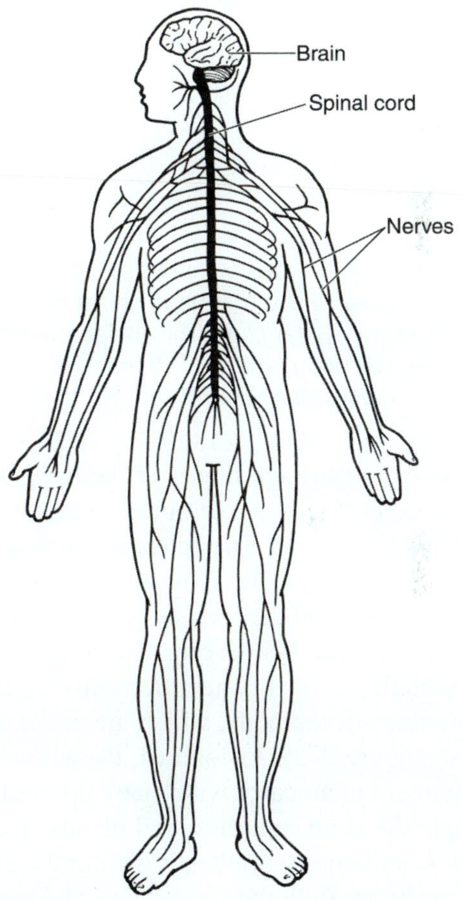

Figure 9–1. The nervous system. The nervous system is comprised of the brain, the spinal cord, and an extensive network of nerves. The system controls many activities of the body by transmitting electrical signals via neurons and the release of chemical signals known as neurotransmitters.

Further divisions occur within the peripheral nervous system. The afferent division brings information, such as temperature, from the external environment, as well as information on the status of internal organs, for example heart rate, to the brain. The efferent division delivers signals from

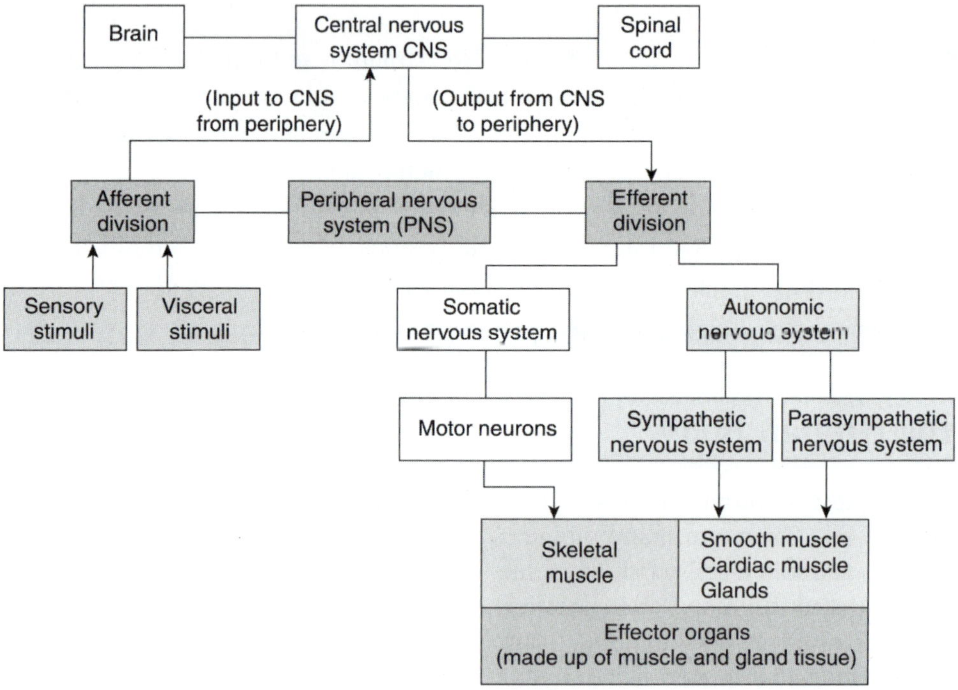

Figure 9–2. The nervous system is a highly organized network. The two major divisions are the central nervous system, which is comprised of the brain and spinal cord, and the peripheral nervous system, which is comprised of a network of nerves outside the spinal cord. The peripheral nervous system is divided into the afferent division, which carries sensory information to the brain, and the efferent division, which carries information from the brain to organs. The efferent division is divided into the autonomic and somatic nervous systems.

the brain to the organs and tissues of the body. The efferent division is further subdivided into the somatic and autonomic nervous systems. The autonomic nervous system is further subdivided into the sympathetic and parasympathetic divisions. Each of the nervous systems in the efferent division is under control of the central nervous system.

The somatic nervous system transmits signals to the skeletal muscles of the body, which are under voluntary control (see figure 9–2). In contrast, the autonomic nervous system communicates with many different organs, for example the heart, muscles, and glands, and it's not under voluntary control—rather, it is controlled automatically by the brain. Both the sympathetic and parasympathetic divisions have, in general, opposing actions in the body. The sympathetic nervous system works when the body is under stress and is best described as that which causes the flight-or-fight response, whereas the parasympathetic system functions when the body is at rest. The actions of the peripheral nervous system are possible because each division releases special chemical messengers called neurotransmitters, which bind to special proteins (receptors) in organs and tissues. For example, the parasympathetic division uses acetylcholine as its chemical messenger and is sometimes referred to as a parasympathetic-cholinergic system. The sympathetic division uses norepinephrine as its chemical messenger and is known as the sympathetic-adrenergic system. All of the divisions of the peripheral nervous system and their actions, whether initiated voluntarily or automatically, are under control of the central nervous system.

✔ The nervous system is the major communication system in the body. It receives signals from organs and transmits them to different organs in order to regulate their activities.

Communication by the nervous system is rapid, and changes in the body can take place quickly. For example, the brain may receive information from special sensors in the skin indicating that the temperature of the skin is too hot. Consequently, the brain transmits a signal to blood vessels near the surface of the skin, informing them to dilate, causing heat to be lost and, as a result, the skin cools. In addition to regulating everyday functions, the central nervous system is the area where information is stored and complex functions are regulated and controlled (for example, forming and storing memories, learning, feeling emotions, feeling motivation, and sleep).

The autonomic (involuntary) nervous system (ANS) is responsible for regulating the internal organs of the body, such as sweat glands, smooth muscle, heart, lungs, eyes, kidneys, and sexual organs. For example, the brain may receive information that the heart is beating too rapidly; it interprets this information and consequently directs the nerve cells of the autonomic nervous system to transmit signals to the heart to slow its rate through the parasympathetic division of the ANS. In contrast, the somatic nervous system, via signaling by the central nervous system, is solely responsible for regulating the contractions of the skeletal muscle.

The ability of the central and peripheral nervous systems to communicate with and regulate the function of organs in the body is possible through the release of neurotransmitters. These messengers are produced and stored in the nerve cells; they are released only when an appropriate signal is transmitted (see figure 9–3).

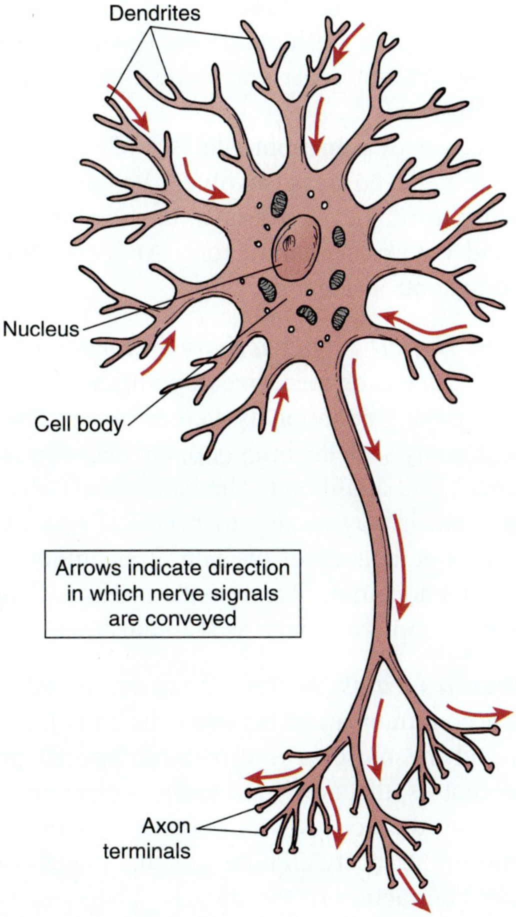

Figure 9–3. The neuron. The neuron is the major cell of the nervous system and is important in communication. It communicates by transmitting electrical signals by way of its axon and releasing chemical messengers from the axon terminal to organs.

Common Diseases and Disorders

Many problems can occur when the communication processes within the nervous system break down or are disrupted. Because many of these conditions are chronic, the technician should expect to see patients returning for refills on a routine basis.

Seizure Disorders. A seizure is a brief, strong surge of electrical activity that affects part of the brain. It can last anywhere between a few seconds and a few minutes; when a seizure occurs, the individual may experience multiple symptoms such as blank staring, strange sensations, confusion, erratic muscle movements, and loss of consciousness. There are many different types of seizures; epilepsy is a medical condition characterized by recurrent seizures. Many causes have been proposed, but it is believed that an imbalance between the brain neurotransmitters GABA and acetylcholine precipitates seizures. Antiepileptic drugs are used to correct the imbalance in the brain's electrical activity.

Parkinson Disease. A condition in which the nerve cells in the brain that control motor function begin to degenerate and gradually lose their ability to release the neurotransmitter dopamine. This leads to an imbalance between dopamine and acetylcholine. The symptoms include difficulty with initiating and controlling the process of movement, for example, a stooped, slow, stiff, and shuffling gait. Muscle tremors at rest are common. Drug therapy for Parkinson disease focuses on restoring the balance between dopamine and acetylcholine.

Alzheimer Disease. A progressive, degenerative neurological disorder in which brain tissue, in specific areas of the brain, begins to shrink and nerve cells are lost. Abnormal tissue formations are present in the brains of people with the disease. The primary nerve cells that are lost are those that produce the neurotransmitter acetylcholine.

Eventually, the condition leads to impairments in memory, thinking, reasoning, and the ability to communicate. These symptoms slowly become more pronounced over time. Other accompanying conditions include depression and paranoia. Drug treatment includes the use of cholinesterase inhibitors, which prevent the breakdown of acetylcholine.

Multiple Sclerosis. In the central nervous system (CNS), the neurons that comprise the somatic nervous system are covered with a fatty substance called myelin. This substance facilitates the correct conduction of electrical activity from the CNS to the skeletal muscle, and thus allows for coordinated voluntary muscle movement. In multiple sclerosis (MS), this myelin sheath is broken down, lesions appear on the nerves, and multiple symptoms develop—for example, speech and swallowing difficulty occurs, muscle weakness develops, balance and gait become affected, and eye muscles become paralyzed. Numbness and tingling in the extremities also occurs. The lesions in the nerves are thought to be the result of an inflammatory response triggered by the immune system in genetically susceptible individuals. Drug treatment is focused on preventing exacerbations and on treating the symptoms.

Pain. There are many forms of pain. Pain can occur in the skin; in the body structures, such as joints, tendons, and muscles; or in the organs or the brain itself when an individual experiences a headache or a migraine. When it involves the nerves, it is called neuropathic pain. It can also last for varying lengths of time. For example, acute pain can last for six months or less. In contrast, chronic pain lasts for months to years and may be accompanied by other symptoms, such as sleep problems, lack of appetite, and depression. Pain is perceived by specialized receptors in the body that transmit signals via neurotransmitters and specialized pain pathways in the spinal cord to specialized areas of the brain. The brain in turn, through a complex system of processes, releases natural opioids to dampen the perception of pain. Drugs known as analgesics are used to treat pain by blocking the transmission of pain impulses.

Mood Disorders. A mood disorder is a type of mental illness involving a disturbance of mood. The two most common mood disorders are depression and bipolar disorder, also known as manic-depressive disorder. Depression is characterized by a loss of interest in pleasurable activities; depressed mood; lack of energy; problems with sleeping; changes in diet (loss of appetite or overeating); difficulty concentrating; feelings of guilt, worthlessness, or helplessness; irritability or restlessness; and suicidal thoughts. Research suggests that one of the causes of depression is an imbalance of the specific neurotransmitters serotonin and norepinephrine, which are involved in nerve transmission within the brain. Antidepressant drugs work by increasing the levels of these neurotransmitters. Bipolar disorder is characterized by extreme mood swings; patients cycle between an agitated or overexcited (manic) state and depression. Treatment is focused on treating the manic and depressed states, as well as preventing the mood swings.

Anxiety Disorders. Anxiety is described as a feeling of being powerless and unable to cope with stressful events. In anxiety disorders, worrying is excessive and out of proportion to the situation so that it interferes with daily functioning. There are several types of anxiety disorders including generalized anxiety disorder, panic disorder, social anxiety disorder, and obsessive-compulsive disorder (OCD). The exact mechanism that causes anxiety disorders is unknown, but it is believed that a number of factors contribute to it, including environmental, genetic, and chemical. Pharmacologic treatment involves drugs that correct the imbalance of neurotransmitters in the brain.

Psychotic Disorders. Psychosis is a mental disorder in which a person's capacity to recognize reality is distorted. Schizophrenia is one type of psychosis. It is a chronic, disabling disorder that alters the way an individual thinks, behaves, expresses emotions, perceives reality, and interacts with people. Common symptoms include hallucinations (hearing or seeing things that are not real) and delusions (fixed beliefs that are false).

The cause of schizophrenia is unclear, but several factors are believed to be involved: heredity (genetics), an imbalance of the neurotransmitter dopamine in the brain, and environmental factors. Antipsychotic drugs are used to control schizophrenia.

Attention Deficit Hyperactivity Disorder (ADHD). A condition that is characterized by difficulty staying focused and paying attention as well as hyperactivity. It is most commonly seen in childhood, but may continue into adolescence and adulthood. The cause of the disorder is unknown, but it may be due to genetics, environmental factors, or a deficiency of the neurotransmitters norepinephrine and dopamine. Treatment consists of behavioral modification and drugs such as stimulants.

Myasthenia Gravis. A chronic neuromuscular disease in which communication between the somatic nervous system and the muscles is disrupted. Special proteins, called receptors, that are found in the skeletal muscle are destroyed by the body's own defense systems, and the neurotransmitter acetylcholine can no longer function to initiate contraction of the muscle. The symptoms are muscle weakness; difficulty speaking, swallowing, and breathing; extreme fatigue; and drooping eyelids. Drug treatment includes the use of acetylcholinesterase inhibitors, drugs that block the enzyme that breaks down acetylcholine.

The Cardiovascular System

Overview of Structure and Function

The cardiovascular system is comprised of the heart, blood vessels called arteries, capillaries and veins, and the blood (see figure 9–4). Blood is a fluid that flows throughout the body and contains blood cells. Blood is a mixture of plasma and cells such as platelets and red and white blood cells (see figure 9–5). The red blood cells (erythrocytes) are responsible for transporting oxygen to, and carbon dioxide away, from the cells of body tissues. Specialized cells, known as white blood cells (leukocytes), are also found in blood, and they help the body fight against invading microorganisms. Blood is also responsible for carrying nutrients to cells, and breaking down products away from them. Blood vessels function to transport blood throughout the body. The heart is a strong muscular organ that pumps blood through the blood vessels to all organs and tissues of the body.

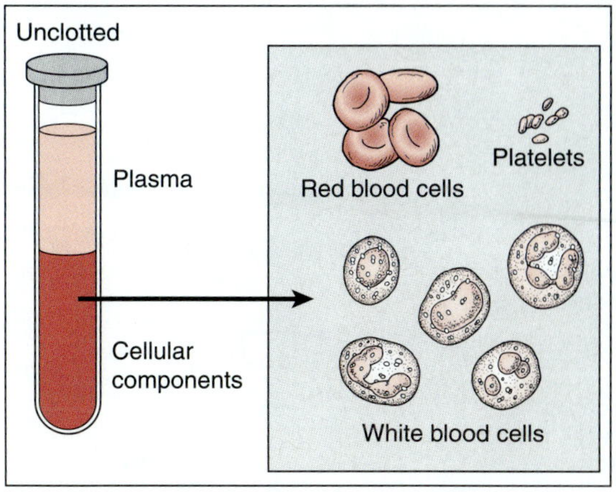

Figure 9–5. Components of blood. Cellular components found in the blood.

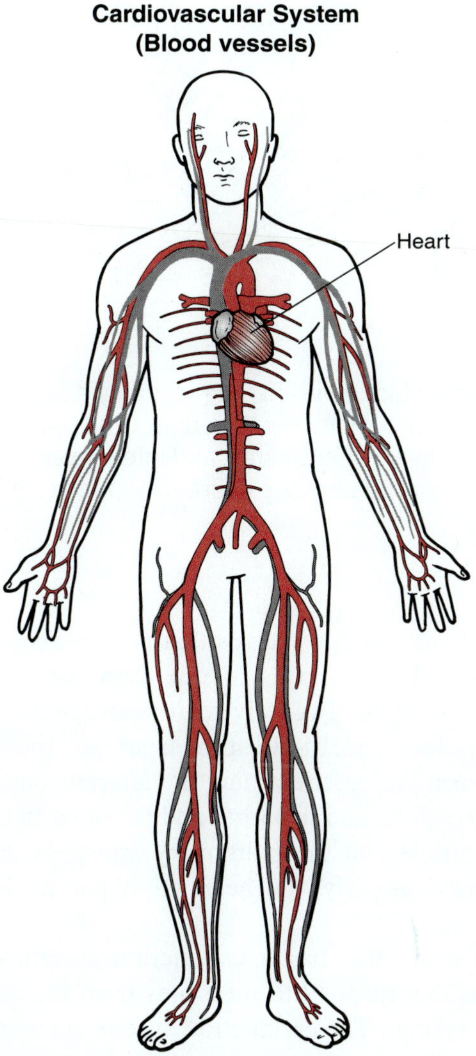

Figure 9–4. The cardiovascular system. The cardiovascular system is comprised of the heart and an extensive system of arteries and veins that transports blood, nutrients, and gases to and from organs. In general, arteries carry blood rich in oxygen away from the heart, except the pulmonary artery, which carries blood low in oxygen to the lungs. In general, veins carry blood low in oxygen to the heart, except the pulmonary vein, which carries oxygenated blood from the lungs.

The heart is a fist-sized, hollow muscular organ, located in the center of the chest (thoracic) cavity between the lungs and behind the breast bone (sternum). In the chest cavity, the bottom (apex) of the heart is tilted toward the left side of the body (see figure 9–6A). Surrounding the heart is a protective covering (the pericardium), which is attached to the chest wall. Beneath the covering is the outside layer of the heart, which contains the blood vessels of the heart (coronary arteries), nerve fibers, and fat. Underneath this is the middle layer of the heart, which consists of specialized muscle cells (the myocardium) that make up the majority of the heart tissue. This muscular tissue is responsible for contracting the heart in response to nerve signals from the autonomic nervous system. The inside of the heart (and its structures) is lined with a special membrane (the endocardium), which allows for the smooth flow of

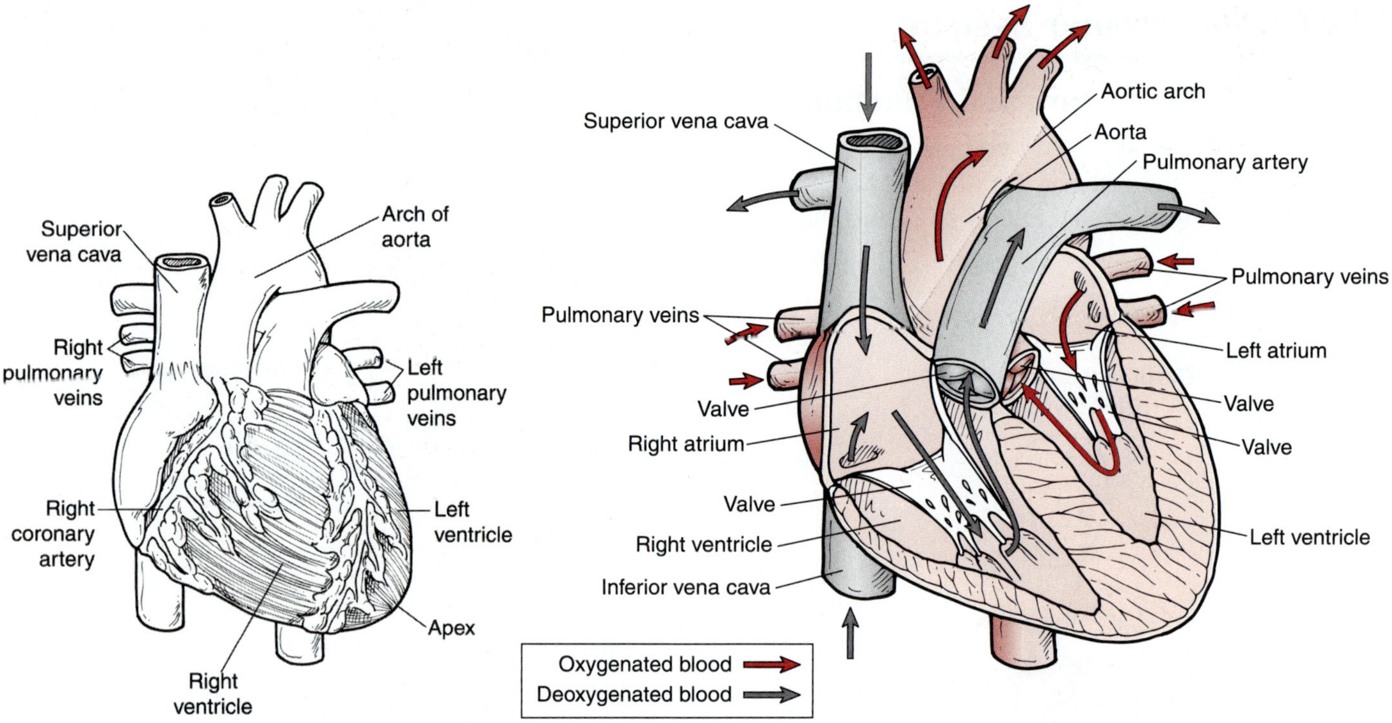

Figure 9–6. A & B. The anatomy of the heart. (A) The heart has its own blood vessels, the coronary artery and veins, which supply blood to and from the heart. (B) The structure is divided into four chambers. The upper chambers are called atria and the lower chambers are called ventricles. On the right side of the heart, the superior and inferior vena cava enter the right atrium, and the pulmonary artery leaves the right ventricle. On the left side of the heart, the left and right pulmonary veins enter the left atrium, and the aorta leaves the left ventricle.

blood. Throughout the heart muscle is a fibrous network of special connective tissue, which adds structure to the heart.

The heart is separated into four chambers. Two upper chambers are called the atria, which are found on the left and right side of the heart; below them are the two ventricles. The right and left sides of the heart are separated into two functional pumps—the right atria and the right ventricle function together as a low-pressure pump that pumps blood into the lungs, and the left atria and left ventricle work as a high-pressure pump responsible for pumping blood throughout the body.

Blood is brought to and away from the heart by blood vessels. Veins deliver blood to the right and left atria of the heart. These veins are called the superior and inferior vena cava when they come into the right atrium, and they are called pulmonary veins when they enter the left atrium. Arteries take blood away from the heart and they exit from both ventricles: the pulmonary artery exits from the right ventricle, and the aorta exits from the left ventricle.

The heart has four valves that prevent backflow and ensure that blood travels in one direction as it flows through the organ. Two valves are between the atria and the ventricles on each side of the heart, and the other two are between the ventricles and the arteries: one between the left ventricle and the aorta and the other between the right ventricle and the pulmonary artery. When valves don't work properly, the heart can't pump blood efficiently.

The heart also has a conduction system of nerve pathways that respond to messages from the autonomic nervous system. The conduction system ensures that the heart muscles contract at a controlled rate in a regular rhythm.

The cardiovascular system functions to pump oxygenated blood (high in oxygen, low in carbon dioxide) to every part of the body, and it transports deoxygenated blood (low in oxygen, high in carbon dioxide) from the cells (see figure 9–6B). Blood that is low in oxygen enters the right atrium from the superior and inferior vena cava and flows through the valves separating the

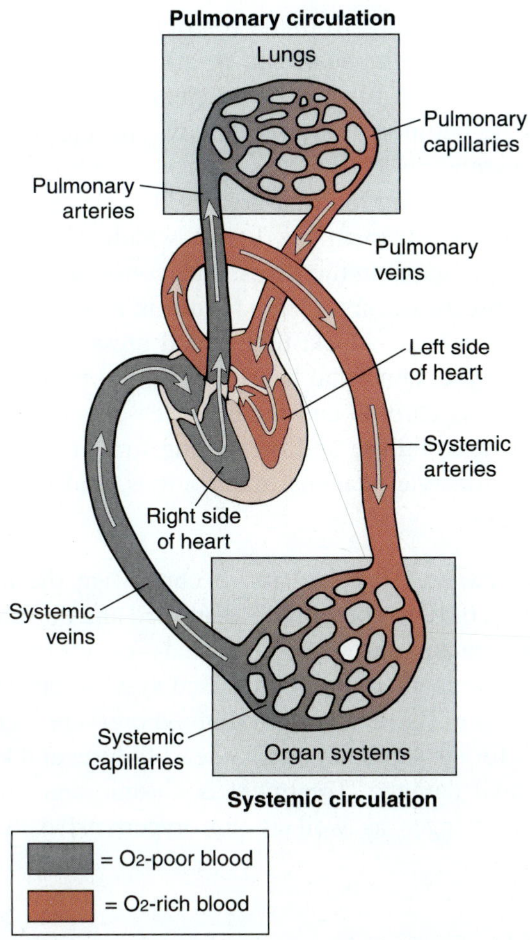

Figure 9–7. How blood flows through the circulatory system. There are two major divisions that transport blood throughout the body. In the pulmonary circulation, blood is pumped between the heart and the lungs to carry out gas exchanges. In the systemic circulation, blood is pumped between the heart and the organs and tissues of the upper and lower body.

two chambers into the right ventricle; from there, it is pumped through the pulmonary veins into the right and left lungs. In the lungs, carbon dioxide is exchanged for oxygen (see figure 9–7). The oxygen-rich blood then returns to the left atrium, and flows through the valve into the left ventricle where it is pumped throughout the body to organs and tissues via a network of blood vessels known as arteries, which branch into smaller vessels called arterioles. Eventually they branch into tiny, thin-walled vessels called capillaries. At the capillary level, nutrients, hormones, oxygen, and drugs are delivered to cells of all organs and tissue, and waste products and carbon dioxide are transported away by venules and veins back to the right side of the heart.

The cardiovascular system maintains blood pressure. Flow of blood through the chambers of the heart is pumped in a continuous and repetitive cycle. The two atria contract to push blood into their respective ventricles. Then the two ventricles contract to pump the blood out of the heart. As each set of chambers is contracting (**systole**), the other set of chambers is relaxing (**diastole**). Diastole allows the chamber to refill with blood. During this cardiac cycle, the pressure in the heart rises and falls. When the ventricles of the heart contract, and consequently eject blood from the heart, the pressure in the arteries rises. This creates the systolic blood pressure. Conversely, when the ventricles are relaxed and filling with blood, the pressure falls. This creates the diastolic blood pressure. The pressure changes can be measured by a **sphygmomanometer**, and these two measurements are an indication of blood pressure. Figure 9–8 illustrates the technique for measuring blood pressure.

Part 2

✔ Normal systolic blood pressure in adults is less than 120 millimeters of mercury (mmHg). Normal diastolic blood pressure in adults is less than 80 mmHg. Blood pressure is written as systolic over diastolic pressure: 120/80

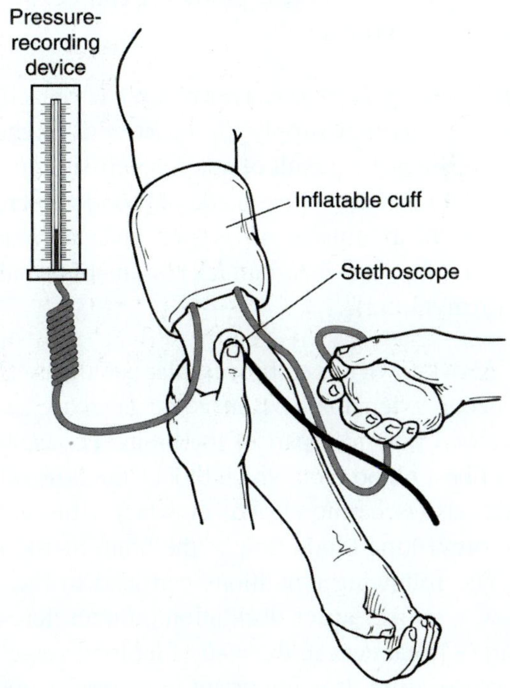

Figure 9–8. The sphygmomanometer. This instrument accurately measures arterial blood pressure. The inflatable cuff is placed over the brachial artery and the pressure in the cuff is varied to determine systolic and diastolic readings of blood pressure.

The heart contains specialized cells, called pacemaker cells, which generate electrical signals that trigger contraction of the heart and set the heart rhythm. The electrical activity of the heart can be traced using a test called an electrocardiogram (ECG or EKG). When the electrical activity of the heart is abnormal, a condition known as an arrhythmia develops. Drugs can be used to return the abnormal electrical activity to normal. In addition, the rate and force with which the heart pumps blood is regulated by the two divisions of the autonomic nervous system: the sympathetic and parasympathetic divisions. The sympathetic division increases the heart rate and the force with which the heart contracts. In contrast, the parasympathetic division slows the heart rate. Alteration of the rate and force of contraction of the heart can also affect blood pressure. The heart, in conjunction with the ability of arterioles to contract and dilate, can further alter blood pressure in the short term. Long-term control of blood pressure is also controlled by the kidney through its ability to alter blood volume.

Common Diseases and Disorders

When the regulation of the cardiovascular system is disrupted, a number of clinical problems can occur. Some examples are described below.

Coronary Artery Disease. This disease is caused when the blood vessels that supply the heart with oxygen become narrowed as the result of atherosclerosis, caused by fatty deposits (plaque) in the inside of blood vessels. This deprives the heart muscle of oxygen and can lead to a myocardial infarction (heart attack) or an abnormal heart rhythm (arrhythmia).

Stroke. Also known as cerebrovascular accidents (CVAs), strokes occur when there is an acute decrease or stoppage of blood flow to a part of the brain. The cause of a stroke can be a blood clot, which blocks the flow of blood in the vessels (ischemic stroke) or when a blood vessel ruptures, preventing blood flow to the brain (hemorrhagic stroke). The following conditions can lead to the development of a stroke: atrial fibrillation, atherosclerosis, an aneurysm (a weakness in the wall of a blood vessel), and high blood pressure. It is important to recognize and treat a stroke right away to prevent and/or minimize permanent changes in speech, language, vision, and memory.

Heart Failure. Also called chronic or congestive heart failure (CHF), heart failure occurs when the heart cannot eject adequate blood from the ventricles of the heart. One or both sides of the heart can be affected. If this occurs in the left side of the heart, sufficient oxygenated blood cannot be pumped around the body, and the individual shows symptoms of tiredness, shortness of breath, lower extremity swelling, and an increased heart rate (pulse). Fluid can build up in the lungs, which decreases the exchange of gases in the lungs, and, consequently, shortness of breath occurs. Heart failure is most commonly caused by a heart attack, high blood pressure, coronary artery disease, abnormal heart valves, and heart defects. Treatment is chronic and aimed at lessening the symptoms of heart failure and preventing further damage. It includes lifestyle changes, medications, and surgery in some cases.

Hypertension. Hypertension occurs when the normal regulation of blood pressure is disrupted and the diastolic pressure remains chronically elevated—over 90 mmHg—and is accompanied by an increased systolic pressure of over 140 mm Hg. Uncontrolled blood pressure increases the risk for stroke, heart attack, heart failure, and kidney and retinal damage. Treatment is chronic and involves lifestyle changes as well as anti-hypertensive medications.

Rx for Success

A healthy lifestyle is critical to preventing heart disease and stroke, and includes activities such as quitting smoking, maintaining a healthy weight, practicing good nutrition, and exercising.

Venous Thromboembolism. In this condition, a clot forms in the veins of the body, for example, in the legs. Small portions of the clot can break away and travel to the lungs, causing a pulmonary (lung) embolism. This condition requires urgent treatment with anti-clotting drugs (anticoagulants).

Arrhythmias/Dysrhythmias. Abnormal rhythms of the heart. Some can cause the heart to beat too slowly (bradycardia) or too rapidly (tachycardia), while others produce abnormal electrical activity. Common arrhythmias originating in the atria include atrial fibrillation and atrial flutter. Premature ventricular contractions (PVCs), ventricular tachycardia, and ventricular fibrillation originate in the ventricles. Symptoms include dizziness, fatigue, and palpitation (forcible and rapid heartbeats). Drug treatment is usually chronic and is aimed at controlling the heart rate and maintaining a normal rhythm.

The Respiratory System

Overview of Structure and Function

The respiratory system consists of the upper airways, the respiratory tract, and the lungs. When air is breathed in, it enters the body through the upper airways—the nasal and oral cavities—into a muscular tube called the pharynx (see figure 9–9). From there, it moves into the voice box (larynx), which also contains the vocal cords and the epiglottis, a flap-like structure at the opening of the larynx that prevents food and water from entering into the respiratory tract. From the larynx, air enters the trachea, which is a rigid tube held open by C-shaped rings of cartilage, and then into smaller airway passages called bronchi.

There are two major bronchi that conduct air to the left and right lungs. Inside each of the lungs, the bronchi divide many more times; as they divide, they become progressively smaller until they become tiny tubes that have no cartilage, called bronchioles. Finally, they terminate in single-layered cell structures called alveoli, where the exchange of gases takes place between the lungs and the blood. Breathing—and therefore the exchange of gases—can occur because movement of the muscles of the chest wall create pressure changes that are responsible for air

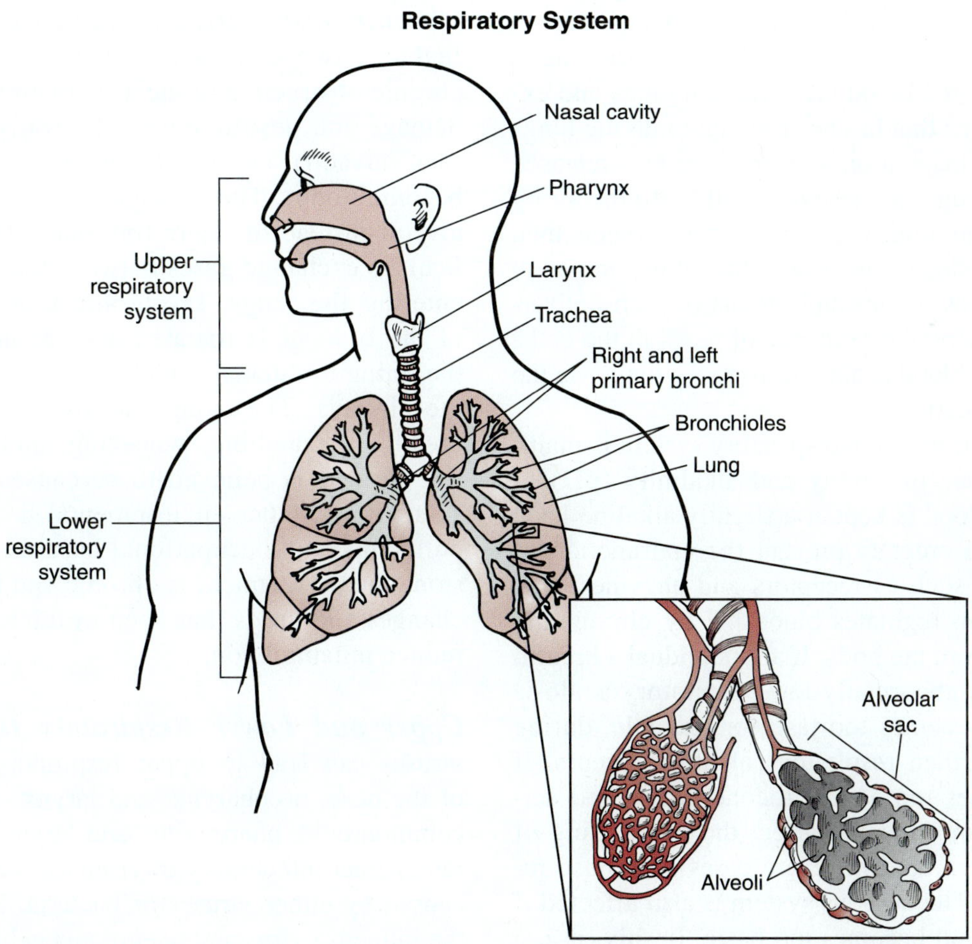

Figure 9–9. Anatomy of the respiratory system. The upper respiratory system is comprised of structures that bring air into the lungs. The lower respiratory system contains the bronchi, bronchioles, and the lungs. At the terminal end of the bronchioles are the alveolar sacs where the exchange of gases takes place.

moving into the lungs (inspiration) and out of the lungs (expiration).

Lining the larynx and trachea are specialized cells that **secrete** mucus, which traps particles and dust from the air breathed in to the lungs. The mucus and trapped particles are then propelled toward the pharynx by the beating action of cilia (hair-like projections), where they are swallowed.

The respiratory system is responsible for gas exchange, which ultimately allows oxygen to be taken to cells in the body and carbon dioxide to be removed from the same cells. Gas exchange occurs at two levels: in the lungs between the alveoli and the blood, and at the cellular level between blood and the tissues. In red blood cells (erythrocytes), a molecule called hemoglobin is responsible for carrying oxygen. Carbon dioxide is transported in the blood, some attached to hemoglobin and the rest dissolved in the blood.

Deoxygenated blood (low in oxygen and high in carbon dioxide) travels from the right side of the heart to the lungs; at the level of the alveoli, carbon dioxide is released from the red blood cells into the lungs and exchanged for oxygen that has been brought into the lungs by the process of inspiration. Carbon dioxide is released by the lungs (through the nose or mouth) into the air by the process of expiration. The blood, rich in oxygen, then travels to the left side of the heart where it is pumped to cells of the various tissues and organs oxygen delivering to the cells. After the exchange of gases in the cells, the deoxygenated blood again returns to the lungs via the right side of the heart.

Another function of the respiratory system is maintaining the balance of acidity and alkalinity (**pH**) of the blood. The blood is kept at a slightly alkaline level (its pH is 7.4) in order to prevent the malfunction of critical proteins, such as receptors and enzymes. The respiratory system regulates blood pH by eliminating carbon dioxide from the body. If an individual's breathing rate becomes abnormally low, respiratory acidosis can occur; if it becomes too fast, for example, during hyperventilation, then respiratory alkalosis occurs. If the blood becomes too acidic, a condition called acidosis develops, and this can affect the functioning of the nervous system, and in severe cases can cause respiratory failure. The nervous system is also affected if the pH of the blood becomes too basic. In this case, a condition called alkalosis develops and the nervous system becomes overactive, which results in seizures and convulsions.

Other functions of the respiratory system involve filtering out irritants in the air breathed and protecting the body from invading pathogens.

Common Diseases and Disorders

Asthma. Asthma is a disease of the lungs characterized by inflammation of the bronchioles, increased mucus secretion, and abnormal contractions of the smooth muscles in the bronchioles, which leads to the narrowing of the airway passages. The symptoms are difficulty breathing, wheezing, and coughing. The cause of the disease is often an allergic response to pollen, molds, dust mites, or pet dander. Other factors can also induce asthma, such as exercise, cold air, and stress. Treatment of asthma involves the use of drugs that can open and relax the airways of the lungs and decrease the inflammation that is associated with this disease.

Chronic Obstructive Pulmonary Disease (COPD). Includes two conditions known as emphysema and chronic obstructive bronchitis. In emphysema, there is damage and destruction of the walls between the air sacs (alveoli), causing them to lose their shape and become floppy. The damage leads to fewer and larger alveoli instead of many tiny ones. This makes it difficult to exchange gases between the blood and the air entering the lungs. In chronic bronchitis, the lining of the bronchi is irritated and inflamed. This causes the lining to thicken. Thick mucus forms, which plugs the airways. The symptoms of COPD are difficulty breathing, coughing, wheezing, and chest tightness. The disease is believed to be caused by factors such as smoking, other environmental hazards such as air pollutants, and occupational hazards such as coal and stone dust. Treatment is chronic and includes lifestyle changes and drugs that open or dilate the airways and reduce inflammation.

Upper and Lower Respiratory Infections. Many viruses can lead to upper respiratory tract infections of the nose, oropharynx, and larynx—for example, the common cold, pharyngitis, and laryngitis. Lower respiratory tract infections (lower airways and lungs) can be caused by either viruses or bacteria. Examples include the influenza virus and pneumonia, which can be caused by either bacteria or viruses. Supportive treatment is used for viral infections, and antibiotics are used to treat infections caused by bacteria.

The Musculoskeletal System

Overview of Structure and Function

This system consists of a framework of individual bones called the skeleton. The skeleton is made up of 206 bones, each of which varies in size and shape (see figure 9–10). Bones are connected by ligaments, and the points of connection are joints. Some bones, such as those in the skull, are fixed to hold the structure together and prevent movement. Others are partially moveable to allow some flexibility, such as the spine. Additionally, some joints are freely moveable, such as those found in the hipbones, arms, and legs.

The skeleton of a man and woman are almost identical, with only small differences between the sexes. For example, the density of the bones in the arms and legs are heavier in males, and the hip bones of females are wider.

Covering the skeleton are the skeletal muscles, most of which are connected to the bones by tendons. Some muscles, such as the facial muscles, are attached to the skin. There are more than 600 muscles in the body, which vary in mass and length (see figure 9–11). Each muscle consists of numerous individual muscle cells called muscle fibers that are highly elongated in shape, and, in many cases, these muscle fibers can run the length of the bone they are covering (see figure 9–12).

The muscle fibers are made up of thick and thin filaments that contain specialized proteins, called actin and myosin. Actin and myosin are responsible for making a muscle contract and relax. The orderly arrangement

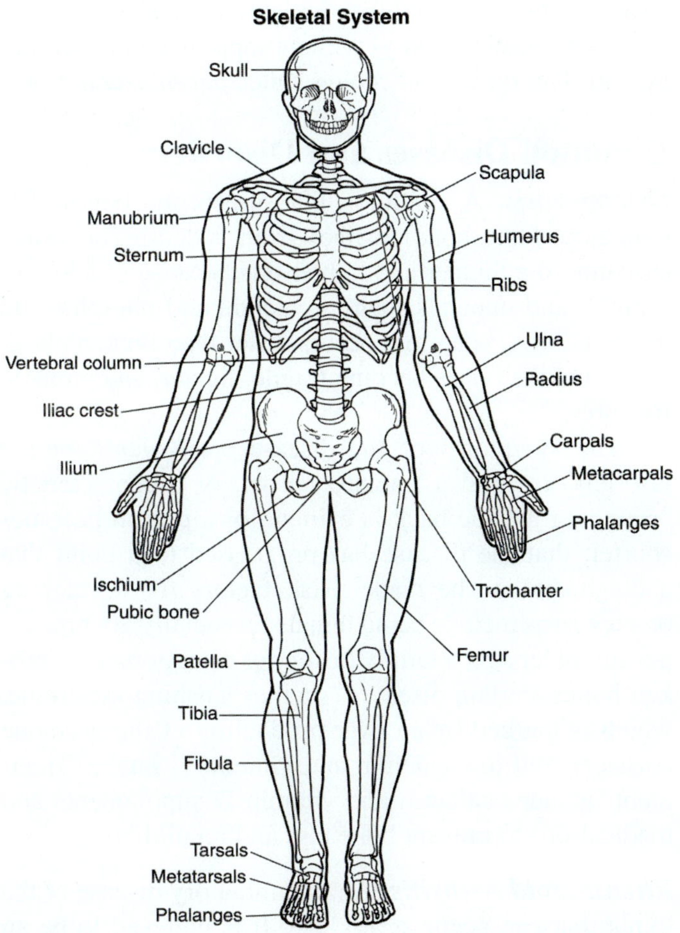

Figure 9–10. The skeletal system anterior view. The skeletal system is an extensive system of large and small bones that supports the muscle and protects the internal organs.

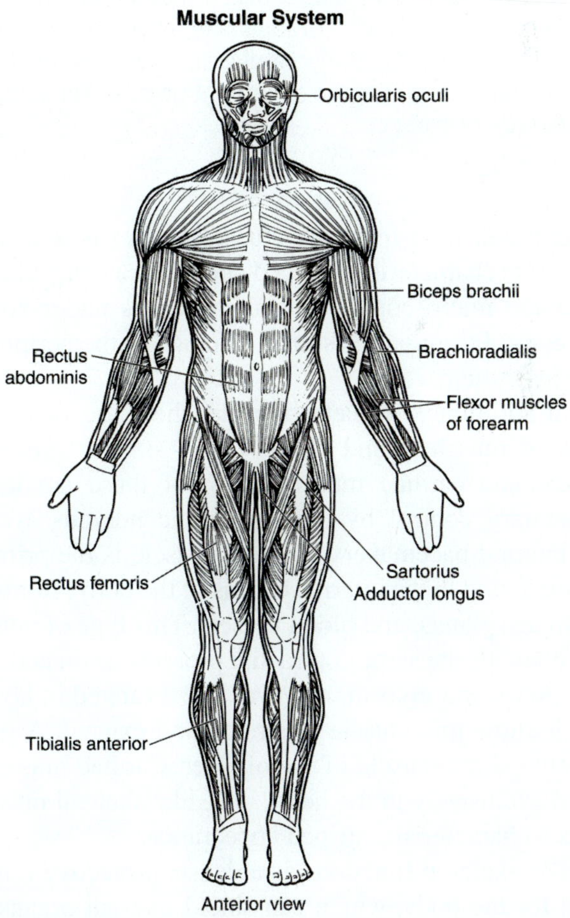

Figure 9–11. The skeletal muscles of the body. The skeletal muscles of the body attach to the skeleton via ligaments and tendons. When they contract, they can move or restrain parts of the body.

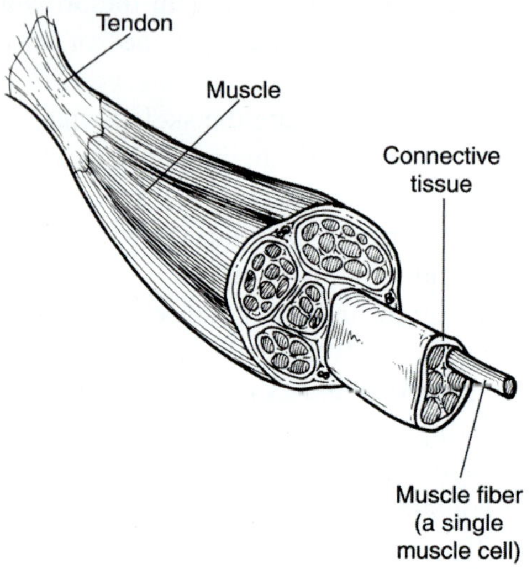

Figure 9–12. The structure of skeletal muscle. Each muscle is comprised of single muscle cells known as muscle fibers. The muscle fiber is formed from bundles of myofibrils that are surrounded by a specialized membrane known as the sarcolemma, which contains the sarcoplasmic reticulum and T-tubules. Each myofibril is composed of thick and thin filaments, and their arrangement gives skeletal muscle its striated appearance.

of actin and myosin in the muscle fibers gives skeletal muscle its characteristic striped appearance when viewed under the microscope. Skeletal muscle is under voluntary control through the somatic branch of the peripheral nervous system.

In addition to skeletal muscle, there are two other types of muscle found in the body: smooth (visceral) muscle and cardiac muscle. Both of these are under involuntary control by the autonomic nervous system and internal pacemakers. Smooth muscle is the primary muscle found in the internal organs of the body: stomach, intestines, glands, and blood vessels. This type of muscle also contains the same contractile proteins, actin and myosin. Actin and myosin, however, are arranged in layers, which allow this muscle to stretch and expand. A good example is the muscle of the bladder. Cardiac muscle is found exclusively in the heart, and, like skeletal muscle, it has a characteristic striped appearance.

The skeleton functions as a dense, protective framework for the body, which can shield internal organs, in addition to forming a structure to which other tissues, such as muscle, can attach. The skeleton also supports the weight of the body. Moreover, most bones of the body contain red bone marrow inside their structure. The red bone marrow is essential for the production of all blood cells.

The skeletal muscles function to move the body by their ability to contract and relax in a synchronized fashion. When the somatic nervous system sends a signal to the muscle, it contracts. Some muscles contract and relax quickly, such as the eyelid muscles, whereas others contract for a longer period of time, such as the muscles in the back that control posture.

✔ The proper functioning of muscles allows an individual to carry out a wide range of complex movements, from gross motor control movements required for running to fine motor control movements required for playing the piano.

Skeletal, smooth, and cardiac muscles are regulated by the nervous system. Smooth and cardiac muscles, however, have their own ability to initiate electrical signals (and therefore muscle activity) without input from the nervous system. This type of function is called *pacemaker activity*.

Common Diseases and Disorders

Osteoporosis. A condition that affects the bones. The structure of the bone changes from a dense and heavy structure to a thinner and lighter one because of a loss of proteins and minerals such as calcium and phosphate. In this condition, bone loss occurs faster than bone replacement, and the bones become fragile, lighter, and prone to fractures.

The symptoms of the disease are "silent," and it is often not until a fracture occurs, or a characteristic "rounding" of the back is evident, or a person becomes shorter, that the disease has progressed to a point that a diagnosis can be made. Risk factors for developing osteoporosis include being female (especially after menopause), older age, a family history of osteoporosis or broken bones, certain diseases (such as Cushing syndrome, which is marked by an over production of the hormone cortisol), and low calcium and vitamin D intake. Treatment includes calcium and vitamin D supplements and medications to prevent bone loss and rebuild bone.

Rheumatoid Arthritis. An inflammatory disease of the joints that can occur at any age. It is believed to be an autoimmune disease whereby the body produces specific proteins called antibodies that cause inflammation of a special membrane around the joints. In the early stages of the disease, the person may complain of a low-grade fever, lack of energy, loss of appetite, or a general feeling of malaise. As the disease advances, the joints become swollen, red, painful, and stiff. Joint destruction can occur rapidly in rheumatoid arthritis. Treatment involves drugs that decrease the inflammation in the joints and prevent further destruction of the joint tissue.

Osteoarthritis. A condition whereby the cartilage of the joint deteriorates. This starts to affect the bone underneath, which eventually begins to thicken and distort. It generally affects the weight-bearing joints (i.e., the hips, knees, and spine) of the body. Pain, swelling, and stiffness of the joints are characteristic symptoms of this condition. This type of arthritis most often occurs as a result of aging. The joint damage occurs slowly as the joints wear out. Drug treatment is focused on relieving pain and joint swelling.

Muscle Sprain and Strain. When a muscle or a tendon becomes injured, for example, during a sport activity or overwork, it is called a strain injury.[12] If the ligament becomes injured, it is called a sprain injury.[12] Sprains and strains can happen in a number of regions in the body, such as the back, wrist, ankle, knee, and hamstring muscles. Over-the-counter drugs such as ibuprofen are commonly prescribed to reduce the pain and swelling associated with these injuries.

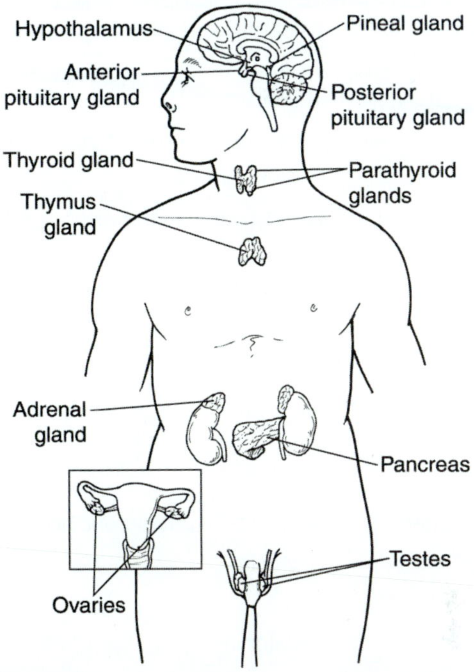

Figure 9–13. The major glands of the endocrine system. The endocrine system is made up of a group of glands that secrete chemical substances, known as hormones, into the bloodstream. The endocrine glands are widely dispersed throughout the body and are not structurally related to each other.

The Endocrine System

Overview of Structure and Function

The **endocrine** system is made up of a group of glands that release chemical substances into the blood. The glands that make up the endocrine system are widely dispersed throughout the body and are not structurally related to each other. Even though the **endocrine glands** are not connected to each other, they make up a system in a functional sense by performing the same role: they secrete chemical messengers called **hormones** into the bloodstream. The hormones circulate in the bloodstream and affect many types of body cells. The major endocrine glands are shown in figure 9–13.

The endocrine system is made up of the endocrine glands and the hormone(s) they secrete into the bloodstream. The hormone, together with the target tissue or cells, functions to relay information and instructions throughout the body.

The purpose of the secreted hormones is to bring on a specific response in *other* cells of the body, which are in another location. Some hormones function only to regulate the production of other hormones, whereas others exert their effects on the target tissues themselves. The hormones are secreted into the bloodstream, giving them access to all other cells of the body.

The endocrine system works to

- Maintain the body's normal internal balance (homeostasis)
- Help the body deal with stressful situations
- Regulate growth and development
- Control reproduction
- Produce, use, and store energy

The endocrine glands are characterized by the hormone(s) that they secrete and the target tissue(s) that the hormone affects (see table 9–1).

Common Diseases and Disorders

Because there are so many endocrine glands, hormones, and target cells throughout the body, when something in

Table 9–1. Endocrine Glands and Hormonal Physiologic Effects on the Body

Endocrine Gland	Principal Hormone(s) Secreted	Target Tissue(s)	Physiologic Effect of Hormone
Hypothalamus	Releasing and inhibiting hormones	Anterior pituitary	Controls release of anterior pituitary hormones
Anterior pituitary	Thyroid-stimulating hormone (TSH)	Thyroid	Production of thyroid hormone
	Adrenocorticotropic hormone (ACTH)	Adrenal cortex	Secretion of cortisol
	Growth hormone	Bones; soft tissues	Stimulates growth of bones and soft tissues
	Follicle-stimulating hormone (FSH)	Females: ovary	Promotes growth of ovarian follicle; stimulates estrogen secretion
	Luteinizing hormone (LH)	Males: testes	Stimulates sperm production
		Females: ovary	Stimulates ovulation; stimulates estrogen and progesterone secretion
	Prolactin	Males: testes	Stimulates testosterone secretion
		Females: breast	Promotes breast development; stimulates milk secretion
Posterior pituitary	Vasopressin (antidiuretic hormone)	Kidney	Causes water retention
	Oxytocin	Uterus	Causes contractions
		Breasts	Causes ejection of milk
Pineal	Melatonin	Brain; anterior pituitary; reproductive organs; possibly other sites	Sets the body's "time clock;" causes sleep in response to darkness
Thyroid	Thyroid hormones (T_3 and T_4)	Most cells	Increases the metabolic rate; necessary for normal growth and development
Parathyroid	Parathyroid hormone	Bone; kidney; intestine	Increases amount of calcium in the bloodstream; decreases amount of phosphate in the bloodstream
Thymus	Thymosin	T lymphocytes	Enhances the production of T lymphocytes
Pancreas	Insulin	Most cells	Promotes use and storage of nutrients, particularly glucose, after eating
	Glucagon	Most cells	Maintains glucose levels in the bloodstream during periods of no food
	Somatostatin	Digestive system	Inhibits digestion and absorption of nutrients
Adrenal medulla	Epinephrine and norepinephrine	Nervous system sites throughout the entire body	Reinforces the nervous system; "fight or flight" system
Adrenal cortex	Aldosterone	Kidney	Increases sodium retention and potassium secretion
	Cortisol	Most cells	Increases glucose in the bloodstream
	Androgens	Females: bone and brain	Puberty growth spurt and sex drive in females
Testes (male)	Testosterone	Male sex organs; body as a whole	Stimulates production of sperm; responsible for development of sex characteristics; promotes sex drive
Ovaries (female)	Estrogen	Female sex organs; body as a whole	Stimulates uterine and breast growth; responsible for development of sex characteristics
	Progesterone	Uterus	Prepares for pregnancy

one of the endocrine glands goes wrong, it can have a profound impact on a number of other bodily functions. Generally, problems within the endocrine system are due to one of two things: either too little or too much of a hormone is produced. Thus, disorders resulting from decreased production of hormones by the endocrine glands are treated by giving the patient a replacement hormone. When too much of a hormone is produced, drugs are used to inhibit hormone production. Disturbances within the endocrine system may also occur from damage done directly to the endocrine gland, or, less commonly, from a decreased sensitivity of the target tissue to the hormone. Because the actions of hormones are so extensive, this review will focus only on the most common endocrine disorders.

Diabetes Mellitus. Diabetes is the most common endocrine disease, characterized by high levels of glucose (sugar) in the bloodstream and urine. Symptoms include frequent urination, unusual thirst, extreme hunger, and frequent infections. Type 1 diabetes (previously known as juvenile diabetes) is characterized by a lack of insulin production from the pancreas. It is most commonly diagnosed in children and young adults and it is treated with insulin. Type 2 diabetes is the most common type of diabetes, and it is characterized as either decreased production of insulin or an abnormal sensitivity of the tissues to the insulin that is present. Type 2 diabetes is treated with diet alone, oral hypoglycemic agents, insulin, or a combination of those remedies.

Diabetes Insipidus. This condition occurs when the pituitary gland doesn't produce antidiuretic hormone (ADH, or vasopressin), or if the kidneys do not respond to the hormone ADH. As a result, the kidneys are unable to reabsorb water, which leads to high volumes of urine excreted and extreme thirst. It is treated with the replacement hormone vasopressin.

Thyroid Disease. Thyroid disease can result from the production of too little thyroid hormone (hypothyroidism), which is characterized by weakness, fatigue, muscle cramps, intolerance to cold, dry skin, and lethargy. Production of too much thyroid hormone causes hyperthyroidism, which is characterized by weakness, sweating, weight loss, nervousness, moist skin, and intolerance to heat. An individual suffering from hypothyroidism can be treated with thyroid hormone replacement. Hyperthyroidism is not as easily treated. Depending upon the cause of increased thyroid levels, treatment may range from using a thyroid hormone blocker to treatment of the thyroid gland with radioactivity to destroy part of the gland.

The Immune System

Overview of Structure and Function

The body is equipped with a complex defense system—the immune system—which provides constant protection against invasion by foreign substances or organisms. The immune system is the name of a collection of molecules, cells, and organs whose complex interactions form an efficient system that is usually able to protect an individual from both outside invaders and its own altered internal cells, and also able to rid the body of unwanted cellular debris.

Part 2

The immune system is composed of the cells in our bone marrow, the thymus gland, the lymphatic system of ducts and nodes, the spleen, and the blood that all work together to protect the body from invasion (see figure 9–14).

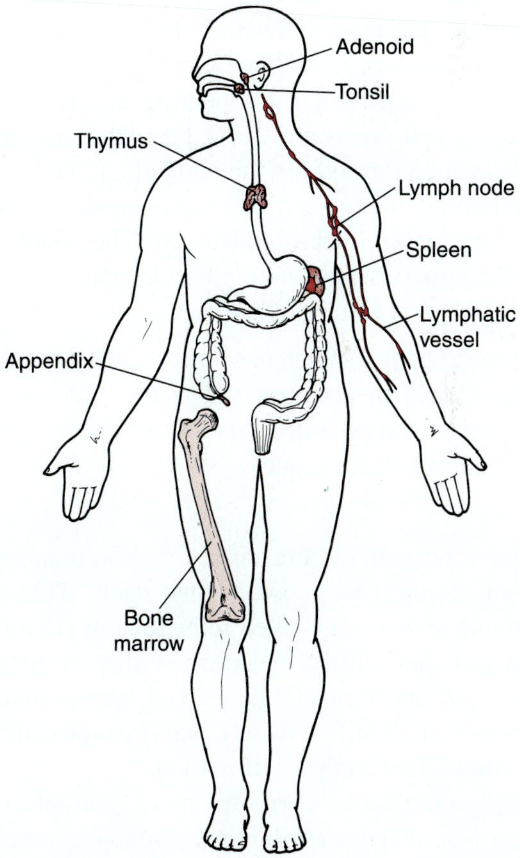

Figure 9–14. Tissues of the immune system. The immune system is composed of the cells of the bone marrow, the thymus, and the lymphatic system of ducts and nodes, spleen, and lymphoid tissue (tonsils, adenoids, appendix), which protect the body against foreign materials. Note that the components of the immune system are widely dispersed throughout the body.

The "worker" cells of the immune system, which are responsible for the various immune defenses, are found in the bloodstream and known as white blood cells (leukocytes). Several different types of leukocytes circulate in the blood stream. There are numerous other cells that contribute to the function of the immune system including phagocytes (such as monocytes, macrophages, and neutrophils), granulocytes (eosinophils and basophils), and lymphocytes. The two types of lymphocytes are called B cells and T cells.

The organs of the immune system are located throughout the body, and they are known as lymphoid organs because they are concerned with the growth, development, and deployment of lymphocytes. The organs of the immune system are connected with one another and with other organs of the body by a network of lymphatic vessels similar to blood vessels. Immune cells and foreign particles are transported through the lymphatic vessels in lymph, a clear fluid that bathes the body's tissues. The major lymphoid organs of the immune system are lymph nodes, tonsils, adenoids, the appendix, the spleen, and the thymus. Lymph nodes are small, bean-shaped structures that are located throughout the body along the lymphatic routes. Lymph nodes function to remove any cellular debris before it enters the bloodstream. They contain specialized compartments where immune cells congregate.

✔ When the body is threatened by microorganisms, viruses, or cancer cells, the immune system goes into action to provide protection by destroying the threatening organisms. This is known as the immune response.

Under normal circumstances, the immune system does not mount a response against itself. This lack of an immune response is called **tolerance**. It is vitally important that the immune response is able to distinguish between *self* and *nonself*. Every cell carries distinctive molecules that identify it as self, and immune cells do not attack tissues that carry a self marker.

Foreign molecules carry distinctive markers as well: characteristic shapes that allow the immune system to recognize them as foreign and initiate an immune response. Any substance capable of triggering an immune response (and carrying a distinctive nonself marker) is known as an **antigen**. An antigen can be a bacterium or a virus, or even a portion or product of one of these organisms. Antigens also trigger the production of antibodies by the immune system, and this is the mechanism by which immunity, or resistance, to a disease is acquired. Tissues or cells from another individual also act as antigens; that is why transplanted tissues are rejected as foreign without preventive drug therapy.

Invading microorganisms attempting to get into the body must first get past the body's first line of defense: the skin and mucous membranes. If the invader gets past these initial physical barriers, the immune system "players" are called to duty.

The Immune Response. The immune response is engineered to rid the body of unwanted invaders, and it can occur in a number of different ways. These mechanisms, known all together as immunity, include both innate (naturally occurring) and also adaptive or acquired immune responses. Innate immune responses are nonspecific responses that defend against foreign material nonselectively, even the first time the body is exposed to it. Adaptive or acquired immune responses are specific responses that target specific invaders, because the body has been exposed to the invader at least once before. In an adaptive immune response, the body is ready because it has been specially prepared for the invader to return.

The immune response is initiated once the immune system recognizes a foreign molecule. The first immune system cells the invader encounters are cells circulating in the bloodstream that attack all invaders, regardless of the antigens they carry. One example of an innate immune response is the inflammation response. Inflammation is a nonspecific response to foreign invasion or tissue damage that occurs when neutrophils and macrophages destroy foreign or damaged cells. The ultimate goal of inflammation is to bring more help from the immune system to destroy the invaders, remove the dead cells, and begin the process of tissue healing and repair. These actions are responsible for the signs and symptoms of inflammation: swelling, redness, heat, and pain.

Common Diseases and Disorders

A number of clinical problems can occur when something within the immune system goes wrong. If the immune system is deficient in the number of T cells it produces, the immune system fails to defend itself against viral infections. Similarly, if the immune system is deficient in its ability to make B cells, the immune system fails to defend itself against bacterial infections.

Allergy. One of the most well-known disorders of the immune system is allergy. Allergies occur when the body mounts an immune response against a normally harmless substance such as grass pollen. In this case, the offending agent is called an allergen. The first time an allergy-prone individual is exposed to an allergen (such as grass pollen), the individual's B cells make large amounts of grass pollen IgE antibody. These IgE molecules attach to granule-containing cells known as mast cells, which are plentiful in the lungs, skin, tongue, and linings of the nose and gastrointestinal tract. The next time the individual is exposed to grass pollen, the IgE-primed mast cells release powerful chemicals, including histamine, that cause the wheezing, sneezing, itching, and other symptoms of allergy. Drugs called antihistamines are commonly used to treat and prevent allergies.

Autoimmune Disease. Characterized by the body's immune system destroying its own normal cells. When the body loses its ability to correctly identify body cells belonging to self, it can mount immune responses directed against its own cells and organs. In this event, antibodies produced by B cells against its own body are called autoantibodies, and they are responsible for many diseases. **Autoimmunity** can cause a broad range of human illnesses. For instance, T cells that attack pancreas cells contribute to diabetes, and an autoantibody known as rheumatoid factor is common in persons with rheumatoid arthritis.

Acquired Immune Deficiency Syndrome (AIDS). Caused by infection with the human immunodeficiency virus (HIV). This virus is passed from one person to another through blood-to-blood and sexual contact. HIV destroys T-helper cells, which are essential to the normal function of the immune system. Infection with HIV can weaken the immune system to the point that it has difficulty fighting off infections. These types of infections are known as opportunistic infections because they take the opportunity a weakened immune system provides to cause illness. Many of the infections that cause illness or may be life threatening for people with AIDS usually do not cause illness in those with a normal immune system.

Most people infected with HIV carry the virus for years before enough damage is done to the T-helper cells and the immune system for AIDS to develop. There is a strong connection between the amount of HIV in the blood and the decline in T-helper cells, and the development of AIDS. Therefore, drug therapy has been targeted at reducing the amount of virus in the body with anti-HIV medications to slow the immune system destruction and progression of the disease.

The Gastrointestinal System

Overview of Structure and Function

At its simplest, the gastrointestinal (GI) tract is a hollow tube running through the body from the mouth to the anus. The adult gastrointestinal tract (also known as the digestive tract) is about 30 feet long. The basic components of the gastrointestinal system are described below (see figure 9–15):

Part 2

- **Mouth**: The mouth, or oral cavity, is the entrance to the digestive tract. Food is broken down mechanically by chewing. Saliva is added as a lubricant, and it also contains enzymes that begin the digestion of starch.

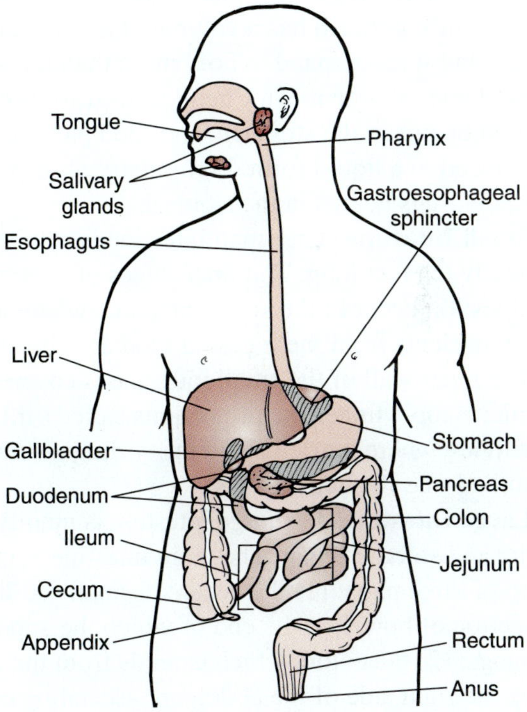

Figure 9–15. Anatomy of the major components of the gastrointestinal tract. The gastrointestinal tract can be thought of as a long, hollow tube running through the body from the mouth to the anus. Shown are the basic components of the gastrointestinal tract, which function to transfer energy from ingested food to the internal cells of the body and rid the body of undigested waste.

- **Pharynx**: The pharynx is about five inches long, and it is a cavity located at the rear of the throat. It serves as a shared passageway for food and air. A flap called the epiglottis reflexively closes the trachea while food is being swallowed.
- **Esophagus**: The esophagus is a fairly straight muscular tube that extends between the pharynx and the stomach; it serves simply to connect the mouth with the stomach. It is the least complex section of the gastrointestinal tract. The esophagus is guarded at both ends by sphincters, rings of muscle that control passage of contents through an opening into or out of a hollow organ. When the sphincter is closed, it prevents passage through the tube it guards.
- **Stomach**: The stomach is a pouch-like chamber located in the upper middle of the abdominal cavity; it lies between the esophagus and the small intestine. The stomach stores food while thoroughly mixing it with acids and enzymes, breaking it into much smaller digestible pieces. When it is empty, an adult's stomach has a volume of one-fifth of a cup, but it can expand to hold more than 8 cups of food after a large meal. Chemical **digestion** of most food begins in the stomach, and food particles are reduced to a liquid form. Preliminary absorption of some drugs begins in the stomach.
- **Small Intestine**: The small intestine is a coiled tube nearly ten feet long. The final stages of chemical digestion occur in the small intestine, where almost all nutrients from the ingested food are absorbed. The inner wall of the small intestine is covered with microscopic fingerlike projections called villi. The villi are where nutrients and many drugs are absorbed into the body.
- **Large Intestine**: The large intestine is mainly a drying and storage organ. The large intestine is made up of three parts: (1) the cecum, a small sac-like section of bowel, at the end of which the appendix hangs; (2) the colon, which extends from the cecum, up the right side of the abdomen (ascending colon), across the upper abdomen (transverse colon), and then down the left side of the abdomen (descending and sigmoid colon); (3) the rectum, which is connected to the last part of the colon ultimately terminates at the anus. The cecum and colon are about five feet long, whereas the rectum is only five inches long. The anal sphincter controls flow out of the GI tract.
- **Liver**: The liver is located beneath the ribcage in the right upper part of the abdomen. It is the center of metabolic activity in the body, and it also plays a large role in the digestion and absorption of nutrients by producing bile, which emulsifies dietary fat.
- **Gallbladder:** This is located near the liver and stores bile. When dietary fat passes into the small intestine, bile is released to emulsify fat and aid in the absorption of fat-soluble vitamins.
- **Pancreas**: The pancreas is located beneath the stomach. It serves an important role because it provides a potent mixture of digestive enzymes to the small intestine, which are critical for digestion of food. The pancreas also serves as an endocrine organ by secreting hormones such as insulin and glucagon.

✔ The gastrointestinal tract functions to transfer energy from the food we eat to the cells in the internal environment of the body. This system also functions to eliminate undigested food residues to the external environment.

Plants are capable of transforming the energy from the sun into usable forms of energy to survive; humans are not. Humans must rely on ingested food as an essential energy source for the cells of the body to use to carry out vital energy-dependent activities. The breakdown of food is accomplished through a combination of mechanical and chemical (enzymatic) processes. To accomplish this breakdown, the digestive "tube" requires considerable assistance from accessory digestive organs, such as the salivary glands, liver, and pancreas, which dump their secretions into the tube. The main function of the digestive tube is to break down the food we eat (proteins, fats, and carbohydrates), which cannot be absorbed whole, into smaller molecules (amino acids, fatty acids, and glucose) that can be absorbed across the tubular and into the circulatory system for distribution throughout the entire body. Some of the molecules are used for energy, some are used as building blocks for tissues and cells, and some are stored for future use.

The first step in the digestive process is the chewing and mixing of ingested food by the teeth. The purposes of chewing are (1) to tear, grind, and break down food particles into smaller pieces to facilitate swallowing, and (2) to mix food with saliva. Saliva is produced by salivary glands located outside of the mouth, and it is secreted into the mouth by small ducts. The mass of chewed, moistened food (known as a bolus) is moved to the back of the mouth by the tongue. In the pharynx, the bolus triggers an involuntary swallowing reflex that prevents food from entering the lungs and directs the bolus into the esophagus.

Muscles in the esophagus propel the bolus by waves of involuntary contractions (**peristalsis**) of the muscle lining the esophagus (see figure 9–16). The bolus passes through the lower esophageal sphincter (LES) into the stomach. The stomach provides four basic functions that assist in the early stages of digestion and prepare the ingested food materials for further processing in the small intestine: (1) it serves as a short-term storage site, allowing a rather large meal to be consumed quickly and dealt with over an extended period of time; (2) it is in the stomach that substantial chemical and enzymatic digestion is started; (3) vigorous contractions of the stomach muscles mix and grind food with acidic stomach secretions, resulting in liquefaction of food, which must occur before it can be delivered to the small intestine; and (4) once food is liquefied in the stomach, it is slowly released into the small intestine for further processing.

By the time food is ready to leave the stomach it has been processed into a thick liquid called chyme (see figure 9–17). The outlet of the stomach—a small sphincter muscle called the pylorus—keeps the chyme in the stomach until it reaches the right consistency to pass into the small intestine. Chyme is then forced down into the duodenum of the small intestine by the action of peristalsis. In the small intestine, where the majority of nutritional and drug absorption occurs, digestive chemicals work on the partially digested food.

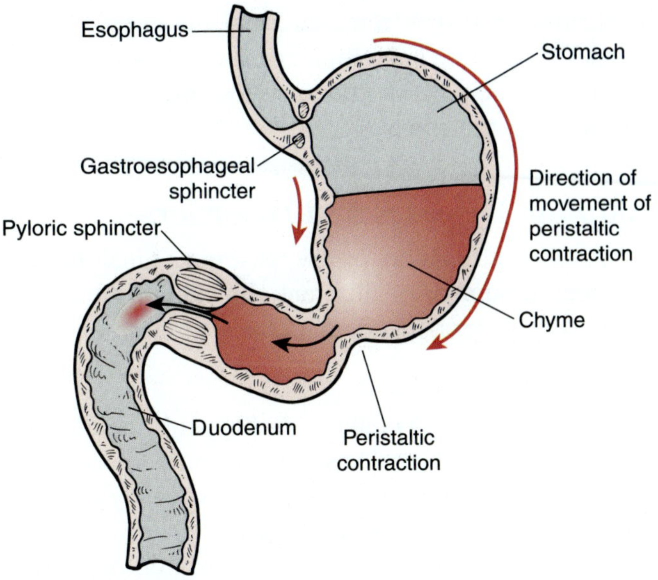

Figure 9–17. Gastric emptying. Peristaltic contractions originate in the upper portions of the stomach and gain strength as they near the pyloric sphincter. These contractions function to mix and propel chyme (liquid stomach contents) toward the pyloric sphincter and are responsible for pushing small quantities of chyme through the sphincter into the duodenum.

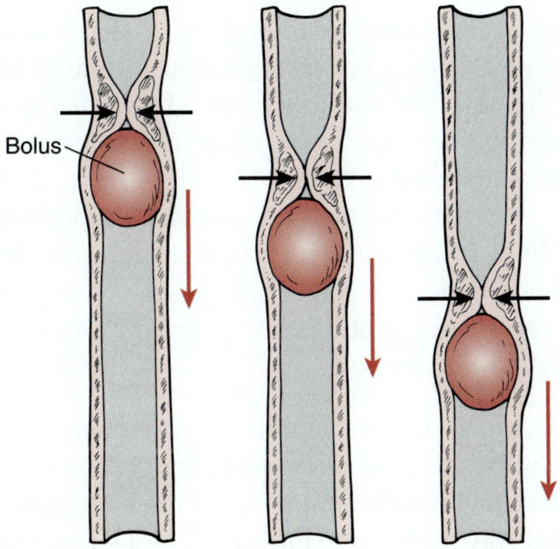

Figure 9–16. Peristalsis. Waves of involuntary muscular contractions propel boluses of food along the esophagus down toward the stomach.

The pancreas and liver connect with the small intestine and send secretions into it to aid in the process of digestion. These include pancreatic juice, which contains enzymes that help digest carbohydrates, proteins, and fats; and bile, which breaks down and aids in the absorption of fat. Although bile is produced in the liver, it is stored in the gallbladder and sent into the small intestine through the bile duct. Once broken down, these now-soluble food products are dissolved and absorbed directly into the bloodstream through the walls of the small intestine, along with vitamins and minerals. This process is called absorption.

By the time the food reaches the large intestine, the work of digestion is almost finished. The main function of the large intestine is to remove water from the undigested matter and form it into stool, which will be eliminated from the body by excretion. Bacteria in the colon aid digestion of the remaining food products. The final waste product, the feces, is then stored in

Part 2

the rectum until it is released from the body through the anal sphincter. The elimination of feces is called a bowel movement (BM), because the intestinal tract is referred to as the bowel.

Common Diseases and Disorders

If the normal function of the gastrointestinal tract is disrupted, a number of different clinical situations may occur. They differ depending on the site of the malfunction or disease.

Ulcers. The stomach contains strong acids to aid in the breakdown of food products. Under normal conditions, the stomach and small intestines are extremely resistant to irritation by the strong acids they contain. A bacterium (most commonly *helicobacter pylori*), or the chronic use of certain medications or alcohol, may weaken the protective coating of the stomach and duodenum and allow acid to get through to the sensitive lining beneath. Both the acid and the bacteria can irritate and inflame the lining (a condition known as gastritis) or cause peptic ulcers, which are sores or holes that form in the lining of the stomach or the duodenum and cause pain or bleeding. Medications that block the production of acid are used to treat these conditions; a course of antibiotics may be given if *helicobacter pylori* is involved.

Esophageal Disorders. Inflammation of the esophagus (esophagitis) can be caused by complications of certain medications or infection. Esophagitis is also commonly caused by a condition in which the lower esophageal sphincter is weakened and thus allows the acidic contents of the stomach to move backwards, or reflux, up into the esophagus. The result is inflammation and tissue damage of the esophagus. This condition is known as gastroesophageal reflux disease (GERD). Medications that reduce the production of stomach acid are used to protect the tissue lining the esophagus.

Gastrointestinal Infections. Infections of the gastrointestinal tract are quite common and are caused most commonly by viruses (such as enterovirus or rotavirus), by bacteria (such as *salmonella, shigella,* or *E. coli*); or by parasites or protozoan organisms. The microorganisms that cause GI infections often increase the muscle contractions (peristaltic) activity of the gastrointestinal tract; this results in vomiting and diarrhea. When a gastrointestinal infection is present, vomiting and diarrhea often occur, a protective response to rid the body of the harmful organisms or toxins. GI infections may be treated with anti-infective medications, depending on the causative organism.

Inflammatory Bowel Disease. Inflammatory bowel disease is a chronic inflammation of the intestines. There are two primary types: ulcerative colitis, which affects just the rectum and the large intestine, and Crohn disease, which can affect the whole gastrointestinal tract, from the mouth to the anus. The most common symptoms of inflammatory bowel disease are chronic abdominal pain, and intermittent, severe diarrhea, which may be bloody, and weight loss. Flare-ups of inflammatory bowel disease can occur at any time, but they are especially common during times of stress. Drug therapy is aimed at reducing inflammation and preventing flare-ups of the disease.

Irritable Bowel Syndrome. Irritable bowel syndrome is a chronic condition in which the bowels are especially sensitive to certain foods and stress. It can also be triggered by anxiety. The cause is unknown. Symptoms include abdominal pain, bloating, and abdominal discomfort. Some people have constipation as the predominant symptom and mucous may cover the feces. Others have diarrhea as the predominant symptom, whereas others may alternate between the two. Treatment depends on the predominant symptoms and may include changes in diet in addition to drug therapy.

Diarrhea. Diarrhea is a condition in which bowel movements are abnormally frequent and feces are loose and watery. It occurs when the muscle contractions (peristalsis) of the intestines move the fecal material along too quickly and there is not enough time for the water content to be absorbed into the body. If diarrhea is severe, the body can lose too much water and electrolytes and become dehydrated. In addition to bacterial and viral infections, diarrhea can also be caused by food poisoning (when food is infested with harmful bacteria), drinking contaminated water, lactose intolerance, some medications, and stress. Anti-diarrheal drugs are commonly used if diarrhea is severe.

Constipation. In this condition, the contents of the intestines do not move along fast enough, and there is an infrequent and painful emptying of the intestines. Waste materials stay in the large intestine so long that too much water is removed and the feces become too hard and difficult to pass. Fiber and stool softeners are taken to prevent constipation.

The Urinary System

Overview of Structure and Function

The structures of the urinary system are the kidneys, ureters, the bladder, and the urethra. The kidneys are fist-sized, bean-shaped organs that produce urine and are located in the mid-abdominal cavity, toward the back (see figure 9–18). Each of the kidneys receives a large supply of blood which enters the organs via the renal arteries. The blood supplies oxygen to the kidney tissue and it is filtered by the kidneys to remove waste products (urine). Once the blood has been filtered, it leaves the kidneys via the renal veins and returns to the right side of the heart. Each kidney has a tube called a ureter that is responsible for transporting the urine to the bladder. The bladder is a small, muscular sac that can expand to a large volume to store urine until it is ready to be excreted from the body, via the urethra.

The kidney itself has highly specialized anatomy, which allows it to filter huge volumes of blood and produce urine. The outermost layer of the kidney is called the cortex, the inner layer is called the medulla, and the innermost region is called the renal pelvis. Contained in the cortex and medulla are the functioning units of the kidney, called nephrons; each kidney contains tens of thousands of nephrons. A tiny blood vessel called an arteriole delivers blood to each nephron to be filtered, with the end result being the formation of urine (see figure 9–19). All of the urine that has been formed by the nephrons is collected into the renal pelvis and then transported to the ureter.

The kidneys perform many important functions. One such function is to filter the blood as it passes through the nephrons and remove waste products, such as products from protein breakdown, while reabsorbing important substances, such as glucose and protein, and returning them to the circulation for use by the cells of the body. In the process of filtering the blood, urine is formed. The kidney also plays a critical role in regulating the volume of the plasma, and therefore the blood volume, which affects blood pressure. Another function is regulating the

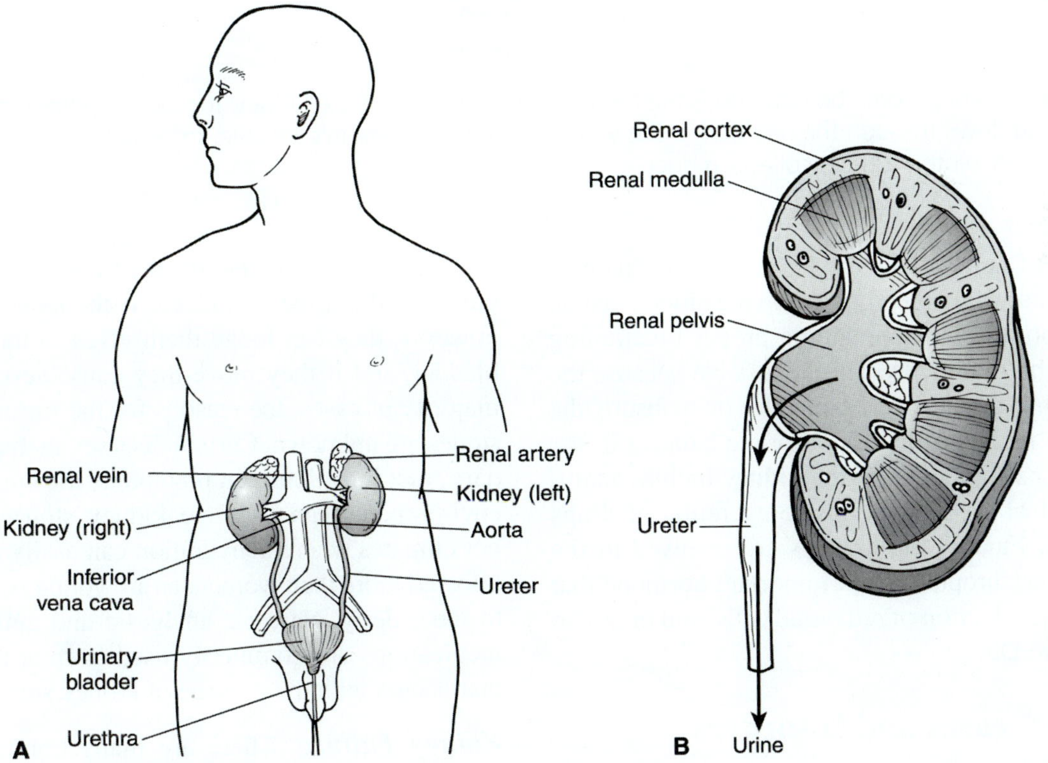

Figure 9–18. The anatomy of the urinary tract system. The urinary tract system is comprised of the right and left kidney and ureters, the bladder, and the urethra. The kidney has two major layers of tissue—renal cortex and renal medulla—and an inner structure—renal pelvis. Urine collects in the renal pelvis and flows from the kidneys, via the ureters, to the bladder, where it is stored until emptied outside the body by way of the urethra.

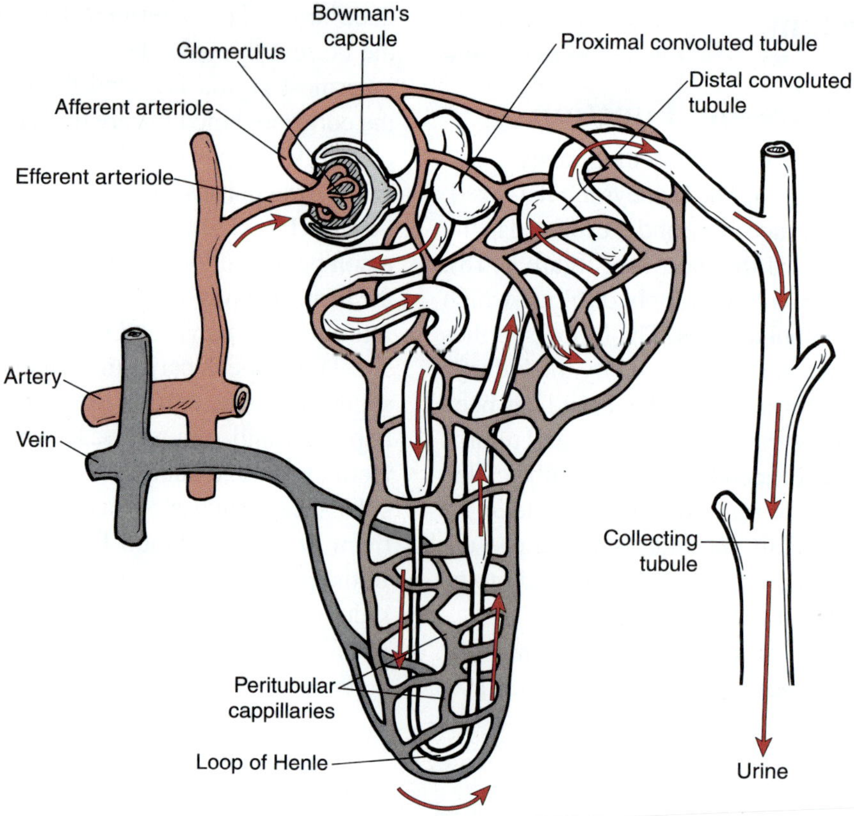

Figure 9–19. The nephron. The nephron is the basic functioning unit of the kidney. It processes blood plasma and produces urine. Fluid flows through the nephron in the following order: Bowman's capsule, proximal convoluted tubule, loop of Henle, distal convoluted tubule, collecting duct.

concentration of certain electrolytes (chemicals such as sodium, potassium, and bicarbonate) in the blood plasma, which are important for maintaining proper functioning of cells throughout the body. This is possible because the kidneys are able to selectively excrete, or reabsorb the electrolytes to maintain their appropriate balance in the blood. Additional functions of the kidney include maintaining the pH of the blood and the excretion of drugs and pesticides. Finally, the kidneys are involved in the production of erythropoietin, an important hormone that stimulates the production of red blood cells, and they also activate vitamin D3.

Common Diseases and Disorders

Kidney Stones. In a condition known as nephrolithiasis, kidney stones are formed when the substances that are to be excreted in the urine instead crystallize in the pelvis of the kidney and form into small stones. They can be formed from substances such as calcium, phosphate, or uric acid. Many stones, if small enough in size, are excreted in the urine unnoticed. If the stones are too large, however, they can lodge themselves in the kidney or the bladder, and if they move they cause severe pain. In the majority of cases, the reasons for the formation of kidney stones are unknown. Certain diseases such as gout and urinary tract infections can precipitate the condition. Certain environments can promote kidney stones, for example, hot climates where dehydration can easily occur. Men are affected more than women, as are young people compared to the elderly. Narcotic analgesic and anti-inflammatory medications are commonly used to treat the severe pain that occurs with the passage of kidney stones.

Kidney Failure. There are many conditions that can seriously damage the kidneys and cause them to fail either acutely or chronically. Most kidney diseases attack the nephrons, causing them to lose their ability to filter the blood. Damage to the nephrons can happen quickly, with the kidney function recovering after a few weeks.

For example, in acute nephritic syndrome, which can occur after tonsillitis or a certain type of streptococcal bacterial infection, damage to the filtering component of the nephron occurs. This can progress to acute failure of the kidneys if left untreated. However, most kidney diseases (such as diabetic nephropathy, uncontrolled high blood pressure, and polycystic kidney disease) destroy the nephrons slowly and, ultimately, the kidneys fail. This is known as chronic renal failure, and dialysis or kidney transplant is the only cure.

Safety First Many drugs are removed by the kidneys; the dosage of these drugs usually needs to be reduced in the event of kidney failure to prevent harmful effects. Pharmacists often monitor kidney function and recommend dosage adjustments in these cases.

Overactive Bladder. This is also referred to as urge incontinence, which is the sudden need to urinate. Normally, when urine is stored in the bladder, the detrusor muscle is relaxed. Contraction of the muscle causes urine to move through the urethra. For those with an overactive bladder, the detrusor muscle contracts involuntarily, causing urine loss. Symptoms include a sudden urge to urinate, uncontrollable leakage of urine, and urinating frequently. The detrusor muscle may have involuntary contractions caused by neurologic disorders such as multiple sclerosis, Parkinson disease, Alzheimer disease, spinal cord injuries, or stroke. Medications available to treat this condition include anticholinergic agents, which decrease the muscle contractions.

Other Body Systems

In order for an individual to maintain a stable internal environment (homeostasis), it must be equipped to deal with fluctuations in its external environment and continually adapt to ever-changing circumstances. Somehow, information from the external environment (the outside world), must be communicated to the internal environment (the brain) of a human being in order for the individual to perceive the world and its surroundings.

The skin and special senses make up a functional system of **perception** that allows the individual to perceive its surroundings for the purpose of adaptation to its environment. There are specialized organs, known as sensory organs, responsible for sensing information on the exterior of the body and transmitting it to the brain in the central nervous system. There, that information can be processed and a response can be sent via the autonomic and/or the somatic-nervous system (see figure 9–20). Each of the sensory organs has receptors that are able to detect changes in the exterior environment and transmit this information to the brain.

Part 2

The general manner in which the signals from the outside are transmitted to the inside involves a number of players: **receptors**, nerve cells, and the brain. There are different types of receptors, characterized by what they are capable of detecting. For example, receptors on the skin that are sensitive to temperature changes are called thermoreceptors. Receptors have been identified that are responsive to changes in light (photoreceptors), mechanical energy (mechanoreceptors), chemicals (chemoreceptors), joint angle and muscle length (proprioceptors), and pain and damage to tissue (nociceptors).

The sensory organs of primary importance that possess these receptors are the skin, the eyes, the ears, and the nose and tongue. From the actions of these sensory organs we have the abilities we know as the senses:

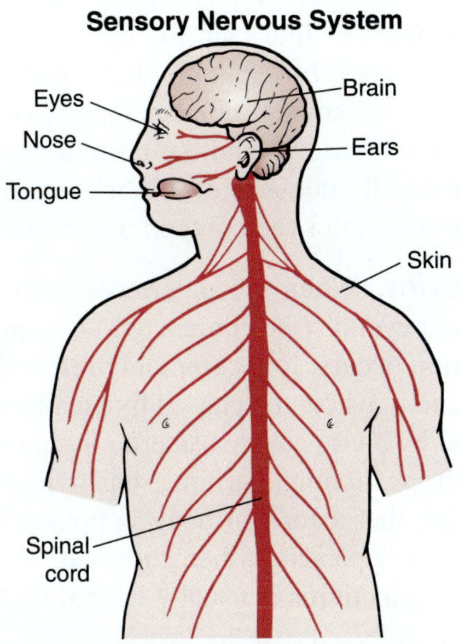

Figure 9–20. The sensory nervous system. The sensory organs of primary importance are the skin, eyes, ears, nose, and tongue. From the actions of these sensory organs, individuals have the abilities known as the *senses*: vision, hearing, taste, smell, and touch.

vision, hearing, taste, smell, and touch. In this section, the eyes, ears, and skin will be presented.

Section I: The Eyes

Overview of Structure and Function

The eyes are fluid-filled, round structures enclosed by three layers. The outermost layer is the sclera/cornea, the middle layer is the choroid/ciliary body/iris, and the innermost layer is the retina. Our ability to see requires at least one functional eye. The anatomy of the eye is designed to allow light to pass through to the back of the eye where it reaches a structure called the retina. Light must then pass through several layers of the retina before it reaches the rods and cones, the functional parts of the eye that contain the light receptors (photoreceptors). The main function of the eye is to focus light rays from the environment onto the photoreceptors. The photoreceptors then change the light energy into energy capable of being carried on a nerve cell. Once this energy change occurs, the nerve cell carries information collected from the eye to the brain where the information is processed.

Common Diseases and Disorders

Dry Eyes. Sometimes referred to as dry eye syndrome, dryness is one of the most common eye problems. This occurs when the tear glands around the eye produce insufficient tears to lubricate the eye. There are many causes of dry eyes: for example, heat, wind, air-conditioning, cigarette smoke, contact lenses, certain drugs and medical conditions, and the normal aging process. Treatment usually consists of a lubricant solution (eye drops) that resembles the composition of natural tears.

Conjunctivitis. When the outermost layer of the eye and the inner eyelids (the conjunctiva) become inflamed, this condition occurs. It is commonly referred to as pink eye. Conjunctivitis can be caused by an allergic reaction or infection by a virus or by bacteria. Symptoms include redness, tearing, itching, burning, sensitivity to light, and the sensation that a foreign body is present in the eye. The treatment depends on the cause and the symptoms. Bacterial conjunctivitis is usually treated with antibiotic eye drops.

Glaucoma. A leading cause of blindness and vision loss, glaucoma is a group of diseases that cause damage to the optic nerve in the eye. The optic nerve is a bundle of nerve fibers that connects the retina to the brain. The most common type of glaucoma is called open-angle glaucoma. The eye continuously makes fluid (aqueous humor) to deliver nutrients to the cornea and lens. The aqueous humor needs to be drained into a special drainage channel to prevent excess accumulation of this fluid. When the drainage of fluid is blocked, the pressure inside the eye rises, causing damage to the optic nerve, open-angle glaucoma, and loss of vision. Those at high risk for this type of glaucoma include African Americans who are older than 60 and who have a family history of glaucoma. There may be no symptoms, but as the disease progresses, vision gradually gets worse, especially peripheral (side) vision. Medications are used to lower the pressure in the eye and/or to lessen the amount of fluid produced by the eye.

Section II: The Ears

Overview of Structure and Function

The ear is comprised of three sections: the external ear, which contains the pinna of the ear, the auditory canal, and the ear drum (tympanic membrane); the middle ear; and the inner ear, which contains three small bones, the vestibular apparatus and the Organ of Corti. The anatomy of the ear allows an individual to hear. Sound waves are captured by the pinna of the ear and are then transmitted through the auditory canal to the fluid-filled middle ear and to the Organ of Corti in the inner ear. Sound waves are then converted to electrical signals and transmitted to the brain, which senses them as sounds. The vestibular apparatus in the inner ear detects changes in position and movement of the head, and it is responsible for maintaining balance and equilibrium.

Common Diseases and Disorders

Otitis Externa. Sometimes called swimmer's ear, otitis externa is inflammation of the outer ear and auditory canal. The most common cause is excessive moisture, which leads to removal of the protective earwax and subsequent bacterial or fungal infection. Trauma to the delicate ear canal is also a common cause. Ear drops that contain drugs to fight the infection and decrease the inflammation are typically prescribed.

Otitis Media. Infection or inflammation of the middle ear. It is a common infection in children and usually follows a cold or sore throat. Symptoms include fever, fluid in the ear, severe ear pain, and trouble hearing. If there is too much fluid in the ears, the pressure in the ear can build up and lead to perforation of the eardrum. Antibiotics are often prescribed to treat this condition.

Section III: The Dermatologic System

Overview of Structure and Function

The skin is the largest organ in the body with many functions. These include regulation of temperature, preventing damage from ultraviolet (UV) radiation, synthesis of vitamin D, and protecting the body against excess fluid loss and penetration by invading microorganisms.

Anatomically, the skin is a layered structure composed of two layers: the epidermis and dermis. The epidermis synthesizes vitamin D, serves to protect an individual from the effects of excess radiation from the sun, and prevents germs from penetrating the body. This is possible because there are specialized cells called melanocytes in the innermost layer of the epidermis that produce a protective pigment called melanin when exposed to the sun. Additionally, the cells of the epidermis produce keratin as they mature. This keratinized layer, which is on the outermost layer of the epidermis, forms a protective layer that serves as a barrier to invading microorganisms and helps to prevent fluid loss from the body.

The inner layer is known as the dermis. This contains hair follicles, pressure receptors, blood vessels, sebaceous glands, and sweat glands. The blood vessels in this layer contract to help prevent heat loss during cold conditions. They help with cooling by dilating during hot conditions and allowing heat loss. Sweat glands in this layer help to cool during hot conditions through evaporation of the sweat on the skin.

Common Diseases and Disorders

Dry Skin. A common condition in which the skin loses excess sebum from the sebaceous glands. This can be caused by excess heat, cold, medications, and some medical conditions. Moisturizing creams and lotions are used to treat dry skin.

Sunburn. Overexposure of the skin to ultraviolet radiation from the sun causes damage to the epidermal layer of the skin. Depending on the degree of sun exposure, the sunburn can be mild and cause the skin to turn red and inflamed, or it can be severe, causing blistering and damage to the lower skin layer. Excess exposure to the skin has been shown to cause melanoma and other types of skin cancer. The use of sunscreen has been shown to prevent sunburn.

Contact Dermatitis. When the skin of an individual becomes exposed to an allergen, chemicals, metals, or plants, a red rash, blisters, or wheals, as well as itching and burning, may occur. Barrier creams, topical antihistamines, and anti-inflammatory agents are often used to decrease the symptoms associated with this condition.

Eczema. Inflammation of the epidermis. Patches of inflammation usually cover the skin, and the condition can affect any part of the body. The areas of inflammation are usually red, dry, and cause crusting, flaking, and itching of the skin. The inflammation can cause isolated skin areas to develop raised, fluid-filled bumps, resulting in blistering, cracking, and oozing of the skin, or bleeding, especially when scratched. Causes of the condition are variable and include a family history of allergies, asthma, or eczema; foods; chemicals; weather conditions; and other environmental factors. Drug treatment includes topical anti-inflammatory creams, lubricants, and antihistamines.

Acne. A common condition when adolescents, especially boys, go through puberty. The changes in hormone levels cause the sebaceous gland associated with the hair follicles in the skin to produce excess sebum. The follicles can become inflamed, and spots and pimples occur. If the inflammation is severe, it can result in damage to the skin and cause scarring. There are many over-the-counter and prescription products that are used to treat acne. Drug treatment is used topically and even orally to reduce inflammation, decrease bacteria, and keep pores open.

Women's Health

Overview of the Female Reproductive System

The primary reproductive organs, or **gonads**, in females are the ovaries. Mature gonads perform two functions: (1) the production of reproductive cells, called gametes (eggs), and (2) the production of the sex hormones estrogen and progesterone.

The female reproductive system consists of those organs which enable a woman to produce eggs (ova), to have sexual intercourse, to nourish and house the fertilized egg until it is fully developed, to give birth, and to be the sole source of nutrition for a newborn baby. Unlike the male, the female sexual organs are almost entirely internal. The female organs are made up of the vulva, the vagina, the uterus (or womb), the fallopian tubes, the ovaries, and the breasts.

The reproductive capability of an individual depends upon a complex relationship between glands in the brain (hypothalamus and anterior pituitary), reproductive organs, and target cells of sex hormones.

Estrogen and progesterone in the female are responsible for the development of secondary sex characteristics when an individual reaches puberty. The ultimate consequence of sexual development is the production of reproductive cells that will pass genes on to the next generation. In the female, the reproductive cells are known as the ova (eggs). Each individual produces an enormous number of reproductive cells; the female possesses all of her several million reproductive cells at birth; only several hundred will develop to the point at which they will have the chance to be fertilized—the rest will degenerate along the way. She will not produce any more during her lifetime.

Common Diseases and Disorders

Infertility. Women who are unable to get pregnant or stay pregnant are considered to be infertile. In order to get pregnant, several steps must occur: the ovaries must release an egg (ovulation), the egg must travel through the fallopian tube toward the uterus (womb), the sperm must fertilize the egg, and then the fertilized egg must attach to the inside of the uterus (implantation). Infertility results when there are problems during any of these steps. Some of the most common causes of infertility in women include not ovulating properly, blocked fallopian tubes, structural problems in the uterus, and being greater than 35 years of age. Treatment of infertility depends on the cause and often includes the use of medications and surgical procedures. Medications are commonly used to help women who have problems with ovulation.

Hormone Deficiencies. Alteration in the levels of the sex hormones in females can cause conditions such as menstrual disorders and polycystic ovarian syndrome (PCOS). As a woman ages, the levels of sex hormones (estrogen and progesterone) decrease, menstruation becomes irregular, and the period of menopause begins. Typically, this begins between the ages of 48 and 55. Symptoms may include changes in menstruation, hot flashes, vaginal dryness, sleep problems, and mood changes. If symptoms are bothersome, they may be treated with small doses of estrogen or progesterone.

Endometriosis. When the tissue that lines the uterus, called the endometrium, forms in areas outside of this organ, for example, the ovaries or the abdomen.[13] The tissue responds to estrogen and progesterone during the menstrual cycle, just like it does normally in the uterus. During the menstrual cycle, this tissue can expand, adding extra tissue and blood. When the tissue and blood are shed in the body, it can cause inflammation, scarring, and pain. Symptoms include painful menstruation, pain during or after intercourse, urination, and bowel movements. Pain medication and hormone therapy are often prescribed for this condition.

Sexually Transmitted Diseases (STDs). The female is susceptible to a sexually transmitted disease when she has unprotected intercourse with an infected partner. There are many types of STDs that are caused by viruses (e.g., HIV-AIDS, genital herpes, hepatitis C, human papillomavirus [HPV] and genital warts) or bacteria (e.g., chlamydia, gonorrhea, syphilis, trichomoniasis, and pelvic inflammatory disease). Each of the conditions presents with different symptoms, and drug therapy is determined by the infecting organism, susceptibility patterns, and individual patient characteristics.

Men's Health

Overview of the Male Reproductive System

The primary reproductive organs, or gonads, consist of a pair of testes in males. In males, the mature gonads perform two functions: (1) the production of reproductive cells, called gametes (sperm), and (2) the production of the sex hormone, testosterone.

The male reproductive system enables a man to have sexual intercourse and to fertilize eggs (ova) with sperm (male sex cells). Sperm, along with male sex hormones, are produced in the testes, a pair of oval-shaped glands that are suspended in a pouch called the scrotum. The sexual organs of males are partly external and partly internal. The visible parts are the penis and the scrotum. Inside the body, the prostate gland and tubes that link the system together reside. In the male, the prostate gland has the primary function of producing part of the fluid that makes up semen. The male organs produce and transfer sperm to the female for fertilization.

The reproductive capability of a male depends on a complex relationship between glands in the brain (hypothalamus and anterior pituitary), reproductive organs, and the target cells of sex hormones.

The hormone testosterone is responsible for the development of secondary sex characteristics when an individual reaches puberty. The ultimate consequence of sexual development is production of reproductive cells that will pass genes on to the next generation. In the male, the reproductive cell is sperm. Each male produces an enormous number of reproductive cells. Sperm is produced continuously after the male has reached sexual maturity, and each ejaculation releases perhaps one hundred million sperm.

Common Diseases and Disorders

Benign Prostatic Hyperplasia (BPH). As men get older, the prostate gland enlarges. In some men, especially those greater than 60 years of age, the gland expands so much that it presses against the urethra, causing bladder problems such as frequent urination, a weak stream of urine, and urgency or leaking of urine. The cause is unknown, but may be related to age-related changes in the hormones testosterone, estrogen, and dihydrotesterone (DHT). Medications are used to shrink the prostate gland and improve the flow of urine.

Erectile Dysfunction. When a male cannot achieve or maintain an erection, it is known as erectile dysfunction or impotence. Common causes of this condition include diseases, such as diabetes, atherosclerosis, and neurologic disease; injury or damage to the nerves and arteries, such as from surgery; psychological factors; and side effects of drugs. There are a variety of different medications available in various dosage forms, such as tablets or medications that are directly injected or inserted into the penis.

Sexually Transmitted Diseases. The male is susceptible to a sexually transmitted disease when he has unprotected intercourse with an infected female or male. There are many types of STDs that are caused by either a virus, for example HIV-AIDS, genital herpes, hepatitis C, human papillomavirus (HPV), and genital warts; or bacteria, for example, chlamydia, gonorrhea, and syphilis. Each of the conditions presents with different symptoms, and drug therapy depends on the infecting organism, susceptibility patterns, and individual patient characteristics.

Summary

Although each of the body systems has different functions, for example, the cardiovascular system pumps deoxygenated blood to the lungs, whereas the lungs are responsible for exchanging gases in the deoxygenated blood, each is dependent on the others to maintain normal physiological balance in the body. When damage takes place in one of the systems and disrupts normal function, disease states can occur. Some disease states develop rather quickly, such as Type I diabetes, whereas others can take years to develop, as in hypertension. When pathophysiological conditions occur, this imbalance can affect other body systems as well, further illustrating the interdependence of the body systems. For example, hypertension can cause problems with the kidneys, blood vessels, and the heart; diabetes can cause malfunctions in the kidneys, eyes, circulation, and nerves.

Therefore, one can understand how normal functioning of the organ systems is required to bring about a balanced internal environment.

Self-Assessment Questions

1. Which of the following statements is true regarding the nervous system?
   a. The autonomic nervous system is under voluntary control.
   b. The somatic nervous system is under voluntary control.
   c. The central nervous system consists of the brain, spinal cord, and nerves that leave the spinal cord.
   d. The somatic nervous system includes the sympathetic and parasympathetic nervous systems.
2. What is a common symptom of Parkinson's disease?
   a. Tremor
   b. Delusional thoughts
   c. Seizures
   d. Pain
3. What is the right ventricle of the heart responsible for?
   a. Generating electrical signals that trigger the contraction of the heart
   b. Pumping oxygen-rich blood to the body
   c. Pumping oxygen-rich blood to the lungs
   d. Pumping deoxygenated blood to the lungs
4. Where is smooth muscle found in the body?
   a. Arms
   b. Face
   c. Stomach, bladder
   d. Heart
5. What is the physiologic effect of the hormone aldosterone?
   a. Promotes growth of the ovarian follicle and stimulates estrogen secretion
   b. Causes contractions of the uterus
   c. Increases sodium retention and potassium secretion
   d. Produces thyroid hormone
6. Which bacteria can cause peptic ulcer disease?
   a. *Helicobacter pylori*
   b. *Salmonella*
   c. *E. coli*
   d. Rotavirus
7. Where does gas exchange occur in the respiratory system?
   a. Bronchi
   b. Bronchioles
   c. Capillaries
   d. Alveoli
8. What is diabetes insipidus?
   a. Decreased production of insulin, which causes high levels of glucose in the blood and urine
   b. Insufficient vasopressin leading to losses of large volumes of urine
   c. Swelling and inflammation in the kidney due to damage of the filtering component of the nephron
   d. Increased systolic pressure in the kidney
9. What is the term for the primary reproductive organs?
   a. Chyme
   b. Prostate
   c. Gonads
   d. Ovaries
10. Which of the following is a true statement?
    a. An antibody can be a bacterium, a virus, or a cancer cell
    b. A lymphocyte is a type of red blood cell
    c. The lack of an immune response to self is called autoimmunity
    d. T lymphocytes attack viruses.
11. With which of the following disorders would patients most likely be prescribed medications on a long-term basis (chronically)?
    a. Glaucoma
    b. Bacterial conjunctivitis
    c. Sunburn
    d. Otitis Media

Self-Assessment Answers

1. b. The somatic nervous system is under voluntary control and is responsible for regulating the contractions of skeletal muscle. The autonomic nervous system is not under voluntary control. The actions are carried out without us being consciously aware of the changes. The central nervous system consists of the brain and spinal cord. Nerves that leave the spinal cord are in the peripheral nervous system. The autonomic nervous system contains the sympathetic and parasympathetic nervous systems.
2. a. Parkinson disease is a disease that affects movement and does not affect the way a person thinks. Delusional thoughts are part of the symptoms of schizophrenia. Seizures are associated with epilepsy. Pain is not a common symptom of Parkinson disease.
3. d. The right ventricle of the heart is responsible for pumping deoxygenated (low in oxygen) blood to the lungs to allow gas exchange and oxygenation of the blood. Oxygen-rich blood returns to the left atrium, through the valve into the left ventricle, and then is pumped throughout the body. Pacemaker cells generate electrical signals that trigger contraction of the heart and set the heart rhythm.
4. c. Smooth (visceral) muscle is found in the internal organs of the body, such as the stomach, intestines, bladder, and blood vessels. Cardiac muscle is found in the heart and skeletal muscle is found in the face and arms.
5. c. Aldosterone is secreted by the adrenal cortex; its target tissue is the kidney where it increases sodium retention and potassium secretion. Follicle-stimulating hormone (FSH) promotes growth of the ovarian follicle and stimulates estrogen secretion. Oxytocin causes contractions of the uterus. Thyroid-stimulating hormone (TSH) produces thyroid hormone.
6. a. Bacterial infection with *helicobacter pylori* can result in the formation of peptic ulcers. Rotavirus, *salmonella,* and *E. coli* are common causes of infection in the gastrointestinal tract, but they do not cause peptic ulcer disease.
7. d. Gas exchange occurs between the blood and the alveoli which are located at the ends of the smallest bronchioles in the lungs.
8. b. Diabetes insipidus is where the kidneys do not respond to vasopressin or there is insufficient secretion of vasopressin from the pituitary gland, resulting in large losses of urine. Diabetes mellitus is due to decreased production of insulin, resulting in high blood and urine levels of glucose. Nephritic syndrome is swelling and inflammation in the kidney due to damage of the filtering component of the nephron (the glomeruli).
9. c. The gonads are the primary reproductive organs; they are known as the testes in males, and the ovaries in females. Chyme is a thick liquid composed of partially digested food. The prostate is a gland in the male that produces and secretes the fluid in semen.
10. d. T lymphocytes attack viruses, whereas B lymphocytes attack bacteria. B and T lymphocytes are a type of white blood cell that is produced outside of the bone marrow. An antigen can be a bacterium, a virus, or a cancer cell. Antibodies indirectly destroy invaders by binding to antigens and intensifying the immune response that has been initiated against the invader. The lack of an immune response to self is called tolerance. Autoimmunity is an immune response against the self.
11. a. Glaucoma is a chronic disease that is treated with medications to prevent further optic nerve damage and vision loss. Bacterial or viral conjunctivitis and otitis media (ear infections) are treated with short courses of anti-infective medications. Sunburn is not generally treated with medications.

References

1. Sherwood L. *Human Physiology: From Cells to Systems.* 4th ed. Pacific Grove, CA: Brooks Cole Publications; 2001.
2. Germann WJ, Stanfield CL. *Principles of Human Physiology.* 1st Ed. San Franscisco, CA: Benjamin Cummings Publications; 2002.
3. WebMD. Mental Health Center: Schizophrenia. http://www.webmd.com/schizophrenia/default.htm. Accessed April 2010.

4. WebMD. Alzheimer's Disease Health Center. Alzheimer's Disease–Topic Overview. http://www.webmd.com/alzheimers/tc/alzheimers-disease-topic-overview. Accessed April 2010.
5. WebMD. Kidney Stones Health Center. Understanding Kidney Stones—the Basics. http://www.webmd.com/kidney-stones/understanding-kidney-stones-basics. Accessed April 2010.
6. Harley JP. *Study Guide for Sherwood's Human Physiology: From Cells to Systems*. 4th ed. Pacific Grove, CA: Brooks Cole Publications; 2001.
7. Moffett DE, Moffet SB, Schauf CL. *Human Physiology: Foundations and Frontiers*. 2nd ed. St. Louis MO: Mosby-Year Book, Inc., 1993.
8. Crimando J "Anatomy and Physiology Tutorials" Web-Site images and text created and © GateWay Community College; Phoenix, AZ; Orig. created: Fall, 1997. http://www.gwc.maricopa.edu/class/bio201/index.html Accessed April 2010.
9. Austgen L, Bowen RA, Rouge M. Pathophysiology of the Digestive System. http://arbl.cvmbs.colostate.edu/hbooks/pathphys/digestion/index.html. Accessed April 2010.
10. Stedman TL. *Stedman's Medical Dictionary for the Health Professionals and Nursing*, 6th ed. Philadelphia: Wolters Kluwer Health/Lippincott, Williams & Wilkins; 2008.
11. MedicineNet.com. MedTerms Medical Dictionary. http://www.medterms.com/script/main/hp.asp. Accessed April 2010.
12. Iannelli V. Treating Sprains and Strains. About.Com: Pediatrics. http://pediatrics.about.com/od/hometreatmenttips/a/05_sprains.htm Accessed April, 2010.
13. Endo-Online. What is endometriosis? Endometriosis Association. http://www.endometriosisassn.org/endo.html. Accessed April 2010.

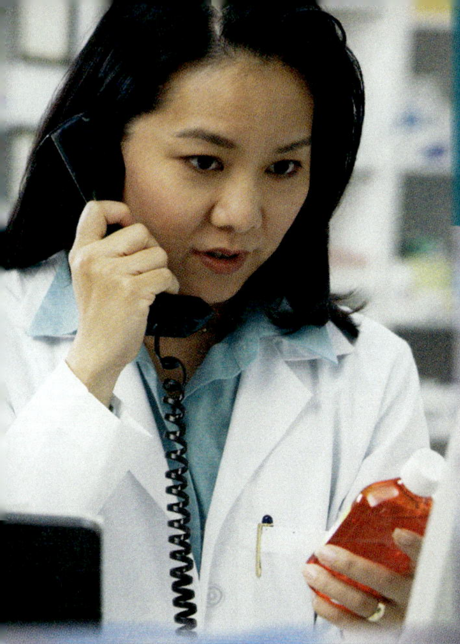

Chapter 10

Drug Classifications and Pharmacologic Actions

Sheri Stensland

Learning Outcomes

After completing this chapter you will be able to

- Identify the common drug names for each classification.
- Describe the important actions and/or therapeutic uses for the major classes of drugs.
- Describe the most common or most serious adverse effects for the major classes of drugs.
- List special precautions for the major classes of drugs.

Key Terms

agranulocytosis A dramatic decrease in white blood cells.

antiproliferative A substance used to prevent the spread of cells into surrounding tissue.

arthralgia Joint pain.

cross-sensitivity Sensitivity to one substance that predisposes an individual to sensitivity to other substances that are related in chemical structure.

expectorate To cough up or spit.

myalgia Muscle pain.

myelosuppression The suppression of white blood cell and platelet production from the bone marrow.

peripheral neuropathy Damage of nerves other than the brain and the spinal cord.

rhinitis Inflammation of the nasal lining.

A drug can be defined as any substance that, when introduced into the body, alters the body's function. An ideal drug has several characteristics: effectiveness for its therapeutic use, safety even if large quantities are ingested, and no adverse effects. Unfortunately, the ideal drug does not exist. All drugs have some adverse effects and many drugs are toxic when more than the recommended dose is taken. Therefore, the decision to use any drug therapy is made after weighing the benefits of the drug against the risks involved with its use.

There are many different ways to classify medications. They can be classified by medical conditions, by body organ systems, or by type of action. Drugs often have actions in more than one part of the body and may be mentioned in several areas. The major actions or uses of drugs, their major adverse effects, and important characteristics particular to specific drugs, especially where these characteristics are important in dispensing activities, will be discussed. Many of the drugs discussed are listed in tables with both the generic name and the trade name listed. The United States Adopted Names Council (USAN) has approved stems for generic names that help to classify medications according to their mechanism of action. For example, the medication metoprolol has an -olol ending and is classified as a beta-blocking agent, which is commonly used to treat high blood pressure. Learning to recognize these stems will help in identifying the classifications for different medications.

Rx for Success

A link to the top 200 drugs can be found at www.ashp.org/techmanual.

Section 1: Body Systems

Drugs that Affect the Nervous System

Antiepileptic Agents. There are several types of seizures, and some of the medications discussed here may be used alone to treat one or more types of seizures, whereas others may need to be used in combination with other antiepileptics to control certain types of seizures. Some antiepileptic drugs have other therapeutic uses, such as migraine prevention, psychiatric disorders, a painful facial nerve condition called trigeminal neuralgia, and other types of nerve pain.

Antiepileptic agents, also called anticonvulsants, are used to reduce the frequency of seizures.[1] They do this by reducing the excitability of the nerve cells in the brain.[2] All antiepileptics have adverse effects, so they are only used when the risk of recurrent seizures is more worrisome than the adverse effects of the drugs. Therapy is usually started with one medication in order to minimize the adverse effects and improve patient compliance.

In approximately 50–70% of patients, seizures can be controlled with one agent.[1] Medications should be started with low doses and then titrated up, allowing for the dosage to be individualized for each patient. Once therapy is started, patients need to be monitored for treatment success or failure. Monitoring may include blood levels or the number of seizures and side effects. If therapy is considered a failure, either due to lack of seizure control or adverse effects, the medication may be changed or an additional medication may be added.[1]

Antiepileptic agents should not be discontinued abruptly.[2] Some patients may experience seizures if the medication is suddenly stopped. Ideally, agents should be slowly tapered over one to three months.[2]

The major drugs used to control seizures are phenytoin (Dilantin), carbamazepine (Tegretol), levetiracetam (Keppra), and divalproex sodium (Depakote). Other drugs

Table 10-1. Antiepileptics

Generic Name (Brand Name)	Dosage Forms	FDA Approved Indications
Carbamazepine (Tegretol, Tegretol XR)	capsules, suspension, tablets, extended-release	Tonic-clonic, partial seizures
Clonazepam (Klonopin)	tablets, oral-disintegrating tablets, wafers	Absence, myoclonic seizures
Diazepam (Valium, Diastat)	Injection, rectal gel	Status epilepticus
Divalproex sodium (Depakote, Depakote ER)	capsules (sprinkle), delayed-release tablets, extended-release tablets	Absence, partial seizures
Fosphenytoin (Cerebyx)	injection	Status epilepticus, prevention and treatment of seizures during neurosurgery, short-term administration when unable to take oral phenytoin
Gabapentin (Neurontin)	capsules, solution, tablets	Tonic-clonic, partial seizures
Lacosamide (Vimpat)	Tablets, injection	Adjunctive to partial
Lamotrigine (Lamictal, Lamictal XR)	tablets, oral-disintegrating tablets, extended-release tablets	Partial seizures
Levetiracetam (Keppra)	injection, solution, tablets, extended-release tablets	Adjunctive to partial
Lorazepam (Ativan)	injection	Status epilepticus
Oxcarbazepine (Trileptal)	suspension, tablets	Partial seizures
Phenobarbital	Tablets, injection	Generalized tonic-clonic, partial seizures, status epilepticus
Phenytoin (Dilantin)	extended-release capsules, chew-tabs, suspension, injection	Generalized tonic-clonic (grand mal), complex partial seizures, prevention and treatment during or following neurosurgery, status epilepticus (IV)
Pregabalin (Lyrica)	tablets	Adjunctive to partial
Tiagabine (Gabitril)	tablets	Adjunctive to partial
Topiramate (Topamax)	capsules (sprinkle), tablets	Adjunctive to tonic-clonic, partial
Valproic acid (Depakene), valproate sodium (Depacon)	capsules, syrup, injection	Absence seizures, complex partial, simple
Zonisamide (Zonegran)	capsules	Adjunctive to partial

available are listed in table 10-1, along with the types of seizures they treat. Older agents require stricter monitoring and are often taken more frequently, reducing patient compliance. Some of these medications are now available as generic formulations. It should be noted that there may be differences in the bioavailability (extent of absorption) of the generics versus brand-name drugs. This may correlate to an increase in adverse effects/toxicities or an increase in seizure frequency. Therefore, patients should be closely monitored when switching between products.[2]

Status epilepticus is a condition of repetitive seizures with little or no interruption between them. This is a life-threatening condition that must be treated immediately using IV medications. These agents are generally used only by emergency personnel or in an institutional setting. Injectable forms of the benzodiazepines diazepam (Valium) and lorazepam (Ativan) are commonly used initially to stop the repetitive seizure activity. Longer-acting drugs, such as phenytoin (Dilantin) or fosphenytoin (Cerebyx), are given to prevent the recurrence of seizures.[2]

Phenytoin has been available for many years and effectively prevents many types of seizures. Dosing of phenytoin is complicated, and blood levels are usually measured to ensure that enough phenytoin is present to prevent seizures but not enough to cause side effects. This drug is known to have a narrow therapeutic index, which means small changes in the dose results in large changes in the drug's effects. Side effects that are dose-related include double vision, loss of muscle coordination, and sedation. Side effects that are common but are not related to the dose are overgrowth of the gums (gingival hypertrophy) and excessive hair growth (hirsutism). Phenytoin also has many drug interactions. Patients should be warned not to take extra doses or other drugs without checking with their doctor or pharmacist first.[2]

Fosphenytoin (Cerebyx) is an injectable medication that is converted to phenytoin in the body. An advantage of fosphenytoin is that it can be mixed in either normal saline or dextrose, whereas phenytoin IV must be mixed only in normal saline. If phenytoin is mixed with dextrose, a precipitate will form. Fosphenytoin also causes less damage to veins, it can be infused over a shorter period of time, and it causes less hypotension (low blood pressure) compared to phenytoin.[2] Fosphenytoin is preferred over phenytoin in many institutions.

Like phenytoin, blood levels of some antiepileptics are measured to ensure that the dose is producing therapeutic blood levels but not levels high enough to result in adverse effects. Newer agents do not need this additional monitoring. Liver function and blood cell counts must be monitored with several of the antiepileptic drugs. Carbamazepine (Tegretol) can cause a rare, serious adverse effect called pancytopenia, which is a depression of the production of all types of blood cells (red cells, white cells, and platelets). Liver toxicity is a serious side effect of divalproex sodium (Depakote) use, but is reversible if the drug is stopped. Other side effects of antiepileptic agents may include dizziness, fatigue, nausea, vomiting, headache, weight gain, increased appetite, and hair loss. Phenobarbital is effective against a number of different seizure types, but the adverse effects of phenobarbital, mainly excessive sedation and the potential for dependence and withdrawal symptoms, limits its usefulness today.

✔The antiepileptic drugs increase the risk of suicidal thoughts or behavior; therefore, it is important that patients are monitored for unusual changes in mood or behavior. An FDA-approved Medication Guide must be dispensed with all prescriptions for antiepileptic drugs warning patients about this potential risk.

Parkinsonian Agents. Parkinson disease (PD) is a progressive disease, and the goals for treatment are to maintain function and quality of life, as well as to avoid drug-induced complications. Drug therapy is focused on decreasing acetylcholine and increasing dopamine (table 10-2). Drugs affecting dopamine levels include levodopa, dopamine agonists, catechol-O-methyl transferase (COMT) inhibitors, and selegiline. Drugs used to restore the balance between acetylcholine and dopamine include anticholinergics and amantadine.

Table 10–2. Drugs Used to Treat Parkinson Disease

Classifications and Medications	Available Dosage Forms
Anticholinergics	
Benztropine (Cogentin)	Tablets, injection
Trihexyphenidyl (Artane)	Tablets, sustained-release capsules
Amantadine (Symmetrel)	Tablets, capsules, solution
Carbidopa/levodopa products	
Carbidopa/levodopa (Sinemet, Sinemet CR)	Tabets, extended-release tablets
Carbidopa/levodopa/entacapone (Stalevo)	Tablets
MAO-B inhibitors	
Rasagiline (Azilect)	Tablets
Selegiline (Eldepryl, Zelapar ODT, Emsam patch)	Capsules, oral-disintegrating tablets, transdermal patch
COMT inhibitors	
Entacapone (Comtan)	Tablets
Tolcapone (Tasmar)	Tablets
Dopamine agonists	
Bromocriptine (Parlodel)	Tablets, capsules
Pramipexole (Mirapex)	Tablets, extended-release tablets
Ropinirole (Requip)	Tablets, extended-release tablets
Apomorphine (Apokyn)	Subcutaneous injection

The main therapies for PD include levodopa plus carbidopa, dopamine agonists, and the monoamine oxidase (MAO-B) inhibitors.[3] The most commonly used treatment is the combination of levodopa and carbidopa. Levodopa is converted to dopamine in the body, but it must move into the brain to be helpful for Parkinson's treatment. Unfortunately, once it is converted peripherally, only a small amount is able to enter the central nervous system (CNS). The remainder stays in the periphery and causes side effects such as nausea, vomiting, arrhythmias, and orthostatic hypotension.[4]

Carbidopa is a dopa decarboxylase inhibitor and keeps levodopa from being converted to dopamine in the periphery. By getting the levodopa into the brain for conversion to dopamine, it decreases the side effects in the body and increases its effectiveness for the treatment of PD. Akinesia (loss of normal motor function), tremor, and rigidity often improve with the use of levodopa and carbidopa, but balance and gait (the rate of moving, especially walking) may not. Medication compliance may be an issue with these agents because the tablets need to be taken three or more times a day. An extended-release formulation is also available to decrease the frequency of administration to two or three times a day.

Dopamine agonists are thought to work by binding to and stimulating the dopamine receptors. This class of medications appears to improve movement or motor functions. Pramipexole (Mirapex) and ropinirole (Requip) are indicated for monotherapy or adjunct therapy with levodopa/carbidopa. The most common side effects include depression, confusion, insomnia, anxiety, hypotension, and arrhythmias. These agents are more selective for the dopamine receptors, leading to fewer side effects than some of the other classes. Pramipexole and ropinirole have extended release formulations available for once-a-day dosing.[2]

Apomorphine (Apokyn) is a dopamine agonist that can be used to treat the "off" periods of movement. It is a subcutaneous injection that is generally given as needed. It is considered adjunct therapy to other agents. In some patients, apomorphine may cause orthostatic hypotension, so patients should receive a test dose and have their blood pressure monitored closely prior to starting therapy. The most common side effects are nausea and vomiting. Patients should be treated with the antiemetic agent trimethobenzamide (Tigan) prior to receiving a dose of apomorphine.[2]

Anticholinergic agents and MAO-B inhibitors have an important role in PD. Anticholinergic agents are known for their drying effects. Because of these side effects, they have been found to be useful in improving the drooling effects seen in patients as well as some improvement in the tremor of early disease. MAO-B inhibitors may also be used in mild symptoms. Rasagiline (Azilect) has been approved to be used as monotherapy.

The COMT inhibitors are generally considered third- or fourth-line therapy and should be used as adjunct therapy with levodopa/carbidopa. These agents work by limiting the breakdown of dopamine, thus allowing for a lower dose of levodopa to be used. The combination levodopa/carbidopa/entacapone (Stalevo) was developed to improve patient compliance so patients don't have to take two separate agents. Tolcapone (Tasmar) can cause severe liver failure, which limits its use.

Alzheimer Disease Agents. Alzheimer disease is a progressive neurodegenerative disorder. Signs and symptoms include memory impairment as well as behavioral changes in social and functional capacities. The main neurotransmitter thought to be associated with the decline in memory function is acetylcholine.[6] At this time, there is no cure for Alzheimer disease. Pharmacologic treatments available are not able to reverse the devastating consequences, but may slow the progression of the disease to allow patients to have a better quality of life.[7] The two classes of medications available for Alzheimer disease are the cholinesterase inhibitors and the N-methyl-D-aspartate (NMDA) receptor antagonists (table 10-3).

Other agents that may be used are antidepressants and antipsychotic agents. Patients with Alzheimer often experience depression as part of the disease, so the selective serotonin reuptake inhibitors (SSRIs) may be used to help with this.[2] The antipsychotic agents haloperidol (Haldol), risperidone (Risperdal), and olanzapine (Zyprexa) may be used to decrease hallucinations, suspiciousness, agitation, and aggression.[2]

The cholinesterase inhibitors are first-line therapy for mild-to-moderate dementia of Alzheimer disease; in addition, donepezil (Aricept) has been approved for use in severe Alzheimer disease.[8] These agents work by preventing the breakdown of acetylcholine. Increasing the amount of acetylcholine in the brain is thought to result in stabilizing or improving of memory function.[6] Choosing the best agent for the patient is based on efficacy, adverse effects, available dosage forms, ease of titration, and cost.[2]

Table 10-3. Alzheimer Disease Agents

Classifications and Medications	Available Dosage Forms
Cholinesterase inhibitors	
Donepezil (Aricept)	Tablets, oral disintegrating tablets (ODT)
Galantamine (Razadyne)	Tablets, extended release tablets, solution
Rivastigmine (Exelon)	Capsules, solution, patch
Tacrine (Cognex)	Capsules
N-methyl-D-aspartate (NMDA) receptor antagonists	
Memantine (Namenda)	Tablets, oral solution

Adverse effects of these agents include nausea, vomiting, diarrhea, dizziness, and fatigue.[8] These effects can be minimized by starting with a low dose and titrating up. Tacrine (Cognex), which was the first available agent, has been associated with liver toxicity. Due to this adverse effect and because it must be given four times a day, it is now a last-line agent in the cholinesterase inhibitor class.[8]

The titration of these agents should be slow to minimize gastrointestinal adverse effects. Initial doses are low and then gradually increased every four to six weeks until the target dose is achieved. It is important to note that if rivastigmine (Exelon) or galantamine (Razadyne) are stopped for more than a couple of days, the dose needs to be retitrated back to the maintenance dose.[8]

Rivastigmine (Exelon) is the only agent available as a topical patch. Titration to maintenance dose is still required with this dosage form. The patch is to be changed every twenty-four hours and recommended placement is on the upper or lower back, although the upper arm and chest may be used if the patient is unable to reach the back. Patients or their caregivers need to be counseled that a new patch should not be applied to the same location for at least two weeks.[9]

The new class that is now available is the N-methyl-D-aspartate (NMDA) receptor antagonists. The only agent currently approved in this class is memantine (Namenda), and it has been approved for the treatment of moderate to severe Alzheimer disease. NMDA receptors are stimulated by a neurotransmitter known as glutamate, which is thought to play a role in learning and memory.[6] In Alzheimer disease, some patients may have excess amounts of glutamate that can overstimulate these NMDA receptors, leading to a dysfunction in the storage of information. Blocking these receptors with memantine will reduce the overstimulation, potentially leading to the normal functioning of the system.[6] Memantine may be used as monotherapy or as adjunct therapy with the cholinesterase inhibitors. Adverse effects include constipation, dizziness, fatigue, and headache. Slowly titrating the dose every four weeks should alleviate these adverse effects.[10]

Multiple Sclerosis Agents. Multiple sclerosis (MS) is a progressive neurological disorder affecting the brain and the spinal cord. Its onset is generally between the ages of eighteen and forty-five and affects women more often than men.[11] In MS, the myelin sheath that covers neurons degenerates, causing a disruption of nerve transmission.[2] An inflammatory response occurs that forms lesions or plaques. These lesions are found on the nerves in the brain, spinal cord, and the eye. Symptoms may include visual disturbances, muscle spasms, weakness, balance problems, and difficulty with speech, as well as bowel, bladder, and sexual dysfunction.[2] The disease is characterized by exacerbations and remissions. Drug therapy is focused on preventing exacerbations and treating the symptoms (table 10-4). Due to the complexity of the disease, symptoms are treated as they appear. Corticosteroids are often used to reduce inflammation in acute exabercations. Muscle relaxers (e.g., baclofen [Lioresal], tizanidine [Zanaflex]) are used to decrease muscle spasms. Urinary antispasmodics (oxybutynin [Ditropan], tolterodine [Detrol]) treat overactive bladder symptoms, and pain is often treated with neuropathic pain medications such as lamotrigine (Lamictal) or gabapentin (Neurontin).

The most common agents used in MS patients are those that are used for the prevention of relapses and

Table 10-4. Multiple Sclerosis Agents

Medications' Generic (Brand) Names	Available Dosage Forms	Indications
Glatiramer acetate (Copaxone)	Subcutaneous injection	To reduce the frequency of relapses in relapsing-remitting MS
Interferon—1a (Avonex)	Intramuscular injection	Treatment of relapsing forms of MS to slow disease progression and prevent exacerbations
Interferon-ß-1b (Betaseron)	Subcutaneous injection	Treatment of relapsing forms of MS and to prevent exacerbations
Natalizumab (Tysabri)	Intravenous infusion	Treatment of relapsing forms of MS to delay disease progression and prevent exacerbations; used when an inadequate response or intolerance to other agents
Mitoxantrone (Novantrone)	Intravenous infusion	To reduce neurologic disability and frequency of relapses in secondary, chronic progressive, relapsing-remitting MS

disease progression. The agents used for this treatment have become known as the ABC therapy (Avonex, Betaseron, Copaxone).[2] Interferon-β-1b (Betaseron) was the first agent available for reducing the relapses of MS. It is a subcutaneous injection given every other day. Studies show that patients treated with this interferon had no significant increases in lesions during treatment time.[12]

Interferon-β-1a (Avonex) is an intramuscular injection administered once a week to patients with MS. Studies of this agent have shown a reduction in relapse rates as well as a slowing of disease progression.[13] It is unknown how the interferons reduce the relapses of MS. Side effects can be somewhat limiting. The most common side effect seen is flu-like symptoms following the injection. Fever, chills, and muscle aches can occur for up to twenty-four hours after the injection is given. Pre-treatment with acetaminophen (Tylenol) or ibuprofen (Advil) may help to alleviate the flu-like symptoms. Glatiramer acetate (Copaxone) is a daily subcutaneous injection that is thought to help reduce inflammation, demylination, and nerve damage. The side-effect profile is more favorable than for the interferons. Injection-site reaction is the most common side effect seen with glatiramer acetate (Copaxone). Injection-site reactions are common among all three agents; these include pain, itching, redness, and swelling.[2]

Drugs to Treat Headaches/Migraines. In 2001, the number one over-the-counter (OTC) recommendations made by pharmacists were for headache products.[14] Headache pain can be described as constant, throbbing, dull, or severe, and may be only on one side or throughout the head.[12] They may be classified as migraines, tension, cluster, or others. Some criteria used to classify headaches include the number and length of headaches, level of pain, location of the headache, and presence of nausea, vomiting, photophobia, or phonophobia.[17] Treatment of headaches includes acute (abortive) therapy, which involves treating the current headache pain, and preventive therapy. Treatments available do not cure chronic headache, but can help to manage the condition. Goals of therapy include[17]

- Ability to maintain normal activities
- Provide quick relief of headache pain
- Reduce frequency of attacks
- Minimize the amount of medications needed

Acute/abortive treatment is used to stop an attack. These medications should be used only two to three times per week. Overuse of these medications can lead to a medication-induced headache. Drug classes used to treat headaches include non-steroidal inflammatory drugs (NSAIDs), triptans, butalbital-containing products, opioids, steroids, and others (table 10-5).

The most common class of medications used for the treatment of migraines is the serotonin 5-HT_1 receptor agonists, or the "triptans." These medications work by binding to vascular 5-HT_1 receptors and causing vasoconstriction. Onset of action is generally within thirty minutes to one hour. Most of the drugs in this class are dosed so that if the patient does not have relief after two hours, he/she may repeat the dose. These drugs should not be used to treat more than four headaches per

Table 10–5. Drugs Used to Treat Headaches

Classifications and Medications	Available Dosage Forms
Triptans	
Almotriptan (Axert)	Tablets
Eletriptan (Relpax)	Tablets
Frovatriptan (Frova)	Tablets
Naratriptan (Amerge)	Tablets
Rizatriptan (Maxalt)	Tablets, orally disintegrating tablets
Sumatriptan (Imitrex)	Tablets, nasal spray, injection
Zolmitriptan (Zomig)	Tablets, orally disintegrating tablets, nasal spray
Sumatriptan and naproxen (Treximet)	Tablets
Butalbital-containing products	
Butalbital and acetaminophen (Phrenilin)	Tablets
Butalbital, acetaminophen, caffeine (Fioricet, Esgic, Esgic-Plus)	Tablets
Butalbital, acetaminophen, caffeine, codeine (Fioricet with codeine)	Tablets
Butalbital, aspirin, caffeine (Fiorinal)	Capsules, tablets
Butalbital, aspirin, caffeine, codeine (Fiorinal with codeine)	Capsules
Ergotamine derivatives	
Ergotamine, caffeine (Cafergot, Migergot, Ergomar)	Suppositories, tablets, sublingual tablets
Dihydroergotamine (D.H.E. 45, Migranal)	Injection, nasal spray

month. Overuse of these products may lead to "rebound" headaches.[18]

Side effects most commonly seen with these agents include asthenia, dizziness, nausea, fatigue, and dry mouth. Some patients using triptans have experienced some cardiac-like symptoms such as chest, jaw, or neck tightness. These occurrences are rare.[19] Non-responders to triptans do occur; that is, the medication does not work for some patients. In these patients, it is possible to try another triptan agent before moving on to another class of drugs.[20]

Butalbital-containing products are often used, but no studies show that they are effective for the treatment of migraines. These agents belong to the barbiturate classification. Its exact mechanism of action is unknown. It is combined with caffeine and either aspirin or acetaminophen and sometimes codeine to enhance its pain-relieving capabilities. Butalbital-containing products can cause dependency in patients and may also cause withdrawal symptoms. Side effects include drowsiness, dizziness, GI problems, confusion, and nervousness.[21]

Ergotamine derivatives work on headaches by constricting peripheral and cranial blood vessels. Dihydroergotamine (DHE) is the drug most commonly used in this class. DHE should not be used with certain drugs, such as the protease inhibitors (discussed later in this chapter). In addition, DHE should not be used within twenty-four hours of triptans.[18]

There are some OTC agents available for the treatment of headaches; in fact, some brands have started to market their OTC products specifically for "migraines." These agents often contain ibuprofen, naproxen, or combinations of aspirin, acetaminophen, and caffeine. A review of studies on the use of OTCs for migraine management shows mixed results. Most showed these products to be more effective than placebo without causing serious adverse reactions. The ability to return to normal daily functions two hours after administration increased for those whose migraines were mild to moderate in nature.[16]

Patients who have recurring migraines (four or more per month), who are not having adequate relief from other agents, or who have headaches that are disabling should consider preventive therapy. Medications used for preventive therapy are taken on a daily basis. Many medications are used as preventive therapy, but the most common are topiramate (Topamax), propranolol (Inderal), amitriptyline (Elavil), and divalproex (Depakote ER).[21]

Drugs to Treat Neuropathic Pain. Neuropathic pain may be due to the persistent stimulation of nerve fibers, or nerve damage in the central or peripheral nervous system. This overstimulation can cause the patient pain even without the presence of pressure or being touched. Symptoms of neuropathic pain include spontaneous shooting pain, or a burning or tingling sensation. Often patients describe the pain as pins-and-needles sensation. Unlike for pain in the traditional sense, opioid analgesics are not traditionally used first line for the treatment of neuropathic pain.[2] Instead, other classes of agents are used (table 10-6).

Table 10–6. Agents to Treat Neuropathic Pain

Classifications and Medications	Available Dosage Forms
Topical agents	
Capsaicin (Zostrix)	Lotion, cream, gel, patch, roll-on stick
Lidocaine (Lidoderm)	Patch
Antidepressants	
Amitriptyline (Elavil)	Tablets
Duloxetine (Cymbalta)	Capsules
Fluoxetine (Prozac)	Tablets, capsules, oral solution
Paroxetine (Paxil)	Tablets, oral suspension
Venlafaxine (Effexor)	Tablets, capsules
Antiepileptics	
Carbamazepine (Tegretol)	Tablets, capsules, oral suspension
Divalproex, valproic acid (Depakote, Depakene)	Capsules, tablets, syrup
Gabapentin (Neurontin)	Tablets, capsules, oral solution
Lamotrigine (Lamictal)	Tablets
Pregabalin (Lyrica)	Capsules
Topiramate (Topamax)	Tablets, capsules

One of the topical agents used for the treatment of neuropathic pain is capsaicin (Zostrix), which is a substance found in hot peppers. It works by depleting substance P from the nerves, thus stopping the transmission of pain from one nerve to another. Patients may complain of burning at the application site, and it should not be used with heat or heating pads. Onset of pain relief is about two to four weeks. Capsaicin is found in over-the-counter creams.

Lidocaine (Lidoderm) is available in a patch formulation for neuropathic pain due to a condition called post-herpetic neuralgia. Lidocaine is an anesthetic and numbs the area where it is applied. The patch should be applied to the site of pain, and up to three patches may be applied at a time. The patch should remain in place for twelve hours and then be removed for twelve hours.[22]

Antidepressant medications are often used in the treatment of neuropathic pain. Tricyclic antidepressants, such as amitriptyline (Elavil), cause pain inhibition by blocking reuptake of norepinephrine and serotonin. Amitriptyline is prescribed at a lower dose for neuropathic pain than for the treatment of depression. Elderly patients are more prone to adverse effects, which include sedation, sweating, sexual dysfunction, nausea, and vomiting. Used more often in younger patients, these medications are typically given at night because they cause sedation. Other antidepressants include selective serotonin reuptake inhibitors (SSRIs) and serotonin-norepinephrine reuptake inhibitors (SNRIs). These work by blocking serotonin and/or norepinephrine, thus enhancing pain inhibition. Common SSRIs include paroxetine (Paxil) and fluoxetine (Prozac). Common SNRIs used include venlafaxine (Effexor) and duloxetine (Cymbalta). Side effects include headache, nausea, diarrhea, insomnia or somnolence, and sexual side effects. These types of antidepressants are not as effective in treating neuropathic pain as the tricyclic antidepressants. Currently, the only antidepressant FDA approved for the treatment of neuropathic pain is duloxetine.[23]

Another class of medications commonly used includes antiepileptic agents such as gabapentin (Neurontin), pregabalin (Lyrica), carbamazepine (Tegretol), and divalproex (Depakote). Antiepileptics are effective in treating neuropathic pain by decreasing nerve excitability, thus decreasing pain sensations. Common side effects of these medications include dizziness and headaches. Valproic acid may cause liver injury, so liver function tests should be performed periodically. Pregabalin can cause peripheral edema (ankle and leg swelling), so caution should be used in patients with congestive heart failure and hypertension.[2]

Drugs to Treat Mood Disorders. The drugs used in the treatment of the mood disorders work by altering the various chemicals, called neurotransmitters, found at the nerve junctions in the brain. Norepinephrine, epinephrine, serotonin, and dopamine are examples of neurotransmitters. The following types of drugs are discussed in this section: antidepressants, anti-anxiety (anxiolytics), antipsychotics, sedatives, hypnotics, and stimulants.

Antidepressants. Antidepressants (table 10-7) are divided into several classes based on their chemical structures and chemical actions in the brain. There are many classes of antidepressants, such as tricyclic antidepressants, monoamine oxidase inhibitors (MAOIs), selective serotonin reuptake inhibitors (SSRIs), and serotonin norepinephrine reuptake inhibitors (SNRIs). The most frequently used drugs today are the SSRIs. Several of the drugs, such as bupropion (Wellbutrin), nefazodone (Serzone), trazodone (Desyrel), and mirtazapine

Table 10-7. Antidepressants

Classifications and Medications	Available Dosage Forms
Tricyclic antidepressants	
Amitriptyline (Elavil)	Tablets
Nortriptyline (Pamelor)	Capsules
Imipramine (Tofranil, Tofranil-PM)	Tablets, capsules
Protriptyline (Vivactil)	Tablets
Desipramine (Norpramin)	Tablets
Clomipramine (Anafranil)	Capsules
Doxepin (Sinequan)	Capsules
MAO-Is	
Phenelzine (Nardil)	Tablets
Tranylcypromine (Parnate)	Tablets
Isocarboxazid (Marplan)	Tablets
SSRIs	
Fluoxetine (Prozac, Sarafem)	Capsules, tablets
Paroxetine (Paxil)	Tablets
Sertraline (Zoloft)	Tablets
Citalopram (Celexa)	Tablets
Escitalopram (Lexapro)	Tablets
Fluvoxamine (Luvox)	Tablets
SNRIs	
Venlafaxine (Effexor, Effexor XR)	Tablets, extended-release tablets
Desvenlafaxine (Pristiq)	Tablets
Duloxetine (Cymbalta)	Tablets
Misc. agents	
Trazodone (Desyrel)	Tablets
Nefazodone (Serzone)	Tablets
Bupropion (Wellbutrin, Wellbutrin-SR Wellbutrin XL, Zyban)	Tablets, extended-release tablets
Mirtazapine (Remeron)	Tablets

(Remeron), do not fit into these classifications. All of the antidepressants are effective treatments for depression, and they are also used to treat other conditions, such as anxiety disorders, obsessive-compulsive disorder, post-traumatic stress disorder, pain, and other conditions. Generally, SSRIs, SNRIs, or bupropion (Wellbutrin) are used as an initial treatment choice. The choice of an agent for a patient is dependent on several factors:[2]

- Symptoms the patient is experiencing
- Prior medication use
- Adverse effects
- Cost

A rare adverse effect that may occur with these agents is the serotonin syndrome. Any medication that can increase the serotonin level in the body can cause this syndrome. Symptoms include confusion, agitation, fever, hypertension, tachycardia, seizures, and coma.[24] Other medications that may increase serotonin levels include triptans, opioid medications such as meperidine (Demerol), and weight loss medications such as sibutramine (Meridia).

Many medications now contain "black box warnings," which are strong warnings that need to be considered carefully prior to prescribing the medication to a patient. The patient should be carefully monitored for these potential effects during the time they are on the medication. Antidepressant medications contain a black box warning regarding an increased risk of suicidal ideations and behavior. Patients should be monitored for any change in their behavior, mood, or thought processes. During the initial start of an antidepressant medication, the patient should be seen by a health care professional more often to monitor for these potential changes.[2] Antidepressants are usually started at low doses and gradually increased. It may take four to six weeks of therapy or more before a patient will respond fully to antidepressants.[2] Caution must be used when discontinuing one antidepressant and starting another so that adverse effects are minimized. Antidepressants should be discontinued over a period of several weeks. During this time the dose should be tapered gradually. Drug interactions are common with most antidepressants. Patients should be warned to check with their doctor or pharmacist before taking other prescription or nonprescription medications.

Tricyclic Antidepressants. Tricyclic antidepressants (TCAs) were the most widely used antidepressants for many years and have the recognizable stem of –triptyline on some of their names. The mechanism of action is unclear, but they are thought to enhance the action of norepinephrine, serotonin, and dopamine in the brain. They are effective but have a number of bothersome side effects that include dry mouth, blurred vision, constipation, difficulty urinating, dizziness upon standing, sedation, and sexual dysfunction. These side effects may be so bothersome that patients stop taking their medication.[2]

There is also a higher risk of patients with pre-existing heart disease to have a higher incidence of cardiovascular events. These agents also tend to be more lethal in overdose situations than other antidepressants.[25]

Monoamine Oxidase Inhibitors (MAO-I). These drugs are thought to work by preventing the natural breakdown of neurotransmitters. MAO-Is are effective antidepressants, but are not commonly used because they have drug-diet interactions with tyramine-containing foods and many drug-drug interactions. If an interaction occurs, hypertensive crisis, an extreme rise in blood pressure that can be fatal or produce organ damage, can occur. Patients must be fully informed of the foods (e.g., aged cheeses, sausages, and red wine) and medications (e.g., pseudoephedrine in decongestants, meperidine [Demerol]) that must be avoided. The most common side effect of MAO-Is is postural hypotension, which is a drop in blood pressure upon rising (moving from a sitting or lying position to a standing position) that results in dizziness.

> **Rx for Success**
>
> Pharmacy technicians should always notify the pharmacist when there is a drug interaction alert. The pharmacist will determine the seriousness of the interaction and decide what action to take for the specific patient

Selective Serotonin Reuptake Inhibitors (SSRIs). The selective serotonin reuptake inhibitors are FDA approved not only for depression, but also for obsessive compulsive disorder (OCD), anxiety, panic disorders, post-traumatic stress disorder, and to help treat the eating disorder bulimia.[2] These drugs gained quick acceptance because the side effect profile is more tolerable when compared with the older classes of antidepressants, and the SSRIs are less dangerous in overdose situations.

The side effects that are common with the SSRIs are headache, nausea, anorexia, diarrhea, anxiety, nervousness, and insomnia. Sexual dysfunction occurs frequently.[25] Paroxetine (Paxil), fluoxetine (Prozac), and fluvoxamine (Luvox) have the most drug-drug interactions and should be used with caution in patients taking antiarrhythmic agents, TCAs, and phenytoin (Dilantin).[25]

Serotonin Norepinephrine Reuptake Inhibitors (SNRIs). The serotonin norepinephrine reuptake inhibitors are potent inhibitors of the reuptake of serotonin and norepinephrine, but work only weakly on dopamine. Like the SSRIs, these agents are better tolerated than some of the other antidepressant medications. Examples include venlafaxine (Effexor) and duloxetine (Cymbalta). Duloxetine is FDA approved for neuropathic pain as well as for the treatment of fibromyalgia. Side effects are similar to those for the SSRIs, but patients should also be monitored for a potential increase in blood pressure.[25]

Miscellaneous Agents. Nefazodone (Serzone), trazodone (Desyrel), bupropion (Wellbutrin), and mirtazapine (Remeron) do not fit into the usual classes of antidepressants. Nefazodone and trazodone share some of the adverse effects of the tricyclic antidepressants, such as sedation and postural hypotension, but they are less likely to cause heart rhythm disturbances or anticholinergic effects, such as dry mouth, blurred vision, constipation, and difficulty urinating. Trazodone is more often used as a sedative hypnotic agent than for depression. Nefazodone has a high incidence of liver toxicity and is rarely used at this time. Like the tricyclic antidepressants, bupropion (Wellbutrin) can cause constipation and dry mouth, although it does not cause the weight gain that many of the other agents cause. The most serious adverse reaction of bupropion is that it can lower the seizure threshold. Bupropion is unique in that it also approved for smoking cessation and is marketed under the brand name Zyban. Mirtazapine (Remeron) is not likely to cause heart rhythm disturbances or seizures, but it can cause **agranulocytosis**, a decreased production of all types of blood cells, and neutropenia, a decreased production of white blood cells.[2]

Drugs for Bipolar Disorder. Bipolar disorder, also called manic-depressive disorder, is characterized by extreme mood swings. Patients cycle between an agitated or overexcited state and a depressed state. Treatment is focused on treating the manic and depressed states, but there is also a maintenance phase that needs to be treated in hopes of controlling the relapses. Manic episodes have traditionally been treated with lithium, although some of the medications in the antiepileptic and atypical antipsychotic classes may also be used (table 10-8).[27] Lithium (Lithobid), olanzapine (Zyprexa), and lamotrigine (Lamictal) are appoved to be used as maintenance drugs to prevent relapses.

Table 10-8. Drugs Used to Treat Bipolar Disorder

Classifications and Medications	Dosage Forms
Lithium carbonate (Lithobid)	Capsules,tablets, controlled-release tablets, syrup
Antiepileptics	
Carbamazepine (Tegretol)	Capsule, suspension, tablets, extended-release tablets
Divalproex sodium (Depakote)	Capsule(sprinkle), injection, delayed-release tablets, extended-release tablets
Oxcarbazepine (Trileptal)	Suspension, tablets
Lamotrigine (Lamictal)	Tablets, oral-disintegrating tablets
Atypical antipsychotics	
Risperidone (Riserdal)	Injection, solution, tablets, oral-disintegrating tablets
Olanzapine (Zyprexa)	Injection, tablet, oral-disintegrating tablets
Quetiapine (Seroquel)	Tablets, extended release tablets
Ziprasidone (Geodon)	Capsules, injection
Aripiprazole (Abilify)	Injection, solution, tablets, oral-disintegrating tablets

The mechanism of action of lithium is unclear. Lithium affects many of the salts in the blood, leading to adverse effects such as increased thirst and urination. Other adverse effects include GI problems, fatigue, and weight gain. Tremors are a common side effect of lithium and may be alleviated with propranolol (Inderal). Lithium also decreases thyroid function in a high percentage of patients and may cause kidney toxicity. The amount of lithium in the blood is measured to ensure that the dose is high enough to be effective but still low enough to avoid adverse effects.[2]

The antiepileptics are often used in patients with "mixed mania" with better results than lithum. This state is when the patient has both manic and depression symptoms occurring at the same time. The antipsychotic agents are often added to lithium or an antiepileptic agent in severe manic phases, or as adjunct therapy in other manic phases if monotherapy is not working for the patient.[28]

Anti-Anxiety Agents (Anxiolytics). Drugs used for anxiety (anxiolytics) include the SSRIs, benzodiazepines, SNRIs, TCAs, and buspirone (Buspar). Over the years the first-line agents for the treatment of anxiety have changed. Many years ago barbiturates were the preferred class; these agents are rarely, if ever, used anymore. Since then, the benzodiazepines became first-line agents, but those have also fallen out of favor due to their potential for adverse effects and abuse. Currently, the SSRIs are the preferred first-line agents for anxiety disorders.

Benzodiazepines may be used for anxiety or sleep (table 10-9).[2] It should be noted that the characteristic ending to the benzodiazepines used for anxiety is -azepam, whereas those that are used for sleep often end in -azolam. Other uses for the benzodiazepines include muscle spasms and seizures. The most common side effects of the benzodiazepines are drowsiness, confusion, slurred speech, and slowed reactions. These effects are enhanced when drugs such as alcohol or narcotics are used simultaneously. All patients taking benzodiazepines should be warned about possible impairment of driving abilities, ability to operate machinery, and judgment. An auxiliary label should be placed on the prescription vial (See figure 10-1).[29]

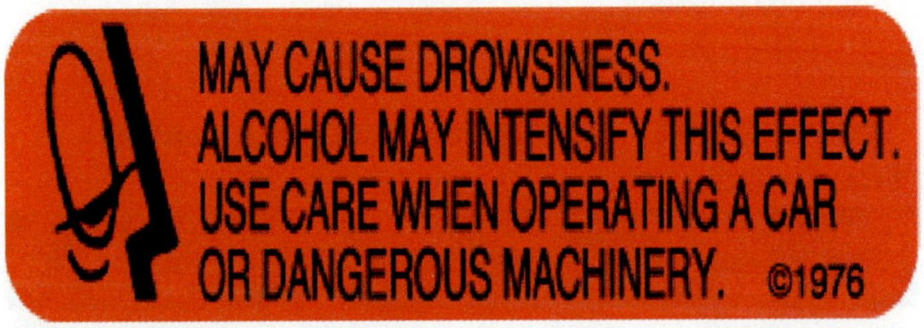

Figure 10-1. An example of a warning label that should be placed on prescription vials containing benzodiazepines.

Withdrawal symptoms can occur when benzodiazepines are taken for a long time and then abruptly stopped. In cases of overdose, a drug called flumazenil (Romazicon) is used as an antidote to reverse some of the effects, such as sedation and respiratory depression.[2]

Buspirone is chemically different from the benzodiazepines. Its advantage over benzodiazepines is that it is less likely to cause drowsiness and slowed reactions. It also has a low potential for abuse and no withdrawal symptoms. The most common adverse effects seen with this agent are dizziness, nausea, and headaches. Although the benzodiazepines may be used on an as-needed basis for anxiety, it is important to note that buspirone must be taken on a scheduled basis in order to achieve the anti-anxiety effect desired.[2]

Table 10–9. Agents Used to Treat Anxiety

Classifications and Medications	Available Dosage Forms
Benzodiazepines	
Alprazolam (Xanax)	Tablets, intensol solution, extended release tablets, oral-disintegrating tablets
Diazepam (Valium)	Injection, intensol solution, solution, tablets
Lorazepam (Ativan)	Tablets, injection, intensol solution
Clonazepam (Klonopin)	Tablets, oral-disintegrating tablets, wafers
Chlordiazepoxide (Librium)	Capsules, injection
Clorazepate (Tranxene)	Tablets
Non-benzodiazepine	
Buspirone (Buspar)	Tablets

Antipsychotic Agents. Psychosis is a mental disorder in which a person's capacity to recognize reality is distorted. Schizophrenia is one type of psychosis. Common symptoms include hallucinations (hearing or seeing things that are not real), delusions (fixed beliefs that are false), and thought processes that are not logically connected. Antipsychotic agents are classified as conventional and atypical agents (table 10-10). Although the precise mechanism of action is not known, conventional antipsychotics are thought to act by blocking the action of the neurotransmitter dopamine. The newer agents, classified as atypical or second-generation antipsychotic agents, developed in the 1990s, appear to block not only dopamine, but also serotonin. Orally disintegrating tablets are available for patients who refuse tablets. Fluphenazine decanoate (Prolixin), haloperidol decanoate (Haldol), risperidone (Risperdal Consta), and paliperidone (Invega Sustenna) are available as long-acting injections for patients who may not be compliant with daily medication regimens. The long-acting injections are usually given intramuscularly (IM) every two to four weeks.[2]

Adverse effects of the antipsychotics differ by classification and potency. The low-potency conventional agents tend to produce more sedation and anticholinergic effects, whereas the high-potency agents produce extrapyramidal effects. Extrapyramidal symptoms (EPS) include abnormal muscle contractions and restlessness. Some muscle contractions can be life-threatening (such

Table 10–10. Antipsychotics

Classifications and Medications	Available Dosage Forms
Conventional antipsychotics	
Chlorpromazine (Thorazine)	Tablets, injection
Fluphenazine (Prolixin)	Tablets, injection, liquid, elixir
Haloperidol (Haldol)	Tablets, conc. liquid, injection
Perphenazine (Trilafon)	Tablets
Thioridazine (Mellaril)	Tablets
Trifluoperazine (Stelazine)	Tablets
Atypical antipsychotics	
Aripiprazole (Abilify)	Tablets, solution, oral-disintegrating tablets, injection
Clozapine (Clozaril)	Tablets
Olanzapine (Zyprexa, Zyprexa Zydis)	Tablets, oral-disintegrating tablets, injection
Paliperidone (Invega, Invega Sustenna)	Extended-release tablets, long-acting injection
Quetiapine (Seroquel)	Tablets, extended-release tablets
Risperidone (Risperdal, Risperdal Consta)	Tablets, oral-disintegrating tablets, solution; long-acting injection
Ziprasidone (Geodon)	Capsules, injection

as when the throat muscles contract). Anticholinergic side effects include dry mouth, blurred vision, constipation, difficulty urinating, and increased heart rate.[30]

The atypical antipsychotic agents have not been shown to be more effective than the older agents; however, they do tend to have less EPS and may also have some mood stabilizing effects because of their serotonergic effects. Clozapine (Clozaril) was the first agent in this class approved. It has several black box warnings associated with its use, including the potential for agranulocytosis, myocarditis, seizures, and respiratory depression. Patients are required to have their blood drawn every one to four weeks to monitor for a serious condition called agranulocytosis, a decrease in the white blood cell count that could lead to an increase risk of infections and other problems. Newer agents approved after clozapine (Clozaril) do not have this problem.[2] The most pronounced adverse effects of the atypical agents is low blood pressure upon standing. Patients should be counseled on rising slowly from a lying or sitting position. Other adverse effects include drowsiness, constipation, weight gain and even increases in cholesterol or glucose levels.[30]

Sedatives and Hypnotics. Sedative-hypnotic drugs are used for the treatment of sleep disorders (table 10-11). Sedatives are often defined as drugs that reduce anxiety or produce a calming effect. Hypnotic drugs are used to produce sleep or drowsiness. Some drugs have sedative effects at lower doses and hypnotic effects at higher doses.

Hypnotics may be used to treat a variety of sleep problems: difficulty in falling asleep, frequent awakening during the night, early morning awakening, and not feeling rested even after what should be an adequate amount of sleep. Nondrug therapies are usually tried first, such as establishing a regular bedtime and wake-up time and reducing the use of alcohol, caffeine, and nicotine. General guidelines for the use of hypnotics include using the lowest effective dose for the shortest duration possible.[31]

Hypnotic drugs, like sedatives, include barbiturates, benzodiazepines, and nonbarbiturate, nonbenzodiazepine drugs. Because of their potential for the development of tolerance, fatality in overdose, dependence, withdrawal symptoms, and drug interactions, barbiturates are rarely used as hypnotics.[2]

Table 10–11. Sedative and Hypnotic Medications

Classifications and Medications	Available Dosage Forms	Use as Sedative or Hypnotic
Diazepam (Valium)	Injection, intensol solution, solution, tablets	Sedative
Flurazepam (Dalmane)	Capsules	Hypnotic
Midazolam (Versed)	Injection, syrup	Sedative
Temazepam (Restoril)	Capsules	Hypnotic
Triazolam (Halcion)	Tablets	Hypnotic
Estazolam (Prosom)	Tablets	Hypnotic
Quazepam (Doral)	Tablets	Hypnotic
Other agents (nonbenzodiazepines)		
Choral Hydrate	Capsules, syrup, suppository	Sedative
Eszopiclone (Lunesta)	Tablets	Hypnotic
Zaleplon (Sonata)	Capsules	Hypnotic
Zolpidem (Ambien, Ambien CR)	Tablets, extended-release tablets	Hypnotic

The effects of some hypnotics carry over into the daytime. This carryover of drowsiness and decreased concentration, called a "hangover effect," is an important consideration in the use of hypnotics. Elderly patients tend to metabolize drugs at a slower rate, tend to exhibit more confusion and disorientation upon waking, and are at greater risk for falls. Hypnotics with a hangover effect like flurazepam (Dalmane) should be used with caution in these patients. Benzodiazepines that are metabolized and excreted rapidly, such as triazolam (Halcion), are less likely to produce a hangover effect.[2] Tolerance, a loss of effectiveness over time, may occur with all benzodiazepines.

Some of the benzodiazepines are used for sedation purposes before procedures in a hospital setting. Injectable forms of midazolam (Versed) and diazepam (Valium) are frequently used for sedation for procedures such as a colonoscopy or minor surgical procedures. Amnesia, or memory loss, is an adverse effect but is desirable when these drugs are used for sedation during painful medical procedures.[2]

Nonbenzodiazepine hypnotics have the ability to induce sleepiness and/or to reduce the number of nighttime awakenings; that is, they may help the patient fall asleep and/or stay asleep. Zolpidem (Ambien) has the ability to help patients fall asleep and stay asleep for six to eight hours. Zaleplon (Sonata) has a fast onset of action, which allows patients to fall asleep quickly, but because it does not last long, it may not assist patients who tend to wake up in the middle of the night. Eszopiclone (Lunesta) also allows patients to fall asleep quickly, and it increases total sleep time and sleep quality.[31]

Other classes of medications may also be used as hypnotics because drowsiness is one of their most common side effects. The antihistamine diphenhydramine is found in many over-the-counter (OTC) sleep aids, such as Tylenol PM, which also contains acetaminophen. Although diphenhydramine effectively causes drowsiness, some patients may experience a hangover effect the next day and should use caution. Antidepressants such as amitriptyline and trazodone are sometimes used for patients who have depression and difficulty sleeping.

Drugs to Treat Attention Deficit Hyperactivity Disorder (ADHD). ADHD is a common childhood psychiatric disorder that affects behavioral, social, and emotional function and the development of the child.[32] There is no cure and up to 75% of the children still suffer from ADHD into adulthood.[33] ADHD is thought to occur due to a deficiency of norepinephrine and dopamine. Norepinephrine is thought to affect attention and mood while dopamine is thought to influence behavior and impulsivity.[32] Overall treatment consists of behavior-modification and pharmacotherapy.[33]

Table 10-12. Agents to Treat ADHD

Classifications and Medications	Available Dosage Forms
Stimulants	
Dexmethylphenidate (Focalin)	Tablets, extended-release capsules
Dextroamphetamine (Dexedrine)	Tablets, extended-release capsules, solution
Lisdexamfetamine (Vyvanse)	Capsules
Methylphenidate (Ritalin, Metadate, Methylin, Concerta, Daytrana)	Tablets, extended-release tablets, capsules, patch
Mixed amphetamine salts (Adderall, Adderall XR)	Tablets, extended-release capsules
Non-stimulants	
Atomoxetine (Strattera)	Capsules

Several classes of medications may be used in the treatment of ADHD. First-line therapy includes the stimulants (table 10-12). If these don't work or are contraindicated, the patient may be switched to atomoxetine (Strattera), bupropion (Wellbutrin), venlafaxine (Effexor), or other psychotropic medications.[2]

The stimulants are thought to work by increasing the release of norepinephrine and dopamine and blocking the reuptake of these neurotransmitters. The immediate release agents are typically dosed two to three times a day. Twice daily dosing is given in the morning and at lunch; if dosed three times daily, a dose is also given after school. Doses are given early in the day so the medication does not interfere with sleep at night.[32]

In recent years, longer-acting formulations have been developed that allow for once-daily dosing. The methylphenidate (Daytrana) patch is worn for nine hours a day and allows for continuous administration of the medication during that time period.[32] Lisdexamfetamine (Vyvanse) is a prodrug of dextroamphetamine, meaning that it has no action until it is converted to dextroamphetamine by the liver. By delaying its action, it is possible to lessen adverse effects as well as reduce the potential for abuse and toxicity.[33]

Adverse effects with the stimulants include headache, decreased appetite, nausea, insomnia, and increased blood pressure or heart rate. With the patch, skin irritation and rash may occur. To help prevent long-term adverse effects in children, "drug holidays" are often done, in which the drugs are not taken on weekends and/or during the summer or other breaks when the child is not in school.[32,33]

The nonstimulant medication atomoxetine (Strattera) blocks the reuptake of norepinephrine in the brain. It is taken once or twice a day on a regular basis with no "drug holidays." Atomoxetine has a black box warning regarding the possibility of suicidal ideations and behavior in adolescents. The adverse effects are similar to those of the stimulant medications and it has an additional warning regarding possible increase in liver enzymes.[2]

Drugs that Affect the Cardiovascular System

Cholesterol-lowering Agents. Cholesterol and triglycerides are the fats implicated in heart disease. Cholesterol is measured as total cholesterol, which is a combination of low density lipoprotein (LDL), the so-called "bad" cholesterol, and high density lipoprotein (HDL), the "good" cholesterol. Ideally, drugs should be able to reduce LDL levels and/or increase HDL levels. Current drugs have differing effects on these various components of blood cholesterol and triglycerides (TG). Drugs are selected based on the type of fats that are elevated as well as the side effect profiles of the drugs.

Initially, high cholesterol is treated with diet and exercise. If these methods fail, drugs often are added (table 10-13). These agents, called antihyperlipidemics, may be used alone or in combinations to lower cholesterol. Some of the agents have been combined into single dosage forms to improve patient compliance. When initiating pharmacologic therapy, the main lipid targeted is LDL. High levels of LDL are a main cause of clogged arteries, also known as coronary artery disease (CAD). Patients should have their cholesterol levels checked after six to twelve weeks, and medication is adjusted if needed. Once patients are stabilized on a lipid regimen, they should continue to have their levels checked every four to six months.[34]

Table 10–13. Cholesterol Lowering Agents

Classifications and Medications	Available dosage forms
Bile acid sequestrants	
Cholestyramine (Questran)	Powder, packets
Colestipol (Colestid)	Granules, packets, tablets
Colesevelam (Welchol)	Tablets
HMG-CoA reductase inhibitors (statins)	
Atorvastatin (Lipitor)	Tablets
Fluvastatin (Lescol)	Capsules, extended-release tablets
Lovastatin (Mevacor)	Tablets
Pravastatin (Pravachol)	Tablets
Simvastatin (Zocor)	Tablets
Rosuvastatin (Crestor)	Tablets
Fibrates	
Gemfibrozil (Lopid)	tablets
Fenofibrate, fenofibric acid (Antara, Fenoglide, Lofibra, Lipofen, Triglide, Trilipix,Tricor)	Tablets, capsules
Misc. and combination agents	
Amlodipine/atorvastatin (Caduet)	Tablets
Ezetimibe (Zetia)	Tablets
Ezetimibe/Simvastatin (Vytorin)	Tablets
Niacin/lovastatin (Advicor)	Tablets
Niacin/simvastatin (Simcor)	Tablets
Nicotinic acid (Niacin, Niaspan)	Tablets, capsules, sustained-release capsules
Omega-3 fatty acids (Lovaza)	Capsules

HMG-CoA Reductase Inhibitors. The HMG-CoA reductase inhibitors, also known as "statins," prevent the formation of cholesterol from fats in the liver and are often considered first-line therapy for lowering LDL. They decrease LDL and increase HDL, as well as decrease total cholesterol and triglycerides. The most common side effects are muscle and joint pain, headache, and gastrointestinal distress. The most serious effects include abnormalities of liver function tests, although liver damage does not usually occur. A more serious muscle disease, rhabdomyolysis, can occur, usually in patients taking high doses or in combination with the fibrates and possibly other drugs. Pravastatin (Pravachol) is the agent that has the fewest drug-drug interactions associated with its use; the other agents, although differing in potency, are similar with respect to drug interaction potential and adverse effects.[2]

Bile Acid Sequestrants. Bile aids the absorption of fats in the intestines. The bile secreted into the intestine is reabsorbed back into the blood. The body uses cholesterol to make more bile, which is then bound and excreted; this cycle leads to a decrease in LDL and total cholesterol. Bile acid sequestrants bind the bile in the intestines and prevent it from being reabsorbed. Instead, it is excreted in the feces. The most common side effects with these drugs are constipation, aggravation of hemorrhoids, abdominal cramping, gas, nausea, vomiting, diarrhea, and heartburn.

Tablet forms of these drugs are available, but for convenience, these drugs are also available as powders to be mixed in juice or water. If enough fluid is not given with the bile acid sequestrants, they can form a solid mass in the esophagus or the intestines, resulting in blockage of these parts of the digestive tract. Patients often complain that these formulations are not very palatable and are gritty when in liquid.

In the same way that these drugs bind bile acids, they can also bind other medications. Other drugs should be taken one hour before or four to six hours after the bile acid sequestrants. Because of these drawbacks, the bile acid sequestrants are used infrequently.[34]

Fibrates. Fibrates lower LDL and raise HDL, and are very useful for their triglyceride-lowering effects. The mechanism of action is unknown. The most common side effects are nausea and other gastrointestinal symptoms, muscle and joint aches, skin rash, fatigue, taste disturbances, and weakness. More serious effects include a possible increased risk of liver cancer, gallstones, and decreased white and/or red blood cells.[2]

Other Lipid-lowering Agents. Ezetimibe (Zetia) works in the intestines to decrease the absorption of cholesterol. It may be used as monotherapy, but is more often used in conjunction with other cholesterol lowering agents to lower LDL and triglycerides and raise HDL. The most common adverse effects include back and joint pain, GI problems, and an increase in liver function tests and hepatotoxicity.[2]

Nicotinic acid (Niacin, Niaspan) is a form of vitamin B that reduces serum cholesterol and triglycerides. Another form of this vitamin, nicotinamide (niacinamide), does not affect blood cholesterol levels. Niacin is beneficial in lowering triglyceride (TG) levels, is the best agent available in raising HDL levels, and has a lesser effect on lowering LDL. The most bothersome adverse effect of niacin is a flushing sensation or a feeling of warmth, as well as itching, tingling, or headache. An aspirin tablet thirty minutes before the niacin dose can alleviate this effect. GI upset can also occur. Using a sustained release formulation can also alleviate these bothersome effects. Niacin may also raise blood sugar levels and needs to be used with caution in patients with diabetes. More serious effects include abnormal liver function tests, which tend to occur with high doses and with the sustained-release products.[2]

Omega-3 fatty acids (Lovaza), commonly found in fish oil, have been shown to reduce triglyceride levels in patients with very high triglycerides in their blood (hypertriglyceridemia). Although there are over-the-counter versions of fish oils available, they are not approved by the FDA and are not standardized to ensure the proper amount of the ingredient is in the product. The most common side effects of the fish oils are fishy taste and fishy burps, GI upset, and increased liver function tests. These agents may also increase bleeding time, so patients who are receiving anticoagulation therapy need to be monitored closely.[2]

High Blood Pressure Agents (Antihypertensives). There are many classes of drugs used to treat high blood pressure. Diuretics and beta-blockers have been shown in clinical studies to reduce the risk of death from heart attacks and strokes. Angiotensin-converting enzyme inhibitors (ACE inhibitors), angiotensin receptor blockers (ARBs), and calcium channel blockers are other drugs that have advantages in certain types of patients. Central alpha-2-agonists, peripheral adrenergic antagonists, and direct vasodilators are other agents that are available, although they are used when the other agents have failed.[35]

Diuretics. Diuretics decrease blood pressure by decreasing the blood volume. They are commonly called "water pills" and work on the kidneys to increase urinary excretion of sodium, chloride, and water. Since all diuretics increase urination, they should be taken as early in the day as possible so that urination does not interrupt the patient's sleep.[35]

There are three types of diuretics used to treat hypertension (table 10-14): thiazides, loop diuretics, and potassium-sparing diuretics. Thiazide diuretics (e.g., hydrochlorothiazide) in low doses are usually effective for high blood pressure. Loop diuretics (e.g., furosemide [Lasix]) are more effective in patients with mild kidney failure. Both the thiazide and loop diuretics can decrease potassium in

Table 10-14. Diuretics

Classifications and Medications	Available Dosage Forms
Thiazide diuretics	
Hydrochlorothiazide – HCTZ (Microzide)	Capsules, tablets
Chlorothiazide (Diuril)	Injection, suspension, tablets
Metolazone (Zaroxolyn)	Tablets
Loop diuretics	
Furosemide (Lasix)	Injection, solution, tablets
Bumetanide (Bumex)	Injection, tablets
Torsemide (Demadex)	Injection, tablets
Ethacrynic acid (Edecrin)	injection
Potassium-sparing diuretics	
Eplerenone (Inspra)	Tablets
Spironolactone (Aldactone)	Tablets
Triamterene (Dyrenium)	Capsules
Combination agents	
Triamterene/HCTZ (Dyazide, Maxzide)	Tablets, capsules
Spironolactone/HCTZ (Aldactazide)	Tablets

the body, and patients may need to take potassium supplements. Potassium-sparing diuretics are weak diuretics but are often added to other diuretics (e.g., triamterene/hydrochlorothiazide [Dyazide]) to prevent potassium loss.[2]

Although the thiazide diuretics are well tolerated by patients, certain precautions should be noted. Blood glucose control in patients with diabetes may be altered by thiazide diuretics. Patients who are taking thiazide diuretics may be more sensitive to sun, so they should be warned to avoid exposure or use sunscreen (See figure 10-2). Patients allergic to sulfonamides may also be allergic to thiazide diuretics.[2]

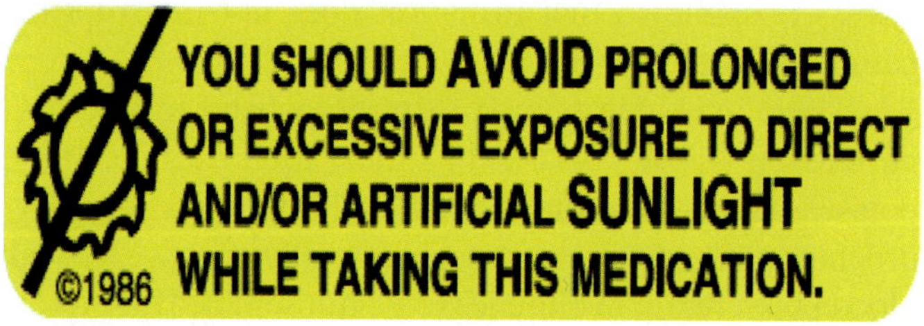

Figure 10-2. A warning label that should be placed on prescription vials containing thiazide diuretics.

Loop diuretics are more potent diuretics and may affect electrolytes such as sodium, potassium, chloride, calcium, and magnesium to a greater degree than the thiazides. Adverse effects are similar to those of the thiazides, including altered blood glucose control in diabetics, sun sensitivity, and allergic reactions in sulfonamide-allergic patients. Ethacrynic acid (Edecrin) does not contain a sulfa group, so it may be used in patients allergic to sulfonamides.[35]

Potassium-sparing diuretics used alone do not cause potassium loss like the other diuretics. In fact, they may increase potassium levels in patients and should be used with caution in patients using ACE inhibitors, or other medications that may increase potassium levels. Potassium-sparing diuretics are often used with other diuretics to combine the greater potency of a loop or thiazide diuretic with their potassium-sparing effects.[2] Some diuretics have been combined with other diuretics or antihypertensive drugs to make convenient dosage forms.

Beta-blockers. Beta-blockers block the action of certain nerves in cardiac muscle, lungs, and the smooth muscles of the blood vessels. There are two types of beta receptors: β_1-receptors are found in the heart and kidney, and β_2-receptors are found in the lungs, arterioles, pancreas, and liver. When the β_1-receptors are stimulated, there is an increase in heart rate and contractility. When the β_2-receptors are stimulated, vasodilation and bronchodilation occur. Beta-blockers lower blood pressure by decreasing the volume of blood pumped by each contraction of the heart, thus slowing heart rate; however, they may also cause bronchoconstriction.[2]

Beta-blockers are further classified as cardioselective if they are more selective for the receptors in the heart (β_1), or noncardioselective (β_1 and β_2). They typically have an –olol ending (table 10-15). Because beta-blockers may constrict the airways, they should be used with caution in patients with asthma or COPD; however, agents that are cardioselective are a better choice for these patients since there should be little to no β_2-receptor stimulation. Beta-blockers are first-line drugs for the treatment of hypertension and, like diuretics, have been shown to reduce the risk of death from heart attack or stroke. They may be used in the treatment of other conditions, including angina, abnormal heart rhythms, prevention of heart attack, prevention of migraine headache, and tremor.[35]

Beta-blockers also block the symptoms of low blood sugar and should be used cautiously in patients with diabetes. Undesirable side effects include central nervous system effects such as dizziness, tiredness, and depres-

Table 10–15. Beta-blockers

Medications	Cardioselective or Nonselective	Available Dosage Forms
Atenolol (Tenormin)	Cardioselective	Tablets
Bisoprolol (Zebeta)	Cardioselective	Tablets
Carvedilol (Coreg)	Nonselective	Tablets
Labetalol (Trandate)	Nonselective	Tablets, injection
Metoprolol tartrate (Lopressor)	Cardioselective	Injection, tablets
Metoprolol sodium succinate (Toprol-XL)		Extended-release tablets
Nadolol (Corgard)	Nonselective	Tablets
Nebivolol (Bystolic)	Cardioselective	Tablets
Propranolol (Inderal LA)	Nonselective	Solution, extended-release capsules, tablets, injection
Sotalol (Betapace)	Nonselective	Tablets
Combination agents		
Bisoprolol/HCTZ (Ziac)	Cardioselective	Tablets
Metoprolol/HCTZ (Lopressor HCT)	Cardioselective	Tablets
Atenolol/chlorthalidone (Tenoretic)	Cardioselective	Tablets

sion. Some patients may develop tingling, loss of sensation, or intolerance to cold in the hands and feet.[2]

ACE Inhibitors and Angiotensin Receptor Blockers (ARBs). Angiotensin-converting enzyme inhibitors (ACE inhibitors) prevent the production of certain chemicals in the blood that cause the constriction of blood vessels and retention of sodium and water. By blocking blood vessel constriction and salt and water retention, these drugs can lower blood pressure. Like the beta-blockers, they have other uses. ACE inhibitors may slow or prevent the development of kidney disease in diabetic patients and increase survival, alleviate symptoms, and decrease hospitalization in patients with heart failure.[2] The ACE inhibitors have a –pril ending on the name (table 10-16).

A unique side effect of the ACE inhibitors that may lead to discontinuation of the drug is a bothersome dry cough. Some patients experience dizziness when they begin therapy. ACE inhibitors can also cause skin rashes, abnormal taste in the mouth, and high potassium levels.[35]

The angiotensin receptor blockers (ARBs) lower blood pressure in the kidneys by blocking the angiotensin

Table 10–16. ACE Inhibitors and ARBs

Classifications and Medications	Available Dosage Forms
ACE-Inhibitors (ACE-Is)	
Benazepril (Lotensin)	Tablets
Captopril (Capoten)	Tablets
Enalapril, enalaprilat (Vasotec)	Injection, tablets
Fosinopril (Monopril)	Tablets
Lisinopril (Prinivil, Zestril)	Tablets
Moexipril (Univasc)	Tablets
Quinapril (Accupril)	Tablets
Perindopril (Aceon)	Tablets
Ramipril (Altace)	Capsules, tablets
Trandolapril (Mavik)	Tablets
Angiotensin II receptor blockers (ARBs)	
Candesartan (Atacand)	Tablets
Eprosartan (Teveten)	Tablets
Losartan (Cozaar)	Tablets
Irbesartan (Avapro)	Tablets
Olmesartan (Benicar)	Tablets
Telmisartan (Micardis)	Tablets
Valsartan (Diovan)	Tablets
Combination products	
Amlodipine/olmesartan (Azor)	Tablets
Amlodipine/valsartan (Exforge)	Tablets
Amlodipine/valsartan/HCTZ (Exforge HCT)	Tablets
Benazepril/HCTZ (Lotensin HCT)	Tablets
Candesartan/HCTZ (Atacand HCT)	Tablets
Enalapril/HCTZ (Vaseretic)	Tablets
Eprosartan/HCTZ (Teveten HCT)	Tablets
Irbesartan/HCTZ (Avalide)	Tablets
Lisinopril/HCTZ (Zestoretic)	Tablets
Losartan/HCTZ (Hyzaar)	Tablets
Moexipril/HCTZ (Uniretic)	Tablets
Olmesartan/HCTZ (Benicar HCT)	Tablets
Quinapril/HCTZ (Accuretic)	Tablets
Ramipril/HCTZ (Altace HCT)	Tablets
Telmisartan/HCTZ (Micardis HCT)	Tablets
Trandolapril/verapamil (Tarka)	Tablets
Valsartan/HCTZ (Diovan HCT)	Tablets

II receptors and blood vessel constriction. These agents tend to have a –sartan ending on the generic names. The side effects are similar to those of the ACE inhibitors except there is less incidence of dry cough.[2]

Calcium Channel Blockers. The movement of calcium in and out of cells is essential for nerve conduction and muscle contraction. Calcium channel blockers inhibit this movement, resulting in a decreased force of contraction of the heart, blocked contraction of smooth muscle in the blood vessels resulting in dilation of blood vessels, and slowed conduction of nerve impulses throughout the heart resulting in a slowed heart rate. The drugs in this class vary in the selectivity of their actions on heart rate, blood vessel dilation, and heart contraction.[2]

Calcium channel blockers are used for chest pain (angina pectoris), heart rhythm disturbances, migraine headache, and diseases of the heart muscle. One drug, nimodipine, has a special indication for reducing nerve damage caused by bleeding in the brain, which is called subarachnoid hemorrhage. Nimodipine is not used for hypertension.[2]

The drugs in this class are listed in table 10-17. In general, these drugs have similar side effects. Drugs such as diltiazem (Cardizem) and verapamil (Calan, Verelan) are more efficacious in patients with arrhythmias, and have constipation and slow heart rate as adverse effects associated with their use. The other calcium channel blockers tend to be used more often for hypertension, and the adverse reactions of these agents include dizziness, headache, constipation, and, occasionally, swelling of the legs or feet.[35]

The immediate release formulations of this class are indicated for use in patients with chest pain. Many of these agents have sustained-release formulations available which are indicated for the treatment of high blood pressure allowing for once or twice daily dosing, which increases patient compliance.

Table 10–17. Calcium Channel Blockers

Medications	Available Dosage Forms
Amlodipine (Norvasc)	Tablets
Nifedipine (Procardia, Adalat CC)	Capsules, extended-release tablets
Felodipine	Tablets
Isradipine (DynaCirc)	Capsules, tablets
Nicardipine (Cardene)	Capsules, sustained-release capsules, injection
Nislodipine (Sular)	Extended-release tablets
Clevidipine (Cleviprex)	Injection
Nimodipine (Nimotop)	Capsules
Diltiazem (Cardizem, Tiazac)	Extended-release capsules, injection, tablets, extended-release tablets
Verapamil (Calan, Verelan)	Sustained-release caplets, extended-release capsules, injection, tablets
Combination agents	
Amlodipine/atorvastatin (Caduet)	Tablets
Amlodipine/benazepril (Lotrel)	Tablets
Amlodipine/olmesartan (Azor)	Tablets
Amlodipine/valsartan (Exforge)	Tablets
Amlodipine/valsartan/HCTZ (Exforge HCT)	Tablets
Trandolapril/verapamil (Tarka)	Tablets

Vasodilators. The alpha-2 agonists, direct renin inhibitors, and direct vasodilators are other classes of drugs used to treat high blood pressure. They act through various effects on nerve pathways to dilate the blood vessels and reduce blood pressure. Aliskiren (Tekturna) inhibits the enzyme renin, which is produced by the kidney, and can cause the blood vessels to constrict.[36] Because these drugs block the ability of blood vessels to constrict, people who take them often get dizzy or feel faint when they stand up after sitting or sit up after lying down, which is referred to as postural hypotension. Because of the high incidence of side effects with the alpha-2 agonists and direct vasoilators, these agents are not often used.

The alpha-2 agonists include clonidine (Catapres) and methyldopa. Common side effects, in addition to postural hypotension, are drowsiness, sedation, dry mouth, and fatigue. Clonidine is available as a patch that is changed weekly. The Catapres-TTS® patch system consists of an active patch containing drug and an inactive overlay; both patches must be dispensed.

The direct vasodilators hydralazine and minoxidil can cause headache, rapid heartbeat, and fluid retention. Minoxidil was found to increase the growth of body hair in patients and is now available as a topical product (Rogaine®) for stimulating hair growth in people with balding or thinning hair.

Nitrates. Angina pectoris is chest pain of short duration that is due to a lack of oxygen in the cardiac muscle cells. The pain subsides when the imbalance between the amount of oxygen needed by the cells and the amount of oxygen supplied to the cells is corrected. The nitrates are the most commonly used medicines for treating angina pectoris. Nitrates increase the amount of oxygen delivered to the heart and decrease the oxygen needs of the heart. They also dilate the arterial and venous blood vessels.[2] Nitrates are available in many dosage forms. For acute attacks, sublingual tablets or a translingual (on or under the tongue) spray is used. Nitroglycerin is available as an intravenous infusion. The oral sustained-release tablets and capsules, topical ointment, and transdermal patches are used for prevention of angina. Other classes of drugs that may be used for prevention of angina are the beta-blockers and the calcium channel blockers, which are discussed in other sections of this chapter. The nitrates available are nitroglycerin, isosorbide dinitrate (Isordil), and isosorbide mononitrate (Ismo, Imdur).[2]

An important concern in choosing dosage forms and dosage regimens for nitrates is the development of tolerance. After twenty-four hours of continuous therapy, nitrates no longer work. Increasing the dose does not restore efficacy, but a nitrate-free period does. For this reason, nitrates are not usually dosed around the clock. Long-acting tablets and capsules may be given orally once daily or twice daily at 8:00 a.m. and 2:00 p.m. Isosorbide mononitrate regular release is frequently given as two doses seven hours apart during the day. Nitroglycerin patches are often applied in the morning and removed at night. All of these schedules provide a nitrate-free period at night.

Common side effects of nitrates include headaches, postural hypotension, dizziness, or flushing. Headache may be an indicator of the drug's activity and may be treated with aspirin or acetaminophen.[2]

Digoxin. As with many cardiac diseases, diet modification is part of the treatment for heart failure. Fluid restriction and a low sodium diet are often prescribed to reduce the amount of fluid retention. Drug therapy includes several types of drugs: ACE inhibitors, diuretics, beta-blockers, and cardiac glycosides (digoxin). The choice of drugs is based on the severity of disease and the patient's symptoms.[35]

The role of digoxin is not well defined presently, but it has been shown to increase the force of heart muscle contraction in selected patients.[2] Digoxin acts on both the heart muscle and the nerve conduction system of the heart. It decreases the rate and force of heart muscle contractions, resulting in improved pumping of blood and a slower heart rate.[2]

Digoxin has a narrow therapeutic index and can have serious toxicities. Therefore, digoxin blood levels are monitored to help ensure safe dosing. Patients and caregivers should be aware of the early symptoms of toxicity: loss of appetite, nausea, vomiting, diarrhea, headache, weakness, confusion, and visual disturbances (particularly blurred vision, yellow or green vision, or a halo effect). An antidote, digoxin immune fab (Digibind, DigiFab), is administered intravenously to treat life-threatening digoxin intoxication.[2]

Part 2

Digoxin is available as an injection, a tablet, and an elixir. The amount absorbed from the different preparations varies, so the dose may need to be adjusted when dosage forms are switched.

Antiarrhythmics. Common arrhythmias (irregular heartbeats or abnormal heart rhythms) include atrial fibrillation, atrial flutter, and premature ventricular contractions. Rare but serious arrhythmias include ventricular tachycardia, ventricular fibrillation, and torsades de pointes. Many of the drugs used to treat arrhythmias can also cause arrhythmias (table 10-18). Common side effects, which may be severe, are GI disturbances such as nausea, vomiting, abdominal pain, and diarrhea. Some beta-blockers, calcium channel blockers, and digoxin are also used to treat arrhythmias.[2]

Class I antiarrythmic drugs, quinidine and disopyramide (Norpace), are used for both atrial and ventricular arrhythmias. Quinidine is given by IM or IV injection or orally. Disopyramide (Norpace) is given orally. Side effects include dry mouth, difficulty urinating, dizziness, constipation, and blurred vision. The most serious side effects are low blood pressure and heart failure.[22]

Another subset of class I antiarrhythmics, class IB, includes lidocaine (Xylocaine) and mexilitine (Mexitil). Class IB drugs are useful for ventricular arrhythmias. Lidocaine is given intravenously. Its side effects are related to its effects on the central nervous system: dizziness, confusion, mood changes, hallucination, drowsiness, vision disturbances, muscle twitching, and seizures. The side effects of mexilitine are similar to those of lidocaine.

Flecainide (Tambocor) and propafenone (Rythmol) are class IC antiarrhythmics. These drugs are now used only to treat life-threatening ventricular arrhythmias and some life-threatening atrial arrhythmias. Propafenone is also used to treat atrial fibrillation. Both of these drugs are available only as oral dosage forms and have mild

Table 10–18. Antiarrhythmic Agents

Class	Medications	Available Dosage Forms
IA	Quinidine	Tablets, injection
	Procainamide (Pronestyl, Procanbid)	Tablets, capsules, injection
	Disopyramide (Norpace)	Capsules
IB	Lidocaine (Xylocaine)	Injection
	Mexiletine (Mexitil)	Capsules
IC	Flecainide (Tambocor)	Tablets
	Propafenone (Rythmol)	Tablets, capsules
	Moricizine (Ethmozine)	Tablets
II	Atenolol (Tenormin)	Tablets
	Esmolol (Brevibloc)	Injection
	Metoprolol (Lopressor, Toprol XL)	Tablets, injection
	Propranolol (Inderal)	Tablets, capsules, oral solution, injection
III	Amiodarone (Pacerone)	Tablets, injection
	Dofetilide (Tikosyn)	Capsules
	Ibutilide (Corvert)	Injection
	Sotalol (Betapace)	Tablets, injection

side effects that are similar: dizziness, tremor, and blurred vision.[22]

The class III antiarrhythmics include amiodarone (Pacerone) and sotalol (Betapace). They are used to treat ventricular arrhythmias as well as atrial fibrillation. Adverse reactions are common with amiodarone. A unique side effect with amiodarone is a blue-gray discoloration of the skin, which is irreversible. Other side effects are visual disturbances, increased sensitivity to sunlight, fatigue, tremor, and changes in thyroid gland function. More serious side effects are microdeposits in the cornea of the eye resulting in visual halos or blurred vision, lung toxicity, and liver toxicity. Amiodarone is available both orally and intravenously, and dosing of both forms involves an initial loading dose followed by a lower maintenance dose. Sotalol is a beta-blocking drug with antiarrhythmic properties similar to those of amiodarone.[2]

Drugs that Affect the Respiratory System

Two common diseases of the respiratory system are asthma and chronic obstructive pulmonary disease (COPD). Asthma is a condition in which there is a reversible narrowing of the air passages caused by over-responsiveness

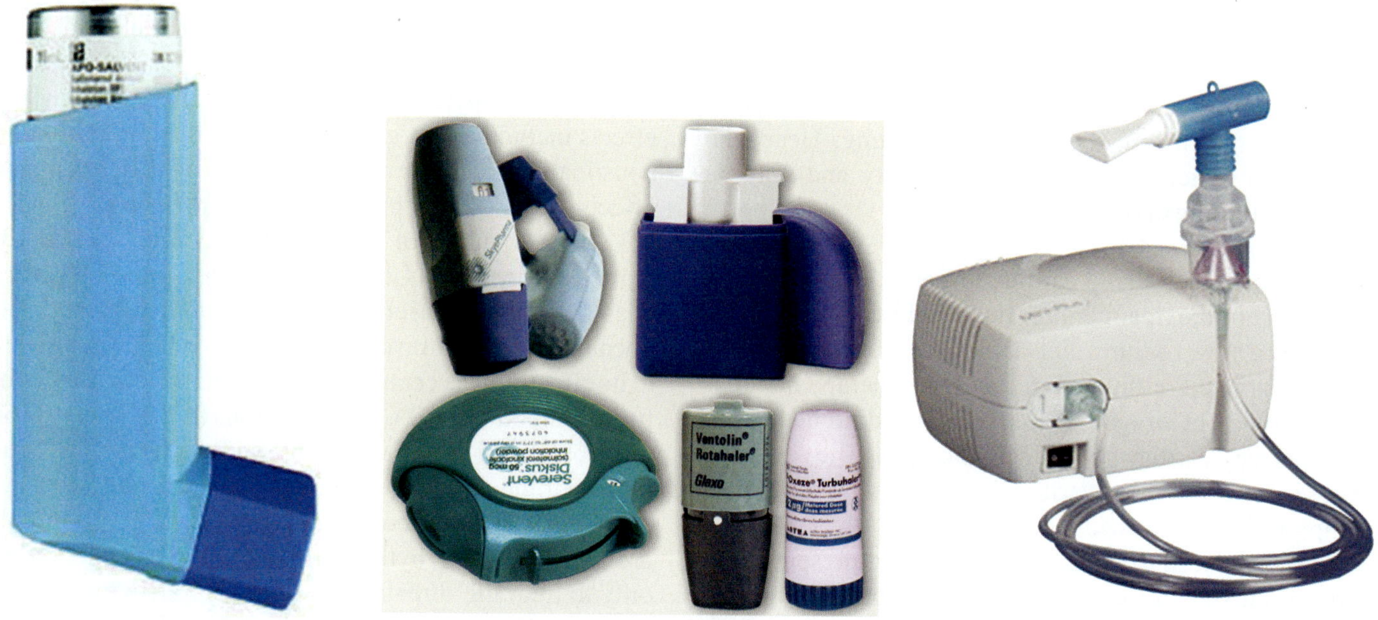

Metered dose inhaler[37] Dry powder inhalers[38] Nebulizer machine[39]

Figure 10-3. Three examples of available dosage forms for bronchodilators such as beta$_2$-agonists.

of the airways to various stimuli and inflammation of the airways. Examples of stimuli that can cause inflammation and airway narrowing include viruses, cold air, exercise, pollens, dust, cigarette smoke, and animal dander. Chronic obstructive pulmonary disease is an irreversible chronic obstruction of the airways. Emphysema and chronic bronchitis are examples of COPD. The symptoms of asthma and COPD are similar: wheezing, difficulty breathing, and coughing. These diseases differ in their cause, development, and reversibility. The agents discussed in this section may be used to treat both asthma and COPD.

Bronchodilators. Medications that work to open up the airways and make it easier to breathe are called bronchodilators. There are three types of bronchodilators: beta$_2$-agonists, anticholinergics, and methylxanthines (table 10-19).

The beta$_2$-agonists are bronchodilators that act by relaxing the smooth muscles in the bronchial airways. These agents are available in several dosage forms: oral tablets and liquids, inhalers (metered-dose [MDI], HFA, dry powder [DPI]), and solutions for inhalation via a nebulizer machine (see figure 10-3).

Most patients use inhalers or nebulizer forms. By delivering the medication directly to the lungs, the patient is able to feel relief quicker and there is less systemic absorption of the medication, leading to fewer adverse effects. The proper use of inhalers is critical to the success of treatment with these drugs. An important patient counseling point should always include proper use of inhalers.[40]

Common side effects of beta$_2$-agonists are a rapid heartbeat, tremors, anxiety, and nausea. Most of these side effects will lessen as the body adjusts to the medication. Overuse of beta$_2$-agonists can result in decreased effectiveness of the agents. Beta$_2$-agonists differ in their duration of action. Short-acting beta$_2$-agonists (e.g., albuterol, levalbuterol) work quickly and are used to stop an attack, whereas long-acting beta$_2$-agonists (e.g., salmeterol, formoterol) are used on a daily basis to prevent attacks.

Epinephrine and ephedrine are drugs that produce bronchodilation similar to the beta$_2$ agonists, but they are not specific for the lungs and also affect the heart. This lack of selectivity increases the number of side effects, including an increase in heart rate and blood pressure. Overuse of these products has led to death in some patients. Epinephrine (Primatene Mist) and ephedrine/guaifenesin (Primatene Tablets) are available in over-the-counter formulations but should not be used without medical supervision.[41]

Table 10–19. Agents to Treat Asthma and COPD

Classifications and Medications	Available Dosage Forms
Short-acting bronchodilators	
Albuterol (Proventil, Ventolin, ProAir)	Inhaler, nebulizer solution, extended-release tablets, oral liquid
Levalbuterol (Xopenex)	Inhaler, nebulizer solution
Pirbuterol (Maxair)	Inhaler
Metaproterenol (Alupent)	Syrup
Long-acting bronchodilators	
Salmeterol (Serevent)	Inhaler
Formoterol (Foradil)	Inhaler
Methylxanthines	
Theophylline (Theo-24, Uniphyl, Theochron)	Injection, elixir, extended-release capsules/tablets
Aminophylline	Injection, tablets
Mast cell stabilizers	
Cromolyn sodium (Intal)	Inhaler, nebulizer solution
Anticholinergics	
Ipratropium (Atrovent)	Inhaler, nebulizer solution
Tiotropium (Spiriva)	Inhaler
Leukotriene modifiers	
Zafirlukast (Accolate)	Tablets
Montelukast (Singulair)	Chewable tablets, tablets, granules
Zileutin (Zyflo, Zyflo CR)	Tablets, extended-release tablets
Combination agents	
Salmeterol/fluticasone (Advair)	Inhaler
Formoterol/budesonide (Symbicort)	Inhaler
Ipratropium/albuterol (Combivent, Duoneb)	Inhaler, nebulizer solution

Anticholinergic drugs (e.g., ipratropium, tiotropium) are also bronchodilators. These drugs also relax the

Part 2

muscles in the airways. The anticholinergic drugs are more useful in COPD than in asthma. They have a longer duration of action than the $beta_2$-agonists, and because of their anticholinergic "drying" effects, they can help to dry the excess mucus production that occurs in patients with COPD. Combined use with a $beta_2$-agonist may increase the benefit. Common side effects include dizziness, headache, nausea, dry mouth, cough, hoarseness, or blurred vision.[2]

The methylxanthines are another class of bronchodilators. The exact mechanism of action of these drugs is not known but may be related to an anti-inflammatory effect. The most common methylxanthines are theophylline and aminophylline. Aminophylline is a salt of theophylline. If theophylline is substituted for aminophylline, the dose should be 80% of the aminophylline dose.[18]

Theophylline has a high incidence of side effects that often occur at therapeutic doses. Nausea and vomiting are common. Other side effects include irritability, restlessness, headache, insomnia, muscle twitching, and rapid heartbeat. Age, diet, smoking, other medications, and illnesses are all factors that can change the amount of theophylline a patient needs to achieve and maintain therapeutic blood concentrations. Blood levels are measured periodically to ensure that patients achieve and maintain therapeutic concentrations. Due to the monitoring and side effect profile, the xanthines are no longer commonly used.[40]

Corticosteroids. Corticosteroids are commonly used to suppress inflammation and the immune response, and are useful in a wide spectrum of diseases including asthma, allergic reactions, lupus, ulcerative colitis, psoriasis, rheumatoid arthritis, bursitis, and organ transplantation.

The inhaled route of administration is useful in pulmonary diseases to provide local effects and prevent the numerous side effects these drugs can cause when given orally (table 10-20). Inhaled corticosteroids were previously avoided in children due to reports that they affect growth. More recent studies have disproven this theory, and current guidelines support the use of corticosteroids in children to control asthma. The most common side effects of inhaled corticosteroids include thrush (fungus of the throat and mouth) and hoarseness. These effects can be prevented by using a spacer device with the inhaler and rinsing the mouth with water after use. Ciclosenide (Alvesco) is a new inhaled corticosteroid that is activated by the tissues in the lungs. Since the drug is not active when inhaled, it is thought to reduce the incidence of oral thrush in patients.[18] Oral corticosteroids are often used to treat exacerbations and may be required on a regular basis in patients with severe asthma.[40]

Short-term use of corticosteroids carries little risk of adverse effects, but long-term use is indicated only when the benefits outweigh the risks. Long-term oral corticosteroid use can lead to Cushing syndrome, which is characterized by a rounded, puffy face; thinning of the skin; osteoporosis (bone weakening); muscle loss; and high blood glucose. Therapeutic use of corticosteroids suppresses natural adrenal gland function, which is essential to the body in times of physi-

Table 10–20. Oral/Inhaled Corticosteroids

Medications	Available Dosage Forms	Comments
Oral corticosteroids		
Prednisone	Solution, intensol, tablets	Bitter taste
Methylprednisolone (Medrol, Solu-Medrol)	Injection, long-acting injection, tablets, dosepak	
Prednisolone (Orapred)	solution, oral-disintegrating tablets, tablets	Orapred liquid must be refrigerated
Inhaled corticosteroids		
Beclomethasone (QVAR)	MDI	
Budesonide (Pulmicort)	Inhaler (DPI)	
Ciclesonide (Alvesco)	MDI	
Flunisolide (Aerobid, Aerobid-M)	MDI	M formulation contains menthol as a flavoring agent
Mometasone (Asmanex)	DPI	
Fluticasone (Flovent HFA, Flovent Diskus)	HFA, DPI	
Triamcinolone (Azmacort)	MDI	Has a built-in spacer

cal stress. The dose of oral corticosteroids must be tapered when they are to be discontinued so that the adrenal gland can recover and begin to secrete natural hormones.[40]

Other Agents for Treating Asthma. Two other classes of medications that may be used to treat asthma are the leukotriene modifiers and the mast cell stabilizers. The leukotriene modifiers cause the muscles in the bronchioles to relax, and tend to reduce inflammation. These agents are taken orally so they are not used in the treatment of acute exacerbations. Some patients who have difficulty using the inhaled products may prefer these dosage forms, but they are not considered first-line agents in the treatment of asthma. Montelukast (Singulair) is also FDA approved for the treatment of seasonal and perennial (year-round) allergies. Zileutin (Zyflo), which is the oldest agent in this class, has been shown to increase liver enzymes and patients need to be monitored while on this medication.[40] The leukotriene modifiers tend to be well tolerated, with headache and GI upset being the main adverse effects noted.

Mast cell stabilizers may reduce the need for the use of beta$_2$-agonists and may reduce asthma symptoms. They work by stabilizing the cell wall of the mast cells. This prevents the release of histamine and other mediators, which can cause bronchoconstriction. Cromolyn (Intal) is not used as much today because it must be taken several times a day, which is associated with poor patient compliance.[40]

Patients with asthma often use combinations of bronchodilators and corticosteroids. Patients should be able to identify which inhalers are meant to prevent an attack (i.e., "controllers") and which inhalers are used to treat an acute attack (i.e., "quick-relief"). It is important that the patients are counseled on the importance of using their controller medications on a regular basis. Patients sometimes believe that these agents are not necessary since they don't feel any different after taking them, but being compliant with these medications will decrease the need for quick-relief medications.

Cough and Cold Products. The common cold remains one of the most bothersome illnesses. More than 120 strains of viruses are responsible for causing the common cold. Most colds are self-limiting and can be self-treated. Treatment is aimed at reducing the symptoms: runny nose, sore throat, and cough. These symptoms are produced by an inflammatory response of the lining of the nose, throat, and lungs to the virus. Each of these symptoms may be treated individually or with combination agents when more than one symptom is present.

Safety First Over-the-counter (OTC) cough and cold products are constantly changing ingredients and formulations. Always check the active ingredients and their strengths on the product to avoid dosing errors and drug duplication.

Part 2

Rhinitis also occurs during infections such as the common cold or the flu. Symptoms of rhinitis may include nasal congestion, runny nose, postnasal drainage, sneezing, itching, redness of the membrane lining the nose, watery eyes, dark circles under the eyes, and inability to breathe through one's nose.

Similar products are used to treat symptoms of all of these conditions. Decongestants (e.g., phenylephrine, pseudoephedrine) are used to reduce the swelling of the lining of the nose. Antitussives (e.g., dextromethorphan, codeine) reduce the frequency of cough. Expectorants (e.g., guaifenesin) are used to decrease the thickness and ease the expulsion of sputum from the lungs (table 10-21).[41]

Decongestants can be used topically in the nose (nasal sprays) or taken orally. They constrict blood vessels in the nose, which decreases nasal swelling and congestion. Topical decongestants deliver the medication directly to the nasal mucosa, which may be preferred because they reduce congestion better, last longer, and have fewer side effects than oral decongestants. However, topical agents are associated with rebound congestion when used for more than three to five days. Essentially, the nasal lining becomes more congested as the effect of the drug wears off. This increased stuffiness may cause the patient to increase the use of the decongestant, creating a cycle that is difficult to break. Xylometazoline and oxymetazoline (Afrin) are available in long-acting formulations and can be used every eight to ten hours and every twelve hours, respectively. Reactions such as stinging, burning, and sneezing may occur. Oral decongestants include pseudoephedrine (Sudafed) and phenylephrine (Sudafed PE). Side effects include tremors, nervousness, fast heart rate, and

Table 10–21. Cough and Cold Agents

Classifications and Medications	Available Dosage Forms
Decongestants	
Pseudoephedrine (Sudafed)	Tablets, extended-release tablets, liquid
Phenylephrine (Sudafed PE, Triaminic Cold PE)	Tablets, extended-release tablets, chewable tablets, oral-disintegrating strip, liquid, nasal spray/drops
Topical decongestants	
Oxymetazoline (Afrin, 4-Way, Neo-Synephrine)	Intranasal gel, intranasal spray
Xylometazoline	Intranasal drops, intranasal spray
Antitussives	
Dextromethorphan (Delsym, Mucinex DM, Robitussin DM)	Syrup, suspension, oral-disintegrating strips, lozenges, tablets
Expectorants	
Guaifenesin (Robitussin, Mucinex)	Granules, syrup, tablets, extended-release tablets

nausea. As stated earlier, decongestants will constrict blood vessels in the nose; however, the oral agents can also cause vasoconstriction thoughout the body. Patients with hypertension, heart disease, overactive thyroid, diabetes mellitus, or an enlarged prostate gland should use caution if taking decongestants. There are restrictions on the quantity of pseudoephedrine that may be purchased because pseudoephedrine has been used to make illegal drugs such as methamphetamine. To deter this from occurring, the drug is kept behind the pharmacy counter and records must be kept on the sale of pseudoephedrine.[41]

Cough can be classified as productive or nonproductive depending on whether or not phlegm is **expectorated** with the cough. A productive cough is helpful if it removes phlegm from the airways. This type of cough should only be treated if the coughing is frequent enough to disturb sleep or is unbearable to the patient. A nonproductive cough without chest congestion can be treated with an antitussive (cough suppressant). Chest congestion can be treated with an expectorant to try to facilitate the expectoration of phlegm. Persistent cough or any cough with chest congestion could indicate a serious condition such as asthma or pneumonia.[42]

Antitussives are drugs that reduce the frequency of cough. Codeine, hydrocodone, dextromethorphan, and diphenhydramine suppress the cough center in the brain. Codeine and hydrocodone are narcotics that can depress breathing and have addiction potential. Their most common side effects are nausea, drowsiness, lightheadness, and constipation. Dextromethorphan is chemically related to codeine and has similar antitussive efficacy but does not have pain-relieving properties, cause respiratory depression, or have addictive potential when used as directed. It is widely used in over-the-counter cough medicines. Drowsiness and gastrointestinal upset are the most common side effects. Diphenhydramine is also an effective cough suppressant that is used in many over-the-counter cough and cold remedies.[42]

Expectorants are controversial because there is little scientific evidence to show that they effectively decrease the thickness of phlegm and thus aid in its expectoration, which may indirectly treat a cough. Guaifenesin is the only expectorant recognized as safe and effective by the FDA. Increased intake of fluids and humidification of air may also be effective in treating cough. Guaifenesin is available in over-the-counter and prescription entities as a single drug or in combination with antihistamines, decongestants, and antitussives. It is available in liquid forms and as regular- and sustained-release capsules and tablets. There are no absolute contraindications to the use of guaifenesin. Nausea and vomiting, dizziness, headache, and rash are rare side effects.[41]

Drugs that Affect the Musculoskeletal System

Osteoporosis Agents. Osteoporosis is a disease that affects both women and men and is characterized by a loss of bone, resulting in misshapen bone, such as curvature of the backbone seen in the elderly, or in easily broken bones.[50] Drugs used to treat osteoporosis can be grouped into those that decrease the reabsorption of calcium and phosphorus and those that increase the deposition of calcium and phosphorus. Drugs that decrease reabsorption of calcium and phosphorus are estrogens, calcium, calcitonin, vitamin D, and bisphosphonates (table 10-22).[51]

Adequate calcium intake is essential for the prevention and treatment of osteoporosis. The various calcium salts provide different amounts of elemental calcium, which is the active part of the drug. Calcium carbonate

Table 10-22. Osteoporosis Agents

Classifications and Medications	Available Dosage Forms
Calcium supplements	
Calcium carbonate (Caltrate, Os-Cal, Viactiv, Tums)	Tablets, chewable tablets, chews
Calcium carbonate + vitamin D (Caltrate +D, Os-cal + D, Viactiv + D)	Tablets, chewable tablets, chews
Calcium citrate (Citracal)	Tablets
Bisphosphonates	
Alendronate (Fosamax)	Tablets, solution
Alendronate/cholecalciferol (Fosamax + D)	Tablets
Risedronate (Actonel)	Tablets
Risedronate/calcium (Actonel and Calcium)	Tablets
Ibandronate (Boniva)	Tablets, injection
Zoledronic acid (Reclast)	Injection
Parathyroid hormone analog	
Teriparatide (Forteo)	Injection
Misc. agents	
Raloxifene (Evista)	Tablets
Calcitonin (Miacalcin, Fortical)	Intranasal

is the most commonly used supplement given orally. Calcium carbonate has a high elemental calcium content and a low cost. Taking calcium carbonate with meals may increase calcium absorption. Constipation is the most common side effect. A deficiency of vitamin D can also lead to bone loss, so many calcium supplements also contain vitamin D.[50]

Bisphosphonates are drugs that work by inhibiting the resorption of calcium from bone, thus allowing the formation of new bone. These agents have become the treatment of choice for osteoporosis and are potent inhibitors of reabsorption of calcium from bone. Alendronate (Fosamax) and risedronate (Actonel) are usually given by mouth once weekly. Risedronate and ibandronate (Boniva) can be dosed by mouth once monthly. To prevent damage to the esophagus and increase absorption, the oral agents must be taken immediately upon arising with a full glass of water. Patients need to remain upright and not eat for at least thirty minutes after taking alendronate and risedronate, and at least sixty minutes after taking ibandronate. Ibandronate and zoledronic acid (Reclast) have injectable formulations available. Ibandronate is injected every three months and zoledronic acid needs to be administered only yearly.[50]

Teriparatide (Forteo) stimulates bone formation and increases bone strength and is indicated for use in patients with severe osteoporosis who have failed or can't tolerate bisphosphonate therapy.[51] It is administered by subcutaneous injection every day. It may cause orthostatic hypotension, arthralgias, leg cramps, and nausea. This is one of the most expensive therapies available for osteoporosis.[50]

Other agents that may be used are raloxifene (Evista) and calcitonin nasal spray (Miacalcin, Fortical). These agents are not as effective as the bisphosphonates and are reserved for patients who are unable to take bisphosphonates.[51]

Anti-Inflammatory Agents. Inflammation is the body's response to infection or trauma. The blood vessels send fluid, dissolved substances, and cells into areas of tissue injury or death. This reaction is intended to protect and aid in the healing of tissue. However, a prolonged or unneeded response produces unnecessary pain or discomfort.[2]

Signs of inflammation include redness, heat, pain, swelling, and altered function of the involved tissue. These signs of inflammation are common symptoms of diseases such as osteoarthritis, rheumatoid arthritis, systemic lupus erythematosus (SLE), tendonitis, bursitis, and gout. Anti-inflammatory agents do not cure these diseases; they just relieve the symptoms.

Nonsteroidal anti-inflammatory drugs are a large class of medications commonly abbreviated NSAIDs. The term nonsteroidal is used to differentiate these agents from corticosteroid hormones, which also have anti-inflammatory properties. NSAIDs also have analgesic (pain-relieving) and antipyretic (fever-reducing) properties. Aspirin is the oldest agent in this class of drugs. Many of the lower strength NSAIDs are available over-the-counter (OTC), such as aspirin, ibuprofen (Advil, Motrin), and naproxen sodium (Aleve). For other drugs in this category see table 10-23.

All NSAIDs can cause serious bleeding and ulcers in the stomach. Many of the drugs used to treat ulcers can be given to prevent damage to the stomach lining while using an NSAID. Diclofenac/misoprostol (Arthrotec) is a combination of an NSAID with an agent to prevent an NSAID-induced gastric ulcer. Misoprostol is a prostaglandin E_1 agent

Table 10–23. Nonsteroidal Anti-inflammatory Agents (NSAIDs)

Medications	Available Dosage Forms
Diclofenac (Voltaren, Cataflam)	Tablets, gel, delayed-release tablets
Fenoprofen (Nalfon)	Capsules
Ibuprofen (Motrin, Advil)	Caplets, capsules, gelcaps, suspension, oral concentrate, drops, tablets, chewable tablets
Indomethacin (Indocin)	Capsules, extended-release capsules, injection, suppository, suspension
Ketorolac (Toradol)	Tablets, injection
Ketoprofen	Capsules, extended-release capsules
Meloxicam (Mobic)	Tablets
Nabumetone (Relafen)	Tablets
Naproxen (Naprosyn, Naprelan, Aleve, Anaprox DS)	Caplets, capsules, gelcaps, suspension, tablets, delayed-release tablets, extended-release tablets
Oxaprozin (Daypro)	Tablets
Piroxicam (Feldene)	Capsules
Sulindac (Clinoril)	Tablets
Diclofenac/misoprostol (Arthrotec)	Tablets
Cox-2 inhibitors	
Celecoxib (Celebrex)	Tablets

that lines the stomach to protect it against the NSAIDs. It has a black box warning regarding its abortifacient effect. Misoprostol has been shown to cause abortions, fetal death, or congenital defects in pregnant patients.[18] NSAIDs have also been shown to cause kidney dysfunction. Due to an inhibition of platelets, NSAIDs can cause bleeding problems, especially in patients taking anticoagulants. Patients receiving anticoagulant therapy should be counseled to monitor for bleeding while taking aspirin or NSAIDs.[2]

Celecoxib (Celebrex) belongs to the class of anti-inflammatory agents called the Cox-2 Inhibitors. Celecoxib has the same indications as the NSAIDs and most of the same side effects. The benefit of the Cox-2 inhibitors is thought to be less GI-adverse effects and less incidence of ulcer development; however, studies have not conclusively shown the GI problems to be significantly different than those of the other NSAIDs. An increased risk of cardiovascular events with these agents caused the removal of the popular drug rofecoxib (Vioxx) from the market. Celecoxib is the only agent remaining in this class.[49]

Because of the potential for Reye syndrome associated with the use of aspirin, it should be avoided in children. Reye syndrome can result in liver disease and central nervous system damage when aspirin is used to treat fever in children with viral infections such as chicken pox and influenza.[2]

Skeletal Muscle Relaxants. Muscle relaxants are a group of medications used to treat muscle pains and spasms. They can be prescribed for a variety of reasons such as back pain, neck pain, fibromyalgia, and acute muscle spasms. These medications work by decreasing the neuronal response from the central nervous system to tense muscles, thus helping to relax muscle tone. Other medications such as baclofen (Lioresal), dantrolene (Dantrium), and diazepam (Valium) treat spasticity as well (see table 10-24).[43]

Although there are a variety of medications used to treat muscle pain and spasm, one muscle relaxant has not been proven superior to another. Therefore, clinicians select muscle relaxants based on adverse effects, patient preference, and abuse potential. All muscle relaxants cause sedation. In fact, it is not known whether these drugs actually relax muscles or relieve pain as a result of their sedative properties.[43] Some agents, such as tizantidine (Zanaflex), can cause more sedation than others. Also, muscle relaxants are commonly given with pain relievers, which may add to the drowsiness.[45] Patients should be warned about driving and other activities that require them to be alert prior to beginning these

Table 10–24. Skeletal Muscle Relaxants

Medications	Available Dosage Forms
Baclofen (Lioresal)	Tablets, intrathecal injection
Carisoprodol (Soma)	Tablets
Chlorzoxazone (Parafon Forte)	Tablets
Cyclobenzaprine (Flexeril)	Tablets
Dantrolene (Dantrium)	Tablets, injection
Diazepam (Valium)	Tablets, oral solution, injection
Metaxolone (Skelaxin)	Tablets
Methocarbamol (Robaxin)	Tablets
Orphenadrine (Norflex)	Tablets, injection
Tizanidine (Zanaflex)	Tablets

medications. Metaxalone (Skelaxin) and methocarbamol (Robaxin) are less sedating and are alternatives for patients who are unable to tolerate tizanidine (Zanaflex) or cyclobenzaprine (Flexeril). Carisiprodol (Soma) is also another common muscle relaxant; however, there have been case reports of drug dependence and withdrawal symptoms when it has been discontinued abruptly after prolonged use.[44]

Diazepam (Valium), baclofen (Lioresal), and dantrolene (Dantrium) are used for muscle spasticity, which is seen in diseases such as cerebral palsy, multiple sclerosis, and following a stroke. Diazepam can cause sedation, psychological and physical dependence.[46] Baclofen causes less sedation and is an appropriate alternative for some patients.

Over-the-counter products that may be used for muscle pain and spasms are available but are less efficacious. These products contain magnesium salicylate (Momentum, Doan's), which acts as an anti-inflammatory medication. They are indicated for minor aches and muscle pains, such as strains.[41]

Analgesics. According to the International Association for the Study of Pain, pain is defined as "an unpleasant sensory and emotional experience associated with actual or potential tissue damage, or described in terms of such damage." It is important to treat pain in order to promote quicker recovery so the patient spends less time debilitated. Analgesics are drugs that relieve pain by altering the way the brain receives and interprets the sensation of pain from the nerves.[47]

Due to the subjective nature of pain, assessment is determined using pain scales. Patients are asked to rate their scale on a scale from 1-10, with 1 being little to no pain and 10 being the worst possible pain. For children, visual analog scales are used in which the child can point to the picture that shows how much pain they are in. These help give the clinician a better idea of how the patient is feeling and to decide which medications to administer to the patient. The choice of drug, dose, and route depends on factors such as the site, duration, and severity of pain.[47]

Opioid analgesics, also called narcotics (table 10-25), act on receptors that are located in the brainstem, spinal cord, and limbic system of the brain to help control pain. Narcotics act at the receptor sites to help alter the perception of pain to the brain. These drugs do not reduce inflammation or lower fever but do have other therapeutically useful properties such as the suppression of cough and antidiarrheal.[2]

Table 10–25. Opioid Analgesics

Medications	Available Dosage Forms
Buprenorphine (Buprenex, Subutex)	Sublingual tablets, injection
Butorphanol (Stadol)	Injection, nasal spray
Codeine	Tablets
Fentanyl (Sublimaze, Duragesic, Fentora, Actiq)	Injection, patch, buccal tablets, transmucosal lozenge
Hydromorphone (Dilaudid)	Tablets, solution, injection, suppository
Meperidine (Demerol)	Tablets, solution, injection
Morphine (Avinza, Kadian, MS Contin, Oramorph SR, Roxanol)	Tablets, capsules, extended-release tablets, solution, injection, suppository
Nalbuphine (Nubain)	Injection
Oxycodone	Tablets, extended-release tablets, solution
Propoxyphene (Darvon)	Capsules
Tramadol (Ultram)	Tablets
Combination products	
Acetaminophen with codeine (Tylenol #3)	Tablets, elixir
Acetaminophen with hydrocodone (Lorcet, Lortab, Norco, Vicodin, Zydone)	Tablets, solution
Acetaminophen with oxycodone (Percocet, Roxicet)	Tablets
Acetaminophen with propoxyphene (Darvocet-N)	Tablets
Acetaminophen with tramadol (Ultracet)	Tablets
Buprenorphine with naloxone (Suboxone)	Sublingual tablets

Similar adverse effects occur with all opioid analgesics. Respiratory depression, the slowing of the breathing reflex, is the most serious side effect, which is a sign of an overdose. Respiratory depression can lead to coma or death. Combining analgesics with other drugs that depress breathing or with alcohol increase this effect. If given in correct doses, these medications should not cause respiratory depression or unconsciousness. These medications do, however, cause sedation. Therefore, patients should be warned about driving and other activities that require them to be alert. Other common side effects include nausea, constipation, and urinary retention. With long-term use, nausea lessens for most patients. However, patients on several days of therapy need to take a stool softener or laxative to prevent constipation.[2]

Since opioids have the potential for abuse, it is important to carefully monitor patients for signs of abuse. Some agents are specially formulated to prevent abuse. For example, buprenorphine is available in a tablet formulation with a medication called naloxone (Suboxone). If abusers attempt to crush the tablet and inject it, naloxone blocks buprenorphine's euphoric effects. Suboxone is not used for pain management but for the treatment of opioid dependence.[47]

The most popular non-opioid analgesic is acetaminophen. This drug is similar to aspirin in its ability to relieve pain and reduce fever, but it has no anti-inflammatory properties. It is a useful alternative to aspirin in children with chicken pox or other viral illnesses, in patients with stomach or intestinal ulcers, in patients with conditions likely to cause bleeding, and in patients with aspirin allergies. In usual doses, acetaminophen rarely causes side effects, but in larger doses it can cause liver damage. The risk of liver damage is increased in patients overusing the medication or drinking alcohol daily. Patients should be reminded of the appropriate acetaminophen dosing and how often to use the medication. Acetaminophen is available over-the-counter and is widely used in oral and rectal dosage forms.[41] There are a variety of topical analgesics used to treat pain that will be discussed in other sections of this chapter.

Drugs that Affect the Endocrine System

Insulin. Insulin is the mainstay of treatment for many patients with diabetes mellitus. Insulin can be given only by subcutaneous or intravenous injection. There are many types of insulin (table 10-26), but only regular insulin can be given intravenously. Most insulin requires a prescription, but the following types of insulin are available over the counter: isophane (NPH), regular (R), and isophane/regular mix (70/30). The types of insulin differ in the time that they take to work (onset of action) and the length of time after the injection that the effects last (duration of action). Vials and pens that are refrigerated expire on the labeled expiration date as long as they remain unopened. Once opened, whether kept refrigerated or at room temperature, most insulin vials expire within twenty-eight to thirty days of opening and pens expire anywhere from ten to fourteen days of opening. Be sure to check the package insert of the specific product to determine the correct expiration date. Insulin doses are measured in units. Special insulin syringes should be used to properly measure the dose (figure 10-4).[52]

Table 10-26. Insulins

Insulin Type	Onset of Action	Duration of Action
Rapid-acting		
Aspart (Novolog)	15 min	3-4 hr
Glulisine (Apidra)		
Lispro (Humalog)		
Short-acting		
Regular (Humulin R, Novolin R)	30-60 min	4-6 hr
Intermediate-acting		
NPH (Humulin N, Novolin N)	2-4 hr	12-18 hr
Long-acting (basal)		
Detemir (Levemir)	3-4 hr	16-20 hr
Glargine (Lantus)	2-4 hr	24 hr

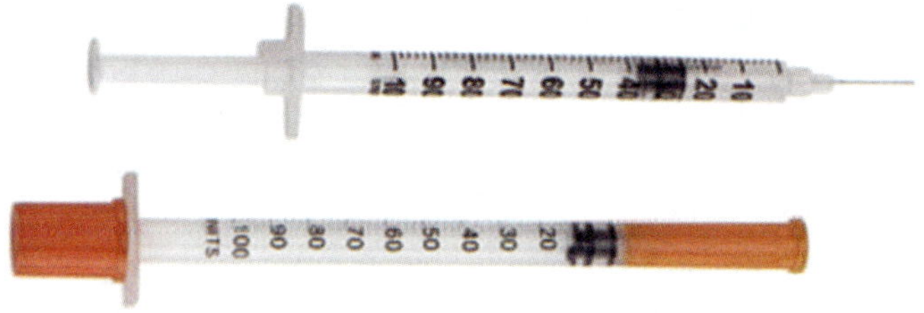

Figure 10-4. Insulin syringes.

Insulin dosing is based on three methods: basal-bolus dosing (most common), split-mix dosing, and insulin pump-based dosing. Basal-bolus dosing mimics the way the body releases insulin from the pancreas. It is a combination of long-acting (basal) insulin given once or twice daily along with rapid/short-acting insulin boluses given two to three times daily at meal time. Split-mix dosing is used in patients who prefer fewer injections per day, and is a combination of intermediate and very rapid/short acting insulin given in a ratio of 2:1 at the same time, given twice daily.

Safety First Insulin is involved in many medication errors every year. Before you dispense insulin, be sure you have the right patient, drug, and dose. Patients need to understand how to correctly use their insulin.

Insulin pump therapy is indicated in patients who desire tighter control of their blood glucose or would like a more flexible lifestyle. However, patients need to be motivated to monitor their food intake, blood glucose, and insulin adjustments and to follow up with their health-care team regularly. Pump therapy involves a continuous infusion of rapid-acting insulin along with bolus doses given prior to meals and snacks based on carbohydrate amounts in the meals. Both the basal and bolus doses are programmed by the patient. Blood glucose monitoring is an important part of insulin therapy and must be done several times daily.[53]

Oral Antidiabetic Agents. Oral hypoglycemic agents (table 10-27) are used to lower blood sugar in Type 2 diabetes. There are several classes of oral hypoglycemics, and each has a different mechanism of action. The sulfonylureas are the oldest agents available. They work by increasing the secretion of insulin from the pancreas. The sulfonylureas are further classified into first and second generation, with the first-generation agents having more side effects associated with them. The most common side effect is low blood sugar (hypoglycemia). Other side effects include weight gain, GI upset, and skin rash. Another class of agents, the secretagogues (e.g., nateglinide [Starlix], repaglinide [Prandin]) work similarly to the sulfonylureas but have a lower incidence of hypoglycemia. The secretagogues are taken with each meal because they work only in the presence of glucose, so if a patient does not eat, he or she should not take the dose.

The biguanides (e.g., metformin [Glucophage]) lower blood sugar by decreasing the amount of glucose produced by the liver, which may increase the sensitivity of insulin receptors, allowing for more sugar to be used by the body. Metformin may cause weight loss, which is a benefit to many patients with diabetes who need to lose weight. Metformin does not cause hypoglycemia when used alone. Nausea, vomiting, and diarrhea are common side effects. Use of metformin is contraindicated in patients with kidney impairment.

The thiazolidinediones, also known as the "glitazones," increase insulin sensitivity, allowing for muscle and fat to utilize glucose. These agents are used as adjunct therapy to other agents. Edema and weight gain are common. There is a warning regarding the potential risk of ischemic cardiovascular events in patients taking rosiglitazone (Avandia).[18]

Exenatide (Byetta) is in a class known as the incretin mimetics, which work by increasing insulin secretion

Table 10–27. Oral Hypoglycemics

Classifications and Medications	Available dosage forms
Sulfonylureas	
Glyburide (Micronase, Diabeta, Glynase)	Tablets
Glipizide (Glucotrol)	Tablets, extended-release tablets
Glimepiride (Amaryl)	Tablets
Meglitinides (secretagogues)	
Nateglinide (Starlix)	Tablets
Repaglinide (Prandin)	Tablets
Biguanides	
Metformin (Glucophage)	Tablets, extended-release tablets
Thiazolidinediones (glitazones)	
Pioglitazone (Actos)	Tablets
Rosiglitazone (Avandia)	Tablets
Alpha-glucosidase inhibitors	
Acarbose (Precose)	Tablets
Miglitol (Glyset)	Tablets
Incretin mimetics	
Exenatide (Byetta)	Injection
Amylin analog	
Pramlintide (Symlin)	Injection
Dipeptidyl peptidase-4 inhibitors (DPP-4)	
Saxagliptin (Onglyza)	Tablets
Sitagliptin (Januvia)	Tablets
Combination agents	
Glyburide/metformin (Glucovance)	Tablets
Glipizide/metformin (Metaglip)	Tablets
Pioglitazone/metformin (Actoplus Met)	Tablets
Repaglinide/metformin (Prandimet)	Tablets
Rosiglitazone/ metformin (Avandamet)	Tablets
Sitagliptin/metformin (Janumet)	Tablets
Pioglitazone/glimepiride (Duetact)	Tablets
Rosiglitazone/glimepiride (Avandryl)	Tablets

from the pancreas when the blood sugar increases. This drug mimics the effects of the incretin hormones in the body. It is a subcutaneous injection given twice daily. It has been associated with an increase in weight loss in patients, partly due to its side effects of nausea, vomiting, and diarrhea. Some patients also indicate they have a feeling of fullness while using this medication, resulting in eating smaller portions of food during meals.

The amylin analog, pramlintide (Symlin), works by decreasing the amount of glucose in the blood after eating. It slows the rate of emptying in the stomach, decreases glucagon secretion, and increases the feeling of fullness so the patient eats less. These mechanisms prevent the spike in blood glucose after eating and promote a steady release of glucose into the blood.[18]

The dipeptidyl peptidase-4 (DPP-4) inhibitors, saxagliptin (Onglyza) and sitagliptin (Januvia), increase and prolong the action of the incretin hormones. Keeping these hormones active leads to an increase in insulin secretion and better control of blood sugar levels. Saxagliptin and sitagliptin are oral medications and are used with other antidiabetic agents. They are well tolerated with few to no side effects.[18]

The last class is the α-glucosidase inhibitors (e.g., acarbose). Acarbose lowers blood sugar levels by delaying the breakdown of sugar and carbohydrates in the intestine, thus slowing the absorption. Abdominal cramping and gas are common with acarbose and limit its use. These medications are taken prior to each meal and should not be taken if the patient does not eat.[18]

Thyroid Agents. The thyroid gland influences the rate of metabolism in the body and the development of the body from youth to maturity. Diseases of the thyroid gland include hypothyroidism (underproduction of thyroid hormone) and hyperthyroidism (overproduction of thyroid hormone).[2]

Hypothyroidism is treated with administration of thyroid hormone (table 10-28). Naturally produced thyroid hormone consists of several substances, including triiodothyroxine (T_3) and levothyroxine (T_4). Levothyroxine (Synthroid, Levoxyl) is the most commonly prescribed drug for hypothyroidism. Thyroid USP is dried animal thyroid gland that contains both T_3 and T_4. Thyroid USP tends to have more variability and unpredictable stability, which limits its use. Since it is considered a natural hormone, some patients prefer it to synthetic agents. Thyroid USP is often prescribed in grains, whereas all the other preparations are prescribed in milligrams or micrograms.

Table 10-28. Thyroid Agents

Medications	Available Dosage Forms
Agents to treat hypothyroidism	
Levothyroxine (Synthroid, Levoxyl, Unithroid)	Tablets, injection
Thyroid USP (Armour Thyroid)	Tablets
Liothyronine (Cytomel)	Tablets, injection
Liotrix (Euthyroid, Thyrolar)	Tablets
Agents to treat hyperthyroidism	
Propylthiouracil (PTU)	Tablets
Methimazole (Tapazole)	Tablets
Iodides (SSKI, Lugol's soln)	Solutions

Liotrix is a combination of T_3 and T_4. All of these drugs are usually given once daily.[54]

Adverse effects related to thyroid hormone replacement include increased heart rate, nervousness, heat intolerance, heart palpitation, and weight loss. These effects indicate that the patient should have a blood test to evaluate whether the dose needs to be adjusted.[54]

Hyperthyroidism is most often caused by an immune system disorder such as Graves disease. Hyperthyroidism is most often treated with nondrug therapies, surgery, or radioactive iodine to remove the gland. Often, hypothyroidism will occur after removal of the gland, and thyroid hormone replacement will be necessary.[54]

Antithyroid drugs block the synthesis of thyroid hormones. They are used most often in children and young adults who do not need permanent removal of the gland. Methimazole and propylthiouracil (PTU) are the primary antithyroid drugs. The most common adverse effect associated with these drugs is a rash. A rare but serious side effect is agranulocytosis, which is a pronounced decrease in white blood cells. This effect is reversible if the drug is discontinued. Other agents may be used as adjunct therapy to the antithyroid agents discussed above. Iodides (SSKI, Lugol's) may be used to block hormone release in the treatment of thyroid storm, which is a life-threatening condition of excessive thyroid release. Beta-blockers are also used as adjunctive therapy in thyroid storm. Propranolol has been shown to block the conversion of T_4 to T_3 to help alleviate symptoms such as heat intolerance, palpitations, and tremors.[55]

Drugs that Affect the Immune System

Antihistamines. Antihistamines block the body's response to histamines and thus reduce or prevent symptoms of allergic rhinitis, such as sneezing, nasal congestion, mucus secretion, itching, and watery eyes. Older antihistamines have many side effects. The side effect that concerns most people is drowsiness. This effect varies among antihistamines and is the reason they are sometimes used as sleep aids, but the newer antihistamines cause less sedation (table 10-29). In children and the elderly, a paradoxical reaction, excitation rather than drowsiness, is sometimes seen. Anticholinergic effects such as dry mouth, blurred vision, difficulty urinating, and constipation occur with many of the older antihistamines. Antihistamines are often included in cold products because of their drying effects on mucosal secretions; however, they have not been shown to effectively shorten the duration of the common cold. Patients with glaucoma, peptic ulcer disease, or an enlarged prostate gland should use antihistamines with caution to avoid exacerbating their disease. Many antihistamines are available over the counter and are available in combination with decongestants, expectorants, and antitussives.[2]

Table 10–29. Antihistamines

Medications	Available Dosage Forms
Older antihistamines	
Chlorpheniramine (Chlor-Trimeton)	Tablets, solution
Diphenhydramine (Benadryl)	Caplets, capsules, solution, syrup, oral-disintegrating tablets, chewable tablets, injection
Clemastine (Tavist)	Syrup, tablets
Newer antihistamines	
Azelastine (Astelin)	Intranasal
Cetirizine (Zyrtec)	Syrup, tablets, chewable tablets
Desloratadine (Clarinex)	Tablets
Fexofenadine (Allegra)	Tablets, oral-disintegrating tablets
Levocetirizine (Xyzal)	Solution, tablets
Loratadine (Claritin, Alavert)	Capsules, solution, syrup, tablets, chewable tablets, oral-disintegrating tablets

Diphenhydramine (Benadryl) is still one of the most commonly used antihistamines, even though it is an older agent with many side effects. It has a high sedation effect and is the active ingredient in many OTC sleep aids. It is also the preferred antihistamine to be administered for drug-induced allergic reactions and anaphylaxis.

Anaphylaxis is a life-threatening reaction that causes itching, hives, bronchoconstriction, cardiovascular collapse, and death if not treated. Although diphenhydramine (Benadryl) is used in the treatment of these reactions, it is not the primary treatment. Diphenhydramine is available in an injectable formulation that makes it available in the bloodstream quickly. The oral formulations also quickly help reverse the effects of many allergic reactions.[2]

Nasal Corticosteroids. Intranasal corticosteroids are used for rhinitis and other allergic or inflammatory conditions of the nose. Intranasal corticosteroids are very effective agents, but it takes regular use to achieve benefit. They are not effective for immediate resolution of symptoms. The aqueous (water-based) preparations sting less than other preparations. Long-acting formulations are available which allow for once daily administration and improved compliance.[2]

Beclomethasone (Beconase AQ), budesonide (Rhinocort Aqua), ciclesonide (Omnaris), fluticasone (Flonase, Veramyst), mometasone (Nasonex), flunisolide (Nasarel), and triamcinolone (Nasacort AQ) are the available products. The systemic absorption is minimal and side effects are mainly localized, including sneezing, dryness, nasal irritation, headaches, nose bleeds, and upper respiratory infections.[18]

Vaccines. The body's response (immunity) can occur in two ways, by active or passive immunity. Passive immunity is when the body is given the protection in the form of antibodies. This type of immunity is often given as a treatment or after exposure to a disease. For example, after someone has been bitten by a rabid animal, they are injected with rabies immune globulin, which contains antibodies against rabies infection, thereby providing passive immunity. This protection works quickly but is short-lived, so the patient must also receive rabies vaccine, which stimulates the body's own immune response (active immunity) against the infection.[2]

Vaccines generally provide active immunity, that is, when a vaccine is administered, it makes a person's own immune system work to provide the immunity. The

Table 10-30. Vaccines

Vaccines	Available Dosage Form	Disease Prevented
Influenza (Fluzone, Fluvirin, Afluria, FluLaval, Flumist)	IM injection, intranasal	Influenza
Meningococcal (Menactra, Menomune)	IM injection	Meningitis
Pneumococcal (Pneumovax)	IM or SubQ injection	Pneumonia
Poliomyelitis (IPOL)	IM injection	Polio
Human Papillomavirus (Gardisil)	IM injection	Cervical cancer, genital warts
Tetanus/diphtheria (Decavax)	IM injection	Tetanus and diphtheria
Tetanus/diphtheria/pertussis (Adacel, Boostrix – adult) (Daptacel, Infanrix – children)	IM injection	Tetanus, diphtheria, pertussis
Hepatitis A (Havrix, Vaqta)	IM injection	Hepatitis A
Hepatitis B (Recombivax HB, Engerix-B)	IM injection	Hepatitis B
Measles, mumps, rubella (MMR II)	SubQ injection	Measles, mumps, rubella
Varicella (Varivax)	SubQ injection	Chicken pox
Herpes Zoster (Zostavax)	SubQ injection	Shingles
Rotavirus (RotaTeq, Rotarix)	Oral suspension	Rotavirus gastroenteritis

immunity that develops takes a few weeks to peak, but the immunity against the disease will last for years.[2]

Vaccines are categorized as either live/attenuated or inactivated (see table 10-30). Live vaccines tend to produce more persistent immunity and more specific antibodies. They must live in the body to work and may cause a mild form of the disease. The varicella (chicken pox) vaccine is an example of a live vaccine. Patients receiving this vaccine may develop a mild case of chicken pox. Up to fifty lesions may develop on the body after receiving the vaccine. Inactivated vaccines are killed proteins that will provoke an immune response. Most vaccines are inactivated and do not cause disease in the body. Inactivated influenza vaccine (flu shot) is an example of an inactivated vaccine. It cannot cause the flu in a patient, but it will protect against getting the flu strains that are in the vaccine.[2]

There are vaccines for infants, children, adolescents, and adults. Some of the childhood vaccines include hepatitis A and B, measles-mumps-rubella (MMR), diphtheria-tetanus-pertusis (DTaP), polio, varicella, and more. Adolescent vaccines include meningococcal vaccine, human papilomavirus (HPV) vaccine, and tetanus-diphtheria-pertussis (Tdap) vaccine. Adult vaccines include tetanus-diphtheria (Td), pneumococcal, and herpes zoster (shingles) vaccine. Each of these vaccines has recommendations for what age, how often, and how many of these vaccines each person should receive. It is important for the recommendations to be followed to eliminate the effects these diseases have on our society.[56]

Safety First

Many vaccines have packages that look alike. Some vaccines also have sound-alike names, like Daptacel and Adacel, Varivax and Zostavax. Some of the vaccines are also available in pediatric and adult doses. Use caution when filling orders for vaccines.[56]

Drugs that Affect the Gastrointestinal System

The most common disorders of the gastrointestinal system are peptic ulcer disease (PUD), gastroesophageal reflux disease (GERD), nausea and vomiting, diarrhea, constipation, and inflammatory bowel disease.

Peptic ulcer disease and gastroesophageal reflux disease are both related to the acid secretion in the stomach. Most gastrointestinal ulcer treatments work by reducing the acid content in the stomach. The most commonly used agents are antacids, histamine-2 receptor antagonists, and proton pump inhibitors.

Antacids. Antacids neutralize existing acid in the stomach. They do not reduce the secretion of acid. Sodium bicarbonate (baking soda) has been a household heartburn remedy for generations. It reacts with acid to create sodium chloride (ordinary table salt), water, and carbon dioxide, which reduces stomach acid. The production of carbon dioxide, a gas, may result in flatulence and distention of the abdomen (bloating).[41]

Calcium carbonate (Tums, Rolaids, Titralac) reacts with acid in the stomach to produce calcium chloride, water, and carbon dioxide. The calcium is not absorbed as well as sodium, so systemic effects are less likely. High doses of calcium-containing antacids can result in milk-alkali syndrome, which consists of high blood levels of calcium, a low blood acid content, irritability, headache, vertigo, nausea, vomiting, weakness, and muscle aches.[41]

Aluminum hydroxide is another ingredient in antacids (e.g., Alternagel). It reacts with acid to produce aluminum chloride and water. Aluminum antacids commonly cause constipation. Magnesium hydroxide is also used as an antacid (e.g., milk of magnesia [MOM]). It reacts with stomach acid to form magnesium chloride and water. Magnesium products commonly cause diarrhea. Therefore, combinations of aluminum and magnesium hydroxides (e.g., Mylanta, Maalox, and Gelusil) are used to try to avoid either constipation or diarrhea. The diarrheal effect tends to predominate with this combination.[41]

There are many over-the-counter antacid products available in a variety of formulations, including tablets, chewables, suspensions, and capsules. They all contain one or more of the ingredients described above. Antacids must be taken in adequate amounts to treat peptic ulcer disease or gastroesophageal reflux disease. Timing of doses is important because the duration of effect of antacids is only fifteen to thirty minutes. They are often given before and after meals and at bedtime.[41]

Antacids are implicated in many drug interactions. For the most part, antacids affect how well drugs are absorbed. Either they react with the drug itself or the changes in the acidity of the stomach inhibit the absorption of other drugs.[41]

Histamine-2 Receptor Antagonists. The histamine-2 receptor antagonists (H_2 antagonists) block a different histamine receptor than the antihistamines used for allergic conditions. When histamine binds to the H_2 receptors on cells in the stomach, it stimulates the secretion of acid. H_2 antagonists reduce the output of acid from stomach cells by blocking this receptor.[2]

The H_2 antagonists (table 10-31) are similar in action and side effects. Their generic names have the –tidine ending on them. They are safe and well-tolerated drugs. The most common side effects are gastrointestinal disturbances. Central nervous system effects such as drowsiness and headache may occur. All products are available over the counter as well as in prescription-only strengths. Patients need to read the labels of the OTC products because some come in multiple strengths. Some of the strengths are lower than the original prescription strengths. Many of the OTC "extra strength" products are the old prescription strength. Drug interactions are most common with cimetidine.[2]

Table 10-31. H_2 Antagonists

Medications	Available Dosage Forms
Cimetidine (Tagamet)	Injection, solution, tablets
Ranitidine (Zantac)	Injection, capsules, syrup, tablets
Famotidine (Pepcid)	Gelcaps, injection, suspension, tablets
Nizatidine (Axid)	Capsules, solution, tablets

Proton Pump Inhibitors. Proton pump inhibitors (table 10-32) act within the stomach cells to prevent the production of acid. They can lower the stomach's acid output more than the H_2 antagonists. Adverse reactions are similar to those of the H_2 antagonists, with nausea, diarrhea, and headache predominating. If a patient cannot swallow the whole capsule, the capsule may be opened and the pellets can be administered with a tablespoon of applesauce. Patients need to be counseled that the applesauce needs to be swallowed and not chewed. If the pellets are crushed, the coating will break down and the drug will be destroyed by the acid in the stomach. The generic names have a –prazole stem allowing for easy recognition of the class.[2]

Current findings suggest that bacteria common to the lining of the stomach, *Helicobacter pylori*, cause peptic ulcer disease. These bacteria produce an enzyme that

Table 10-32. Proton Pump Inhibitors

Medications	Available Dosage Forms
Omeprazole (Prilosec)	Delayed-release capsules, granules for suspension, delayed-release tablets
Pantoprazole (Protonix)	Granules for suspension, delayed-release tablets, injection
Lansoprazole (Prevacid)	Delayed-release capsules, delayed-release tablets, oral-disintegrating tablets
Rabeprazole (Aciphex)	Delayed-release tablets
Esomeprazole (Nexium)	Delayed-release capsules, granules for suspension, injection

degrades the mucosal barrier and allows acid to come in contact with the stomach lining. Treatment of peptic ulcer disease is now directed at elimination of these bacteria if present. Drug regimens directed at eradicating *H. pylori* include various combinations of antibiotics such as amoxicillin, metronidazole, tetracycline, and clarithromycin plus histamine-2 receptor antagonists or proton pump inhibitors and/or bismuth subsalicylate. Bismuth subsalicylate has an antibacterial effect as well as a gastroprotective effect, which makes it beneficial in eradicating *H. pylori*.[18] Prevpac is the only commercially available combination product for *H. Pylori* and it contains lansoprazole, amoxicillin, and clarithromycin.[18]

Anti-Nausea (Antiemetic) Agents. Nausea and vomiting often occur in patients with GI disorders. It also commonly occurs with motion sickness, some forms of chemotherapy, and general anesthesia. In some patients, GI tract motility is reduced, as in GERD and gastroparesis. Gastroparesis generally occurs in patients with diabetes and causes symptoms of nausea, vomiting, and abdominal distention. Nausea and vomiting adversely affect the patient's quality of life, and antiemetics can prevent it. The antiemetic drug and route that is used depends on the cause and how often and how severe the nausea and vomiting are (table 10-33).

Motion sickness is a common cause of nausea and vomiting in patients who are traveling. Motion sickness occurs when there is an imbalance in the inner ear that causes the patient to experience dizziness that may lead to nausea and vomiting. The OTC agents dimenhydrinate (Dramamine) and meclizine (Bonine) are antihistamines that are used to prevent the nausea and vomiting associated with motion sickness. The main side effects with these agents are drowsiness and dry mouth, although meclizine produces fewer of these effects.[41] For longer trips or patients with inner ear imbalances, scopolamine (Transderm Scop) patches may be used to prevent nausea and vomiting. The patch is placed behind the ear and worn for three days. This is an anticholinergic agent, so the side effects associated with this product are dry mouth, blurred vision, constipation, and urinary retention.[18]

Table 10–33. Antiemetic Agents

Medications	Available Dosage Forms
Aprepitant (Emend)	Capsules
Dimenhydrinate (Dramamine)	Injection, tablets, chewable tablets
Meclizine (Antivert, Bonine)	Tablet, chewable tablets
Metoclopramide (Reglan)	Injection, solution, tablets
Prochlorperazine (Compazine)	Injection, suppository, tablets
Promethazine (Phenergan)	Injection, suppository, syrup, tablets
Scopalamine (Trans-Derm Scop)	Patch
Trimethobenzamide (Tigan)	Capsules, injection
$5HT_3$ antagonists	
Dolasetron (Anzemet)	Injection, tablets
Granisetron (Kytril, Sancuso)	Injection, solution, tablets, patch
Ondansetron (Zofran)	Injection, solution, tablets, oral-disintegrating tablets
Palonosetron (Aloxi)	Injection

Metoclopramide (Reglan) is a gastrointestinal stimulant. It works by increasing the motility of the GI tract. Metoclopramide has other effects, which make it useful as an antiemetic drug but also account for some side effects. Metoclopramide can cause drowsiness, nervousness, fatigue, dizziness, weakness, depression, diarrhea, and rash.[18]

Promethazine (Phenergan) and prochlorperazine (Compazine) work by blocking the dopamine receptors in the chemoreceptor trigger zone. These agents are older but just as effective as the newer agents. However, they tend to cause drowsiness and extrapyramidal side effects such as tremors, rigidity, muscle contractions, and other involuntary movements.[18] Dolasetron (Anzemet), granisetron (Kytril), and ondansetron (Zofran) and palonosetron (Aloxi) are agents used for more severe cases of nausea and vomiting. These agents are given either orally or intravenously. They work by inhibiting the serotonin receptor 5-HT_3, which, when stimulated, can cause nausea and vomiting. The main side effects seen with these agents are headache, diarrhea, dizziness, weakness, and fatigue.[18]

Aprepitant (Emend) is thought to work on substance P and the neurokinin receptors to prevent, but not treat, nausea and vomiting. Although it appears to be quite effective in the prevention of chemotherapy-induced nausea and vomiting, its high cost and numerous drug interactions limit its use. Adverse effects include headache, weakness, fatigue, and diarrhea.[18]

Agents to Treat Inflammatory Bowel Disease (IBD). Inflammatory bowel disease (IBD) includes ulcerative colitis and Crohn disease. Goals of treatment include the resolution of abdominal pain, diarrhea, inflammation, and other symptoms. This is generally accomplished with the use of multiple medications

Table 10-34. Agents to Treat Inflammatory Bowel Disease

Classifications and Medications	Available Dosage Forms
Aminosalicylates	
Mesalamine (Asacol, Lialda, Pentasa, Rowasa)	Capsules, suppository, enema, delayed-relese tablets
Sulfasalazine (Azulfidine)	Tablets, delayed-release tablets
Immunosuppressive agents	
Azathioprine (Imuran, Azasan)	Injection, tablets
Mercaptopurine (Purinethol)	Tablets
Monoclonal antibodies	
Infliximab (Remicade)	Injection
Adalimumab (Humira)	Injection

(table 10-34).[2] Aminosalicylates work by blocking the production of some of the inflammatory mediators along with some other processes that are not completely understood. These agents cannot be used in patients with aspirin allergies. The main side effects include belching, abdominal pain, diarrhea, fever, and rash. The agent sulfasalazine (Azulfidine) combines an aminosalicylate with a sulfonamide antibiotic. This agent is only effective if the inflammation is limited to the colon. It may cause nausea, headache, and possibly agranulocytosis. This agent is contraindicated in patients with aspirin or sulfa allergies.[2]

Other agents such as antidiarrheals, corticosteroids, immunosuppressive agents, some antibacterial agents, and antidepressants may also be added. These agents are not used alone but in conjunction with other medications. Oral corticosteroids are used to decrease inflammation. Budesonide (Entocort EC) is a corticosteroid that is designed to release in the ileum so it delivers its action to the site needed; it appears to have lower systemic absorption. Metronidazole (Flagyl) and ciprofloxacin (Cipro) are antibiotic agents and are discussed later in this chapter. The immunosuppressive agents are used in patients who do not respond to the steroid agents. These medications have serious side effects, including **myelosuppression**, liver toxicity, infections, and pancreatitis.[2]

The most expensive agents available for moderate to severe disease are the monoclonal antibodies. These agents have the –mab suffix to their generic names. They work by binding to tumor necrosis factor alpha (TNF-α) and can reduce inflammation in the gut. They are administered by intravenous or subcutaneous routes, depending on the agent. Side effects include headache, nausea, abdominal pain, and upper respiratory infection. Patients must be given a tuberculosis skin test prior to starting therapy because these medications could reactivate a tuberculosis infection in patients who previously had or were exposed to tuberculosis. If the skin test comes back positive, these agents should be avoided.[18]

Antidiarrheals. The frequency of normal bowel movements varies from one stool every two or more days to greater than three stools per day. Therefore, diarrhea is hard to define but is usually considered to be an increased frequency of loose, watery stools. Diarrhea can be acute or chronic and a symptom of another disease. Diarrhea accompanied by fever may have a bacterial cause. Persistent diarrhea should be referred to a physician.[2]

Antiperistaltic drugs treat diarrhea by inhibiting the propulsive movements of the intestine. Slowing passage of the intestinal contents allows absorption of water and electrolytes. Cramping and stool frequency are reduced. Loperamide (Imodium AD) and diphenoxylate/atropine (Lomotil) are antiperistaltic drugs. High doses of diphenoxylate have some narcotic effects, including euphoria. Atropine is added to diphenoxylate to discourage, through unpleasant side effects, the abuse of large doses of diphenoxylate. Antiperistaltic agents should not be used to treat diarrhea caused by bacteria because doing so may result in prolonged diarrhea.[2]

Bismuth subsalicylate (Pepto Bismol, Kaopectate) has been used for indigestion, nausea, diarrhea, and as adjunct treatment for *H. Pylori* infections as previously discussed. Bismuth appears to have an antisecretory action that blocks the copious fluid flow in diarrhea. It has been used to treat infectious diarrhea, including diarrhea common in travelers to foreign countries. Bismuth subsalicylate does contain salicylate, so patients taking aspirin, which also contains salicylate, may inadvertently take too much salicylate. The signs of high levels of salicylate are ringing in the ears, nausea, and vomiting. It should also be avoided in patients with an allergy to aspirin and in children due to the possibility of causing Reye syndrome. There is a specific children's formula available that does not contain a salicylate.[41]

Laxatives. As mentioned previously, the normal frequency of bowel movements varies from person to person. The common misconception that daily bowel movements are necessary for good health leads to the misuse of laxatives and worsens bowel problems. A wide range of diseases, as well as drugs and diet, may cause constipation. Laxatives should be used only after the cause of the constipation has been identified and dietary adjustments have been tried.[2]

Laxatives are used to increase patient comfort and also to prevent complications. Hemorrhoids may be aggravated by constipation. In some cases of constipation, the bowel may become so distended with fecal content that perforation of the bowel or loss of blood supply to the bowel may occur. Laxatives are also commonly used to empty the bowel before various diagnostic procedures. There are several different classes of laxatives (table 10-35).[41]

Table 10–35. Laxatives

Classifications and Medications	Available Dosage Forms
Bulk-forming laxatives	
Psyllium (Metamucil, Konsyl)	Capsules, powder, wafers
Methylcellulose (Citrucel)	Caplets, powder
Polycarbophil (FiberCon, Equalactin)	Caplets, tablets, chewable tablets
Emollient laxatives	
Docusate Sodium (Colace, Correctol)	Capsules, liquid, enema, syrup
Docusate Calcium (Surfak)	Capsules, liquid
Lubricant laxatives	
Mineral Oil (Fleet Mineral Oil Enema, Kondremul)	Liquid, oil (rectal)
Saline laxatives	
Magnesium citrate (Citroma)	Solution
Magnesium hydroxide (Phillips Milk of Magnesia)	Suspension, chewable tablets
Hyperosmotic laxatives	
Glycerin	Suppository
Polyethylene glycol 3350 (Miralax)	Powder
Stimulant laxatives	
Senna (Senokot, Ex-Lax)	Liquid, drops, oral-disintegrating strip, syrup, tablets, chewable tablets
Bisacodyl (Dulcolax)	Enema, suppository, tablets
Combination laxatives	
Senna/docusate sodium (Senokot-S, Peri-Colace)	Tablets

Bulk-forming laxatives dissolve or swell as they mix with the fluid in the intestine. The increased bulk in the intestine stimulates the movement of the intestine. Because this is a natural method of stimulating bowel movement, these laxatives are usually the first choice. Bulk laxatives do not act quickly. They take twelve to twenty-four hours or longer to act. They must be given with adequate water to prevent them from forming an obstruction in the esophagus or intestine.[41]

Emollient laxatives are also known as "stool softeners." They facilitate the mixing of fatty and watery substances in the intestine to soften the fecal contents. They are not fast-acting in treating constipation; they may take up to five days to act. As with bulk laxatives, fluid intake should be increased. These drugs are commonly used in patients who should avoid straining with stool passage. Mineral oil is the only agent in the class of laxatives known as lubricants. It works by coating the stool to allow passage with no straining.[41]

Saline laxatives contain salts that are not absorbed. These salts draw water into the intestines. The increased pressure in the intestine from this water stimulates movement in the intestine. These drugs are indicated for acute evacuation of the bowel because they act within thirty minutes to several hours. Hyperosmotic laxatives draw water into the intestine and work within thirty minutes. Glycerin suppositories are a hyperosmotic laxative. Their effect may be enhanced by the irritant effect of sodium stearate in the suppository.[2]

Stimulant laxatives irritate the lining of the intestine or the nerves in the wall of the intestine, which causes the intestines to excrete their contents. They also increase the amount of water and electrolytes the body secretes into the intestine. These drugs produce thorough evacuation of contents within hours of administration orally and within fifteen minutes if used rectally. They also may produce cramping, colic, mucus secretion, and excessive loss of fluid. Bisacodyl (Dulcolax) tablets are coated to prevent action in the stomach. Administering these tablets with antacids or milk of magnesia may cause the coating to dissolve, which may result in vomiting.

Drugs that Affect the Urinary System

Overactive Bladder Agents. Anticholinergic (antimuscarinic) drugs block detrusor muscle contractions that are responsible for the symptoms of overactive bladder

Table 10-36. Agents Used to Treat Overactive Bladder Disorder

Medications	Available Dosage Forms
Darifenacine (Enablex)	Extended-relase tablets
Oxybutynin (Ditropan, Ditropan XL)	Tablets, syrup, patch, gel, extended-release tablet
Solifenacin (VESIcare)	Tablets
Trospium (Sanctura, Sanctura XR)	Tablets, extended-release capsules
Tolterodine (Detrol, Detrol LA)	Tablets, extended-release tablet

(table 10-36). There are five subtypes of muscarinic (M) receptors, and blockade of detrusor contraction occurs only with M2 and M3 subtypes of anticholinergic receptors. However, muscarinic agents are located in the brain, heart, eyes, salivary glands, and gastrointestinal tract; therefore, the side effects of these agents include dry mouth, constipation, urinary retention, dry eyes, blurry vision, increased heart rate, and confusion.[57]

Drugs that Affect the Other Body Systems

Ophthalmics. Diseases on or near the surface of the eye can often be treated with topical medications. The most common ophthalmic diseases are conjunctivitis, glaucoma, and dryness of the eyes. Drugs used to treat these conditions are listed in table 10-37. Topical treatment of eye diseases is advantageous because the side effects that might occur with systemic (oral) medications can be avoided.

Eye drops and ointments must be used properly to obtain the desired benefit. Drops and ointment should be placed in the lower lid pouch (see Figures 10-5 and 10-6). Ophthalmic solutions and suspensions can cause a burning or stinging sensation upon initial use. If eye products are not used correctly or too many drops are placed in the eye, the drug can drain out of the eye without producing the desired effect. Ointments tend to allow the medication longer contact with the eye, but may cause blurry vision. Ointments are usually used at night to alleviate complaints of blurred vision.[2]

Medications for Treating Conjunctivitis. Conjunctivitis, which is an inflammation of the conjunctiva (the membrane lining the eyelid), is a common eye disease that can be caused by bacterial infection, allergy, chemical irritation, or other diseases.[59] Signs and symptoms

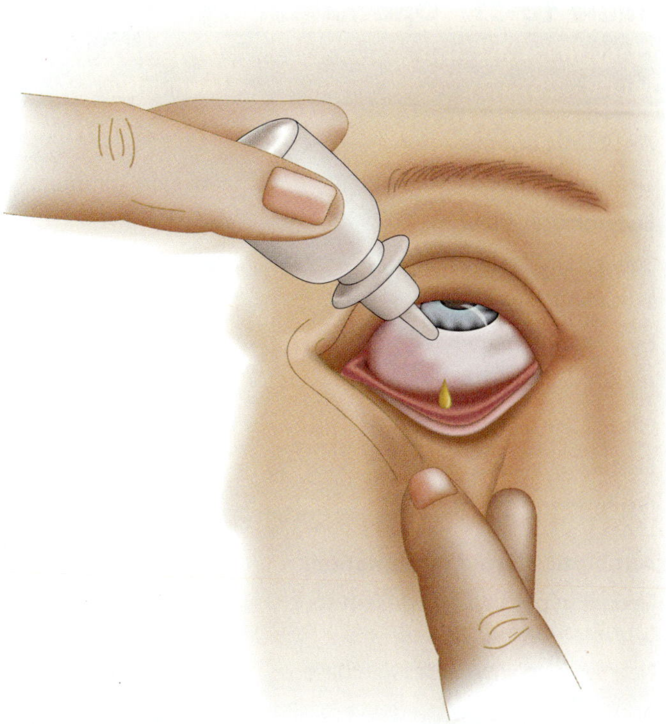

Figure 10-5. Instillation of eye solution[58]

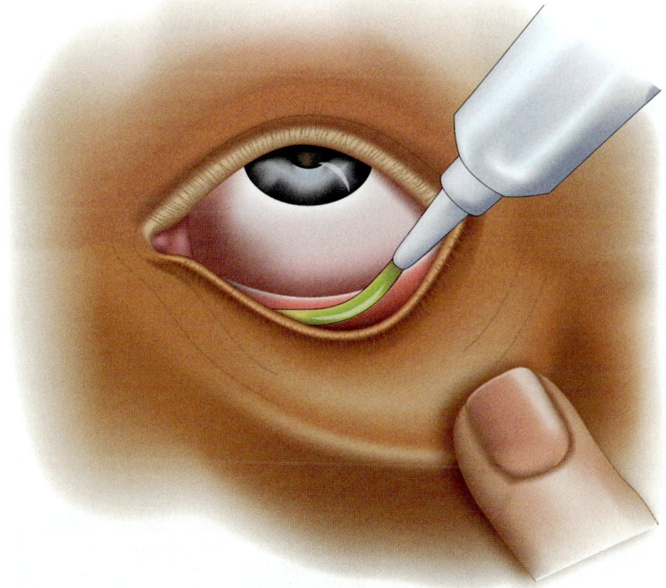

Figure 10-6. Instillation of eye ointment[59]

Part 2

Table 10–37. Ophthalmic Agents

Classifications and Medications	Dosage Forms Available
Antibiotic agents	
Gentamicin (Gentak, Genoptic)	Solution, ointment
Erythromycin (Ilotycin)	Ointment
Sulfacetamide (Sulfacet)	Solution
Tobramycin (Tobrex)	Solution, ointment
Moxifloxacin (Vigamox)	Solution
Ciprofloxacin (Ciloxan)	Solution, ointment
Ofloxacin (Ocuflox)	Solution
Levofloxacin (Iquix, Quixin)	Solution
Gatifloxacin (Zymar)	Solution
Antibiotic/steroid combinations	
Neomycin/polymyxin/hydrocortisone (Cortisporin)	Solution, ointment
Neomycin/polymyxin/dexamethasone (Maxitrol)	Solution, ointment
Tobramycin/dexamethasone (Tobradex)	Solution, ointment
Antiviral agents	
Ganciclovir (Vitrasert, Zirgan)	Gel, implant
Trifluridine (Viroptic)	Solution
Anti-allergy agents	
Azelastine (Optivar)	Solution
Cromolyn (Crolom)	Solution
Ketotifen (Zaditor)	Solution
Naphazoline (Naphcon, Clear Eyes)	Solution
Olopatadine (Patanol)	Solution
Dry eye agents	
Cyclosporine (Restasis)	Emulsion
Phenylephrine (Altafrin, Neofrin)	Solution
Tetrahydrozoline (Visine, Opti-Clear)	Solution
Beta-blockers	
Betaxolol (Betoptic, Betoptic-S)	Solution, suspension
Timolol (Timoptic, Timoptic-XE)	Solution, gel
Sympathomimetics	
Brimonidine (Alphagan P)	Solution
Apraclonidine (Iopidine)	Solution
Carbonic anhydrase inhibitors	
Brinzolamide (Azopt)	Solution
Dorzolamide (Trusopt)	Solution
Prostaglandin analog	
Bimatoprost (Lumigan)	Solution
Latanoprost (Xalatan)	Solution
Travoprost (Travatan)	Solution
Miotics	
Pilocarpine (Pilocar)	Gel, solution

include redness, tearing, secretions, drooping of the eyelid, itching, a scratchy or burning sensation, sensitivity to light, and the sensation that a foreign body present in the eye. The treatment of conjunctivitis depends on the cause and the symptoms.[2]

Conjunctivitis that is caused by infection can be treated with antibiotics or antiviral eye drops. Antibiotics work by harming or killing invading bacteria. Newborn infants are routinely given erythromycin ophthalmic ointment to prevent conjunctivitis caused by bacteria that might have entered the eye during birth. Patients with intense itching and inflammation in addition to an infection may benefit from combination products. Combination products have antibiotics combined with corticosteroids (e.g., dexamethasone, prednisolone, hydrocortisone) to fight the infection as well as to provide an anti-inflammatory action. An example of this is Ciprodex, a combination of ciprofloxacin, a quinolone antibiotic, and dexamethasone, a corticosteroid.[2]

Agents available for the treatment of allergic conjunctivitis depend on the symptoms present. Artificial tear eyedrops soothe itchy, watery, and red eyes. If artificial tears do not work, an antihistamine (e.g., olopatadine, azelastine, epinastine) may be used. Antihistamines help alleviate itchy, watery eyes. Cromolyn sodium is a mast cell stabilizer that also helps to reduce allergic symptoms.[2]

Medications for Treating Glaucoma. Many drugs are used to treat glaucoma by lowering the intraocular pressure. Prostaglandin analogs reduce the pressure in the eye by increasing the discharge of fluid produced by the eye, called aqueous humor. Prostaglandin analogs have an –oprost ending to the generic names, such as bimatoprost (Lumigan). These are often first agents utilized for glaucoma, and they may be combined with other antiglaucoma drugs, such as sympathomimetics. Sympathomimetic drugs lower pressure in the eye by increasing the fluid drainage from the eye. Beta-blocking drugs work by decreasing the production of aqueous humor in the eye. Although ophthalmic drugs have low systemic absorption, ophthalmic beta-blockers can cause bronchoconstriction and slowed heart rate in some patients. Due to these effects, they should be used cautiously in patients who also take oral beta-blockers or who have lung disease, heart failure, and diabetes.

The carbonic anhydrase inhibitors also decrease the production of aqueous humor. Miotic drugs constrict the pupil size, thus increasing the fluid drainage. The most common adverse effects of these drugs are eye discomfort, stinging, burning, or blurred vision upon administration. The miotic agents can cause poor night vision.[2]

Medications for Treating Dry Eyes. A large number of ophthalmic preparations are available as artificial tear solutions for the relief of dry eyes. These products contain salts in the same concentrations that are found in the tissues and fluids of the eye. They also contain buffers to maintain the same acidity as the eye tissues and thickening agents to prolong the time they stay on the surface of the eye. All of these products are available over the counter. A prescription-only insert, hydroxypropyl cellulose (Lacrisert), provides relief from dryness with once-daily insertion as opposed to application of drops multiple times daily. Cyclosporine (Restasis) eye drops, another prescription product, reduces immunologic reactions that cause dry eyes in patients who have keratoconjunctivitis sicca.[18]

Ophthalmic vasoconstrictors, or "decongestants," are commonly used to reduce redness in the eyes from minor irritations. Several products are available over the counter for this purpose. The over-the-counter products should not be used for more than seventy-two hours without consulting a physician.[41]

Otics. Topical otic medications are effective for treating conditions of the external ear. Conditions involving the middle or inner ear require systemic treatment. Topical ear treatments are most commonly used for impacted ear wax and minor infections or irritation of the auditory canal. Otic preparations should be labeled "For the ear (figure 10-7)."[29]

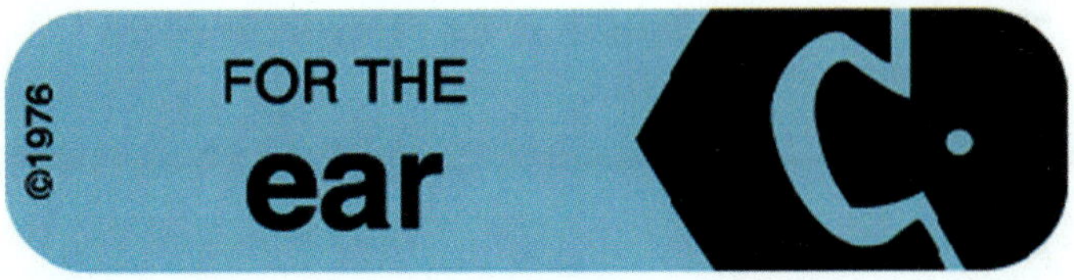

Figure 10-7. Label for otic preparations.

Several products have names similar to ophthalmic products, and care should be taken to avoid confusion and mistakes. Topical otic products should not be used if the ear drum is perforated.

Antibiotic combinations of neomycin and polymyxin B with corticosteroids (Cortisporin) are also used to treat infections. Acetic acid, ciprofloxacin (Ciprodex), and aluminum acetate are antibacterial or antifungal ingredients in ear drops that may also be combined with corticosteroids. Some infections involving the middle ear may necessitate combining an oral antibiotic with one of the otics listed above. Ear infections are painful; a combination product is available that contains antipyrene and benzocaine (A/B Otic) otic solution and is used solely as a pain reliever.[18]

Otic preparations that contain carbamide peroxide/glycerin (Debrox, Murine Ear Wax Removal System) are used to soften and disperse ear wax. After instilling these agents, the wax is removed by irrigating the ear with a bulb-type ear syringe. Any wax not responding to these drugs after four days should be removed by a physician.[41]

Over-the-counter otic agents are available for water-clogged ears. This condition is different from "swimmer's ear." Water-clogged ears occur when water is trapped in the ear by either the ear canal or by excess wax in the ear. Drying agents containing isopropyl alcohol/glycerin (Swim Ear, Auro-Dri) otic drops are approved for this use. This combination allows for the reduction of moisture in the ear without overdrying it.[41]

Topical Agents. Corticosteroid creams, ointments, and lotions are available for a variety of skin conditions involving itching and inflammation such as contact dermatitis, eczema, psoriasis, reactions to insect and spider bites, burns and sunburns, diaper rash, and inflammation associated with fungal infections of the skin. Corticosteroids are available in a variety of different potencies and strengths (table 10-38). Hydrocortisone and hydrocortisone acetate are available over the counter in 0.5% and 1% strengths. Many combinations with antifungals, antibiotics, and antibacterial agents are available. Such products should be applied sparingly.

Table 10-38. Topical Corticosteroids

Corticosteroid Potency Medications	Available Dosage Forms
Low potency	
Desonide (DesOwen)	Cream, ointment, gel, spray
Hydrocortisone (Cortaid, Cortizone-10)	Cream, ointment, gel, spray, solution, lotion
Medium potency	
Mometasone (Elocon)	Cream, ointment, lotion
High potency	
Desoximetasone (Topicort)	Cream, ointment, gel
Fluocinonide (Lidex)	Cream, ointment, gel
Triamcinolone (Aristocort)	Cream, ointment, lotion
Very high potency	
Clobetasol (Temovate, Embeline, Cormax)	Cream, ointment

✔ When topical steroids are being dispensed, the correct formulation (ointment, cream, or lotion) and strength must be carefully selected.

Table 10-39. Topical Agents

Classifications and Medications	Available dosage forms
Agents to treat dandruff, seborrhea, psoriasis	
Acitretin (Soriatane)	Capsule
Adalimumab (Humira)	Injection
Alefacept (Amevive)	Injection
Anthralin (Dritho-Scalp, Dritho-Crème, Psoriatec)	Cream
Calcipotriene (Dovonex)	Cream, solution
Coal tar (DHS, Ionil T, Neutrogena T/Gel)	Shampoo
Etanercept (Enbrel)	Injection
Infliximab (Remicade)	Injection
Salicylic acid (Neutrogena Healthy Scalp, Meted Anti-Dandruff)	Shampoo
Selenium Sulfide (Selsun Blue, Head & Shoulder's)	Shampoo
Tazarotene (Tazorac, Avage)	Cream, gel
Agents to treat fungal/yeast infections	
Clotrimazole (Lotrimin AF, Mycelex)	Cream, lotion, solution
Econazole (Spectazole)	Cream
Ketoconazole (Nizoral)	Cream, shampoo
Miconazole (Micatin, Desenex, Monistat Vaginal)	Cream, powder, spray
Terbinafine (Lamisil AT)	cream
Tolnaftate (Tinactin, Aftatate)	Cream, solution, powder, aerosol
Agents to treat lice/scabies	
Pyrethrins (RID, NIX, A-200, Pronto)	Shampoo, foam, cream
Permethrin (Elimite)	Cream, lotion
Agents to treat acne	
Azelaic acid (Azelex, Finacea)	Cream, gel
Benzoyl peroxide (Stridex, Clearasil, Clean & Clear)	Liquid, wash, pads, gel
Tretinoin (Renova, Retin-A)	Cream, gel

Coal tar and salicylic acid have been used for many years to treat conditions such as dandruff, seborrheic dermatitis (seborrhea), and psoriasis. These products are available as ointments, creams, lotions, shampoos, and bath additives (table 10-39). They have an unpleasant odor and can stain clothing and hair. They should not be applied to broken skin. Salicylic acid is also used to remove warts, calluses, and corns. Since these conditions often have an inflammatory component associated with the condition, the topical corticosteroids may also be used.[41]

Psoriasis is a chronic inflammatory condition of the skin. Several agents are available for the treatment of psoriasis, including topical corticosteroids, coal tar, anthralin (Dritho-creme), calcipotriene (Dovonex), tazarotene (Tazorac, Avage), and psoralen and ultraviolet A (PUVA). Anthralin may stain clothing, skin, hair, and nails a brown to purple color. Calcipotriene and tazarotene have an **antiproliferative** effect and can cause redness, burning, and peeling of the skin. In patients with severe psoriasis, systemic agents are added such as methotrexate, cyclosporine (Neoral, Sandimmune), acitretin (Soriatane), or biologic agents. Acitretin is an oral retinoid that is unsafe in pregnancy. Females who use this drug must use two forms of birth control and cannot become pregnant for three years after treatment. The biologic agents (e.g., etanercept [Enbrel] and alefacept [Amevive]) are generally used as last-line agents due to the high cost and increased risk of infections with these agents. These agents are injections, and alefacept is given in a physician's office due to the potential for hypersensitivity reactions, including anaphylaxis.[61]

Skin may be infected by numerous organisms. Parasites, such as lice and mites, can cause rashes and itching by biting or laying eggs in the skin. Pediculocides (e.g., pyrethins [NIX, RID]) are used to treat these infestations. Fungal and yeast infections are most common in skin folds such as under the breasts and in the groin areas. Fungal infections can also occur on the feet (athlete's foot), on the scalp or body (ringworm), around the nails, or in the mouth. Viral infections that involve the skin include warts, cold sores (herpes simplex), and shingles (herpes zoster). A common bacterial infection that involves the skin is impetigo, a honey-colored crust commonly seen around the mouth and nose in children.

Many topical anti-infective agents are available. Mupirocin (Bactroban), erythromycin, gentamicin, bacitracin, neomycin, and combinations of polymyxin B, neomycin, and bacitracin are commonly used topical anti-bacterial agents. Many of the antifungal agents are marketed for athlete's foot and jock itch. These agents should not be used solely in the treatment of onychomycosis (nail fungal infections); an oral antifungal agent must be used in this condition (see antifungal section of this chapter).[2]

Acne is a chronic condition in which lesions called comedones (whiteheads and blackheads) appear on the skin. It is most common in teenage years. Hormones, friction, sweating, and stress can all cause and influence the severity of acne.[4] A large number of topical products are available for treating acne. Combinations of sulfur drugs, salicylic acid, and resorcinol are also available. Antibiotics such as erythromycin and clindamycin are available to treat acne topically. In more severe cases of acne, systemic treatment with antibiotics or isotretinoin are used. In some cases, both topical and systemic therapies are used.[41]

Sunscreen. Skin cancer is one of the most prevalent cancers being diagnosed. The amount of ultraviolet radiation exposure a person has can place a person at risk for developing skin cancer. There are many medications that can increase a person's sensitivity to the sun. It is important to understand the various sunscreen agents available so patients may be properly counseled on which agent is beneficial.

Ultraviolet (UV) radiation is generated by the sun. The sun is important for warmth and vitamin D synthesis in the body. The damaging effects of the sun include sunburn (caused by UVB rays), premature aging (caused by UVA rays), and skin cancer (caused by UVA and UVB rays). Sunscreen provides the best protection against these effects. To prevent skin cancer and to avoid drug-induced photosensitivity, a broad-spectrum sunscreen should be used. This means it has protection against UVA and UVB rays. These agents come in many different formulations: creams, gels, ointments, sprays, sticks, and lotions. Choice of formulation is a personal choice.[62]

Sunscreen protection is related to its sun protection factor (SPF). SPF measures the length of time a product protects the skin from reddening from UVB rays. Products with SPF between 2 and 11 provide minimal protection, 12 and 29 provide moderate protection, and 30+ provide high protection.

✔ Sunscreens should be applied fifteen to thirty minutes prior to going outdoors. It should be reapplied every two hours or after swimming or perspiring heavily.

There are water-resistant sunscreens, but even those should be reapplied after prolonged exposure to water. Sunscreens should also be applied on cloudy days since UV rays can penetrate through clouds.[63]

Section 2: Women's and Men's Health

Drugs Related to Women's Health

Contraceptives. A female's menstrual cycle is controlled by hormones released in sequence that cause ovulation and prepare the uterus for implantation of a fertilized egg. Manipulating the levels of these hormones can prevent pregnancy (contraception) or make pregnancy more likely. Oral contraceptives are used to prevent pregnancy. Although this is the most common use of these agents, other uses include regulating menstruation and treating endometriosis, polycystic ovary syndrome, and even acne vulgaris.[2]

Oral contraceptives include two types of preparations: estrogen and progestin combinations and progestin-only preparations (table 10-40). There are too many of these agents to list in this chapter, so refer to any drug listing for individual agents. The combination pills work largely by inhibiting ovulation. They also change the lining of the uterus, slow the movement of the egg through

Table 10-40. Contraceptives

Classifications and Medications	Available Dosage Forms
Estrogen and progesterone products	
Low-Ogestrel, Ortho-Tri-Cyclen, Seasonale, Seasonique, Trivora, Yasmin, Yaz	Tablets
Ortho-Evra	Transdermal patch
NuvaRing	Vaginal ring
Progesterone-only products	
Levonorgestrel (Mirena, Plan B, Plan B One-Step)	Intrauterine device, tablets
Medroxyprogesterone acetate (Depo-Provera)	Injection
Norethindrone (Nor-QD)	Tablets

the fallopian tubes to the uterus, and thicken the cervical mucus so that it is more difficult for sperm to penetrate it. These effects make fertilization of the egg and implantation of the fertilized egg less likely should ovulation occur.[2]

The risks associated with these pills occur rarely but are higher for women who smoke or take higher-dose preparations. The greatest risk in smokers is the occurrence of blood clots. The low-dose combinations available have been found not to increase the risk of developing other conditions such as gallbladder disease, strokes, and heart attacks. Side effects that are less serious but bothersome include irregular vaginal bleeding or spotting, headaches, and breast tenderness. Progestin-only pills have a higher incidence of abnormal bleeding but do not have the same risk of blood clots associated with estrogen. Other side effects include nausea and vomiting.[2]

Other formulations of hormonal contraceptives are available. A once-monthly injection with estradiol cypionate (Depo-Estradiol) is available. Medroxyprogesterone acetate (Depo-Provera) is given as an injection every three months. Levonorgestrel (Mirena) is available as an intrauterine device (IUD) providing protection for five years. A transdermal patch containing ethinyl estradiol and norelgestromin (Ortho-Evra) can be worn for seven days. The advantage of these forms is that patients do not have to take a pill every day.[2]

Levonorgestrel is also available as tablets for the use of emergency contraception. Plan B and Plan B One-Step are FDA-approved forms of emergency contraception that do not require prescriptions for women over the age of seventeen. Plan B should be used only in cases of unprotected intercourse or in cases where another contraceptive failed. The patient should be informed that it is not to be used on a regular basis and will not cause an abortion if already pregnant. Plan B must be taken within seventy-two hours from intercourse and is more effective the sooner it is taken. Side effects include nausea, vomiting, lower abdominal pain, fatigue, headache, and breast tenderness.[64]

Fertility Agents. Fertility agents are used to increase the likelihood of pregnancy in patients having difficulty conceiving (table 10-41). A woman is considered to have infertility problems after attempting to conceive for over one year without success. Infertility can occur for many reasons. One of the most common is polycystic ovarian syndrome. Fertility agents stimulate the pituitary hormones that release the egg from the ovary (ovulation). Clomiphene, urofollitropin, and menotropins are drugs used to stimulate ovulation.[65,66]

Clomiphene is a medication commonly used to induce multiple follicular development. This medication can double the rate of pregnancy per cycle to 4–5%. There are certain side effects of clomiphene such as nausea, vomiting, breast tenderness, abdominal distention, headache, and abnormal uterine bleeding. The risk of multiple pregnancies is 8–10%. Patients using clomiphene for greater than twelve cycles increase their risk of ovarian cancer and therefore should not take clomiphene for extended periods of time. Urofollitropin and menotropins also help induce ovulation.[67, 68] They are administered as a subcutaneous or intramuscular injection. Urofollitropin is follicle stimulating hormone (FSH), while menotropin is human menopausal gonadotropin (hMG).[67, 68]

Table 10-41. Fertility Agents

Medications	Available Dosage Forms
Clomiphene (Clomid, Serophene)	Tablets
Urofollitropin (Bravelle)	Injections
Follitropin alfa (Gonal-F) Follitropin beta (Follistim AQ)	Injections
Menotropin (Repronex)	Injection
Chorionic gonadotropin (Pregnyl, Ovidrel)	Injections
Micronized progesterone (Prometrium)	Capsules
Progesterone vaginal (Crinone, Prochieve)	Vaginal gel

An injection of human chorionic gonadotropin (HCG) is given after a cycle of urofollitropin and menotropins. Timing the doses of these drugs to coincide with the woman's cycle is important for success in inducing ovulation. Therefore, pharmacy personnel must ensure that HCG will be available for the patient when she needs it. Progesterone may also be used for infertility to help elongate the luteal phase of a woman's cycle, allowing for greater chances of pregnancy. Progesterone is given in a variety of dosage forms including suppositories, gels, and injections. Prometrium is available in capsules, which can be taken orally or inserted vaginally. Headache, abdominal pain, and breast tenderness are common side effects. Women should be seen frequently by their physicians while taking fertility agents so that adverse effects are noticed early. Multiple births occur more commonly in women who have taken fertility agents.[66]

Hormone Replacement Therapy. Hormone replacement therapy is commonly initiated to treat vasomotor symptoms and vaginal atrophy that occurs during menopause. These symptoms include hot flashes, night sweats, headache, nausea, and dizziness. For prevention, these medications are taken at the time of menopause, either natural menopause or menopause caused by removal of the ovaries. Hormone replacement is also used to prevent and treat osteoporosis, although it is not recommended as first-line therapy.[69]

Hormone replacement therapy (HRT) refers to administration of both estrogen and progesterone (table 10-42). HRT is indicated for patients who have an intact uterus. The combination is given to decrease the risk of cervical cancer. Estrogen therapy is the administration of estrogen alone. Estrogen therapy is indicated for patients who have undergone a hysterectomy. Hormone therapy is available in various dosage forms, including tablets, transdermal patches, creams, gels, intrauterine devices, and others.[69]

Estrogen therapy can cause adverse effects including nausea, headache, breast tenderness, and vaginal bleeding. More serious side effects include venous thromboembolism, stroke, and breast cancer. The most common side effects seen with HRT are irregular bleeding, irritability, depression, headache, bloating, and fluid retention. More serious side effects include an increased risk of coronary heart disease, gallbladder disease, and ovarian cancer.[2]

Drugs Related to Men's Health

Medications to Treat Benign Prostatic Hypertrophy (BPH). Benign prostatic hypertrophy (BPH) is a noncancerous enlargement of the prostate gland that develops in older men. Because the prostate gland encircles the urethra and urine leaves the body through the urethra, enlargement of the prostate can cause difficulties in urinating.[2]

Alpha-adrenergic blocking drugs and androgen hormone inhibitors (table 10-43) are the first-line drugs when a patient presents with urgency to urinate, urination during the night, and soiling of clothes, known as "irritative" voiding symptoms. The alpha-adrenergic blocking drugs

Table 10-42. Hormone Therapy

Classifications and Medications	Available Dosage Forms
Estrogen products	
Estrace, Femtrace, Menest, Premarin	Tablets, Creams
Climara, Estraderm, Vivelle-Dot	Transdermal patches
Estrasorb	Topical Emulsion
Vagifem	Intravaginal tablets
Estring, Femring	Vaginal insert
Estrogen and progesterone products	
Activella, Femhrt, Prefest, Prempo	Tablets
ClimaraPro, CombiPatch	Transdermal patches

Table 10-43. Agents Used to Treat Benign Prostatic Hypertrophy (BPH)

Medications	Available Dosage Forms
Alpha$_1$ adrenergic inhibitors	
Doxazosin (Cardura, Cardura XL)	Tablets, extended-release tablets
Prazoxin (Minipress)	Capsules
Terazosin (Hytrin)	Capsules
Alfuzosin (Uroxatral)	Extended-release tablets
Tamsulosin (Flomax)	Capsules
Androgen hormone inhibitors	
Finasteride (Proscar)	Tablets
Dutasteride (Avodart)	Tablets (film-coated)

are used to relieve the urinary symptoms of BPH but do not affect the growth of the prostate tissue. Doxazosin (Cardura XL) is formulated as a "gastrointestinal therapeutic system" (GITS), a controlled-release system allowing for once daily dosing. Like most modified release drugs, it should not be crushed or chewed. Terazosin (Hytrin) and doxazosin should be taken at bedtime since they cause orthostatic hypotension and the first dose has the potential to cause syncope (fainting). Caution is advised with these agents if patients are on a phosphodiesterase-type V inhibitor (discussed in the erectile dysfunction section) or antihypertensive medications, as these may cause a significant decrease in blood pressure.[2]

Alfuzosin (Uroxatral) should be taken right after a meal at the same time daily. An advantage of this medication is that no dose titration is needed. Tamsulosin (Flomax) should be taken thirty minutes after a meal, which reduces the chances of hypotension. This medication is preferred in someone who has hypertension and takes antihypertensive agents.[2]

The androgen hormone inhibitors, dutasteride (Avodart) and finasteride (Proscar), reduce the size of the prostate by inhibiting the conversion of testosterone to dihydrotestosterone (DHT). DHT is the hormone that causes enlargement of the prostate gland. These agents do not work in all patients and may take up to six months to produce a noticeable effect. The adverse effects include impotence, decreased sex drive, and headache. They may cause abnormalities in a male fetus; therefore, women who are or may become pregnant should not be exposed to this drug, including contact with crushed tablets or with semen from a sexual partner taking these drugs. Whole tablets are film coated to protect against exposure to the drug. These agents reduce the size of the prostate and do not have cardiovascular side effects.[2]

Medications to Treat Erectile Dysfunction. Many drugs have an effect on cholinergic transmission, including antihistamines, dopamine agonists, antipsychotics, and antidepressants. Leuprolide, digoxin, spironolactone, and ketoconazole can decrease serum testosterone, which, in turn, can decrease sexual libido and cause or contribute to erectile dysfunction (ED). Any central nervous system depressant, such as antianxiety, sedative/hypnotics, or opiates, can decrease perception from stimuli of the nerves in the penis. Diuretics (e.g., furosemide, hydrochlorothiazide) and clonidine reduce blood flow to the penis, causing a male to have difficulty producing an erection. When a patient with ED is on any of the above drugs, the clinician must weigh the benefits of the drug and its respective dosage against the consequences of ED on the patient's quality of life.[2]

When ED is not due to psychological factors and is not chemically induced, a phosphodiesterase (PDE) type 5 inhibitor may be used (table 10-44). Prior to initiation of these agents, the patient should be evaluated regarding his cardiovascular health, specifically if he is healthy enough to engage in sexual intercourse.[70]

Of the PDE_5 inhibitors, two are short acting and one is long acting. Sildenafil (Viagra) and vardenafil (Levitra) last approximately four to six hours and should be taken one hour before sexual intercourse is anticipated (two hours if taken with a fatty meal). Since the short-acting agents also inhibit PDE_6, the patient may have difficulty with the following: discriminating blue from green, blurry vision, or adapting to changes in light. Tadalafil (Cialis) may be taken forty-five minutes before intercourse and lasts for approximately thirty-six hours. All of the above agents should not be taken with a nitrate (such as nitroglycerin, isosorbide mononitrate, or isosorbide dinitrate) as this causes severe hypotension. These medications also have the following adverse events: headache, flushing, and priapism. Priapism, a prolonged erection lasting over four hours, is a medical emergency.[2]

If PDE_5 Inhibitors are not effective for ED, alprostadil (Caverject, Edex, prostaglandin E_1) may be utilized. Overall, alprostadil is safe and effective but is available only as an injection to be injected into the shaft of the penis. One must attempt to avoid injection into the vein or artery. An advantage of alprostadil is that vasodilation of the penis (and an erection) will occur five to fifteen minutes after injection. To avoid injection site pain, lidocaine or sodium citrate may be added. Alprostadil should be avoided in sickle-cell anemics, coagulopathy, schizophrenics, unstable angina, and patients with poor dexterity.[2]

Table 10–44. Drugs to Treat Erectile Dysfunction

Medications	Available Dosage Forms
Alprostadil (Caverject, Edex, Prosataglandin E1)	Penile injection
Sildenafil (Viagra)	Tablets
Tadalafil (Cialis)	Tablets
Vardenafil (Levitra)	Tablets

Section 3: Anti-Infectives

The term infection refers to the invasion of tissue by a foreign substance such as a microorganism. In response, the body sends white blood cells to destroy the microorganisms. Invading microorganisms include bacteria, viruses, fungi, protozoa, and parasites such as amoebas, flukes, and worms. The emphasis of this section is on drugs used to treat bacteria, with some discussion of antivirals and antifungals. Tissue damage can occur directly from the invading organisms or from the white blood cells sent to fight the organisms. The body can also increase its temperature to help kill the invaders. Therefore, common symptoms of infection are similar to those of inflammation: fever, pain, heat, redness, and swelling.

Antibiotics

Organisms from the environment invade the body every day. Some of these organisms are not harmful, and some are even helpful, such as the bacteria that normally live in the gastrointestinal tract. When too many organisms are encountered or when the body's defenses cannot overcome the organism, signs of the infection may occur. Antibiotics are used when the body's defenses need help fighting an infection or if there may be serious long-term effects of the infection. Many of the infective organisms acquired by patients in hospitals or long-term care facilities are more difficult to kill than those acquired by patients at home.

Antibiotics are divided into classes based on their chemical structures. Antibiotics may differ between classes and within classes in several ways:

- The bacteria they are effective against
- If they kill bacteria (bactericidal) or just prevent the multiplication of bacteria (bacteriostatic)
- Adverse effects
- The sites of infection they are most effective against (e.g., skin, lungs, kidneys, bone)
- How they are removed from the body
- Routes by which they are given (oral, IV, IM)

The severity, site, and source of infection, characteristics of the antibiotic, and characteristics of the patient are all considered when an antibiotic is selected.[2]

Beta-lactam Antibiotics. Beta-lactam antibiotics have a common chemical structure, but vary widely in the organisms against which they are effective (their "spectrum") and in how easily organisms develop resistance to them. The beta-lactam drugs have relatively few adverse effects and are distributed well into many body tissues. Beta-lactam antibiotics are further broken down into penicillins, cephalosporins, carbapenems, and monobactams.[2]

Penicillins. Penicillin was one of the first antibiotics developed and can be identified by the -cillin ending on the drug name. The original penicillin G was effective against limited organisms. Since penicillin G was introduced, bacteria developed enzymes that destroyed the drug. Therefore, it is of limited use now. The next group of penicillins developed, ampicillin and amoxicillin, are "broad spectrum" because they are effective against both gram-positive and gram-negative organisms, but can also be destroyed by the enzymes some bacteria produce. Oxacillin, dicloxacillin, nafcillin, and methicillin were developed to be stable against the enzymes produced by *Staphylococcus aureus*, a common organism. These antibiotics are used when this organism is suspected. The newest penicillins are called "extended spectrum," meaning that they are effective against many types of bacteria. Extended-spectrum antibiotics include ticarcillin and piperacillin. These penicillins are also combined with a beta-lactamase inhibitor, a substance that inactivates the enzymes bacteria produce to prevent the destruction of the antibiotic. Examples include amoxicillin plus clavulanic acid (Augmentin), ticarcillin plus clavulanic acid (Timentin), and piperacillin plus tazobactam (Zosyn).[18]

Penicillin allergies are estimated to occur in 5 to 8% of the population and can be fatal. All patients should be carefully questioned about their allergy history before they are given any drug of this class. Technicians should be sure to record this information accurately.[2]

Cephalosporins. Cephalosporins are another group of beta-lactam antibiotics. These drugs are resistant to some of the bacterial enzymes that destroy penicillins. Some patients who are allergic to penicillin can also be allergic to cephalosporins. This is called **cross-sensitivity**.

> **Rx for Success**
>
> Always ask about and record patient allergy information. It is important because it may prevent reactions to similar medications.

Cephalosporins are divided into generations based on their spectrum of activity (i.e., how many different types of bacteria they are effective against); see table 10-45. First-generation cephalosporins (e.g., cephalexin [Keflex], cefazolin [Ancef]) have the most limited activity but are effective against many bacteria that cause skin infections and urinary tract infections. Second-generation cephalosporins (e.g., cefuroxime [Ceftin]) have broader activity than first-generation cephalosporins. Third-generation cephalosporins (e.g., cefdinir [Omnicef], ceftriaxone [Rocephin]) have the broadest spectrum of activity. Some of them are used to treat serious hospital-acquired infections. The fourth-generation cephalosporin, cefepime (Maxipime), has extended spectrum activity and is used in moderate-to-severe infections.

Carbapenems and Monobactams. The two other types of beta-lactam antibiotics are carbapenems and monobactams. Imipenem-cilastatin (Primaxin) is a carbapenem with activity against many bacteria that have developed resistance to other antibiotics. Some patients who are allergic to penicillin will also be allergic to the carbapenems. Aztreonam (Azactam) is a monobactam with good activity against some of the hospital-acquired organisms but not as many as the third-generation cephalosporins and carbapenems. Patients who are allergic to penicillin can usually take aztreonam safely.[2]

Table 10–45. Cephalosporins

Classifications and Medications	Available Dosage Forms
First-generation agents	
Cephalexin (Keflex)	Capsules, tablets, suspension
Cefazolin (Ancef, Kefzol)	Injection
Cefadroxil	Capsules, suspension
Second-generation agents	
Cefaclor	Capsules, suspension, chewable tablets, extended-release tablets
Cefoxitin (Mefoxin)	Injection
Cefuroxime (Ceftin, Zinacef)	Tablets, injection
Cefprozil	Suspension, tablets
Cefotetan	Injection
Cefpodoxime (Vantin)	Suspension, tablets
Third-generation agents	
Cefixime (Suprax)	Suspension, tablets
Ceftriaxone (Rocephin)	Injection
Cefdinir (Omnicef)	Capsules, suspension
Ceftizoxime (Cefizox)	Injection
Fourth-generation agent	
Cefepime (Maxipime)	Injection

Macrolides. Macrolides are antibiotics that are especially useful against several organisms that cause respiratory infections. Patients who are allergic to penicillin can safely take the macrolides. Erythromycin, the oldest drug in this group, frequently causes diarrhea and gastrointestinal cramping. Clarithromycin (Biaxin) and azithromycin (Zithromax) are effective against more bacteria and cause less diarrhea. An important counseling point for clarithromycin (Biaxin) is to note that the patient may notice a metallic taste in his or her mouth while on this agent. These agents have gained favor due to once and twice daily dosing, which increases compliance. Azithromycin has a short duration of therapy, often only three to five days.[2]

Sulfonamides. Sulfonamides are effective against many bacteria that cause respiratory, urinary tract, and ear infections. The most frequently used sulfonamide is a combination of sulfamethoxazole and trimethoprim (Bactrim, Septra). Since the two drugs act in different ways to inhibit bacteria, the development of resistance is less likely than it is with a single drug.

Allergic reactions to sulfonamides are common but are usually not fatal. A serious skin reaction occurs rarely. Patients with penicillin allergies can usually take sulfonamides. Sulfonamides can precipitate in the urinary tract, so patients should be told to drink plenty of water while taking them. Also, a patient may sunburn more easily when taking sulfonamides. Patients should be told to avoid sun exposure, use sunscreens, and not use artificial tanning lamps.[18]

Tetracyclines. Tetracyclines have a broad spectrum of activity, but they only inhibit the reproduction of organisms (bacteriostatic). Despite their broad spectrum, their inability to kill organisms limits their usefulness to mild infections. Tetracyclines are useful against some of the organisms involved in sexually transmitted diseases, respiratory infections, and acne. The most commonly used drugs are tetracycline, doxycycline, and minocycline. Tigecycline (Tygacil) is given intravenously and is indicated for the treatment of complicated skin infections, complicated intra-abdominal infections, and community-aquired bacterial pneumonia.[18]

Since tetracyclines combine with metals such as iron, aluminum, calcium, and magnesium, they should not be given at the same time as iron tablets, antacids, or milk products.[29]

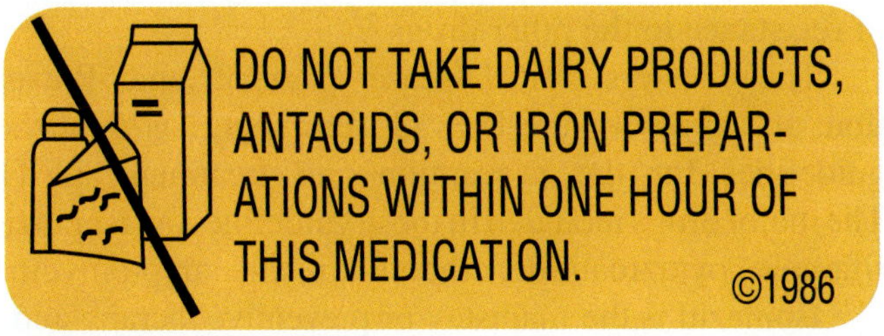

Figure 10-8. A warning label that should be placed on prescription vials containing tetracyclines.

The large molecule formed when they combine with these metals prevents their absorption and renders the drug ineffective. Tetracyclines may discolor tooth enamel, and this discoloration can be permanent. This reaction is of concern in children and the developing fetus because they are actively forming bone and teeth; therefore, this class of medications is generally not given to children or pregnant women.[18]

Allergies are uncommon to tetracyclines, and these drugs can be given to people with penicillin allergies. However, sun sensitivity may occur, and precautions should be followed.

Aminoglycosides. Aminoglycosides antibiotics are able to kill many organisms, including many hospital-acquired organisms. These drugs include gentamicin, tobramycin, and amikacin. They are almost always given intravenously due to their poor oral absorption, but gentamicin and tobramycin are also available as topical ophthalmic medications. These drugs are used for serious infections and often in combination with other antibiotics to broaden the spectrum of bacteria that will be killed and to lessen the development of resistance.[2]

Allergies to aminoglycosides are uncommon, and these drugs can be used in patients with penicillin allergies. Damage to the ear and the kidneys are serious side effects that can be avoided by careful dosing. Many hospitals have pharmacist-managed pharmacokinetic programs to help improve the dosing of aminoglycosides and prevent side effects.[18]

Fluoroquinolones. Fluoroquinolones act by a different mechanism than beta-lactam or aminoglycoside antibiotics and may be useful against bacteria that have developed resistance to other antibiotics. Fluoroquinolones may also be useful in treating infections in penicillin-allergic patients. Note the –floxacin ending to each of the generic names, which help to classify these agents (table 10-46). Ciprofloxacin (Cipro), levofloxacin (Levaquin), and moxifloxacin (Avelox) are available as oral and intravenous preparations. They attain similar blood levels by either route, which allows them to be used orally for some serious infections that are usually treated with intravenous antibiotics. Fluoroquinolones are also used to treat urinary tract infections, respiratory infections, and gastrointestinal infections and as single-dose therapy for some sexually transmitted diseases.[2]

Common side effects of fluoroquinolones are nausea and vomiting, skin rashes, and headache. Fluoroquinolones are contraindicated in pregnant women and children because of possible effects on bone growth. Patients should be cautioned to avoid excessive sun exposure while taking these agents.[18]

Clindamycin. Clindamycin (Cleocin) is effective against many organisms found on the skin and in the mouth. Because of its activity against mouth organisms, it is used in infections that occur in patients who inhale their mouth secretions because of poor swallowing reflexes, also known as aspiration pneumonia. It is also used in combination with other antibiotics for some abdominal infections. There is no cross-sensitivity in penicillin-allergic patients. Diarrhea is a common side effect.[18]

Metronidazole. Metronidazole (Flagyl) is a very effective antibiotic against anaerobic bacteria, bacteria that grow without oxygen. Anaerobic bacteria cause infections primarily in the abdomen and vagina. To cure vaginal infections, both the woman and her sexual partner must be treated. Metronidazole is also used to treat an anaerobic bacterium that frequently causes diarrhea, *Clostridium difficile*. Metronidazole is not effective

Table 10–46. Fluoroquinolones

Medications	Available Dosage Forms
Ciprofloxacin (Cipro)	Injection, suspension, tablets, extended-release tablets
Moxifloxacin (Avelox)	Injection, tablets
Ofloxacin (Floxin)	Tablets
Gemifloxacin (Factive)	Tablets
Levofloxacin (Levaquin)	Injection, solution, tablets
Norfloxacin (Noroxin)	Tablets

against other bacteria, so it is often given in combination with other antibiotics.[18]

Vancomycin. Vancomycin is effective against certain bacteria that are resistant to most of the penicillins. It is also useful for treating infections in patients who are allergic to penicillin. Infections acquired in the nursing home or the hospital are more likely to be caused by bacteria that are resistant to penicillins than are infections acquired at home. Patients, such as cancer patients, who have long-term intravenous lines are also more likely to develop infections that will be resistant to penicillins. Vancomycin is often used in these situations and to treat infections of the heart or heart valves, called endocarditis.

Vancomycin is usually given intravenously. It should be well diluted and given slowly. A reaction referred to as Red Man Syndrome may occur if the drug is given too rapidly. This syndrome is characterized by low blood pressure (hypotension) with or without a rash on the upper trunk, face, and arms. To prevent toxicities, blood levels of vancomycin are measured, and pharmacists usually help dose and monitor vancomycin therapy. Oral vancomycin is not absorbed well enough to treat systemic infections, but is used to treat *Clostridium difficile* infection.

Two other agents that are active against gram-positive bacteria are daptomycin (Cubicin) and linezolid (Zyvox). Both of these agents are active against vancomycin-resistant enterococci (VRE). Daptomycin (Cubicin) is eliminated by the kidneys and the dose is adjusted for patients with kidney impairment. The major side effects with this agent are GI upset and **arthralgias/myalgias**. Linezolid (Zyvox) is available in both injectable and oral formulations. The major side effects include nausea, diarrhea, vomiting, and myelosuppression (which is reversible). With prolonged use of linezolid, **peripheral neuropathy** or lactic acidosis may be seen.[18]

Antitubercular Drugs. Tuberculosis (TB) was a common and dreaded disease prior to the development of effective diagnosis and treatment practices in the 1940s and 1950s. In the United States, drug addicts, patients with end-stage renal disease, homeless shelter residents, nursing home residents, and patients with AIDS are at risk of acquiring active TB.[2]

Antitubercular drugs are used for prevention and treatment of TB. Preventive therapy is used for people with a positive skin test to TB or in people exposed to patients with active cases of TB. Treatment is given to patients with active TB. Because therapy with just one drug often leads to the development of bacterial resistance, TB treatment regimens consist of multiple drugs that are effective against tuberculosis. The use of two or more drugs simultaneously minimizes the development of resistance to the other drugs.[2]

The Centers for Disease Control and Prevention, an agency of the U.S. Government, has published guidelines for the prevention and treatment of TB. The major drugs included in these guidelines are isoniazid, rifampin, pyrazinamide, ethambutol, and streptomycin.[71]

Isoniazid is the mainstay of preventive therapy and is one of the drugs used in treatment when drug resistance is not suspected. Patients receiving isoniazid may also receive vitamin B_6 (pyridoxine) to prevent side effects such as numbness or tingling in the hands or feet. Liver failure is the most dangerous adverse effect, but it rarely occurs.[18]

Rifampin and pyrazinamide are the other drugs recommended for the treatment of tuberculosis and are also given for prevention if isoniazid resistance is suspected. Rifampin is also added to antibiotic therapy associated with other organisms to prevent the development of resistance. Rifampin imparts a harmless orange color to urine, sweat, and tears and can stain contact lenses orange. Patients should be forewarned of this possibility. Rifampin also has many significant drug interactions. Pyrazinamide can cause hypersensitivity reactions such as rash, fever, and joint pain. Like isoniazid, its most serious adverse effect is liver damage.[18]

Antiviral Agents

Until the 1980s, many drugs were available that were effective against bacteria, but few were effective against viruses. The emergence of viral diseases, such as AIDS and genital herpes, and the increased severity of common viral infections like chicken pox in patients with weakened immune systems spurred the development of many new antiviral drugs.

Herpes simplex virus is the cause of fever blisters or cold sores. Another strain of the herpes simplex virus causes genital herpes, characterized by painful lesions on the genitalia that are spread by sexual contact. Several drugs—acyclovir (Zovirax), famciclovir (Famvir), and valaciclovir (Valtrex)—can decrease the symptoms caused by these viruses, and other HIV-related infections. These same drugs are also used to reduce the severity of the symptoms caused by herpes zoster virus. Herpes zoster causes the very painful symptoms of shingles and the potentially serious cases of chicken pox in those with weakened immune systems (e.g., children with leukemia).[2]

Oseltamivir (Tamiflu) is used to prevent and treat both influenza A and influenza B. In order to achieve maximum benefits of the medication, it should be initiated within the first forty-eight hours of the onset of flu-like symptoms. Common side effects include nausea and vomiting. Another medication used for the treatment and prevention of both influenza A and B is zanamivir (Relenza). It is contraindicated in those with airway disorders such as asthma, due to the risk of bronchospasm. It is a powder inhalation, used in the prevention of influenza in persons five years and older. When used as treatment, it should be used in persons seven years and older, who have been symptomatic for less than two days.[2] In addition, it is currently used off-label for the treatment of H1N1 influenza A virus.[18]

Ribavirin (Virazole) is an antiviral drug used for a respiratory virus, called respiratory syncytial virus (RSV),[72] that is common in infants and small children. Ribavirin is administered as an aerosol in an oxygen hood or tent. Ribavirin can cause fetal harm, so women who are or who may become pregnant should avoid contact. Palivizumab (Synagis) is a vaccine that is used for the prevention of RSV. Due to its expense, it is typically used only in high risk infants such as those born premature or with lung disorders.[71]

The emergence of AIDS has prompted the development of several new antiviral drugs (table 10-47). Some of these agents are designed to inhibit the human immunodeficiency virus (HIV) which causes AIDS, while others are designed to treat opportunistic infections. Opportunistic infections occur in patients with abnormally

Table 10-47. HIV Agents[18]

Classifications and Medications	Abbreviation	Dosage Forms
Nucleoside reverse transcriptase inhibitors (NRTIs)		
Zidovudine (Retrovir)	AZT, ZDV	Tablets, capsules, syrup, IV solution
Emtricitabine (Emtriva)	FTC	Capsules, oral solution
Didanosine (Videx)	ddI	Capsules, powder for solution
Zalcitabine (Hivid)	ddC	Tablets, capsules, syrup, IV solution
Stavudine (Zerit)	d4T	Capsules, powder for solution
Lamivudine (Epivir)	3TC	Tablets, oral solution
Abacavir (Ziagen)	ABC	Tablets, oral solution
Tenofovir (Viread)	TFV	Tablets
Non-nucleoside reverse transcriptase inhibitors (NNRTIs)		
Nevirapine (Viramune)	NVP	Tablets, oral suspension
Efavirenz (Sustiva)	EFV	Capsules, tablets
Delavirdine (Rescriptor)	DLV	Tablets
Etravirine (Intelence)	ETV	Tablets
Protease inhibitors (PIs)		
Indinavir (Crixivan)	IDV	Capsules
Ritonavir (Norvir)	RTV	Capsules, oral solution
Nelfinavir (Viracept)	NFV	Tablets, oral powder
Saquinavir (Invirase)	SQV	Capsules, tablets
Amprenavir (Agenerase)	APV	Capsules, oral solution
Atazanavir (Reyataz)	ATV	Capsules
Darunavir (Prezista)	DRV	Tablets
Fosamprenavir (Lexiva)	FPV	Tablets, oral suspension
Tipranavir (Aptivus)	TPV	Capsules, oral solution

weak immune systems (immunocompromised), such as AIDS and leukemia patients.

Anti-HIV antivirals work on different enzymes involved with replication of the virus. Because they work on different enzymes, a combination of drugs from different classes enhances their effectiveness and delays the emergence of resistant strains of HIV. Scientists continue to develop more effective agents or more effective ways to use these agents to treat AIDS.[2]

Zidovudine (Retrovir), a nucleoside reverse transcriptase inhibitor (NRTI), was the first drug available with activity against HIV. It can be used alone but is more often used in combination with other drugs to treat patients with AIDS, to treat patients with HIV infection but no symptoms, and to decrease the likelihood of transmission of the HIV virus from mother to fetus. The major side effect of zidovudine is decreased white blood cells, which increases the likelihood of infection. Other NRTIs include emtricitabine, didanosine, and lamivudine. Precautions of NRTIs are enlarged liver and lactic acidosis.[18]

The protease inhibitors are potent anti-HIV drugs. All the drugs in this class have many drug interactions. Indinavir (Crixivan) can cause nausea, abdominal pain, and elevated liver function tests. To avoid the formation of kidney stones, patients should drink six glasses of water daily. Patients on oral contraceptives should also consider alternative methods while on protease inhibitors.[18]

The non-nucleoside reverse transcriptase inhibitors (NNRTI) are always used in combination with other antiviral drugs. The most common adverse effects of nevirapine (Viramune) are rash, fever, nausea, headache, and abnormal liver function tests. Rash associated with nevirapine can be severe and life threatening. Nevirapine can be taken with or without food. Common adverse effects of the NNRTI class include rash and headaches.[2]

Ganciclovir (Cytovene) and foscarnet (Foscavir) are antivirals used to treat cytomegalovirus (CMV), which can cause infections in the eye, colon, lungs, and liver. These drugs can also be used for the prevention of CMV in patients who have had a kidney or liver transplant. Ganciclovir may decrease white blood cells. Foscarnet's major adverse effect is kidney toxicity. Since foscarnet does not affect white blood cells, it can be useful for treating AIDS patients who have decreased white blood cells. Ganciclovir causes less kidney toxicity than foscarnet, which makes it useful for kidney transplant patients. Because ganciclovir has the ability to cause tumors and changes in cellular chromosomes, it is advisable to handle and dispose of ganciclovir according to guidelines for cancer chemotherapy drugs.[2]

Antifungal Agents

Antifungals are often used for skin, nail, or vaginal infections, as already discussed earlier in the chapter. This section will focus on antifungal agents used for internal (systemic) fungal infections (table 10-48).

Like many other types of infections, fungal infections have increased in recent years because of the increased number of patients whose immune systems are not able to control the growth of fungi (e.g., HIV, cancer, and transplant patients). Additionally, the use of antibiotics kills bacteria that normally control the growth of fungi.[2]

Amphotericin B is capable of resolving a wide array of fungal infections. It is given by intravenous infusion

Table 10–48. Antifungals

Classifications and Medications	Available Dosage Forms
Amphotericin B	
Conventional (Fungizone)	Injection
Liposomal (AmBisome)	Injection
Lipid complex (Abelcet)	Injection
Lipid colloidal dispersion (Amphotec)	Injection
Azole antifungals	
Ketoconazole (Nizoral)	Tablets
Fluconazole (Diflucan)	Tablets, powder for oral suspension, injection
Itraconazole (Sporanox)	Capsules, oral solution
Posaconazole (Noxafil)	Oral suspension
Voriconazole (Vfend)	Tablets, powder for oral suspension, injection
Echinocandins	
Caspofungin (Cancidas)	Injection
Micafungin (Mycamine)	Injection
Anidulafungin (Eraxis)	Injection

and as a bladder irrigation for fungal bladder infections. Amphotericin is available in multiple formulations: conventional, liposomal (AmBisome), lipid complex (Abelcet), and a colloidal lipid dispersion (Amphotec). Although amphotericin B is effective against most of the fungi that cause disease in humans, its usefulness is limited by its adverse effects. Infusion-related adverse effects include fever, chills, vomiting, and headache. Amphotericin B may also cause toxicity to the kidneys. These reactions can be limited by the administration of acetaminophen, diphenhydramine, hydrocortisone, and meperidine before the infusion. More serious reactions include kidney toxicity, decreased potassium, and decreased red blood cells (anemia). Liposomal amphotericin B formulations are less toxic to the kidneys and cause less infusion-related adverse events when compared with conventional amphotericin.[1]

The search for effective agents without the side effects of amphotericin B led to the development of the azole antifungals. Ketoconazole (Nizoral), fluconazole (Diflucan), itraconazole (Sporanox), posaconazole (Noxafil), and voriconazole (Vfend) are used to treat both topical and systemic infections.[2]

Fluconazole is an antifungal that can be given orally and intravenously. It is just as effective orally as intravenously, so IV use is necessary only in patients who cannot take the oral formulation or absorb the oral form reliably. Fluconazole is useful for thrush and esophageal infections but is more effective than ketoconazole for fungal infections in the lungs, blood, abdomen, and urinary bladder. A single dose of fluconazole can be used to treat vaginal yeast infections. Many patients prefer a single oral dose to the use of topical creams.

Itraconazole is indicated for the treatment of onychomycosis (nail fungus) and other types of infections that fluconazole cannot treat. For optimal absorption, itraconazole should be taken with a full meal or with a cola beverage.[73]

Echinocandins are the newest class of antifungal agents and are easy to identify as they all end in –fungin. They work by inhibiting the cell wall formation of fungi, especially *Candida* and *Aspergillus* species. They can cause infusion-related reactions, including headache and fever, so acetaminophen is often given before the infusion. The echinocandins include caspofungin (Cancidas), micafungin (Mycamine), and anidulafungin (Eraxis). These agents require a slow infusion to prevent infusion-related reactions.[73]

Section 4: Hematologic and Oncologic Agents

Drugs that Affect the Hematologic System

Blood Products. For a variety of reasons, patients need exogenous blood products. Blood products may be divided into the following categories: colony-stimulating factors (CSF), erythropoiesis-stimulating agents (ESA), interleukins, stem cell mobilizer(s), thrombopoietin mimetic agents (TMA), thrombopoietin receptor antagonists, and colloids. Each will be discussed individually as to the indication, mechanism of action, and agents available.

Part 2

Colony-stimulating factors are used to increase white blood cells. A decrease in white blood cells may occur due to antineoplastic therapy or in HIV/AIDS. The agents bind to cell-specific receptors in hematopoietic cells and cause new cells to be produced, neutrophils, which are the predominant type of white blood cells needed for immunity. Granulocyte-stimulating factor (G-CSF), or filgrastim (Neupogen) injection, was the first agent in this class. Pegfilgrastim (Neulasta) is a long-acting version of filgrastim with polyethylene glycol (PEG). It is indicated only for antineoplastic therapy-induced decreased neutrophils. Sargramostim (Leukine) helps stimulate production of macrophages and granulocytes (GM-CSF) in addition to neutrophils, which help with the immune response.[18]

Erythropoiesis-stimulating agents (ESA) are used to treat anemia secondary to chronic kidney disease, antineoplastic therapy, and zidovudine, a drug used to treat HIV/AIDS. Erythropoietin is produced in the kidney and stimulates red blood cell formation in the bone marrow. A "black box warning" exists for ESAs, because they may cause serious cardiovascular adverse effects, an increased risk of blood clots, stroke, and tumor progression or recurrence. A solution for injection of recombinant erythropoietin alfa (EPO) is available in multiple strengths under the brand names of Epogen and Procrit. Darbopoietin alfa (Aranesp) is a long-acting erythropoieitin injection.

Interleukins are cytokines that are "messengers" in the immune system. They typically communicate when a pathogen (i.e., bacteria, virus, fungus) is in the body to cells in the immune system. Interleukin 11 (IL-11), along with other cytokines, are responsible for the production of megakaryocytes, which are bone marrow cells that produce platelets. Oprelvekin (Neumega) is recombinant interleukin-11 and is used to prevent severe thrombocytopenia, a state of low platelets, which occurs after certain types of chemotherapy. Oprelvekin can cause allergic or hypersensitivity reactions, including anaphylaxis, so there must be close monitoring for itching, wheezing, swelling of the face, throat, or tongue, and other allergic symptoms after the subcutaneous injection.[74]

Plerixafor (Mozobil) is a stem cell mobilizer that is used for stem cell collection and transplantation in conjunction with filgrastim. Currently, it is approved only for adjunctive use in patients with non-Hodgkin lymphoma or multiple myeloma. Plerixafor basically allows filgrastim to work more effectively.[18]

Romiplostim (Nplate) is a thrombopoietin mimicking agent. This agent increases the production of platelets by binding and activating the thrombopoietin (TPO) receptor. Romiplostim is FDA-approved only for patients with idiopathic (no known cause) chronic immune thrombocytopenic purpura (ITP) who have not responded to other treatments (corticosteroids, immunoglobulins, or spleen removal) and are at high risk of bleeding. Only prescribers enrolled in the NEXUS (Network of Experts Understanding and Supporting Nplate and Patients) program can prescribe and administer romiplostim.[18]

Eltrombopag (Promacta) is an oral thrombopoietin receptor agonist that interacts with the human TPO-receptor, causing production of megakaryocytes from bone marrow progenitor cells. Like romiplostim, this agent is used only in patients with ITP who have not responded to other treatment. Due to the risk of liver toxicity, only prescribers enrolled in the PROMACTA CARES™ program can prescribe the medication, and only pharmacies registered in the program can dispense the tablets to patients registered in the program.[18]

Albumin is a colloidal solution. Albumin is found in the blood plasma and is essential for stabilizing a patient in hypovolemic shock. Other colloids such as normal saline, dextrose in water, lactated ringer's, or any combination of these require a significantly higher amount of fluid and time to stabilize a patient, whereas albumin does not. In hypovolemic shock, 25% albumin products are typically utilized. When the albumin level is acutely low perioperatively, a lower strength (5%) may be given. Common brand names include Albuminar, Albutein, Buminate, Flexbumin, and Plasbumin.[18]

Anticoagulants and Thrombolytics. Coagulation of blood (clot formation) is essential to prevent bleeding to death from injuries. But abnormal blood clot formation within blood vessels can cause heart attack, stroke, or pulmonary embolism (a blood clot in the lung), all potentially fatal conditions. Anticoagulants (blood thinners) are used to prevent these potentially fatal clots from forming. Because anticoagulants slow clot formation, the main concern with anticoagulant therapy is excessive bleeding.[2] Blood tests are used to measure the bleeding time, which helps determine the appropriate dose to prevent clot formation but not allow excessive bleeding.

Table 10-49. Anticoagulants and Thrombolytics

Classifications and Medications	Available Dosage Forms
Heparin	
Unfractionated Heparin	Injection
Low molecular weight heparins	
Dalteparin (Fragmin)	Injection
Enoxaparin (Lovenox)	Injection
Tinzaparin (Innohep)	Injection
Factor Xa inhibitor	
Fondaparinux (Arixtra)	Injection
Direct thrombin inhibitors	
Argatroban	Injection
Bivalirudin (Angiomax)	Injection
Lepirudin (Refludan)	Injection
Vitamin K_1 inhibitors	
Warfarin sodium (Coumadin, Jantoven)	Tablets
Thrombolytics	
Alteplase (Activase, Cathflo)	Injection
Reteplase (Retavase)	Injection
Tenecteplase (TNKase)	Injection

Safety First The anticoagulants are considered high risk medications because if an error is made, the consequences can be life threatening.

For the prevention or treatment of clot formation, unfractionated heparin (UFH) is administered intravenously or subcutaneously, and low-molecular-weight heparins (LMWHs) are administered subcutaneously. Adverse reactions to heparin include a dramatic, rapid, and severe decrease in the number of platelets, called heparin-induced thrombocytopenia (HIT),[2] and bleeding. If the effects of heparin need to be reversed, protamine sulfate is an antidote that can be slowly infused to counteract its effects.

The LMWHs are derived from heparin but have different actions on the clotting cascade and more predictable dosing by subcutaneous injection. They are used to prevent clot formation, especially after orthopedic or abdominal surgeries. The most common LMWH, enoxaparin, is used for the treatment of deep vein thrombosis (DVT), which can be given on an outpatient basis in many patients. Advantages of the LMWHs compared to UFH include simpler dosing, a longer duration of action, and less blood testing.[75] Reductions in platelets are less common with the LMWH, but they can still occur, as can bleeding.

Fondaparinux (Arixtra) is a Factor Xa inhibitor (anticoagulant) that is also given subcutaneously to prevent and treat clotting disorders. It is more expensive compared to the LMWHs and UFH and lacks an antidote, but is often used in patients who have a history of heparin-induced thrombocytopenia. It also causes bleeding, especially in patients with kidney dysfunction.

Warfarin (Coumadin) is the most commonly used oral anticoagulant.[2] The maximal effect of warfarin takes three to five days to occur, so an injectable anticoagulant is usually given until warfarin takes effect. When the full effect of warfarin is present, as measured by a blood test called the INR, the injectable anticoagulant is discontinued. As with other anticoagulants, bleeding is the most serious adverse effect. Many drug interactions and changes in diet can alter the effectiveness of warfarin. Patients should always inform health professionals of all the drugs they take or have taken to avoid drug interactions with warfarin. Patients should be told to watch for signs of bleeding (e.g., bleeding gums, nose bleeds, blood in urine or fecal matter) and bruising; to take their medication at the same time every day; to avoid major diet changes, especially with foods high in vitamin K (e.g., green leafy vegetables); and to have blood tests taken as instructed.[76] The effects of warfarin can be reversed with vitamin K_1 (phytonadione, Mephyton, Aquamephyton).

When a patient suffers from heparin-induced thrombocytopenia (HIT), regardless of whether there is a clotting disorder, a class of drugs called direct thrombin inhibitors (DTIs), are used.[2,75] Argatroban provides a rapid onset of anticoagulation, but its duration of action is less than one hour, so it is given by continuous intravenous infusion. It can be used in patients with poor kidney function. Lepirudin (Refludan) is also a rapid-onset agent that is given by continuous intravenous infusion, but it lasts about eighty minutes. It can be used in patients with a poorly functioning liver. For both argatroban and lepirudin, a lab test that measures the amount of anticoagulation, the aPTT, is used to adjust dosages. Bivalirudin (Angiomax) is another injectable DTI, but is indicated for use only with aspirin when a patient has a cardiac procedure called a percutaneous coronary intervention (PCI).

Thrombolytics. Thrombolytic agents are used to break or lyse blood clots. They are usually used in emergency situations when rapid dissolution of a clot is needed to prevent death or permanent damage, such as in blood clots to the lungs (pulmonary embolism), acute myocardial infarction (AMI), or acute ischemic stroke. They are also commonly used to dissolve blood clots in central intravenous catheters.[2] The available thrombolytics are given intravenously and include alteplase (Activase, Cathflo), reteplase (Retavase), and tenecteplase (TNKase).[18] The thrombolytics can cause bleeding, which can be serious, so care must be taken to select appropriate patients for the drug and ensure correct dosing to prevent excessive bleeding from occurring.

Chemotherapeutic Agents

IV Chemotherapy Agents. Three types of treatment are used for cancer: surgery, radiation, and chemotherapy (drug therapy), or combinations of these. Combinations tailored to specific cancers allow for more successful elimination of cancerous cells and less damage to normal tissue. Chemotherapy is administered to kill cells in large tumors as well as cancer cells that remain after the bulk of the tumor is removed by surgery and/or killed by radiation therapy.[2]

Chemotherapeutic agents are divided into classes on the basis of how they kill cells. Common chemotherapeutic agents are listed below. The toxic effects of these agents on healthy cells can be the limiting factor in the effectiveness of chemotherapy.

✔ Many chemotherapy drugs have several commonly used names, which can lead to confusion and medication errors. Because these drugs have so many dose-related adverse effects, mistakes with chemotherapy (e.g., giving the wrong drug or dose) can be fatal.[2]

Combinations of chemotherapeutic agents usually lead to higher response rates and a longer period of remission than therapy with a single agent. The selection of drugs for combination is based upon different mechanisms of action, responsiveness to dosage schedules, and the toxicity of the agents. Combination therapy often allows decreased doses of each drug, which may decrease the incidence and severity of toxicity. Chemotherapy combinations are called regimens or protocols, and they are abbreviated with the initials of the drug names. The initials stand for trade and generic names, and the same letters do not always stand for the same drugs in different regimens. Orders without the drug names can be confusing. An example of a chemotherapy regimen is the MOPP regimen for Hodgkin disease, the "M" stands for mechlorethamine, "O" stands for vincristine (Oncovin), and the "P"s stand for Procarbazine and Prednisone.

Oral Chemotherapy Agents. There are several chemotherapy agents available in oral formulations, which allow patients to manage their disease and therapy at home rather than having to go into a hospital or clinic for IV therapy. Some oral agents, such as the selective estrogen receptor modulators, are used to maintain a patient in remission. Table 10-50 lists currently available, commonly used oral chemotherapy agents.

These agents can cause certain side effects of which the patient should be made aware. The most common side effects seen with these medications are anemia, diarrhea, nausea, vomiting, fatigue, alopecia, myelosuppression, and abdominal pain. Other agents, such as letrozole (Femara), can cause bone pain and even hot flashes, and lomustine, can cause a loss of appetite. Chemotherapy agents have a wide variety of adverse effects; thus, it very important that the patient be monitored to determine if he or she is able to tolerate the therapy or need to be changed to another medication. Also, monitoring is necessary to determine if the patient needs supportive care therapy, such as antinausea or pain medication, or nutritional support, due to the side effects [2]

Section 5: Nutritional and Dietary Supplements

Vitamins

Vitamins are compounds involved in the cellular chemical reactions that are essential to normal tissue growth, maintenance, and function. Vitamin D can be synthesized by the body upon exposure to sunlight, but the rest of the essential vitamins must be supplied by the diet. The recommended dietary allowance (RDA) is the daily level of intake needed to meet the nutritional needs of most healthy people.[41]

Vitamins are classified as fat-soluble or water-soluble. The fat-soluble vitamins are vitamins A, D, E, and K. These are absorbed with fats in the diet, so very low-fat diets and conditions that impair fat absorption may decrease amounts of these vitamins in the body. Excessive use of mineral oil as a laxative may cause decreased absorption of the fat-soluble vitamins. These vitamins are stored in fats in the body when excess amounts are ingested. Toxic effects may occur when large amounts are taken. The water-soluble vitamins are C, folic acid, and the B vitamins. With normal kidney function, excess of these vitamins is excreted in the urine and toxic levels do not accumulate.[41]

Many vitamins have more than one name. Knowing the alternate names may be helpful for dispensing the correct product. Listed below are some synonyms:

- Vitamin A = Retinol
- Vitamin E = Tocopherol
- Vitamin B_1 = Thiamine
- Vitamin B_2 = Riboflavin
- Vitamin B_5 = Pantothenic acid
- Vitamin B_6 = Pyridoxine
- Vitamin B_{12} = Cyanocobalamin
- Vitamin B_3 = Niacin = Nicotinic acid

Several forms of vitamin D are available but are not substitutable in all patients. These forms include cholecalciferol, 25-hydroxycholecalciferol, 1,25-dihydroxycholecalciferol, and ergocalciferol.[18]

Vitamins are used therapeutically in some situations. Vitamin A may be used for certain skin disorders. Vitamin D analogues are used for patients with bone malformations caused by kidney disease. Vitamin K may be given to reverse the effects of the anticoagulant, warfarin. Niacin (vitamin B3) is used to treat high blood cholesterol. Many of these have been discussed in other sections of this chapter.

Table 10–50. Chemotherapy Agents

Classifications	Medications	Available Dosage Forms
Alkylating agents	Busulfan (Busulfex, Myleran)	Tablets, injection
	Carmustin(BiCNU)	Injection
	Chlorambucil (Leukeran)	Tablets
	Cyclophosphamide (Cytoxan)	Tablets, injection
	Lomustine (CeeNU)	Capsules
	Mechlorethamine (Mustargen)	Injection
	Temozolomide (Temodar)	Tablets
Antibiotics	Bleomycin (Blenoxane)	Injection
	Dactinomycin (Cosmegen)	Injection
	Daunorubicin(Cerubidine, Daunoxome)	Injection, liposomal injection
	Doxorubicin (Adriamycin, Doxil)	Injection, liposomal injection
	Idarubicin (Idamycin)	Injection
	Mitomycin (Mutamycin)	Injection
	Mitoxantrone (Novantrone)	Injection
Antimetabolites	6-mercaptopurine (Mercaptopurine,	Tablets
	Purinethol)	Tablets
	6-thioguanine	Capsules
	Capecitabine (Xeloda)	Injection, liposomal injection
	Cytarabine (Cytosar, Depocyt)	Injection
	Floxuridine	Injection, topical solution, cream
	Fluorouracil (Adrucil)	Injection
	Gemcitabine (Gemzar)	Capsules
	Hydroxyurea (Droxia)	Tablets
	Mercaptopurine (Purinethol)	Tablets, injection
	Methotrexate (MTX, Trexall)	
Aromatase inhibitors	Anastrozole (Arimidex)	Tablets
	Exemestane (Aromasin)	Tablets
	Letrozole (Femara)	Tablets
Biologic response modifiers	Aldesleukin (Interleukin-2,Proleukin)	Injection
	Denileukin (Ontak)	Injection
	Interferon alpha 2b (Intron A)	Injection
Heavy metal compounds (platinums)	Carboplatin (Paraplatin)	Injection
	Cisplatin (Platinol AQ)	Injection
	Oxaliplatin (Eloxatin)	Injection
Hormones	Leuprolide (Lupron, Lupron Depot, Eligard)	Injection, long-acting depot
	Medroxyprogesterone (Provera)	Tablets, injection
	Megestrol Acetate (Megace)	Tablets, oral suspension
Immunomodulators	Lenalidomide (Revlimid)	Capsules
	Thalidomide (Thalomid)	Capsules
Microtubule-targeting agents	Estramustine (Emcyt)	Capsules
Mitotic inhibitors	Vinblastine	Injection
	Vincristine (Oncovin, Vincasar)	Injection
	Vinorelbine (Navelbine)	Injection
Monoclonal antibodies	Alemtuzumab (Campath)	Injection
	Bevacizumab (Avastin)	Injection
	Bortezomib (Velcade)	Injection
	Cetuximab (Erbitux)	Injection
	Ibritumomab (Zevalin)	Injection
	Rituximab (Rituxan)	Injection
	Trastuzumab (Herceptin)	Injection
	Tositumomab (Bexxar)	Injection

Table 10–50. Chemotherapy Agents (continued)

Classifications	Medications	Available Dosage Forms
Retinoids	Bexarotene (Targretin)	Capsules
Selective estrogen receptor modulators (SERMs)	Tamoxifen (Nolvadex)	Tablets
	Toremifene (Fareston)	Tablets
Topoisomerase inhibitors	Etoposide	Injection, capsules
	Topotecan (Hycamtin)	Injection, capsules
Tyrosine kinase inhibitors	Dasatinib (Sprycel)	Tablets
	Erlotinib (Tarceva)	Tablets
	Gefitinib (Iressa)	Tablets
	Imatinib (Gleevec)	Tablets
	Lapatinib (Tykerb)	Tablets
	Sorafenib (Nexavar)	Tablets
	Sunitinib (Sutent)	Capsules
Misc. agents	Asparaginase (Elspar)	Injection
	Dacarbazine (DTIC-Dome)	Injection
	Docetaxel (Taxotere)	Injection
	Paclitaxel (Abraxane,Taxol)	Injection
	Pegaspargase (Oncaspar)	Injection
	Procarbazine (Matulane)	Capsules

Vitamins are also given as supplements. Supplements are indicated when a patient's diet is poor, such as with some elderly patients and alcoholics. Vitamin supplements also may be given during periods of increased metabolic requirements such as pregnancy, major surgery, or cancer. Poor absorption is another indication for vitamin supplementation. Some patients lack a substance necessary for the absorption of vitamin B_{12} and must receive B_{12} by injection. Some drugs may affect absorption or requirements for some vitamins. Patients taking the anti-tuberculosis drug isoniazid may have an increased need for pyridoxine to avoid adverse effects on nerves.[18]

Minerals

Minerals are constituents of enzymes, hormones, and vitamins and are essential to processes such as muscle contraction, nerve conduction, and water and acid balance. The minerals present in the body in larger amounts are calcium, phosphorus, potassium, chloride, magnesium, and sulfur. The minerals present in small amounts (trace elements) are iron, zinc, iodine, chromium, selenium, fluoride, copper, manganese, and others.[41]

Diets may vary in their mineral content to a greater extent than vitamin content. Plants take up minerals from soil, so the mineral content of the soil where they are grown influences the amount of minerals present in foods. Deficiencies of certain food groups in the diet may cause deficiencies in certain minerals. For instance, dairy products are the most important source of calcium. Patients who are intolerant of dairy products or are strict vegetarians may require calcium supplements to get adequate amounts of calcium.[41]

Minerals, like vitamins, may be given individually only when needed. For instance, to prevent the bone disease osteoporosis, postmenopausal women are frequently given calcium supplements. The four minerals that are most commonly administered as single entities are calcium, iron, potassium, and magnesium. Minerals, especially iron, are also added to many multivitamin preparations.[41]

Calcium is available in many different salts that all vary in the amount of calcium provided. Calcium is also available as injectable salts for intravenous use. The oral agents have been discussed in the section on osteoporosis.

Iron-deficiency anemia can result from poor absorption of iron, inadequate intake of iron, or iron loss secondary to bleeding. Iron is administered as many different salts that contain varying amounts of iron. Iron is also available in injectable preparations for intravenous use.[18]

Potassium is the primary mineral found inside cells. Potassium imbalance adversely affects cellular metabolism and nerve and muscle function. Potassium salts are available as tablets and liquids for oral use. The amount of potassium present may be expressed as milli-equivalents (mEq) rather than milligrams (mg). Potassium chloride is the salt most commonly prescribed. Liquid forms tend to have an unpleasant taste, but may be preferred in patients who are unable to swallow the large tablets or capsules. One tablet form, K-Dur, is a tablet of pressed pellets, which can be suspended in liquid to provide a tasteless liquid form. Effervescent potassium tablets are also available to be dissolved in water or juice. Potassium salts are irritating to the stomach, so they are usually given as wax or polymer forms that minimize irritation by slowly releasing potassium in the gut. Potassium chloride and potassium phosphate can also be given intravenously. Overly concentrated intravenous potassium solutions are irritating to veins. Intravenous solutions must be administered slowly to avoid heart rhythm disturbances.[18]

Magnesium is important to many of the body's enzymes, nerves, and muscles. It is the second most abundant mineral found inside cells. Magnesium may be administered as oral tablets, as liquids, or by injection. As with the other minerals, the amount of magnesium in different salts varies. The amount is often expressed as mEq. Magnesium sulfate is the salt used for intravenous administration. Various salts are used for oral replacement. Diarrhea is a common side effect of oral formulations.[41]

Herbals and Other Dietary Supplements

Complementary and alternative medicine (CAM) supplements have become popular alternatives to medications. Many patients believe these products must be safe because they are derived from natural sources instead of being chemically made in a laboratory. The National Centers for Health Statistics have shown that approximately 36% of the population is using some type of alternative medicine. The leading herbal remedy categories are immune system modulators (Echinacea), energy/vitality (ginseng, caffeine), weight loss supplements (caffeine, ginseng, bitter orange), women's health (calcium, soy), depression (St. John's wort), and bone/joint (glucosamine/chondroitin).

Although some of these agents have been shown to be beneficial, what is not always known is how these products will react with other medications or how safe they are. For example, Echinacea has shown some efficacy as an immune system stimulant if taken immediately at the start of a cold; however, patients who have allergies to ragweed should avoid taking this product. St. John's wort may increase mood in patients with mild to moderate depression; however, it has many drug interactions and also drug-food interactions which can limit its use in many patients.

It is important for patients to consult with their physician or pharmacist prior to starting any of type of alternative therapy. Patients tend to believe that, since they are OTC and they are sold in pharmacies, they can do no harm.

Summary

This chapter has focused on the main pharmacological agents that are in use today in the community and institutional settings. The drugs described in this chapter are the most commonly prescribed medications, and many of these agents may be used to treat multiple conditions. For readers who desire more in-depth information or information on less commonly used medications, a list of additional resources is included at the end of the chapter.

Self-Assessment Questions

1. Which of the following statements is false?
   a. Fosphenytoin and phenytoin can be diluted in normal saline or dextrose for IV administration.
   b. Fosphenytoin causes less infusion pain and blood pressure changes than phenytoin.
   c. Phenytoin is a medication in which small changes in the dose can have a large impact on the drug's effects.
   d. Blood levels must be monitored for phenytoin because it has a narrow therapeutic index.
2. Which of the following drugs is used in the treatment of Parkinson disease?
   a. amoxicillin
   b. diazepam
   c. levodopa/carbidopa
   d. enalapril
3. Which of the following is not an anticholinergic medication used to treat Alzheimer disease?
   a. rivastigmine
   b. memantine
   c. galantamine
   d. donezepil
4. Which of the following is classified as an HMG-CoA Reductase Inhibitor?
   a. atorvastatin (Lipitor)
   b. fenofibrate (Tricor)
   c. ezetimibe (Zetia)
   d. gemfibrozil (Lopid)
5. Which of the following medications is considered a preventive medication for migraines?
   a. frovatriptan (Frova)
   b. sumatriptan (Imitrex)
   c. dihydroergotamine (Migranal)
   d. propranolol (Inderal)
6. Which of the statements about beta-blockers is false?
   a. They can cause bronchoconstriction and should be used with caution in patients with asthma or COPD.
   b. They can mask the symptoms of low blood sugar and should be used with caution in patients with diabetes.
   c. They are used for a variety of indications, including high blood pressure, angina, and migraine prophylaxis.
   d. A common side effect is an increased heart rate.
7. Which of the following medications can cause a blue-gray discoloration of the skin as a side effect?
   a. Flecainide (Tambocor)
   b. Propafenone (Rythmol)
   c. Amiodarone (Pacerone)
   d. Diltiazem (Cardizem)
8. Which of the following statements regarding analgesics are false?
   a. Opioid medications have therapeutically useful properties such as the suppression of cough and antidiarrheal
   b. Opioid analgesics act on receptors that are located in the brainstem, spinal cord, and limbic system of the brain, to help control pain
   c. Opioid medications can cause sedation
   d. Opioid medications have anti-inflammatory properties
9. What is the brand name of buprenorphine in tablet form with another medication called naloxone?
   a. Suboxone
   b. Subutex
   c. Darvon
   d. Darvocet
10. Which of the following is a significant adverse effect of muscle relaxants?
    a. Vomiting
    b. Rhinitis
    c. Sedation
    d. Headache
11. Which of the following medications is used to treat depression?
    a. Adderall XR
    b. Ativan
    c. Paxil CR
    d. Valium

Self-Assessment Questions

12. Which class of medications has important dietary restrictions (low tyramine diet)?
    a. Tricyclic antidepressants
    b. Selective norepinephrine reuptake inhibitors
    c. Selective serotonin reuptake inhibitors
    d. Monoamine oxidase inhibitors
13. Which of the following statements is false?
    a. Ambien helps patients fall asleep and stay asleep for 6–8 hours
    b. Sonata is best for patients who need help falling asleep
    c. Sonata helps patients fall asleep and stay asleep for 6–8 hours
    d. Lunesta helps patients fall asleep and stay asleep for 6–8 hours
14. Which of the following agents may be used to treat an asthma attack?
    a. Montelukast (Singulair)
    b. Mometasone (Asmanex)
    c. Fluticasone (Flovent)
    d. Albuterol (Ventolin/Proventil)
15. What is the benefit of using metformin (Glucophage) in patients with diabetes?
    a. It may cause weight loss.
    b. It may cause GI side effects.
    c. It may cause hypoglycemia (low blood sugar).
    d. It may be used in patients with renal problems.
16. Which of the following conditions is not treated with oral contraceptives?
    a. prevention of pregnancy
    b. Acne vulgaris
    c. Irregular menses
    d. stroke
17. Which of the following medications is considered estrogen therapy?
    a. Prempro
    b. Activella
    c. Femhrt
    d. Vivelle-Dot
18. Which of the following statements regarding fertility treatments is false?
    a. Clomiphene (Clomid) is a follicle stimulating hormone (FSH).
    b. Fertility agents increase the likelihood of multiple births.
    c. Clomiphene is used to stimulate ovulation.
    d. Urofollitropin and menotropins are used to stimulate ovulation.
19. Which of the following is *not* a benefit to using a combination of chemotherapy agents?
    a. Combination therapy usually leads to higher response rates.
    b. Combination therapy usually leads to a longer period of remission than compared to therapy with a single agent.
    c. Combination therapy often allows for lower doses of each medication, which may decrease the incidence and severity of toxicity.
    d. Combination therapy is less expensive than single therapy.
20. Which of the following medications can cause significant peripheral vasodilation?
    a. Aldesleukin
    b. Cisplatin
    c. Gemtuzumab
    d. Methotrexate

Self-Assessment Answers

1. a. Phenytoin is compatible only with normal saline and should not be mixed with any other solutions because a precipitate will form. Fosphenytoin can be added to both normal saline and dextrose solutions. Fosphenytoin causes less infusion pain and fewer blood pressure changes and thus is a preferred agent over phenytoin in many institutions. Phenytoin has a narrow therapeutic index, meaning that small changes in the dose can result in large changes in the drug's effects. Since phenytoin has a narrow therapeutic index, blood level testing is necessary to make sure that the concentration of medicine is enough to be effective but not enough to cause side effects.
2. c. Levodopa/carbidopa is the mainstay of therapy for Parkinson disease. Amoxicillin is an antibiotic, diazepam is used as an antiepileptic/antianxiety agent, and enalapril is used to lower blood pressure.
3. b. Memantine (Namenda) is an N- methyl d-aspartate antagonist. All other agents listed are anticholinergic medications used to treat Alzheimer disease.
4. a. Atorvastatin is an HMG-CoA reductase inhibitor, also known as a statin. Fenofibrate and gemfibrozil are fibrates. Ezetimibe decreases the absorption of cholesterol in the body.
5. d. Propranolol is used as a preventive treatment for migraine headaches. Preventive medications are taken on a daily basis to help decrease the occurrence of migraines. Frovatriptan and sumatriptan are triptans, which are used as abortive medications. They are used at the first sign of migraine and not for daily use. Overuse of abortive medications can lead to rebound headaches, which can be even more severe than the initial migraine.
6. d. A common side effect of beta blockers is a decreased heart rate. Beta blockers are commonly prescribed for hypertension and are also used to treat angina and as migraine prophylaxis. They can cause bronchoconstriction in patients with respiratory conditions and can block the symptoms of low blood sugar in diabetics.
7. c. Amiodarone can cause a blue-gray discoloration of the skin that is irreversible. Flecainide and propafenone don't cause blue-gray skin discoloration but can cause dizziness, tremor, and blurred vision.
8. d. Opioid medications do not have anti-inflammatory properties. They also do not have anti-pyretic (fever-reducing) abilities. However, as listed in the other statements, opioid medications have therapeutically useful properties such as the suppression of cough and antidiarrheal. They also commonly cause sedation.
9. a. Suboxone is a combination of buprenorphine and naloxone that is used to treat opioid dependence. Naloxone is added to buprenorphine to prevent potential abusers from crushing the tablet in an attempt to inject the medication. Subutex is the brand name for buprenorphine alone. Darvon is the brand name for propoxyphene. Darvocet is the brand name for propoxyphene and acetaminophen combination.
10. c. All muscle relaxants cause sedation. In fact, it is not known whether these drugs actually relax muscles or cause relief due to their sedative properties. Some agents, such as tizanidine, can cause more sedation than others. Patients should be warned about driving or other activities that require them to be alert prior to beginning these medications. The other answer choices are incorrect and are not common side effects of muscle relaxants.
11. c. Adderall XR is a mixture of amphetamine salts and is used for ADHD. Lorazepam (Ativan) and diazepam (Valium) are benzodiazepines used to treat anxiety. Paroxetine extended release (Paxil CR) is a selective serotonin reuptake inhibitor (SSRI) antidepressant.
12. d. Monoamine oxidase inhibitors (MAOIs) have dietary restrictions. If tyramine-containing foods are taken with an MAOI, a hypertensive crisis can occur. Due to the side effects and multiple interactions, MAOIs are not typically used unless the depression is refractory to other agents.
13. c. Zaleplon (Sonata) lasts approximately four hours. A patient who wakes up in the middle of

the night or has difficulty staying asleep will not have his or her sleep needs met by zaleplon, but rather a longer-acting oral agent like zolpidem (Ambien).

14. d. Albuterol is used to treat an asthma attack. It works by opening up the bronchioles quickly to help the patient breathe easier. The other agents listed are all used to prevent asthma attacks from happening and need to be used on a regular basis.
15. a. Metformin can cause weight loss in patients with diabetes. This is a benefit since patients with Type 2 diabetes are often overweight. Some of the other agents used to treat diabetes commonly cause weight gain.
16. d. Oral contraceptives have different levels of estrogen and progesterone or progesterone alone. They are used to prevent pregnancy, manage acne vulgaris, and regulate menstruation. The most common use for oral contraceptives is to prevent pregnancy by inhibiting ovulation and changing the uterus lining to decrease the chances of fertilization.
17. d. Answer choices a, b, and c are all hormone-replacement therapy products that contain both estrogen and progesterone. Vivelle-Dot is an estrogen-only product that is available as a transdermal patch that is placed on the skin twice weekly.
18. a. Clomiphene helps induce ovulation but is not a follicle-stimulating hormone. Fertility treatments increase the likelihood of multiple births such as twins and triplets. For example, clomiphene can increase the chance of multiple pregnancies by 8–10%. Urofollitropin is a follicle stimulating hormone (FSH) while menotropin is a human menopausal gonadotropin (hMG). They both stimulate ovulation.
19. d. There is no cost savings benefit with combination chemotherapy regimens. Combination chemotherapy usually leads to higher response rates and longer periods of remission compared with single agents. The selection of drugs for combination is based upon different mechanisms of action, responsiveness to dosage schedules, and the toxicity of the agents. Combination therapy often allows decreased doses of each drug, which may decrease the incidence and severity of toxicity.
20. a. Aldesleukin (Interleukin-2) is a biologic response modifier that can cause peripheral vasodilation, necessitating extra fluids and even vasopressors. Though the other medications have many adverse effects, peripheral vasodilation is a significant adverse effect seen with the use of aldesleukin.

Resources

Di Piro JT, et al. *Pharmacotherapy: A Pathophysiologic Approach*. 7th ed. New York, NY: McGraw Hill, 2008.

Handbook of Nonprescription Drugs: An Interactive Approach to Self-Care. 16th ed. Washington, DC: APhA, 2009.

USPDI, Volume II, Advice for the Patient. Rockville, MD: United States Pharmacopeia Convention, Inc; 2005.

USPDI, Volume I, Drug Information for the Health Care Professional. Rockville, MD: United States Pharmacopeia Convention, Inc.; 2005.

Merck Manual of Diagnosis and Therapy. 18th ed. Whitehouse Station, NJ: Merck Sharp & Dohme Corp.

Facts and Comparisons. St. Louis, MO: Facts and Comparisons, Inc.

References

1. Walker M. Status epilepticus: an evidence-based guide. *BMJ*. 2005;331:673–677.
2. DiPiro JT, Talbert RL, Yee GC et al. *Pharmacotherapy: A Pathophysiologic Approach*. 7th ed. New York, NY: McGraw Hill; 2008.
3. Schapira AH. Treatment options in the modern management of Parkinson's disease. *Arch Neurol*. August 2007; 64(8):1083–1088.
4. Lewitt PA. Levodopa for the treatment of Parkinson's disease. *N Engl J Med*. December 4, 2008; 359(23): 2468–2476.
5. Herbert LE, Scherr PA, Bienias JL, Bennett DA, Evans DA. Alzheimer disease in the U.S. population. *Arch Neurol*. 2003;60:1119–1122.
6. Samanta MD, Wilson B, Santhi K, et al. Alzheimer disease and its management: a review. *Am J Ther*. 2006;13:516–26.
7. Cummings JL. Alzheimer's disease. *N Engl J Med*. 2004;351:56–67.
8. Johannsen P. Long-term cholinesterase inhibitor treatment of Alzheimer's disease. *CNS Drugs*. 2004;18:757–768.

9. Exelon Patch (rivastigmine transdermal system) [prescribing information]. East Hanover, NJ: Novartis; July 2007.
10. Namenda (memantine) [prescribing information]. St Louis, MO: Forest Pharmaceuticals, Inc.; July 2005.
11. Anderson DW, et al. Revised estimate of the prevalence of multiple sclerosis in the United States. *Ann Neurol.* 1992;31(3):333–6.
12. The INFB Multiple Sclerosis Study Group and The University of British Columbia MS/MRI Analysis Group. Interferon-β-1b in the treatment of multiple sclerosis: final outcome of the randomized controlled trial. *Neurology.* 1995;45(7):1277–1285.
13. PRISMS-4: long term efficacy of interferon-β-1a in relapsing MS. *Neurology*. 2001;56(12):1628–1636.
14. OTC products: A study of pharmacists' recommendations. *Pharmacy Times.* September 2000 & October 2001 supplements.
15. Lipto, RB, Diamond S, Reed M et al. Migraine diagnosis and treatment: results from the American Migraine Study II. *Headache* 2001 July-August;41(7):638–45.
16. Wenzel RG, Sarvis CA, Krause M. Over-the-counter products for acute migraine attacks: literature review and recommendations. *Pharmacotherapy.* 2003;23(4): 494–505.
17. Silberstein et al. Evidence-based guidelines. *Neurology.* 2000;55:754–762.
18. Facts and Comparisons. Available at http://www.online.factsandcomparisons.com. Accessed September 6, 2009.
19. American Headache Society consensus statement. *Headache.* 2004;44:414–425.
20. Stark S, et al. Naratriptan is effective for the treatment of migraine headache in sumatriptan non-responders (abstract). *Headache.* 1999;39.
21. Wenzel R, Sarvis C. Do butalbital-containing products have a role in the management of migraine? *Pharmacotherapy*. 2002 August;22(8):1029–1035.
22. Facts and Comparisons. Available at: http://www.online.factsandcomparisons.com. Accessed October 7, 2009.
23. Dworkin RH. Recommendations for the diagnosis, assessment, and treatment of neuropathic pain. *Am J Med.* October 01 2009; 122(10suppl):S1–45.
24. American Psychiatric Assocation. Practice guideline for the treatment of patients with major depressive disorder (revision). *Am J Psychiatry.* 2000;157 (suppl):1–45.
25. Adams SM, Miller KE, Zylstra RG. Pharmacologic management of adult depression. *Am Fam Physician.* 2008;77(6):782–792.
26. Stahl SM, Felker A. Monoamine oxidase inhibitors: a modern guide to an unrequited class of antidepressants. *CNS Spectr.* October 2008;13(10):855–870.
27. Zarate CA, Manji HK. Bipolar disorder: candidate drug targets. *Mt Sinai J Med.* 2008;75:226–247.
28. Nandagopal JJ. Pharmacologic treatment of pediatric bipolar disorder. *Child Adolesc Psychiatr Clin N Am.* April 01 2009; 18(2): 455–69.
29. http://www.pharmex.com/.../WarningLabels/wlspa.asp. Accessed October 7, 2009.
30. Schultz SH, North SW, Shields CG. Schizophrenia: a review. *Am Fam Physician.* 2007;75:1821–1829.
31. Schutte-Rodin S, et al. Clinical guideline for the evaluation and management of chronic insomnia in adults. *J Clin Sleep Med.* 2008;4(5):487–504.
32. Rader R, McCauley L, Callen EC. Current strategies in the diagnosis and treatment of childhood attention-deficit/hyperactivity disorder. *Am Fam Physician.* 2009;79(8): 657–665.
33. Manos MJ. Pharmacologic treatment of ADHD: road conditions in driving patients to successful outcomes. *Medscape J Med.* 2008;10(1):5.
34. ATP III Upates: Implications of recent clinical trials for the National Cholesterol Education Program Adult Treatment Panel Guidelines. Available at: http://www.nhlbi.nih.gov/guidelines/cholesterol/atp3upd04.pdf Accessed September 3, 2009.
35. The Seventh Report of the Joint National Committee on Prevention, Detection, Evaluation and Treatment of High Blood Pressure. Available at: www.nhlbi.nih.gov/guidelines/hypertension. Accessed September 5, 2009.
36. Tekturna(aliskiren) [prescribing information]. East Hanover, NJ: Novartis; December 2007.
37. Metered dose inhaler picture. Available at: www.sk.lung.ca. Accessed October 15, 2009.
38. Dry powder inhaler picture. Available at: www.umm.edu. Accessed October 15, 2009.
39. Nebulizer machine picture. Available at: www.gndmoh.com. Accessed October 15, 2009.
40. Expert Panel Report 3 (EPR3): Guidelines for the diagnosis and management of asthma. Available at: www.nhlbi.nih.gov/guidelines/asthma. Accessed September 19, 2009.
41. *Handbook of Nonprescription Drugs: An Interactive Approach to Self-Care* 16th ed. Washington, DC: APhA, 2009.
42. Diagnosis and management of cough: executive summary. *Chest.* January 2006 129:1S-23S; doi:10.1378/chest.129.1_suppl.1S.
43. See S, Ginzburg R. Choosing a skeletal muscle relaxant. *Am Fam Physician.* 2008:78 (3):365-370. Available at: http://www.aafp.org/afp/20080801/365.pdf. Accessed October 16, 2009.
44. Carisoprodol (carisoprodol) tablet [package insert]. Philadelphia, PA: Mutual Pharmaceutical Comp: 2008.
45. Zanaflex (tizanidine) tablet [package insert]. Bachepalli, India: Dr.Reddy's Laboratories:2006.
46. Diazepam (diazepam) tablet [package insert]. Morgantown, WV: Mylan Pharmaceuticals: 2008.

47. Opioid side effects. *International Association for the Study of Pain: Pain Clinical Updates*.15.2. April 2007. Available at: http://www.iaspain.org/AM/AMTemplate.cfm?Section =Home&CONTENTID=7618&TEMPLATE=/CM/ContentDisplay.cfm. Accessed October 16, 2009.
48. Bond M, Btrivik H, Jensen T, et al. Neurological disorders: Public health challenges. Pain associated with neurological disorders. *WHO*.2006. Available at: http://www .iaspain.org/AM/Template.cfm?Section=WHO2&Template =/CM/ContentDisplay.cfm&ContentID=4174. Accessed October 16, 2009.
49. Berenbaum F. New horizons and perspectives in the treatment of osteoarthritis. *Arth Res & Ther.* 2008, 10(suppl 2):S1.
50. Lewiecki EM. Managing osteoporosis: challenges and strategies. *Clev Clin J Med.* Aug 2009,76(8): 457–466.
51. National Osteoporosis Foundation. *Clinician's Guide to Prevention and Treatment of Osteoporosis.* Washington, DC: National Osteoporosis Foundation; 2008.
52. Insulin syringes. picture. Available at: http://www.alibaba.com. Accessed October 4, 2009.
53. American Diabetes Association. Standards of Medical Care 2009. Available at: http://care.diabetesjournals .org/content/32/Supplement_1/S13.full. Accessed October 4, 2009.
54. Singer PA, Cooper DS, Levy EG, et al. Treatment guidelines for patients with hyperthyroidism and hypothyroidism. *JAMA.* 1995;273:808–812.
55. Cooper DS. Antithyroid drugs. *N Engl J Med.* 2005; 352: 905–917.
56. Centers for Disease Control and Prevention. General recommendations on immunization. Recommendations of the Advisory Committee on Immunization Practices (ACIP) and the American Academy of Family Physicians (AAFP). MMWR *Morb Mortal Wkly Rep.* 2009;55:1–47.
57. Fantl JA, Newman DK, Colling J, et al. Urinary incontinence in adults: acute and chronic management. *Clinical Practice Guideline No. 2. 1996 Update*: Rockville, MD: US DHS, PHJS, AHCPR. AHCPR Publication No. 96-0682.
58. Instillation of eye drops picture. Available at: http://www .vote2win.org. Accessed October 18, 2009.
59. How to use eye drops picture. Available at: http://www .glwach.amedd.army.mil. Accessed October 18, 2009.
60. "Conjunctiva." In: *Taber's Medical Dictionary*. 4th ed. 2003.
61. Traub M, Marshall K. Psoriasis: pathophysiology, conventional, and alternative approaches to treatment. *Altern Med Rev.* 2007;12(4):319–330.
62. Sunscreen Drug Products for Over-the-Counter Human Use, Proposed FDA Rule. Available at: http://www .skincancer.org/monograph.html. Accessed: October 20, 2009.
63. Sunscreens Explained—The Skin Cancer Foundation. Available at: http://www.skincancer.org/sunscreens-explained .html. Accessed: October 20, 2009.
64. Plan B [package insert]. Pomona, New York. Barr Pharmaceuticals; 2006.
65. Case AM. Infertility evaluation and management. *Can Fam Physician.* 2003: 49 (11)1465–1472.
66. Homburg R, Insler V. Ovulation induction in perspective. *Human Reprod Update*. 2002: 8 (5):449–462.
67. Repronex [package insert]. Tarrytown, New York. Ferring Pharmaceuticals; 2002.
68. Bravelle [package insert]. Suffern, New York. Ferring Pharmaceuticals; 2004.
69. Morch LS, Lokkegaard E, Andreasen AH, et al. Hormone therapy and ovarian cancer. *JAMA*. 2009;302.3. 298–305.
70. Burnett AL. Phosphodiesterase 5 mechanism and therapeutic application. *Am J Cardiol*. 2005 December 26;96(12B): 29M–31M.
71. WHO Guidelines for Tuberculosis 2009. Available at: http://www.cdc.gov/tb/publications/guidelines/default .htm. Accessed October 24, 2009.
72. Black CP. Systematic review of the biology and medical management of respiratory synctial virus infection. *Respiratory Care.* March 2003; 48: 209–226.
73. Thompson GR, Cadena J, Patterson TF. Overview of antifungal agents. *Clin Chest Med.* 2009; 30:203–215.
74. Shaheen M, Broxmeyer HE. The humoral regulation of hemopoiesis. In: Hoffman R et al., eds. *Hematology: Basic Principles and Practice*. 5th ed. Philadelphia, PA: Elsevier.
75. Hirsh J, Bauer KA, Donati MB, et al. *Parenteral anticoagulants: American College of Chest Physicians Evidence-Based Clinical Practice Guidelines.* 8th ed. *Chest* 2008; 133:141S–159S.
76. Liebman B, Hurley J, Genger T. Vegetables Vitamin K Weighs. *Nutr Action Health Lett.* 2002;29:13–15.

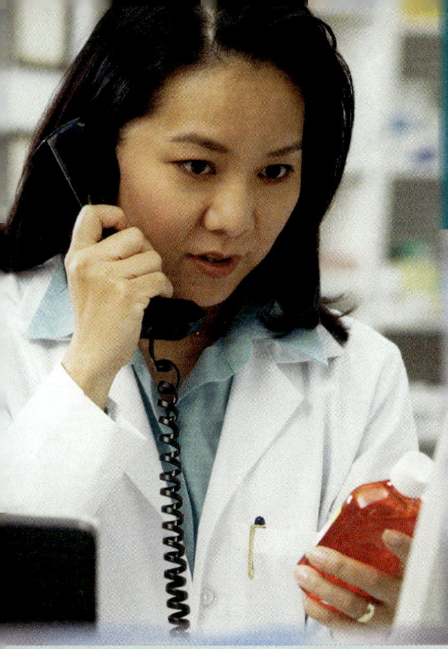

Chapter 11

Basic Biopharmaceutics, Pharmacokinetics, and Pharmacodynamics

Thomas C. Dowling

Learning Outcomes

After completing this chapter, you will be able to

- Define the study of biopharmaceutics.
- List and describe the four major processes that make up the study of pharmacokinetics.
- Describe factors that can alter the absorption of a medication.
- Describe how medications are distributed within the body, including factors that affect medication distribution in the body.
- List and describe the two most common types of drug interactions.
- Define pharmacodynamics.
- Describe how medications are eliminated from the body, including factors (e.g., disease states) that can increase or decrease elimination of a medication.
- Describe the steps that must occur before a medication can exert its effect on the body.
- Describe potential problems that can occur when a product formulation is disrupted or when absorption, distribution, metabolism, or elimination is altered, and how these alterations can affect the pharmacodynamics of a medication.

Key Terms

absorption The amount of medication that enters the bloodstream, or systemic circulation.

bioavailability The percentage of an administered dose of a medication that reaches the bloodstream.

biopharmaceutics The study of the manufacture of medications for effective delivery into the body. It includes the relationships between the physical and chemical properties of a drug, the dosage form in which the drug is given, the route of administration, and the effects of properties and dosage on the rate and extent of drug absorption.

clearance The removal of plasma which is completely cleared of drugs per unit of time. It combines the elimination rate with the flow of a drug through the organs of elimination (i.e., liver and kidneys). It is usually measured in mL/min or L/hr.

cytochrome P450 (CYP) A group of enzymes that metabolize drugs.

disintegration The breakdown of medication from its original solid formulation.

dissolution The dissolving of medication into solution, usually in the stomach and intestinal tract.

drug interaction The impact of a drug or food product on the amount or activity of another drug in the body. This interaction can result in enhanced, reduced, or new activity of the drug in the body.

elimination The removal of a drug from the body, mainly in the urine or feces.

excretion The irreversible removal of a drug or metabolite from a body fluid. The most common location of drug excretion in the body is the kidneys; the biliary tract is another important route of excretion.

first-pass metabolism The metabolism (breaking down) of orally ingested medications by the liver and small intestine before they reach the main bloodstream.

half-life The time that it takes for 50% of a drug to be eliminated from the body.

loading dose A larger first dose given to quickly achieve a high drug concentration in the body.

metabolism The breakdown of medication in the body.

metabolite A breakdown product of a medication that has undergone metabolism.

pharmacodynamics The study of the relationship between the concentration of a drug in the body and the response or outcome observed or measured in a patient.

pharmacokinetics The study of the movement of a drug through the body during the following phases: absorption, distribution, metabolism, and excretion.

therapeutic level The blood level at which most patients receive a medication's desired effect with minimal side effects.

volume of distribution The extent of a medication's outreach to various tissues and spaces throughout the body.

This chapter describes the basic elements of biopharmaceutics, pharmacokinetics, and pharmacodynamics. These concepts are useful in describing how medications exert their effects on body systems, as well as how drugs affect body systems.

The pharmacy technician is often the first person in the pharmacy to handle a patient's medication, often filling multiple prescriptions for a single patient. Thus, the pharmacy technician who prepares prescriptions for dispensing should have a basic understanding of biopharmaceutics, pharmacokinetics, and pharmacodynamics, which collectively describe how a particular medication is prepared, is handled by the body, and affects the body. Having this understanding can help avoid unwanted (adverse) drug events, because the complex interactions of many medications is a risk factor for adverse drug events—especially in older individuals and certain other patient populations, as will be described in more detail in this chapter.

For example, a prescriber may write that a particular prescription medication should be crushed before being taken; however, a knowledgeable pharmacy technician may know that crushing that particular medication results in loss of the slow-release properties of the drug. Likewise, a pharmacy technician knowledgeable about the absorption of a particular medication may know that it should not be taken with certain other medications or dietary agents that could affect its absorption.

An understanding of basic biopharmaceutical, pharmacokinetic, and pharmacodynamic principles can aid the clinician in appropriately monitoring medication therapy, and the pharmacy technician can aid the pharmacist in such surveillance.

Biopharmaceutics

Biopharmaceutics is the study of the manufacture of medications for effective delivery into the body. It includes the relationships between the physical and chemical properties of a drug, the dosage form in which the drug is given, the route of administration, and the effects of properties and dosage on the rate and extent of drug absorption. It has long been recognized that the method by which a medication is prepared and formulated can affect its action. The study of biopharmaceutics has led to the improved design of drug products to enhance the delivery of medication and ultimately to optimize the clinical effects of medication.

Medications can be formulated and administered to the patient in many different ways (see Chapter 12: Medication Dosage Forms and Routes of Administration). Common formulations include tablets, capsules, solutions, suspensions, suppositories, transdermal patches, creams, nasal sprays, and aerosolized medications. Routes of administration include oral, intraocular (in the eye), rectal, sublingual (under the tongue), buccal (cheek), topical, transdermal (through the skin), injectable, and inhaled.

Medications are formulated and administered differently for several reasons. In some case, a particular medication is available via multiple routes, and choosing one over the other may simply be a matter of preference or convenience. For example, the analgesic acetaminophen is available in many different dosage forms, including tablets, capsules, caplets, suspensions, and suppositories. For small children, administration by suspension or suppository will likely be easier than by a tablet. In other cases, different formulations and routes of administration are used because they can influence the rate, duration, or even extent of drug effect. Therefore, using the correct or optimal formulation is important and often has a bearing on the clinical effect of the medication.

Before most medications can exert a pharmacologic response, they need to be absorbed (taken up by the bloodstream), and before they can be absorbed, they need to be released from their formulations. A medication in a tablet formulation, for example, is more than just the active drug. Any given tablet will contain not only active drug but also non-drug ingredients, such as binders that keep the tablet from falling apart, fillers that add bulk to the tablet, and preservatives. Two processes—disintegration and dissolution, in that order—usually need to occur before the medication can be absorbed. **Disintegration** is the breakdown of the medication from its original solid formulation, and **dissolution** is the dissolving of medication into solution, usually in the stomach and intestinal tract. Disintegration aids dissolution, as smaller particles dissolve more easily than larger particles. Once a medication is disintegrated and dissolved, it can be absorbed into the bloodstream (figure 11-1). Some product formulations are disintegrated and dissolved more slowly or more rapidly than others, which may ultimately affect the rate of onset of therapeutic effect. For example, topical creams and ointments may be used to deliver drugs that are dissolved in special vehicles called organogels, such as pluronic lecithin organogel (PLO), which enhance the absorption of the drug across the skin (transdermal). Some injectable products can be designed to dissolve very slowly from the site of injection, such as intramuscular depot injections.

✔ Medications that are given intravenously have a very rapid onset of action because the medications are already in solution (therefore disintegration and dissolution do not need to occur) and are placed directly into the bloodstream.

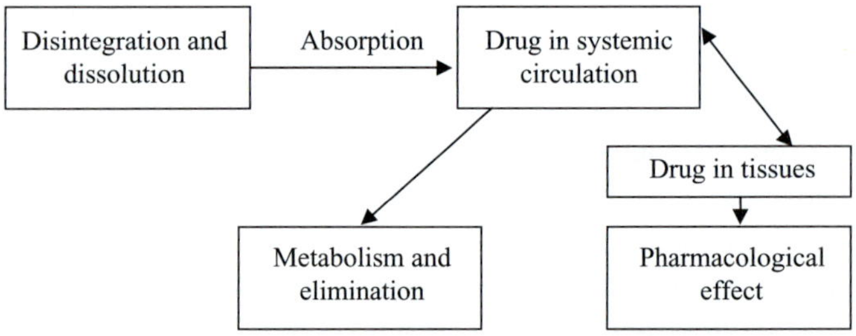

Figure 11-1. Relationship between drug and effect.

Pharmacokinetics

Pharmacokinetics is defined as the study of the movement of a drug through the body during the following phases: absorption, distribution, metabolism, and excretion. These processes are often referred to as "ADME."

Absorption

Absorption refers to the amount of medication that enters the bloodstream, or systemic circulation. Not all the medication in a tablet, capsule, suppository, inhaler, or intramuscular or subcutaneous syringe enters the bloodstream, and therefore not all of it is absorbed. Except for topical products that are applied for a local effect, such as anti-inflammatory creams, only absorbed medication has the potential to exert a systemic pharmacologic effect.

The term **bioavailability** refers to the percentage of an administered dose of a medication that reaches the bloodstream. The bioavailability of an agent depends on many factors, including the amount of drug dissolved, its dosage form, and its route of administration.

Some medications that are ingested orally are metabolized (broken down) before they reach the main bloodstream, which is referred to as **first-pass metabolism.** This often results in a small percentage of the medication being metabolized on the first pass through either the intestine wall or the liver (figure 11-2). Medications that undergo a high first-pass metabolism have a high amount of drug metabolized, and therefore a lower percentage is available to reach the main systemic circulation.

There are some routes of drug administration, such as rectal, inhalation, and sublingual, that avoid first-pass metabolism because they bypass the small intestine and liver and the drugs are absorbed directly into the main bloodstream. For example, drugs such as ergotamine and nitroglycerin are better absorbed when given rectally and sublingually, respectively, than when given orally because if given orally, they are broken down in the small intestine and liver before they can be absorbed into the bloodstream.

Medications given intravenously are administered directly into the vein and therefore enter the bloodstream directly. Thus, they have 100% bioavailability, meaning that 100% of the dose administered is available in the bloodstream and has the potential to exert a pharmacologic effect.

✔ Usually, the dose needed orally is much more than the dose needed intravenously because the bioavailability of the oral formulation is much less than 100%.

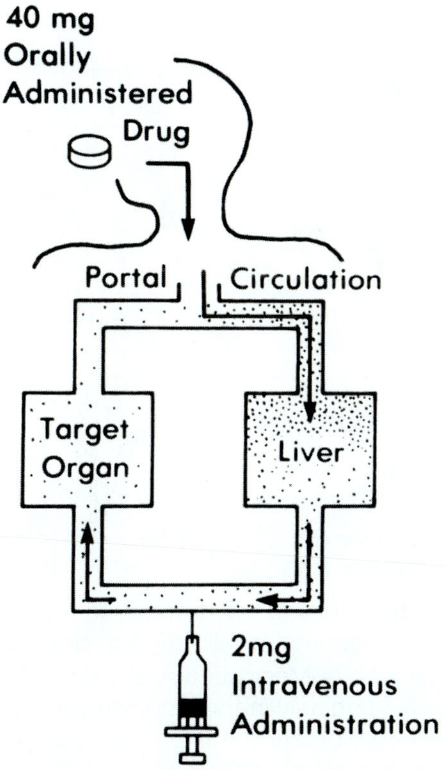

Figure 11-2. First-pass metabolism.

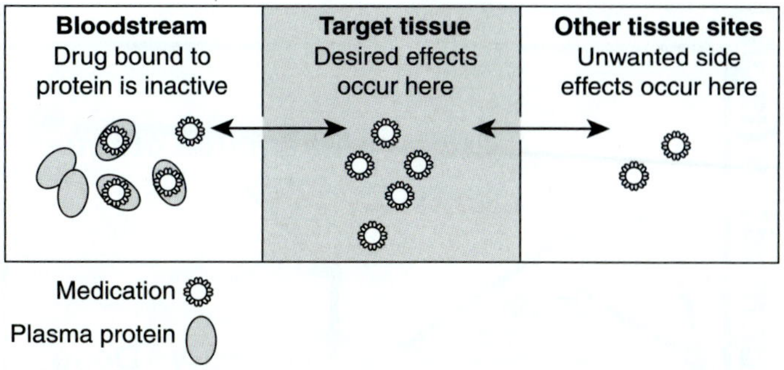

Figure 11-3. Medication distribution. This figure depicts the travel of medication from the bloodstream to the target tissue to other tissues. The double-headed arrows indicate that flow can occur in either direction. Medication bound to protein in the blood is inactive and cannot move (or distribute) to other tissues, but the medication can dissociate or separate from the protein. Once separated, it can move about the body.

For example, levothyroxine, used to treat low thyroid levels, has an intravenous dose that is approximately one-half that of the oral dose, but will produce the same pharmacologic response. In other cases, the oral absorption of an agent is so poor that it must be given intravenously. Vancomycin is an example of an antibiotic that is normally used intravenously to treat serious infections because it is so poorly absorbed orally.

Distribution

Once absorbed into the bloodstream, medication either leaves the bloodstream and enters the tissues—including, but not limited to, the *site of action* (the tissue organ site where the medication is to exert its intended pharmacologic response)—or it remains in the blood, bound to protein components. Therefore, for any given dose of medication, some of it will travel to tissues and some will remain in the bloodstream. Some medications are highly bound to blood proteins, in some cases greater than 90%. The medication bound to blood proteins is inactive and does not exert any pharmacologic effect until it is released from the protein. Only medication that is *free,* or not bound to proteins, can leave the bloodstream and enter the tissues to exert a pharmacologic effect. Of the percentage that is free, or circulating to tissues, only the amount that reaches the target site will exert a pharmacologic effect (wanted or unwanted). This process is reversible; as drug is released from protein, it is distributed into tissues, leading to binding of drug to take its place on the protein (figure 11-3).

Albumin is the main protein that binds medications in the blood. Some diseases, particularly those that damage the liver, can decrease the amount of albumin in the plasma. In such cases, medications that normally bind highly to albumin are unable to do so to the normal extent, and a greater proportion of those medications will be "free" and therefore active. Medications that are highly bound to albumin include phenytoin, which is used to treat seizures, and warfarin, an anticoagulant.

For some drugs, the amount of drug in the bloodstream, typically reported as the concentration of drug in blood (such as mg/L), can be measured in the clinical setting to help guide appropriate therapy. For example, after a drug is ingested orally, the concentration of drug in blood rises slowly, reaches a maximum amount, then drops slowly due to the drug being eliminated or metabolized (figure 11-4). Here, a range of concentrations of drug in the blood is achieved during a specified dosing regimen. For some drugs, the

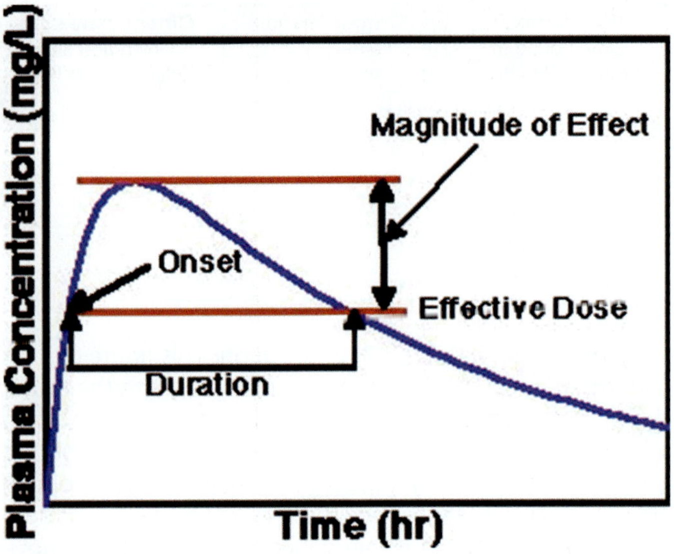

Figure 11-4. Illustration showing the relationship between drug concentration and drug effect, including therapeutic range.

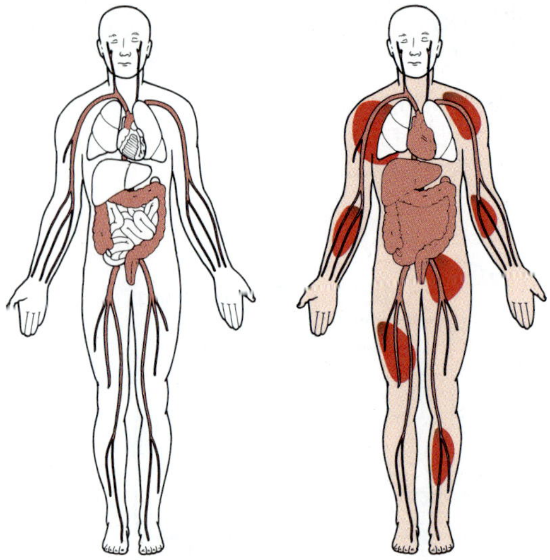

Figure 11-5. Volume of distribution. This schematic hypothetically and simplistically depicts drug distribution throughout the body. Medication A, shown on the left, appears to remain primarily in the bloodstream and is distributed to the target organ, the large intestines. Medication B, shown on the right, appears to be widely distributed throughout the body.

concentration may rise to a level that causes toxicity. These drugs often have side effects that appear with very small dose increments, and researchers have been able to determine the **therapeutic level** for these medications—the level at which most patients receive the desired effect with minimal side effects. Thus, blood levels of these medications can be measured to determine whether a change in therapy is needed on the basis of the laboratory results. Examples of medications whose levels are measured in the blood include many of the antiepileptic agents, such as phenytoin, carbamazepine, valproic acid, and phenobarbital; digoxin for atrial fibrillation; and some antibiotics, including gentamicin, tobramycin, and vancomycin.

The apparent **volume of distribution** for a drug describes the extent of its outreach to various tissues and spaces throughout the body. The space that the drug distributes into is often called a "compartment," which is a hypothetical *pool* to which that drug is distributed. Most medications are distributed throughout the bloodstream and in many organs, fluids, and tissues (fat tissue or lean muscle tissue); other medications are not as widely distributed. In general, medications with a large volume of distribution will have a lower blood concentration, whereas medications with a small volume of distribution will have a higher blood concentration (figure 11-5). A simple way to think of this is to picture a bucket of water. A certain amount of dissolvable red food coloring placed into the bucket will be spread to all areas of the bucket. The same amount of coloring placed in a bucket one-half the size of the first will also spread to all areas of the bucket, but will look more colorful (darker red) because the water volume is smaller. The smaller bucket will appear to contain twice the amount of red color, when actually the same amount of coloring was used in both cases.

Certain other factors can also affect the extent of distribution of a drug throughout the body. Some medications that are highly bound (attracted) to proteins found in the bloodstream often have low volumes of distribution because they tend to stay in the bloodstream. These medications often have very high blood concentrations, and the amount (dose) of medication is relatively small compared with other drugs. Conversely, medications that have a high affinity to body fat and medications that either are bound to proteins in tissue or are not highly bound to plasma proteins tend to have high volumes of distribution—that is, they tend to be widely distributed throughout the body. The doses of these medications can be very high, sometimes upwards of 1–2 grams per day.

How does knowing the volume of distribution of a medication help with drug administration? Knowing the volume of distribution of a certain medication can help the prescriber to approximate the dose of medication needed to attain the desired level of drug in the body for it to be effective or to start working quickly. If a medication is widely distributed through the body and the prescriber wants the medication to start working quickly, sometimes a **loading dose** of the medication (a larger first dose) will be given to more quickly achieve a higher drug concentration in the body. Examples of medications for which a loading dose is sometimes given include phenytoin, digoxin, and some antibiotics.

As a general example, a typical prescription for the antibiotic azithromycin may be written as follows: "Take 2 tablets today (500 mg), then take 1 tablet daily (250 mg) for 4 days." Two tablets are used the first day as a loading dose, to help achieve a certain blood level of the medication to jump-start therapy. If a medication is not widely distributed through the body, a smaller loading dose or no loading dose will be needed. Most medications do not require a loading dose.

Metabolism

The breakdown and elimination of drugs from the body occurs by metabolism and excretion. The **metabolism** of medication is the breakdown of medication in the body. Here, the drug molecule is changed or altered in some way to create a secondary molecule called a **metabolite.** Some drug molecules are not susceptible to metabolic breakdown, and may travel directly to the kidneys to be excreted (explained in more detail below). The liver is the major organ in which drug metabolism occurs, although significant metabolism can occur in the small intestine. Very little metabolism occurs in other organs, such as the kidneys and lungs. Metabolism is most often accomplished by protein substances called *enzymes.* The most common enzymes that metabolize drugs belong to a family of enzymes called the **cytochrome P450 (CYP)** system. These enzymes are very active in converting a drug to its metabolites.

In most cases, metabolism of a drug results in the formation of metabolites (altered chemical forms of the drug) that are not pharmacologically active in the human body. This results in a drop in the concentration of active drug in the body, and usually leads to a loss of drug activity because the metabolites are not binding to the drug receptors. However, in rare cases, metabolism can result in the formation of an *active metabolite* that may be more pharmacologically active than the parent (original) drug, or even toxic. It is therefore important to know whether the active metabolite acts in the same manner as the parent drug. There are also a few examples where a drug is administered in an *inactive* form, which is metabolized or converted to the active component. This inactive form is called a "pro-drug," and examples include enalapril and valacyclovir.

An example of an active metabolite is seen with the drug fluoxetine, used primarily for depression. Fluoxetine is metabolized to norfluoxetine, which is active and exerts an antidepressant effect that is even longer-acting than fluoxetine. This prolonged effect can be good or bad, depending on the situation and specific patient characteristics. An advantage is that a long-acting metabolite allows convenient dosing of the medication once a day, or less frequently with the advent of a once-weekly formulation. A disadvantage is that this long-acting metabolite can remain in the system longer than wanted, so any side effects may occur for a prolonged period, especially in the elderly, who tend to eliminate the drug more slowly.

Excretion

Excretion refers to the irreversible removal of a drug or metabolite from a body fluid. The most common location of drug excretion in the body is the kidneys, with the biliary tract being another important route of excretion. In the kidney, some medications are excreted from the blood by a filtering process whereby drug is eliminated into the urine without being metabolized. After drug metabolism, many metabolites are water soluble, making them very susceptible to excretion by the kidneys. In fact, studies are often conducted to measure the recovery of intact drug and metabolites in urine, to understand the pharmacokinetics of new drugs. Drugs and metabolites may also be excreted from the liver into the bile. Here, drug is transferred from the bloodstream into the liver cell, then into the bile duct. From here, the drug travels through the bile duct and into the small intestine for **elimination.**

The total removal of a drug via metabolism and/or excretion from the blood stream per unit of time can also be referred to as drug **clearance,** which combines elimination rate with the flow of a drug through the organs of elimination (i.e., liver and kidneys). This term is often used to compare various drug pharmacokinetics based on organ blood flow values (in units of mL/min or L/hr).

The **half-life,** often designated by the term "$T_{1/2}$," of a drug is also related to clearance and elimination. Here, half-life refers to the time that it takes for 50% of an amount of drug to be eliminated from the body. A drug with low clearance, meaning one that is not effectively metabolized or excreted, will typically have a long half-life. This means that it will take a long time to eliminate a dose of the drug from the body. Here, drug administration that is too rapid (faster than the drug can be eliminated) can lead to excessive accumulation of the drug in the body. Such drugs have a much higher risk of toxicity than drugs with a short half-life and high clearance.

Drug Interactions

Drugs (and some foods) can compete with other drugs for metabolism within the system or alter the metabolic system altogether, resulting in **drug interactions.** A drug interaction is defined as the impact of a drug or food product on the amount or activity of another drug in the body. This drug-drug (or drug-food) interaction can result in enhanced, reduced, or new activity of the drug in the body. The most common cause of drug interactions is altered drug metabolism in the liver. For example, some medications, foods, and herbal products can *inhibit* (or slow down) enzyme activity, which results in reduced drug metabolism of other medications. Conversely, some drugs can *induce* (or speed up) the metabolism of other medications. These two mechanisms are the most common forms of drug interactions. Thus, knowing the metabolic effects of each medication dispensed to a patient can help determine if a drug interaction is likely to exist.

For example, some antiepileptic medications are referred to as *enzyme inducers,* meaning they up-regulate the metabolism of many other medications. Phenytoin, an antiepileptic agent, is an enzyme inducer, and it is known to increase the metabolism of more than 100 other medications. This can result in lessening the activity of the other medications, because they are broken down and excreted from the body more quickly than normal. Conversely, some medications can inhibit the metabolism of other medications. For example, erythromycin, some antifungal medications, and cyclosporine are all potent *enzyme inhibitors,* or medications that are known to reduce the metabolism of many other medications. This can result in higher, more prolonged blood levels of these other medications, which can lead to prolonged duration of action of the other medications and the development of side effects. An example of a drug-drug interaction is that of erythromycin (a CYP enzyme inhibitor) with the bronchodilator theophylline (metabolized by CYP), resulting in systemic accumulation of theophylline and toxicity. An example of a drug-food interaction is ingestion of grapefruit juice (a CYP enzyme inhibitor) with the antihypertensive nifedipine (metabolized by CYP), resulting in hypotensive episodes.

Patient Variables Affecting Pharmacokinetics

Several factors can affect the normal processes of ADME, leading to altered pharmacokinetics. For example, drug absorption can be altered by a change in the speed of the gastrointestinal tract, such as constipation or diarrhea. The elimination or clearance of a drug can be impacted by diseases of the kidney and liver, such as cirrhosis. Reduced elimination can then lead to a prolonged half-life of the drug when compared with patients without organ dysfunction. Changes in heart function or cardiac output can lead to changes in delivery of drugs via the bloodstream. Severe heart failure, in which there is low cardiac output, can lead to decreased blood flow to the kidneys and liver and therefore to decreased clearance of medications.

✔ Patients who are markedly overweight or underweight may have differing abilities to eliminate medications because kidney and liver size and blood flow are proportional to body weight.

Kidney Disease

The National Institutes of Health has estimated that more than 20 million people in the United States have some form of kidney disease. The progressive worsening of kidney disease can lead to renal failure requiring either hemodialysis or a kidney transplant. Common causes of kidney damage include high blood pressure, high blood cholesterol, and diabetes. It is important to identify individuals with kidney disease because the kidney is a primary organ of drug elimination. The most common way to detect the presence of kidney disease is to measure blood levels of creatinine, a substance that is normally produced in muscles and is cleared from the body by the kidneys. Because creatinine is eliminated by the kidneys similarly to the way medications are excreted, it is possible to estimate how fast a medication can be eliminated by estimating

Table 11-1. Renal Dosing of Amantadine

Renal Function	Initial Dose of Amantadine
CrCl > 60 mL/min	100 mg po, twice daily (monotherapy), 200 mg po per day alternating with 100 mg po per day
CrCl 50–60 mL/min	200 mg/daily alternating with 100 mg po per day
CrCl 40–50 mL/min	100 mg po daily
CrCl 30–40 mL/min	200 mg po twice weekly
CrCl 20–30 mL/min	100 mg po three times weekly
CrCl 10–20 mL/min	200 mg load then 100 mg oral weekly

Notes: CrCl = creatinine clearance
po = by mouth

the creatinine clearance. The creatinine clearance can be easily calculated by using an equation that incorporates the patient's age, sex, body weight, and serum creatinine value. See table 11-1 for an example of a drug dosing regimen that must be adjusted based on the degree of renal impairment. Medications that are eliminated primarily by the kidneys need to be used cautiously in patients with reduced creatinine clearances (table 11-2). Another index of kidney function that is similar to creatinine clearance is the glomerular filtration rate (GFR). Some hospitals automatically report the GFR value in the patient's medical record or chart because it can be quickly calculated by using just age and serum creatinine, and this value is used to help physicians diagnose kidney disease. It is important to note that the GFR value should not be used for dose calculation purposes.

✔The pharmacist is often the health care provider who is responsible for making sure that the drug dose is appropriate for a patient, given the patient's creatinine clearance value.

Table 11-2. Medications That Require Dosage Adjustment for Kidney Impairment

Allopurinol*	Atenolol
Captopril	Ciprofloxacin
Clonidine	Digoxin
Disopyramide*	Enalapril*
Enoxaparin	Famotidine
Gabapentin	Gentamicin
Imipenem-cilastatin	Levofloxacin
Lisinopril	Methotrexate
Pregabalin	Procainamide*
Quinapril	Ranitidine
Tobramycin	Vancomycin

*Drug has major active metabolite that is renally excreted.

Part 2

Liver Disease

It is estimated that liver disease is among the leading causes of death in the United States, resulting in nearly 25,000 deaths each year. In liver disease, the cells in the liver (hepatocytes) become injured and can die. If the injury to the liver is mild, the liver cells can regenerate. However, in cases of more severe injury, irreversible damage can occur, leading to a condition called cirrhosis. As the liver disease progresses, patients have a decrease in liver function and decreased ability to metabolize certain medications. Liver disease is often detected by measuring the blood for enzymes such as aspartate aminotransferase (AST) and alanine aminotransferase (ALT), as well as for bilirubin and albumin.

Patients with liver disease also have reduced blood flow through the liver, resulting in reduced elimination and clearance of some drugs. This is important because reduced elimination can lead to drug accumulation and toxicity. Albumin, a protein in the blood that some drugs bind to, can also be reduced in patients with liver disease. This can lead to reduced protein binding, more distribution of the unbound drug to tissues outside of the bloodstream, and possible drug toxicity. In most cases, the physician and pharmacist will monitor patients with liver disease very closely for side effects resulting from medications.

Advanced Age

Medications must be used very cautiously in elderly individuals. Advanced age can result in reduced liver and kidney function, leading to decreased drug elimination. In such cases, it is very important to estimate the patient's creatinine clearance to determine if dose reduction is needed to avoid drug accumulation and toxicity. The liver may be reduced in size by 20–40% in elderly patients, resulting in lower drug metabolism. For drugs cleared by the liver, it is important to monitor elderly patients very closely for observed toxicity. When giving drugs topically, such as creams or ointments, it has been shown that less drug is absorbed in elderly patients and they may not benefit as well as other patients.

Pregnancy

Very little is known about how a woman's body changes during pregnancy. It is believed that pregnant women have increased blood volume, which forces the heart and kidneys to work harder. Drugs may be cleared through kidneys faster than normal during pregnancy, so pregnant women may need higher doses of some medications, such as antibiotics. In addition to prescription drugs, it is also important to recognize that some over-the-counter (OTC) drugs are unsafe in pregnancy. For example, aspirin should be avoided in the last three months of pregnancy because it may cause problems in the fetus or complications during delivery. Other OTC drugs such as ibuprofen and naproxen carry a similar warning about their use during the third trimester of pregnancy. The safety of herbal, botanical, and dietary supplements during pregnancy remains unknown, and these substances should be avoided.

Safety First All drugs and OTC products should be used with caution in pregnancy, and the risks should be carefully evaluated.

Pediatrics

Pediatrics is another special population for which drugs must be used very cautiously, especially in neonates, infants, and children. Pediatric medications are often dosed based on body weight. Infants and children often have a higher amount of body water than adults, which can lead to a higher relative volume of distribution for some drugs. Therefore, it is very important to know the accurate weight of each child prior to administering medications, and to refer to special pediatric references or manufacturer's guidelines for proper dosing regimens. It is important to note that drug doses must be carefully evaluated by the pharmacist and adjusted based on weight and other factors. This is especially important for neonatal care in hospital settings. The pharmacy technician can play an important role in alerting the pharmacist that a drug is being used in a pediatric patient.

Rx for Success

Drug doses have to be evaluated by the pharmacist and adjusted based on age, weight, and other factors. The pharmacy technician can help alert the pharmacist to doses that may appear to be too high for a given population.

Pharmacodynamics

Just as pharmacokinetics can be thought of as what the body does to the drug, pharmacodynamics can be considered what the drug does to the body. **Pharmacodynamics** refers to the study of the relationship between the concentration of a drug in the body and the response or outcome observed or measured in a patient. Examples of pharmacodynamic responses include an increase in bone mass with a bisphosphonate used for osteoporosis, a decrease in blood pressure with an antihypertensive agent, and a decrease in blood glucose with a sulfonylurea used in the management of diabetes.

For a pharmacologic effect to occur, a drug needs to be absorbed into the systemic circulation and travel to its intended site of action, or target organ, as described earlier. Next, it needs to bind to a specific receptor, like a key fitting into a lock. A receptor is a protein that is embedded on the surface of the cell and that allows communication between the outside and the inside of the cell. Once the drug binds to the receptor, this triggers a cascade of events that leads to the drug's response. The time that it takes to detect a drug's response, whether it be very rapid or delayed, is related to the drug-receptor binding process and to any subsequent chemical reactions that take place inside the target cell or organ.

For example, when a substance called epinephrine binds to specific receptors called beta receptors, the response is an increase in heart rate. Medications mimic these natural substances because they are made to be chemically similar to these natural substances. In this way, medications can "fool" the receptor, bind to it, and exert a similar response. When a medication binds to the receptor, it physically blocks other substances found normally in the body from binding to the receptor. Only by binding to its receptor can a medication exert an effect (figure 11-6). After a medication binds

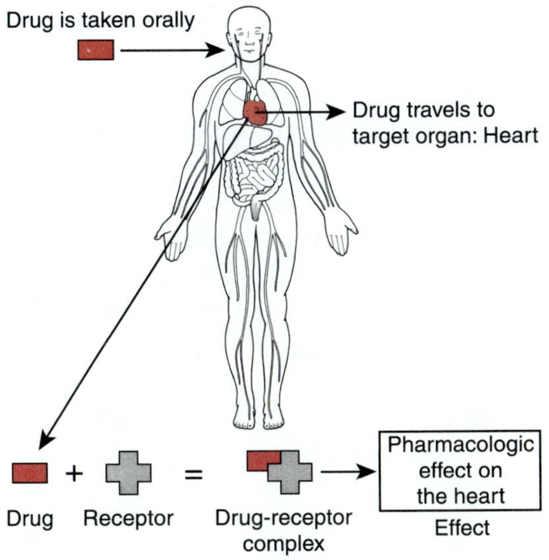

Figure 11-6. Drug-receptor complex. The extent of drug binding to a receptor is dependent on the amount of drug present as well as the affinity or capability of the drug to bind to the receptor.

to a receptor, the receptor helps to communicate specifics about the medication to the inside of the cell by generating a signal in the cell about the medication (figure 11-7).

By binding to the receptor, medications can either promote or block the signal that would ordinarily be generated by binding of the normally occurring substance to the receptor. Medications that augment or enhance a signal normally communicated in a cell are called *agonists*. Medications that block the transmission of a signal normally communicated in a cell are called *antagonists*. As mentioned before, natural beta agonists, such as epinephrine, bind to beta receptors in the heart to increase heart rate. If a beta agonist medication binds to that receptor, the resultant effect is an increase in heart rate, similar to the effect of epinephrine binding to the receptor. An example of a beta agonist is isoproterenol. Conversely, a beta antagonist, such as metoprolol, will prevent epinephrine from binding to a beta receptor, resulting in a drop in heart rate.

The drug-receptor complex forms the basis of medication effects on the body. This drug-receptor interaction is what makes medications work—what makes the antiheartburn medication the technician dispenses soothe the stomach, the antibiotic the technician prepares and dispenses help fight infection, and the pain medication the technician dispenses relieve pain.

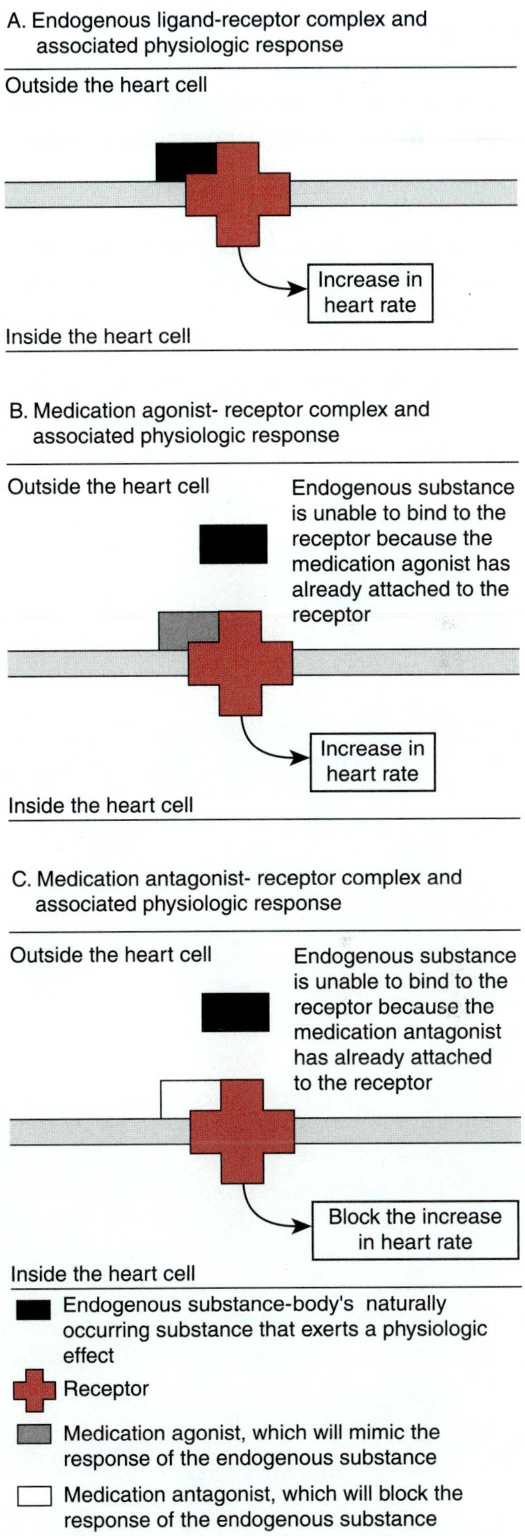

Figure 11-7. A closer look at drug-receptor complexes and pharmacologic response. Note that the medication agonist and antagonist are able to bind to the receptor because they are shaped similarly to the endogenous substance and fit the receptor well. By binding to the receptor as a key fits a lock, the medication prevents the endogenous substance from doing so and exerting its own effect.

Summary

Biopharmaceutics, pharmacokinetics, and pharmacodynamics collectively describe how medications are specially formulated, are handled by the body, and exert their actions in the body. Drugs must be used very cautiously in special cases, such as kidney disease, liver disease, elderly, and pediatric patients, to ensure that the desired clinical effects are achieved and side effects are avoided or minimized. A pharmacy technician must become familiar with the basic principles of these important areas to appreciate their contribution to the clinical effects, drug interactions, and toxicity of medications. When the technician is asked if a medication can be crushed, he or she will know why this seemingly simple question is a very important one with potentially problematic consequences if wrong directions are given. When the computer system alerts the technician to a drug interaction between an enzyme inducer and another medication, he or she will have a basic understanding of the mechanism of the interaction. Knowledge about loading doses will help the technician understand why there might be two doses given in a short period of time for the same drug. Knowledge of differences in dosing in special populations will help the technician assist in recognizing when doses make sense and when they should be questioned.

Self-Assessment Questions

Self-Assessment Questions

1. Which of the following is the FIRST process that a solid dosage form must undergo to exert a pharmacologic effect?
   a. disintegration
   b. dissolution
   c. distribution
   d. metabolism
2. The process of first-pass metabolism occurs in which of the following organs?
   a. kidney
   b. liver and small intestine
   c. heart
   d. pancreas
3. Which of the following pharmacokinetic processes is most impaired in the presence of renal disease?
   a. absorption
   b. distribution
   c. metabolism
   d. excretion
4. Administering a drug by which of the following routes ensures complete (100%) bioavailability into the systemic circulation?
   a. intravenous
   b. subcutaneous
   c. intramuscular
   d. intradermal
5. If a patient has kidney disease, which of the following will need to be adjusted based on creatinine clearance?
   a. route of medication
   b. dose of medication
   c. formulation of medication
   d. number of concomitant medications
6. What does an enzyme inducer do?
   a. It increases the metabolism of other medications.
   b. It increases the absorption of other medications.
   c. It increases the distribution of other medications.
   d. It increases the bioavailability of other medications.
7. A patient is currently taking Drug X to treat high blood pressure. Drug X is known to be metabolized by the CYP enzyme system. After two weeks of taking Drug X, the patient will now begin taking Drug Y, which is known to inhibit CYP enzymes in the liver. Which of the following is likely to occur when the two drugs are given together?
   a. Blood levels of Drug Y will be increased.
   b. Blood levels of Drug Y will be reduced.
   c. Blood levels of Drug X will be increased.
   d. Blood levels of Drug X will be reduced.
8. Which of the following involves studying the effects of medications at a target site?
   a. biopharmaceutics
   b. pharmacoepidemiology
   c. pharmacokinetics
   d. pharmacodynamics
9. Drug binding to ___________is required to produce a clinical effect.
   a. a plasma protein
   b. a receptor
   c. a tissue
   d. a blood cell
10. A patient with liver disease may be expeted to have reduced drug
    a. absorption
    b. distribution
    c. metabolism
    d. renal excretion

Self-Assessment Answers

1. a. Disintegration is the first of several processes that must occur before a medication can exert a pharmacologic effect. Disintegration is the breakdown of the medication from the original solid formulation. The next step is dissolution, or the dissolving of drug into solution. Disintegration makes dissolution easier, as smaller particles are easier to dissolve than large particles.
2. b. Drugs that undergo first-pass metabolism are most often metabolized by CYP enzymes in both the liver and the small intestine.
3. d. The kidneys are responsible for excreting many medications (drugs and metabolites) from the body. When kidney function is poor, the elimination of renally excreted medications is hindered.
4. a. Intravenous medications are administered directly into the vein, and therefore into the bloodstream. Absorption of medications, by definition, is the movement of medication from the site of administration (skin, muscle, subcutaneous fat) into the bloodstream. The other routes administer medication outside the bloodstream, so medication administered by other routes needs to travel to the bloodstream from where it was administered.
5. b. Because kidneys eliminate medication from the body, reduced kidney function can hinder the elimination of medication. Decreased elimination of medication may lead to accumulation of the drug in the body and contribute to prolonged medication effects and side effects. For this reason, patients with kidney disease are often given lower doses of medications that are renally eliminated.
6. a. An enzyme inducer increases the metabolism of other medications that undergo the type of metabolism it induces. For example, phenytoin is an enzyme inducer. It increases the metabolism of other medications, such as phenobarbital, carbamazepine, and valproic acid. Therefore, higher doses of these medications may be needed when given with phenytoin.
7. c. The metabolism of Drug X is inhibited by Drug Y, resulting in an increase in the blood levels of Drug X. This could lead to high blood concentrations of Drug X, resulting in toxicity.
8. d. The study of medication at its target site is the study of pharmacodynamics. Biopharmaceutics is the study of medication formulations and their effects on drug disposition. Pharmacokinetics is the study of medication absorption, distribution, metabolism, and excretion.
9. b. A medication needs to bind to a receptor to produce a clinical effect. Medications can bind to other proteins, such as albumin, or tissue, such as fat tissue, but they are inactive when bound to these components, and therefore do not exert a clinical effect at that time. Medications may affect certain organs and can also affect the blood, but they do not affect them directly; they must bind to a receptor on that organ or to a receptor that will trigger a response to affect the blood.
10. c. Liver disease is associated with impaired hepatocyte function, which leads to reduced metabolism of drugs by the liver.

Resources

Chapron DJ. Drug disposition and response. In: Delafuente JC, Stewart RB, eds. *Therapeutics in the Elderly*. 3rd ed. Cincinnati, OH: Harvey Whitney Books Company; 2001.

Shargel L, Wu-Pong S, Yu ABC. *Applied Biopharmaceutics and Pharmacokinetics*. 5th ed. Columbus, OH: The McGraw-Hill Companies, Inc; 2005.

Winter ME. *Basic Clinical Pharmacokinetics*. 4th ed. Baltimore, MD: Lippincott Williams & Wilkins; 2004.

References

1. Lindley CM, Tully MP, Paramsothy V, Tallis RC. Inappropriate medication is a major cause of adverse drug reactions in elderly patients. *Age Aging*. 1992; 21(4):294–300.
2. Hanlon JT, Gray SL, Schmader KE. Adverse drug reactions. In: Delafuente JC, Stewart RB, eds. *Therapeutics in the Elderly*. 3rd ed. Cincinnati, OH: Harvey Whitney Books Company; 2001.
3. Nolan L, O'Malley K. Prescribing for the elderly, part 1: sensitivity of the elderly to adverse drug reactions. *J Am Geriatr Soc*. 1988; 36(2):142–149.
4. Stewart RB, Cooper JW. Polypharmacy in the aged: practical solutions. *Drugs Aging*. 1994; 4(6):449–61.

5. Montamat SC, Cusack B. Overcoming problems with polypharmacy and drug misuse in the elderly. *Clin Geriatr Med.* 1992; 8(1):143–58.
6. Shargel L, Yu ABC. Biopharmaceutic considerations in drug product design. In: Shargel L, Yu ABC, eds. *Applied Biopharmaceutics and Pharmacokinetics*. 3rd ed. East Norwalk, CT: Appleton and Lange; 1993.
7. Stedman CA, Barclay ML. Review article: comparison of the pharmacokinetics, acid suppression and efficacy of proton pump inhibitors. *Aliment Pharmacol Ther.* 2000; 14 (8):963–78.
8. Drug facts and comparisons (loose-leaf). Facts and Comparisons. St. Louis, MO: A Wolters Kluwer Company; 2010.
9. Humalog [package insert]. Indianapolis, IN: Eli Lilly and Company; 2009.
10. Lantus [package insert]. Bridgewater, NJ: Sanofi-Aventis; 2009.
11. Winter ME. Basic principles. In: *Basic Clinical Pharmacokinetics*. 4th ed. Baltimore, MD: Lippincott Williams & Wilkins; 2004.
12. Hansten PD, Horn JR, eds. Drug interaction analysis and management. Facts and Comparisons. St. Louis, MO: A Wolters Kluwer Company; 2001.
13. Prozac [package insert]. Indianapolis, IN: Eli Lilly and Company; 2009.
14. Cockroft DW, Gault MH. Prediction of creatinine clearance from serum creatinine. *Nephron.* 1976; 16:31–41.
15. Bauer LA. Clinical pharmacokinetics and pharmacodynamics. In: Dipiro JT, Talbert RL, Yee GC, eds. Pharmacotherapy: a Pathophysiologic Approach. 5th ed. New York, NY: McGraw-Hill Medical Publishing Division; 2002.
16. Brody TM, Garrison JC. Sites of action: receptors. In: Brody TM, Larner J, Minneman KP, eds. Human pharmacology: molecular to clinical. 3rd ed. St. Louis, MO: Mosby; 1998.
17. Montamat SC, Cusack BJ, Vestal RE. Management of drug therapy in the elderly. *N Engl J Med.* 1989; 321(5):303–9.

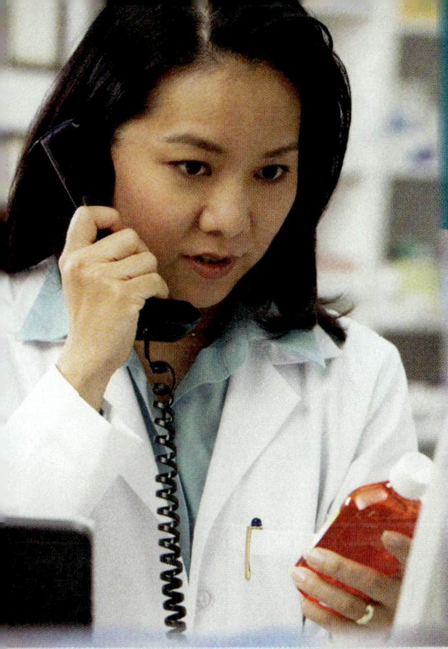

Chapter 12

Medication Dosage Forms and Routes of Administration

Michele F. Shepherd

Learning Outcomes

After completing this chapter, you will be able to

- Explain why medications are often available in more than one dosage form.
- List three advantages of liquid medication dosage forms over other dosage forms.
- List three disadvantages of solid medication dosage forms.
- Outline characteristics of solutions, emulsions, and suspensions.
- Describe two situations in which an ointment may be preferred over a cream.
- Explain the differences in use among various solid medication dosage forms, such as tablets, capsules, lozenges, powders, and granules.
- List six routes of administration by which drugs may enter or be applied to the body.
- Identify special considerations for five routes of administration.
- List five parenteral routes of administration.
- Distinguish between sublingual and buccal routes.

Key Terms

aerosol A suspension of very fine liquid or solid particles distributed in a gas, packaged under pressure, and shaken before use, after which medication is released from the container as a spray.

aqueous solution A liquid solution that contains purified water as the vehicle.

buccal A solid medication dosage form that is placed in the pocket between the cheek and gum and absorbed through the cheek into the bloodstream.

douche An aqueous solution that is placed into a body cavity or against a part of the body (e.g., the internal vaginal cavity) to clean or disinfect.

elixir A clear, sweet, flavored water-and-alcohol (hydroalcoholic) mixture intended for oral use.

emulsion A mixture of two liquids that normally do not mix, in which one liquid is broken into small droplets (the internal phase) and evenly scattered throughout the other (the external or continuous phase) and an emulsifying agent prevents the internal phase from separating from the external phase.

endotracheal Administering a medication into the trachea (windpipe); intratracheal.

enema A solution that is inserted into the rectum to empty the lower intestinal tract or to treat diseases of that area; often given to relieve severe constipation or to clean the large bowel before surgery.

extractive A concentrated preparation of material extracted, or removed, from dried plant or animal tissue by soaking it in a solvent, which is then evaporated, leaving behind the tissue parts containing medical activity; examples include extracts, tinctures, and fluid extracts.

inhalant A fine powder or solution of a drug delivered as a mist through the mouth into the respiratory tract.

intra-arterial Injected directly into an artery and therefore immediately available to act in the body.

intra-articular Injected directly into the articular (joint) space.

intracardiac Injected directly into the heart muscle.

intradermal Injected into the top layers of the skin.

intramuscular Injected directly into a large muscle mass, such as the upper arm, thigh, or buttock, and absorbed from the muscle tissue into the bloodstream.

intraperitoneal Administered into the peritoneal space (abdominal cavity).

intrapleural Administered into the pleural space, which is the sac that surrounds the lungs.

intrathecal Injected into the space around the spinal cord.

intratracheal Administered into the trachea (windpipe); endotracheal.

intrauterine Administered into the uterus.

intravenous Injected directly into a vein and therefore immediately available to act in the body.

intraventricular Injected into the brain ventricles or cavities.

intravesicular Administered into the bladder.

intravitreal Administered into the vitreous space in the eye; intravitreous.

intravitreous Administered into the vitreous space in the eye; intravitreal.

irrigant A solution used to wash or cleanse part of the body, such as the eyes, the urinary bladder, open wounds, or scraped skin.

jelly A semisolid solution with a high liquid content, usually water.

lozenge A hard, disk-shaped solid medication dosage form that contains medication in a sugar base, which is released as the lozenge is held in the mouth and sucked.

nonaqueous solution A liquid solution that uses a solvent or dissolving liquid, other than water, as the vehicle.

oil-in-water (O/W) emulsion An emulsion in which small oil droplets (internal phase) are scattered throughout water (external, continuous phase).

ointment A semisolid medication dosage form, applied to the skin or mucous membranes, which lubricates and softens or is used as a base for drug delivery.

parenteral A route of medication administration that bypasses the gastrointestinal tract, such as intravenous, intramuscular, or subcutaneous administration.

percutaneous Through the skin; transdermal.

solution An evenly distributed, homogeneous (even) mixture of dissolved medication in a liquid vehicle.

subcutaneous Deposited in the tissue just under the skin.

subgingival Administered via the subgingival space, which is the space between the tooth and gum.

sublingual Placed under the tongue, where it dissolves and is absorbed into the bloodstream.

suspension A mixture of fine particles of an undissolved solid spread throughout a liquid or, less commonly, a gas.

topical Applied to the skin, mucous membranes, or other external parts of the body, such as fingernails, toenails, and hair.

transdermal Through the skin; percutaneous.

transdermal patch A patch that contains a drug in a reservoir in the patch, which is delivered through the patch and absorbed from the skin into the bloodstream.

transmucosal Administered through, or across, a mucous membrane.

water-in-oil (W/O) emulsion An emulsion in which small water droplets (internal phase) are spread throughout oil (external, continuous phase).

When most people think about taking a medication, they imagine swallowing a tablet or a capsule. Although this is the most common way people take medications, other forms of medication are used to introduce medicines into the body by routes other than the mouth. Solutions, suspensions, suppositories, and sprays can be used to deliver medications into body areas such as the ears, nose, eyes, rectum, or bloodstream.

This chapter describes many medication dosage forms and routes of administration. It is not intended to be all-inclusive, but rather to serve as an introduction to commonly used and not-so-commonly used dosage forms and administration routes. Pharmacy technicians must be familiar with these concepts, since they are important as the technicians prepare, dispense, store, and otherwise manage medications.

Medication Dosage Forms

The most common medication dosage forms are liquids and solids. Liquid formulations deliver medication in a fluid and may be poured from a bottle or vial; solid medication dosage forms hold their original shape. Both dosage forms are usually administered orally, but may sometimes be administered by other routes. Availability of medications in different dosage forms offers options to prescribers, patients, caregivers, and manufacturers. For example, liquid medications are easier for children to take than solid ones. On the other hand, some medications are degraded by digestive enzymes found in the stomach or have poor absorption, so manufacturers formulate them to be given into a vein, thus bypassing the gastrointestinal tract.

✔ A local *effect* refers to an action of a medication that takes place at the area of contact. Contact may be with the skin, mucous membranes, respiratory tract, gastrointestinal system, eyes, or other organ systems. Absorption of the medication into the bloodstream does not usually occur. In contrast, a *systemic effect* is the result of an action of a medication that affects the whole body or takes place at a location distant from the medication's initial point of contact. Absorption of the medication must occur.

Liquid Medication Dosage Forms

Liquid medication dosage forms deliver medication in a fluid medium. The fluid serves as a carrier, or delivery system, for the medication and is referred to as the *vehicle.* Common medication vehicles are water, alcohol, glycerin, and mineral oil. The medication can be dissolved in the vehicle or can be present as very fine solid particles that are suspended, or floating, in the vehicle. Liquid medication dosage forms may pour as freely as water or may have the thickness of heavy syrup. They may be meant for oral intake or for use in, or on, other parts of the body.

Liquid medication dosage forms offer some advantages over other medication dosage forms, including

- Oral liquid medication dosage forms are usually faster-acting than solid medication dosage forms. Medications are absorbed into the bloodstream in a dissolved state. The medication in a liquid medication dosage form either is already dissolved or is present in small particles which then dissolve in fluids in the gastrointestinal tract, so the medication can be readily absorbed into the bloodstream. In contrast, tablets must first dissolve in the stomach (or other place where they may be administered, such as the vagina) before they can be absorbed, so it takes more time for the medication to be absorbed and to act.

- For patients who have difficulty swallowing, oral liquid medications may be easier to take than oral solid medication dosage forms.
- Liquid doses have more flexibility than some other dosage forms because liquid medications are usually dispensed in bulk containers rather than distinct dosage units. For example, a liquid medication contains 500 mg of a drug in 10 mL of liquid. The same medication is also available in 500 mg tablets. To take a 600 mg dose of the liquid medication, a patient would simply need to measure out 12 mL of liquid. However, to take a 600 mg dose of the tablet, the patient would need to take 1.2 tablets, which would be difficult.
- Liquid medications may be used where solid medication dosage forms are not practical to administer. For example, medications that need to be placed directly into the ears or eyes can be administered more easily as a liquid than as a solid.

There are also some disadvantages to liquid medication dosage forms, such as

- Often, liquid medication dosage forms have shorter times to expiration than other dosage forms.
- Many drugs have an unpleasant taste as the drug dissolves or is chewed into small particles. Drug particles are already present in oral liquid medications and come in contact with the taste buds of the tongue. People often find the taste or sensation of these drug particles unpleasant. Sweeteners and flavoring agents are necessary to make these liquid medications taste better. Even with such sweetening or flavoring, the taste of some liquid medications may remain unpleasant. Tablets and capsules, on the other hand, are often coated and can be swallowed quickly to avoid contact with the taste buds.
- Patients sometimes find liquid medications inconvenient because they may be spilled, require careful measuring before administration, or have special storage or handling requirements, such as refrigeration or shaking before use.

Liquid medication dosage forms are grouped based on several characteristics: the vehicle (e.g., water or alcohol) in which the medication is delivered, whether the medication is dissolved or suspended as particles in the liquid, or the intended use of the medication. Table 12-1 gives examples of solutions, emulsions, and suspensions.

Table 12-1. Liquid Medication Dosage Forms

Dosage Form	Examples

Solutions	■ Aqueous (water-based)
	  ■ Gargles
	  ■ Oral rinses
	  ■ Washes and mouthwashes
	  ■ Douches
	  ■ Irrigants
	  ■ Enemas
	  ■ Sprays
	  ■ Viscous (thick) aqueous
	    ■ Syrups
	    ■ Jellies
	■ Nonaqueous
	  ■ Hydroalcoholic
	    ■ Elixirs
	    ■ Spirits
	  ■ Alcoholic
	    ■ Collodions
	    ■ Spirits
	  ■ Glycerites

Extractives	■ Extracts ■ Tinctures ■ Fluidextracts
Emulsions	■ Oil-in-water ■ Water-in-oil
Suspensions	■ Lotions ■ Magmas and milks ■ Gels ■ Mucilages

Solutions. **Solutions** are evenly distributed, homogeneous (even) mixtures of dissolved medication in a liquid vehicle. Because the medication is already dissolved in the solution, the upper gastrointestinal tract, skin, or other site of administration absorbs it more quickly than other medication dosage forms.

Safety First Solutions should appear clear with no visible particles present. If particles or cloudiness are noted, the solution should not be used.

Solutions may be subdivided on the basis of the characteristics of the vehicle into a) aqueous b) nonaqueous and c) miscellaneous solutions.

Aqueous solutions. **Aqueous solutions** use purified water as the vehicle and can be ingested orally, applied topically (externally), or injected into the bloodstream.

Gargles are solutions that treat conditions of the throat. The gargle is held in the throat as the patient gurgles air through the solution. Although gargles are used in the mouth, they should not be swallowed. A familiar commerical gargle is Cepacol antiseptic mouthwash/gargle. *Oral rinses,* such as chlorhexidine (Peridex), are used to treat conditions inside the mouth. Oral rinses are also not supposed to be swallowed and should be spit out after swishing in the mouth.

A *wash* is a solution used to cleanse or bathe a body part, such as the eyes or mouth. Massengill Feminine Cleansing Wash is a vaginal wash intended to cleanse the external vaginal area. A *mouthwash* is a solution used to deodorize, refresh, or disinfect the mouth, primarily for cosmetic reasons. Although many people use mouthwashes as gargles, the two are technically in different classes of solutions: gargles are used to treat throat conditions, such as a sore throat, while mouthwashes are used to freshen the mouth. Like gargles, mouthwashes should not be swallowed. Common mouthwashes include Advanced Formula Plax and Listerine.

A ***douche*** [doosh] is an aqueous solution placed into a body cavity or against a part of the body to clean or disinfect. Douches are commonly used to cleanse the internal vaginal cavity, but a douche may also be used to remove debris from the eyes or to cleanse the nose or throat. Examples of commercially available vaginal douche products are Massengill and Summer's Eve.

Irrigating solutions, or ***irrigants,*** are used to wash or cleanse part of the body, such as the eyes, the urinary bladder, open wounds, or scraped skin. These solutions often contain medication, such as antibiotics or other antimicrobial agents, and are usually sterile. Irrigating solutions may be used in surgical procedures to clear the body area of blood and surgical debris. A common irrigating solution used in the eye is balanced salt solution (BSS). Although similar to douches, irrigating solutions are usually used in larger volumes and over larger areas of the body for a more general cleaning than douches.

Enemas are solutions that are inserted into the rectum to empty the lower intestinal tract or to treat diseases of that area. Enemas, such as Fleet enema, are often given to relieve severe constipation or to clean the large bowel before surgery.

Sprays are solutions that are applied as a mist to the area to be treated. Some sprays are for use on the mucous membranes of the nose and throat, while other sprays are used on the skin. Nasal decongestants (e.g., oxymetazoline [Afrin 12-Hour Original] and phenylephrine [Neo-Synephrine 4-Hour]) and antiseptic throat solutions (e.g., phenol [Cheracol Sore Throat Spray]) are spray products for the nose and throat.

Viscous aqueous solutions are sticky, thick, sweet solutions that are either liquid or semisolid. A *syrup* is a concentrated mixture of sucrose, or another type of sugar, and purified water. The high sugar content makes syrups different from other types of solutions. Syrups may or may not contain medication or added flavoring agents. Syrups without a medication are called non-medicated syrups. Simple syrup, which contains only sucrose and water, is one such example. Flavored syrups have an added flavoring agent and are often are used as vehicles for unpleasant-tasting medications; the result is a medicated syrup. The amount of sugar present in syrups makes them likely to be contaminated by bacteria, so they often contain a preservative. The high sugar content also makes syrups a poor choice for patients who have diabetes mellitus. Some medications are available as "sugar-free syrups," but they are not true syrups since by definition, syrups are mixtures of sugar and water. They would be more appropriately labeled as "liquids."

The advantage of syrups is that their sweet taste can disguise the unpleasant taste of medications. Because syrups are thicker than aqueous solutions, only a portion of the medication dissolved in the syrup comes in contact with the taste buds. The remainder of the medication is held above the tongue by the thick syrup, so it is not tasted as it is swallowed. For this reason, syrups are commonly used for medications taken by children. The thick nature of syrups also has a soothing effect on irritated tissues of the throat, so syrups are often used for cough formulations. Robitussin is an example of a common line of cough and cold syrup products.

Jellies are semisolid solutions that have a high liquid content, usually water. K-Y Jelly is an example of a commonly used lubricant jelly. It may be used to make insertion of rectal thermometers or other medical instruments into body openings more comfortable, as a sexual lubricant, or to reduce friction and enhance transmission of sound waves during ultrasound procedures. Lidocaine jelly is used as a local anesthetic for patients who are to have endotracheal tubes placed down their throats or urinary catheters (tubes) placed into their urethras. Jellies are also used as vaginal lubricants or as vehicles for vaginal contraceptive agents.

Nonaqueous solutions. **Nonaqueous solutions** are those that use solvents, or dissolving liquids, other than water. Commonly used nonaqueous solvents include alcohol (ethyl alcohol or ethanol), glycerin, mineral oil, and propylene glycol.

Hydroalcoholic solutions differ from aqueous solutions in that they contain alcohol as well as water. Elixirs and spirits are examples of hydroalcoholic solutions.

Elixirs [i-lick-serz] are clear, sweet, flavored water-and-alcohol (hydroalcoholic) mixtures intended for oral use. The amount of alcohol in elixirs varies greatly depending on how well the other ingredients in the elixir dissolve in water. Many drugs do not dissolve easily in pure water but do so in a water-and-alcohol mixture. Some elixirs have as little as 3% alcohol, whereas others may contain almost 25%.

The alcohol content of an elixir is a disadvantage or a reason to avoid use in patients who should not or cannot ingest alcohol. In addition, alcohol can have undesired interactions with other medications the patients may be taking. Elderly and alcoholic patients, as well as parents of children, should be made aware of the alcohol content of elixirs, because these patients may be especially sensitive to even small amounts of alcohol. For this reason, some elixirs have been re-formulated to remove the alcohol and are no longer true elixirs, but may be still be known as such. Phenobarbital elixir and digoxin pediatric elixir are two prescription elixirs.

Aromatic and licorice elixirs are used as flavoring agents. An aromatic elixir is a nonmedicated elixir commonly used as a vehicle for other medications. Simple elixir, which contains orange, lemon, coriander, or anise oils in syrup, water, and alcohol, is one example.

Spirits, or essences, are alcoholic or hydroalcoholic solutions that contain volatile, or easily evaporated, substances. Because the volatile substances dissolve more easily in alcohol, spirits can contain a greater amount of these materials than aqueous solutions can. Perhaps the most familiar spirits administered internally are the alcoholic beverages brandy (*Spiritus Vini Vitis*) and whiskey (*Spiritus Frumenti*). Other spirits may be inhaled (e.g., aromatic ammonia spirits, commonly known as smelling salts and used for fainting), while still others, such as peppermint spirits, are used as flavoring agents.

A *collodion* [kuh-loh-dee-uhn] is a liquid preparation of pyroxylin [pie-rock-suh-lin] (found in cotton fibers) that is dissolved in ethyl ether and ethanol. After the collodion is applied to the skin, the ether and ethanol evaporate and leave a pyroxylin film. Some medicated collodions are used to treat corns and warts (e.g., Compound W). Unmedicated collodions, such as liquid adhesive bandages (e.g., New-Skin) and skin protectants (e.g., BlisterGard), may be applied to the skin for protection or to seal small wounds.

Glycerites are nonaqueous solutions of medication dissolved in glycerin, a sweet oily fluid made from fats and oils. Glycerin can be used alone as a vehicle or in combination with water, alcohol, or both. Because glycerin easily mixes with water and alcohol, it can be used as a solvent for medications that do not dissolve in either alone. After a medication is dissolved in glycerin, the medication/glycerin mixture can then be added to a water vehicle or alcohol vehicle. Glycerin may be used in oral, otic (ear), ophthalmic (eye), topical (on the skin), and parenteral formulations. Most glycerite solutions are very viscous and thick, some to the point of being jelly-like. Debrox Drops, used to remove earwax from ears, is an example of a product formulated in glycerin.

Extractives. **Extractives** are concentrated preparations of materials found in plant or animal tissue. The crude drug is extracted, or removed, from the dried plant or animal tissue by soaking it in a solvent. The solvent is then evaporated, leaving behind the tissue parts containing medical activity. Extracts, tinctures [tingk-cherz], and fluidextracts are examples of formulations prepared in this manner. They differ only in their strength or potency.

Extracts are prepared in the same manner as tinctures and fluidextracts and are two to six times as potent as the crude drug. Vanilla, almond, and peppermint extracts, commonly used in cooking and baking, are examples of extracts.

Tinctures are alcoholic or hydroalcoholic solutions whose potency is adjusted so that each milliliter of tincture contains the equivalent of 100 mg of crude drug. Iodine tincture and opium tincture are two examples.

Fluidextracts are more potent than tinctures; each milliliter of fluidextract contains the equivalent of 1,000 mg of crude drug. Cascara sagrada fluidextract and senna fluidextract are extracts that, in the past, were commonly used to clear the bowels.

Emulsions. **Emulsions** are mixtures of two liquids that normally do not mix. In an emulsion, one liquid is broken into small droplets and evenly scattered throughout the other. The liquid present in small droplets is referred to as the internal phase; the other liquid is called the external, or continuous, phase. To keep the two liquids from separating, an emulsifying agent is added to the formulation to prevent the small particles of the internal phase from coming together and eventually separating from the external phase to form two distinct layers. Oil-and-vinegar salad dressing is a common household emulsion that is formed by shaking the two liquids together. Because no emulsifying agent is added, the oil and vinegar separate within seconds after shaking and the emulsion is broken.

In most emulsions, the two liquids are oil and water. An **oil-in-water (O/W) emulsion** consists of small oil droplets scattered throughout water. O/W emulsions are desirable for oral use for several reasons. Unpleasant oily medications are broken into small particles and dispersed throughout a sweetened, flavored aqueous vehicle. These small particles are carried past the taste buds and swallowed without the patient tasting the oily medication. The small particle size increases medication absorption from the stomach and small intestine into the bloodstream. One formulation of cyclosporine (Neoral), a medication used to prevent rejection of transplanted organs, is such an example.

In **water-in-oil (W/O) emulsions,** water droplets are spread throughout the oil. W/O emulsions are often used on unbroken skin. They spread more evenly than O/W emulsions because the natural oils of the skin mix with the external oil phase of the emulsion. They soften the skin better because they hold moisture and are not easily washed off with water. However, they have a heavy, greasy feel and may stain clothing.

The choice of O/W or W/O emulsion for preparations applied to the skin depends on several factors. As an example, medications that are irritating to the skin feel better when applied as small particles in the internal phase. The external phase keeps them from directly contacting and irritating the skin. O/W emulsions may be more desired in some cases because they are water-washable and do not stain. They feel lighter and nongreasy and have an advantage when the emulsion is to be applied to a hairy part of the body, such as the scalp.

Some emulsions may also be injected into the bloodstream. Intravenous fat emulsion (Intralipid, Liposyn II) and the anesthetic medication propofol (Diprivan) are examples of O/W emulsions that are given intravenously.

Suspensions. **Suspensions** are mixtures of fine particles of an undissolved solid spread throughout a gas or, more commonly, a liquid. The difference between a solution and a suspension is that in a solution the particles are dissolved, whereas in a suspension they are not. Suspensions are useful for administering a large amount of solid medication that would be inconvenient to take as a tablet or capsule. The fine particles dissolve more quickly in the stomach or small intestine and are absorbed into the bloodstream more quickly than the medication of a solid tablet or capsule. Suspensions need to be shaken before use to redistribute particles that may have settled to the bottom or risen to the top of the container after standing.

Most suspensions are for oral use, but some may be taken by other routes, such as the rectal, otic, ophthalmic, or parenteral routes. Suspensions taken by mouth usually use water as the vehicle, although suspensions that are given by parenteral routes, such as into muscles or joints, may use oil as the vehicle. Medication particles suspended in oil dissolve more slowly than in water. This imparts a "depot" effect and gives the medication extended-release properties. Haloperidol decanoate 50 is formulated in sesame oil, which allows it to be given intramuscularly (IM) on a monthly basis.

Safety First Parenteral suspensions should NEVER be given intravenously. Serious adverse effects such as cardiorespiratory (heart and lung) failure, coma, or death may occur.

Lotions are suspensions intended for external application to the skin. They contain finely powdered medications, and cool, soothe, dry, and/or protect the skin. Lotions are usually applied without a lot of rubbing and work easily into large areas of the skin without leaving a greasy or oily feel. Calamine lotion is a common example of a protective lotion.

Magmas and *milks* are thick, viscous suspensions of undissolved drugs in water. Milk of magnesia is the most common example of a magma. Magmas and milks are usually intended for oral administration and should be shaken well before each use.

Gels are similar to magmas and milks except that the suspended particle size in gels is smaller. Gels, too, are often intended for oral administration. Many commercially available antacids are gels. Other gels are intended for application to skin or mucous membranes. Testosterone gel (AndroGel) is a gel that is applied topically to the skin of males who lack adequate amounts of male hormones. Diazepam rectal gel (Dia*stat*) is used to treat epileptic seizures. Gels may also be intended for vaginal use;

progesterone vaginal inserts (Crinone and Prochieve), used for infertility treatment, are such examples.

Mucilages [myoo-suh-lahj-iz] are thick, viscous, gummy liquids. They are composed of water that contains the sticky, pulpy parts of vegetables. Mucilages are useful dosage forms that prevent nondissolving solid particles from settling to the bottom of liquids. Bulk-producing laxative products, such as psyllium (Metamucil), form a mucilage when the powder is added to water or juice.

Solid Medication Dosage Forms

Medications are commonly formulated in solid form. Examples of solid medication dosage forms include tablets, capsules, suppositories, and lozenges. Solid medication dosage forms allow for delivery of medications orally, rectally, or vaginally. Like some liquid medication dosage forms, some solid medication dosage forms may be used by more than one route. For example, tablets are used for oral medications but may also be used to deliver medications into the vagina. Suppositories are usually given rectally (e.g., glycerin rectal suppositories) but may also be used to deliver medications into the vagina (e.g., miconazole [Monistat 3] vaginal suppositories) or, very rarely, into the urethra (e.g., alprostadil [Muse] urethral suppositories). Table 12-2 summarizes the solid medication dosage forms that are discussed in this chapter.

Table 12-2. Solid Medication Dosage Forms

Dosage Form	Examples
Tablets	■ Molded
	■ Compressed
	■ Sugar-coated
	■ Film-coated
	■ Enteric-coated
	■ Sublingual
	■ Buccal
	■ Effervescent
	■ Chewable
	■ Vaginal
Capsules	■ Hard gelatin
	■ Soft gelatin
Caplets	
Lozenges	
Suppositories	■ Rectal
	■ Vaginal
	■ Urethral
Semisolids	■ Ointments
	■ Creams
	■ Pastes

Tablets. Tablets are compacted solid medication dosage forms; they may be further classified by their method of manufacture. *Molded tablets* are made from wet materials placed in molds and then shaped and dried. *Compressed tablets* are formed by die-punch compression of powdered, crystal, or granular substances.

Other ingredients that have no medicinal activity may be included in a compressed tablet. These inactive, or inert, ingredients (e.g., binders, diluents, lubricants, colorants) are necessary for the manufacturing process or to make the tablet more effective (e.g., disintegrators).

- Binders hold the compressed tablet together and keep it from crumbling.
- Diluents are fillers that are added to the active medication to make the tablet a practical size.
- Lubricants help in the removal of the tablet from the die punch.
- Colorants add color to the product.
- Disintegrators help the tablet break apart so it can dissolve more quickly in the stomach, in the small intestine, or elsewhere in the body.

Compressed tablets may have a sugar, film, or enteric coating on the outside. Sugar coating or film coating may be used to mask foul-tasting or foul-smelling drugs, to add color to the tablet, or to protect the drug from exposure to air and humidity. A film coating coats the tablet with a hard shell to make it sturdier and easier to swallow.

Enteric-coated oral tablets have a coating that protects the lining of the stomach from irritation by the drug. The coating delays the dissolution of the tablet as it passes through the stomach and into the small intestine. Effects of enteric-coated tablets are thus delayed, since they must first pass through the stomach and into the intestine before they are absorbed and become active. Thus, the stomach lining is not exposed to the irritating effects of the drug. Medications that cause nausea or bleeding of the stomach mucosa are often enteric coated. Other medications are degraded by stomach acid and so lose their medicinal effects. The enteric coating of these tablets acts as a barrier between the medication and the acid and allows the tablets to pass through the stomach intact. Once they reach the small intestine, they then dissolve without being degraded and are absorbed into the bloodstream.

Rx for Success

Tablets that are enteric coated should not be crushed, chewed, or cut. Doing so destroys the purpose of the coating.

Tablets may be described by a number of other terms as well. **Sublingual** [sub-ling-gwuhl] and **buccal** [buhk-uhl] tablets are useful solid medication dosage forms that dissolve under the tongue (sublingual) or in the pocket between the cheek and gum (buccal). They are small tablets designed to dissolve almost instantly in the mouth. The medication is then absorbed directly into the bloodstream through the lining under the tongue or of the cheek; this allows it to begin to work much faster than if it were swallowed as an oral tablet. For example, nitroglycerin sublingual tablets are administered to treat episodes of chest pain. Medications that are destroyed by stomach acid or that are poorly absorbed into the bloodstream may also be formulated as sublingual or buccal tablets.

Effervescent [ef-er-ves-uhnt] tablets contain ingredients that bubble and release the active drug when placed in a liquid. Their advantage is that they disintegrate and dissolve before administration, so the drug can be absorbed quickly after it is ingested. Alka-Seltzer Effervescent Tablets are an example.

Chewable tablets are those that do not need to be swallowed whole and may, or even should, be chewed. They are softer than other tablets, are pleasantly flavored, and are especially useful for children's medications (e.g., chewable multivitamins). Some adult tablets are also chewable. Antacid tablets (e.g., Rolaids Tablets and Tums) may be chewed before swallowing so that the tablet quickly disintegrates and the medication disperses more quickly in the intestine.

Vaginal tablets are inserted into the vagina. The tablets dissolve, and the medication may either be absorbed through the vaginal mucous lining into the bloodstream or remain in the vagina to exert its local effects within the vaginal cavity. Nystatin vaginal tablets are an example of a vaginal tablet that is not absorbed, but stays within the vagina to treat fungal infections.

Capsules. Capsules are solid medication dosage forms in which a drug, with or without inert ingredients, is contained within a gelatin shell. The gelatin shells are made of animal protein.

Rx for Success

Gelatin capsules are made in a variety of sizes: 000 (largest size), 00, 0, 1, 2, 3, 4, and 5 (smallest size). A size 000 capsule is the largest most people can swallow. Some even larger sizes are made for veterinary medicines.

Hard gelatin capsules are two-piece oblong casings filled with powdered ingredients. Most often they are for oral use and swallowed whole. Some capsules are sealed shut, or banded, to protect the ingredients from leaking out of the capsule, to prevent product tampering, or sometimes to give a product a distinctive appearance. Phenytoin capsules (Dilantin Kapseals) are an example of a banded capsule. However, some capsules may be or should be opened and the powdered ingredients inside sprinkled on food or in water before taking (e.g., divalproex sodium [Depakote Sprinkle] and topiramate [Topamax Sprinkle]).

Safety First

Many over-the-counter capsules are banded to more easily identify capsules that may have been tampered with before purchase by a consumer.

Other capsules contain powders that should be inhaled through the mouth into the lungs where the drug takes effect. These capsules are inserted into a mechanical device that punctures the capsule and releases the powder. Patients then inhale the powder through the device mouthpiece. Formoterol (Foradil), a medication to treat asthma, uses this type of device.

Soft gelatin capsules have ingredients added to the gelatin to give it a soft, squeezable, elastic consistency. The two halves of the capsule are sealed shut and, unlike hard gelatin capsules, cannot be opened. Soft gelatin capsules may be round, egg-shaped, or oblong and filled with liquid, pasty, or powdered medications. Vitamin E and docusate sodium, a stool softener, are available as soft gelatin capsules.

Caplets. Caplets are solid, capsule-shaped tablets that are generally coated for easy swallowing. They were designed to be more tamper-resistant than hard-shelled gelatin capsules.

✔ It is common for patients to refer to tablets and capsules as "pills." However, pills are a distinctly different dosage form. They are small, round, solid medication dosage forms intended for oral use. They are very rarely, if ever, used today.

Lozenges. **Lozenges,** also known as *troches* [troh-kee] or *pastilles* [pa-steel], are hard, disk-shaped solid medication dosage forms that contain medication in a sugar base. Lozenges are used to deliver antiseptic, local anesthetic, antibiotic, analgesic, antitussive, astringent, or decongestant drugs to the mouth or throat. The lozenge is held in the mouth and sucked. As it dissolves, the lozenge releases the medication. Sucrets Sore Throat lozenges contain local anesthetic, antiseptic, and other ingredients useful for treating minor sore throats. Nicotine polacrilex (Commit) lozenges are used to help patients quit tobacco smoking. Clotrimazole (Mycelex) troches treat oral fungal infections.

Suppositories. *Suppositories* are solid medication dosage forms that are inserted into the rectum, the vagina, or, very rarely, the urethra. Most often suppositories are molded from a soft, solid material (called a base), such as cocoa butter or glycerin. The base is melted, medication is added, and the resulting liquid is poured into a mold and allowed to cool and harden. After insertion into the appropriate body opening, the base re-melts and releases the medication. The medication is then absorbed through the thin mucous membrane lining of the body opening and enters the bloodstream.

Rx for Success

Suppositories should be kept in a cool place to prevent them from melting before use. Some may even require refrigeration or freezing. On the other hand, if the suppository is too soft to handle, it may be cooled in a refrigerator for 20 to 30 minutes or held under cold water for a few minutes while it is still in the wrapper.

Suppositories are useful for administering medication to very young children, elderly adults, or those who otherwise may not be able to take medication by other routes, such as patients who have no intravenous (IV) access or who are unable to swallow. Medications that can be destroyed by transit through the gastrointestinal tract may also be formulated in a suppository form.

Suppositories may treat local conditions in the immediate area of administration (e.g., bisacodyl [Dulcolax] rectal suppositories for relief of constipation or miconazole [Monistat-7] vaginal suppositories to treat vaginal fungal infections) or may exert systemic effects elsewhere in the body (e.g., acetaminophen [Tylenol] rectal suppositories for pain relief or prochlorperazine [Compazine] rectal suppositories to relieve nausea).

Safety First Patients should be instructed to allow suppositories to warm to room temperature before use and to remove the wrappers before insertion. Before insertion, the suppository or the insertion area should be moistened with water.

Semi-Solid Medication Dosage Forms

Ointments. **Ointments** are semisolid medication dosage forms that are applied to the skin or mucous membranes. They lubricate and soften or are used as a base for drug delivery. Not all ointments contain medication. Ointments are categorized based on their characteristics. The primary types of ointment bases are oleaginous, anhydrous, emulsion, and water-soluble.

Oleaginous, or *hydrocarbon,* bases are emollients that soothe the skin or mucous membranes. They are occlusive (provide a barrier) and protect the skin or mucous membrane from the air. They are hydrophobic (repel water), so they do not wash off with water and they feel greasy to the touch. Oleaginous bases are used mainly for their lubricating effect, because they do not allow moisture to escape from the skin, do not dry out, and remain on the skin for a long time. Vaseline petroleum jelly is an example of an oleaginous base.

Anhydrous, or *absorption,* bases contain no water and are similar to oleaginous bases, but instead of repelling water, they absorb it. They also soften skin, but not to the same degree as the oleaginous bases. Anhydrous bases absorb aqueous, or water-based, drugs. Anhydrous lanolin and cold cream are widely used anhydrous bases.

Emulsion bases may be water-in-oil (W/O) or oil-in-water (O/W). The W/O emulsion bases are emollient, occlusive, and greasy. They contain water, and some may be able to absorb additional water. Lanolin, mentioned above as an anhydrous base, and cold cream are considered to be W/O emulsions when water is added to them. Emulsion bases of the O/W type, or water-washable bases, are quite different. They are nongreasy and readily wash off with water. They are nonocclusive and may be diluted, or thinned, with the addition of water. In certain skin conditions, O/W emulsion bases are used to absorb watery discharge or to help the skin absorb certain medications.

Water-soluble bases are nongreasy, nonocclusive, and water-washable. They do not contain any fats and usually do not contain any water. Nonaqueous or solid medications are added to this type of ointment base. Polyethylene glycol ointment is one such base.

Ointment bases are chosen primarily on the basis of the characteristics described above. A W/O emulsion base may be used if a liquid medication is to be added to the ointment. Some medications may be more stable or more readily absorbed by the skin when delivered in a particular type of ointment base. The softening or drying characteristics of the ointment base may also influence the choice of a base. For instance, a nongreasy ointment base may be chosen if the ointment is to be applied to the face, because a greasy base may leave an unpleasant feeling.

Creams. *Creams* are semisolid O/W or W/O emulsions that may or may not contain medication. They are easily worked into the skin, or vanish, and feel lighter than ointments. They, too, soften the skin. Creams do not leave a residue on the skin and allow the skin to "breathe." This is an important consideration in the treatment of some dermatologic (skin) conditions.

Creams may be preferred over ointments because they are easier to spread, have a cooling effect on the skin, and, in the case of O/W creams, are easier to wash off with water. Many drug products are available as either creams or ointments to cater to the preferences of patients and physicians. Creams are also widely used in many cosmetic products.

Rx for Success

Creams and ointments are not necessarily interchangeable. If a product is available as a cream and as an ointment, the prescriber will select that which is most appropriate for the patient. A cream cannot be substituted for an ointment nor an ointment substituted for a cream without the prescriber's authorization.

Pastes. *Pastes* are semisolid medication dosage forms that contain medication intended for topical application. Pastes adhere well to the skin and, because of their heavy, thick nature, also protect the skin. They may absorb secretions from oozing wounds or act as a dam around the area of treatment. Amlexanol (Aphthasol) oral paste is used by patients with mouth ulcers (sores), and zinc oxide paste is often used to protect skin.

Miscellaneous Medication Dosage Forms

A number of medication dosage forms do not fit neatly into a specific category. They may be either unique in and of themselves, or may be a combination of dosage forms. Table 12-3 outlines these dosage forms.

Table 12–3. Miscellaneous Medication Dosage Forms

Dosage Form	Examples
Miscellaneous	■ Extended-release ■ Powders ■ Granules ■ Inhalants ■ Aerosols ■ Liniments ■ Shampoos and crème rinses ■ Wipes and scrubs ■ Transdermal patches ■ Implants

Extended-Release Dosage Forms. In some cases, having a medication dosage form that slowly and consistently releases a drug over an extended period of time, instead of all at once, is desirable. These medication dosage forms are called *extended-release, sustained-release, long-acting,* or *controlled-release.* Although the exact

Box 12–1. Common Abbreviations For Extended-Release Medications

CD	Controlled-diffusion
CR	Controlled-release, continuous-release
CRT	Controlled-release tablet
LA	Long-acting
SA	Sustained-action
SR	Sustained-release, slow-release
TD	Time-delay
TR	Time-release
XL	Extra-long
XR	Extended-release

meanings of these terms differ in some respects, each of these terms implies a gradual release of medication over a longer period than standard dosage forms. Box 12-1 lists common abbreviations used for extended-release products. Oral tablets and capsules are the most common dosage forms that are formulated as extended-release. Other extended-release dosage forms, such as implants, transdermal patches, some oral suspensions, and some intramuscular injections, will be discussed later.

Extended-release dosage forms offer several advantages:

- They deliver medication in a slow, controlled, and consistent manner so the patient absorbs the same amount of medication throughout a given time period.
- The risk of drug side effects is reduced because the medication is delivered in smaller amounts over a long period of time, rather than all at once.
- Patients may need to take the medication less frequently, perhaps only once or twice a day, or even as infrequently as once a week, once a month, or even longer.
- Patients are more likely to take their medications properly, and are less likely to experience side effects, if they can take them less often.
- The daily medication cost to patients may be decreased. Although extended-release products may be more expensive on a per-dose basis, the total daily cost may be less because the patient takes fewer doses overall.

There are disadvantages to extended-release dosage forms:

- There may be a delay between the time the patient takes the medication and the time it takes effect. Therefore, extended-release products are not helpful in situations where an immediate effect is required.
- If a patient does experience a side effect, it may take some time for the effect to dissipate, because some of the medication may remain in the body.
- Most extended-release products cannot be cut, crushed, or chewed. This may limit the situations in which the product may be used.
- The medication may be more expensive than an immediate-release product.

Several technologies are available to give medication dosage forms extended-release properties. Many small beads of medication in varying sizes may have varying thicknesses of a coating material. These beads are then put in a hard gelatin capsule, suspended in a liquid vehicle, compressed into a tablet, or put into a soft gelatin shell. In the stomach, the small beads are released and then dissolve and release medication at varying rates over a period of time.

Other extended-release products use a slowly eroding matrix in which a portion of the medication is treated and made into special granules. These granules are combined with an untreated portion of the medication granules and made into a tablet or capsule. The untreated drug granules immediately release the drug in the stomach, while the treated ones slowly wear away to provide a prolonged effect. Some extended-release products are formulated in two or more layers. One layer dissolves immediately, and the remainder dissolves more slowly and releases the drug gradually.

Other products embed the drug in an inactive plastic or wax matrix core that is covered by a controlled-release layer. The drug is released into the body as it slowly trickles out of the matrix. The matrix does not dissolve and is passed through the gastrointestinal tract and excreted in the feces. This remnant matrix is sometimes called a ghost tablet.

Rx for Success

Patients may notice a ghost tablet in their feces and become concerned that the medication has "passed through" without exerting its effect. You can reassure them that this is normal and that the medication has been absorbed as it should have been.

A very sophisticated extended-release system uses an osmotic pump to deliver medication over time. This system uses the principle of osmosis, where fluids flow from areas with a high concentration of a substance to areas with a low concentration. The pump system consists of a special membrane surrounding a core of medication. As fluid in the stomach passes through the membrane, the drug core inside swells and forces medication out of a small hole drilled in the membrane. Nifedipine (Procardia XL) is one product that uses an osmotic pump system.

If it seems necessary to crush, chew, or cut an extended-release product, an immediate-release formulation of the same drug should be used instead or the medication changed to a different one that can be used in the situation.

✔ The extended-release characteristic of most extended-release products is dependent upon the dosage form remaining intact and unbroken. For this reason, they should not be opened, cut, crushed, chewed, or otherwise damaged before taking. If an extended-release product is so damaged, the patient will receive a large dose of the medication and be at risk for adverse side effects.

Lists of extended-release products that should not be cut, crushed, or chewed are available in many pharmacy and nursing drug reference books. Any medication that includes one of the abbreviations listed in Box 12-1 as part of its name should not be cut, crushed or chewed. Products that are likely to be extended-release are products that are given only once or twice a day or even less frequently, tablets that have a special coating, or hard-shell capsules that have a seal around the seam of the two halves. Usually, tablets that are scored (have an indented line running through the middle of the tablet) *can* be cut along the score line.

Powders. *Powders* are finely ground particles of dry medication that can be used externally or internally. Some medications may have short shelf lives or take up a lot of shelf space when formulated as a liquid product. However, when formulated as powders, they may be more chemically stable and thus have longer shelf lives, and since the liquid has been removed, they may take up less storage space.

External powders, or dusting powders, are finely ground mixtures of dry drugs and inactive ingredients that are sprinkled or dusted on the area to be medicated. Johnson's Baby Powder is a familiar example of an over-the-counter external powder. An example of a prescription powder is nystatin (Mycostatin) powder, used to treat fungal skin infections.

Internal powders are reconstituted (dissolved or suspended in a liquid) prior to use. Often, pediatric forms of oral medications are formulated as a powder. Upon dispensing, the pharmacist will reconstitute the powder with water, creating an oral suspension of the medication. This then is more easily taken by a child than a tablet or capsule. Many antibiotics, such as amoxicillin and cefdinir, are available as such powders. Many oral potassium products are available as powders, which the patient dissolves in water or juice just before drinking. Some powders, such as powdered toothpaste, are mixed with water at the time of use and used in the wetted state. Many injectable drugs are also manufactured as powders and must be reconstituted with a sterile fluid (usually water or saline) before they are administered into a patient's bloodstream.

Safety First Powders for injection must always be reconstituted before use. The powder should be thoroughly dissolved in fluid and the resulting product inspected to be sure that no visible particles remain before administration.

Finally, some powders are inhaled into the lungs to treat lung conditions such as asthma. Fluticasone/salmeterol (Advair Diskus) is a medication delivery system that, after inhalation through the mouth, delivers powdered medication directly into the lungs.

Zanamivir (Relenza), used for the prevention and treatment of influenza, is delivered in a similar manner except that the powder is packaged as a powder in a foil blister-pack, which is punctured by a special device before the patient inhales the powdered medication.

Powders are packaged in bulk containers or, when the amount delivered must be accurate, in powder papers. Powder papers are folded paper envelopes that contain enough powder for one dose or application. Goody's Extra Strength Headache Powders and BC Powder Arthritis Strength are analgesics that are packaged as powder papers.

Granules. When powders are wetted, allowed to dry, and ground into coarse pieces, the resulting medication dosage form is called a *granule.* Granules differ from powders in that the particle size is larger and usually more stable. Many antibiotics are formulated as granules. Water is added to form a solution or suspension at the time of dispensing. For example, water is added to clarithromycin (Biaxin) granules before administration.

Inhalants. **Inhalants** are fine powders or solutions of drugs delivered as a mist through the mouth into the respiratory tract. Many drugs used to treat respiratory conditions, such as asthma or chronic obstructive pulmonary disease (COPD), are formulated as inhalants. The prescription drug albuterol (Proventil) is a well-known example.

Aerosols. **Aerosols** are suspensions of very fine liquid or solid particles distributed in a gas and packaged under pressure. These formulations need to be shaken before use, after which medication is released from the container as a spray (e.g., Bactine Antiseptic Anesthetic), foam (e.g., ProctoFoam-HC, RID Mousse), or solid (e.g., Tinactin). Aerosols are conveniently packaged and easy to use.

Aerosols may be used to deliver medications to internal and external sites. Aerosols inhaled through the mouth, such as albuterol (Proventil HFA and Ventolin HFA) are used to treat conditions such as asthma. A device called an *inhaler* aerosolizes the drug, and the patient inhales the drug through a mouthpiece directly into the lungs, where it begins to act immediately. The drug does not first have to be dissolved in the stomach and absorbed into the bloodstream, as it would if it were formulated as a tablet or capsule. The end result is that less drug is needed to produce its effects, so side effects are decreased.

A *nebulizer* works similarly in that it produces a fine mist that is inhaled by a patient. Compressed air is pumped through a liquid to make small droplets. These are then inhaled through a mask or mouthpiece. Nebulizers require a power source and are larger, less portable, and more expensive than inhalers, but are easier to use for infants, very young children, or elderly adults who suffer from cystic fibrosis, asthma, COPD, or other respiratory disorders.

External aerosols, such as Tinactin and Bactine Antiseptic Anesthetic sprays, may be applied topically (externally) for skin conditions. An external aerosol can deliver medication to a hard-to-reach area of the skin and can be applied to inflamed or irritated skin without causing further irritation.

Liniments. A *liniment* is a medication dosage form that is applied to the skin with friction and rubbing. Liniments may be solutions, emulsions, or suspensions. Some liniments contain agents that produce a mild irritation or reddening of the skin. This irritation produces a counter-irritation, or mild inflammation, of the skin that relieves the inflammation of deeper structures, such as muscles. Ben-Gay Original Ointment is a liniment widely used to relieve minor aches and pains of muscles.

Shampoos and Crème Rinses. *Shampoos* and *crème rinses* are used as vehicles for medications to treat conditions of the hair and scalp. Ciclopirox (Loprox) and clobetasol (Clobex) are available as shampoos used to treat seborrhea and psoriasis of the scalp, and permethrin (Nix) is an example of a crème rinse used to treat head lice.

Wipes and Scrubs. Other dosage forms have been developed for user ease and convenience. Bactine Pain Relieving Cleansing Wipes, Stri-Dex pads, and Hibistat towelettes are all similar and are used to directly wipe and clean areas of skin. Scrubs, such as chlorhexidine topical scrub, are abrasive cleansers and also wash and clean skin. Some anti-acne over-the-counter facial cleansing products are scrubs.

Transdermal Patches. Adhesive **transdermal patches,** similar to plastic bandages, contain drugs in a small reservoir. Patches are convenient to use. Depending on the patch, it may be applied to the skin from once a day to once a week or longer.

Transdermal patches are formulated in one of two ways. One type of patch is formulated so that the patch itself controls the rate of delivery of drug to the skin. A special membrane in the patch is in contact with the skin. The membrane controls the amount of drug delivered from a drug reservoir in the patch, through the membrane and skin, and into the bloodstream.

The second type of transdermal patch is designed so that the skin controls the rate of drug delivery. The drug moves from an area of high concentration (the drug reservoir) into an area of low concentration (the skin and bloodstream). The disadvantage of this type of patch is that the release of drug is less controlled, and a large amount of drug could suddenly be released from the patch into the blood.

Medications available in a patch formulation include a narcotic analgesic (fentanyl [Duragesic]), female hormones (estradiol [Estraderm]), and drugs to treat high blood pressure (clonidine [Catapres-TTS]), chronic chest pain (nitroglycerin [Nitro-Dur]), and motion sickness (scopolamine [Transderm-Scop]) and to aid in smoking cessation (nicotine [Nicoderm CQ]). Other patches are designed to produce a local effect by limiting delivery of medication to only the external skin. Synera is a dermal patch that releases local anesthetic medications (lidocaine and tetracaine) to the skin and decreases the amount of pain experienced during minor procedures, such as removal of skin lesions or placement of IV needles.

Implants. An *implant* is a medication pump or device inserted semipermanently or permanently into the body. Medication is released from the implant and delivered in a controlled fashion. Implants are often used to treat chronic (long-term) conditions or diseases. Some diabetic patients have a small pump implanted in their bodies that delivers insulin. Certain types of cancers may be treated with chemotherapeutic agents delivered into the arteries that enter the cancerous organ. A small pump filled with the drug is implanted in the body and infuses the chemotherapy drug into the artery. The contraceptive implant, etonogestrel (Implanon), is another type of implant that is placed under the skin (subcutaneously) of female patients. The implant is inserted into the arm and slowly releases birth control medication for up to three years. Histrelin acetate (Vantas) implants are placed under the skin of male patients. These subcutaneous implants release prostate cancer medication for the duration of one year.

Routes of Administration

Drugs can be administered by several different routes (see table 12-4). Although the oral route is most common, it may not always be the most convenient or practical. Drugs may be administered into or through any body orifice or opening (e.g., mouth or rectum), through the skin (e.g., creams, ointments, or transdermal patches), or into an artificially made opening (e.g., feeding tubes inserted directly into the stomach through the abdominal wall).

Oral

Medications taken by the oral route are introduced into the body through the mouth. The oral route is abbreviated *PO,* from the Latin *per os* (by mouth). Tablets, capsules, solutions, suspensions, and emulsions are some of the medication dosage forms that may be taken orally.

✔ The oral route shares the advantages and disadvantages of oral dosage forms. It is safe, convenient, and generally less expensive than other routes.

Oral dosage forms may be modified to deliver drugs in an extended-release fashion. However, the oral route cannot be used to administer medications to unconscious patients or those who have trouble swallowing. Because an oral medication must be absorbed before entering the bloodstream, there is a lag time between ingestion and the time the drug begins to act. This lag time is a problem if an immediate action is desired. Food, other drugs, and acid or lack of acid in the stomach can interfere with the dissolution or absorption of the drug.

Sublingual, Buccal, Transmucosal, and Subgingival

The terms sublingual (under the tongue) and buccal (inside the cheek) refer not only to types of tablets, but also to routes of oral medication administration. To administer a drug sublingually, the drug is placed under the tongue, where the medication dissolves and is absorbed into the bloodstream through the underlining of the tongue. Nitroglycerin sublingual tablets, used to treat chest pain, are administered under the tongue. Sublingual tablets and sprays are used when a rapid drug effect is desired, such as in the treatment of chest pain. Nitroglycerin spray (Nitrolingual) is a lingual spray that may be sprayed under, or even on, the tongue and is used when a prompt effect is desired.

Buccal tablets are placed inside the pouch of the cheek and stick to the inside lining of the cheek. Medication dissolves and is absorbed over time through the cheek lining (mucosa) into the bloodstream. Testosterone (Striant) buccal tablets are used as a hormone replacement in men who lack adequate amounts of that hormone. Although not formulated as a tablet, nicotine gum (Nicorette) uses the buccal route to deliver nicotine into the bloodstream of people who are trying to quit cigarette smoking.

Rx for Success

Patients should not swallow buccal tablets. They are not designed to be chewed or swallowed. If they are, they lose their extended-release properties and patients get larger doses of medication than intended.

Sometimes, a patient may have difficulty swallowing or may not be alert enough to swallow. In this case, **transmucosal** drug administration, where drug enters the body through, or across, a mucous membrane, may be a practical option. Fentanyl (Actiq) is a transmucosally delivered opioid analgesic that is used for pain relief in cancer patients. The active drug is contained within a core on a handle; the core is placed in the patient's mouth between the cheek and lower gum. The patient sucks on the core, and the medication moves from the core, into saliva, across the mucous membranes within the mouth, and into the patient's bloodstream.

Table 12–4. Routes of Medication Administration

Route	Methods	Definition/Description
Oral	Oral	Through the mouth (PO)
	Buccal	Inside the cheek
	Lingual	On the tongue
	Sublingual	Under the tongue (SL)
	Subgingival	Under the gums
	Transmucosal	Across mucous membranes
Enteral	Enteral	By way of the intestine
	Nasogastric (tube)	A feeding tube inserted through the nose into the stomach (NG or NGT)
	Gastrostomy (tube), percutaneous endoscopic gastrostomy (tube)	A feeding tube inserted through the abdominal wall into the stomach (GT, PEG)
	Jejunostomy (tube)	A feeding tube inserted into the jejunum (small intestine) (JT)
Inhalation	Inhalation	Drawn through the mouth into the lungs
Parenteral	Parenteral	Bypassing the gastrointestinal tract
	Implant	A device inserted into or under the skin
	Intra-arterial	Into an artery (IA)
	Intra-articular	Into a joint (IA)
	Intracardiac	Into the heart muscle (IC)
	Intradermal	Into the top layers of the skin (ID)
	Intratracheal, endotracheal	Into the trachea (IT)
	Intramuscular	Into a muscle (IM)
	Intraperitoneal	Into the peritoneal (abdominal) cavity
	Intrapleural	Into the pleura (sac that surrounds the lungs)
	Intrathecal	Into the space around the spinal cord
	Intrauterine	Into the uterus
	Intravenous	Into a vein (IV)
	Intraventricular	Into the ventricles, or cavities, of the brain
	Intravesicular	Into the urinary bladder
	Intravitreal or intravitreous	Into the eye
	Subcutaneous	Immediately under the skin (SubQ, SC, SQ)
Nasal	Intranasal	Into the nose
Ophthalmic		Into the eye
Otic, aural		Into the ear
Percutaneous		Through the skin
Rectal		Through the anus into the rectum
Topical		Applied to skin or mucous membranes
Transdermal		Through the skin
Vaginal		Into the vagina

Medication that is administered **subgingivally** is deposited into the subgingival space (the space between the tooth and gum) to treat gingivitis (inflammation of the gums). Doxycycline hyclate (Atridox) dental gel is a thick antibiotic liquid that is administered subgingivally. Chlorhexidine chips (PerioChip) are biodegradable chips that contain an antimicrobial medication and are placed subgingivally into the tooth pocket in the gum as a treatment for gum disease.

Enteral

There may be times when a patient cannot swallow a medication—for example, because he or she is mechanically ventilated and has an endotracheal tube in the throat. Medications may then be given enterally, bypassing the patient's mouth. Usually, liquid medication is poured down a tube that is inserted through the nose, throat, or abdomen and threaded into the patient's stomach or small intestine. Although these tubes may be inserted for other reasons, they offer alternatives to the oral route. If a medication is not available in a liquid form, an alternative is to crush an oral solid dose form and add water or another suitable liquid to the crushed medication. The resulting slurry can then be poured and rinsed down the enteral tube.

Rx for Success

Sometimes crushed medications can clog an enteral tube, so proper attention to the administration technique must be paid when giving medication in this manner. Care must be taken to use only products that can be crushed. In some situations, a liquid form may need to be compounded by a pharmacy professional.

The name of the tube offers clues as to where it enters into and ends in the body. Nasogastric tubes (NGT) are inserted through the nose ("naso-") and end in the stomach ("-gastric"). Gastrostomy tubes (GT) are inserted into the stomach ("gastro-") through an opening ("-ostomy") in the abdominal wall. A subtype of gastrostomy tube is the percutaneous endoscopic gastrostomy (PEG) tube. Gastrostomy and PEG tubes are similar to each other but are inserted by using different techniques. Finally, jejunostomy tubes are placed through an opening in the abdominal wall into the jejunum ("jejuno-"), a portion of the small intestine.

Parenteral

Parenteral routes of administration are those that bypass the gastrointestinal tract. Medications administered parenterally are most commonly introduced into the body intravenously, intramuscularly, or subcutaneously. They may be injected over a short period of time (seconds to minutes) with a needle and syringe or infused into the body at a constant rate over hours or days. Drugs that are given parenterally are most commonly formulated as solutions (e.g., potassium chloride, dextrose, many antibiotics, regular insulin), and less often as suspensions (e.g., perflutren microspheres [Definity], penicillin G benzathine) and emulsions (e.g., intravenous fat emulsion).

✔ Parenterally administered drugs are given when patients are unable to take oral medications, when faster drug action is desired, or when a drug is not available in a form that can be administered by another route.

A disadvantage of parenteral routes is that they are invasive—that is, a needle penetrates the skin to enter into veins, arteries, and other areas of the body. This penetration may be painful for the patient and could introduce bacteria or other contaminants into the body, resulting in infection or inflammation.

Intravenous (IV). **Intravenous (IV)** medications are introduced into the body through a needle placed directly in a vein. These drugs are usually given as solutions, which must be sterile and particle-free. Drugs given by the IV route are immediately available to act in the body. Because they act quickly, care must be taken in giving IV medications. If too high a dose is given or if the patient experiences an adverse reaction, quick action may be needed to reverse the drug's effects.

IV drugs may be given as a *bolus,* by *short infusion,* or by *continuous infusion.* A bolus dose is injected into the body over a relatively short period of time—seconds to minutes—to produce an almost immediate effect in the body. The term *IV push* also refers to this administration technique; the drug is pushed into the body by means of a syringe. Heparin, a drug used to prevent and treat blood clots, is often given as a bolus. In contrast, some medications can be infused into veins continuously over hours to days by using an infusion, which provides a constant supply of drug to the body. Bolus doses and continuous infusions are often used together. For example, after heparin is given as an IV bolus, a continuous heparin infusion is usually started to maintain an adequate amount of the drug in the blood.

If some medications are introduced too quickly into the body, patients may experience undesired side effects, such as low blood pressure, feelings of warmth or facial flushing, or pain at the point where the medication enters the veins. To avoid these effects, medications may be administered over longer periods of time than if they were given as IV boluses. Many antibiotics are administered as short infusions over 15 to 30 minutes as IV "piggybacks" to manage their side effects.

Rx for Success

If a patient experiences an undesired side effect from a medication given as a bolus or short infusion, lengthening the infusion time may help.

Intramuscular (IM). **Intramuscular (IM)** administration involves direct injection of medication into a large muscle mass, such as the upper arm, thigh, or buttock. The drug is absorbed from the muscle tissue into the bloodstream. IM drugs may be given as solutions or suspensions. Drugs given by the IM route act more quickly than orally administered drugs, but not as quickly as IV drugs. Some IM drugs may be formulated as extended-release suspensions, often in an oil vehicle, that slowly release drug into the bloodstream over hours, days, or even months. Some types of penicillin are formulated in this manner. Disadvantages of the IM route are that it is difficult to reverse the drug's effects once the injection has been given, that the injection is painful to receive and may cause bruising, and that drug absorption from the muscle into the bloodstream may be erratic and incomplete.

Subcutaneously. Solutions or suspensions injected **subcutaneously** (SubQ, SC, or SQ) are deposited in the tissue just under the skin. Drugs given by the SubQ route are absorbed to a lesser extent and act more slowly than those given by the IV or IM routes. Patients can easily be taught to self-administer SubQ injections. Many diabetic patients, for example, give themselves daily SubQ injections of insulin.

A limitation of both the SubQ and IM routes is the relatively small volume of drug that can be injected under the skin or into the muscle. It may be undesirable to use the SubQ route in patients with little body fat or the IM route in patients with obesity, decreased muscle mass, or bleeding problems.

The IV, IM, and SubQ routes are the most commonly used parenteral routes. However, drugs can be injected into almost any body space, including the epidural space. Several other parenteral medication dosage routes are used for specialized purposes or to limit drug delivery to the immediate area of the injection. These routes include intradermal, intra-arterial, intra-articular, intracardiac, intraperitoneal, intrapleural, intratracheal (endotracheal), intraventricular, intrauterine, intravesicular, intravitreous (intravitreal), and intrathecal.

Intradermal (ID). The **intradermal (ID)** route involves injecting a drug into the top layers of the skin. ID injections are not injected as deeply as SubQ injections. The ID route is used to administer drugs for skin testing, such as tuberculin purified protein derivative (PPD), which is a test for tuberculosis. It is also used for allergy testing to determine if patients are allergic to drugs or other substances, such as dust, pet dander, or pollen.

Intra-arterial. **Intra-arterial** injections involve administering an agent directly into an artery. These injections have the advantage of delivering drugs, such as cancer chemotherapy agents or thrombolytics (e.g., alteplase), directly to the desired location and may decrease some of the side effects caused when the drug acts in other parts of the body.

Safety First

The intra-arterial route involves greater risk than the IV route and is dangerous if a drug not intended for intra-arterial use is administered into an artery.

Intra-articular. The **intra-articular** route involves injecting a drug into a joint, such as a knee or elbow, to treat diseases in the joint. For example, anti-inflammatory steroid drugs (e.g., triamcinolone acetonide [Kenalog], methylprednisolone acetate [DepoMedrol]) are injected intra-articularly to treat the inflammation caused by arthritis or joint injury. Medications for intra-articular use are often formulated as suspensions to provide a long-lasting effect.

Intracardiac. The **intracardiac** route, injection directly into the heart muscle, is used in life-threatening emergencies. This route is not often used because it may rupture the heart.

Intraperitoneal. **Intraperitoneal** injections are given into the peritoneal, or abdominal, cavity. This route is used to administer antibiotics to treat infections in the peritoneal cavity. One method of dialysis, peritoneal dialysis, uses the intraperitoneal route to remove waste products from the blood of patients with kidney failure.

Intrapleural. **Intrapleural** describes the injection of drugs into the sac surrounding the lungs, or the pleura. Drugs are injected intrapleurally to stimulate inflammation and scarring of the pleural tissues so that excessive fluid can no longer accumulate in the pleural sac.

Intratracheal. **Intratracheal,** or **endotracheal,** medications are delivered into the windpipe, or trachea. Poractant alfa (Curosurf) and calfactant (Infasurf) are examples of medications administered through a special tube (catheter) into the tracheas of premature infants to help their lungs mature.

Intraventricular. The **intraventricular** route is used to administer drugs into the ventricles, or cavities, of the brain to treat infections or cancerous brain tumors. Caution must be used when interpreting an order for the intraventricular route, because the heart also has ventricles.

Safety First Caution must be used when interpreting abbreviations that refer to the route of medication administration. The abbreviation IV usually refers to the intravenous route, but it can also refer to the intravitreal or intravitreous (into the eye) or intraventricular (into the brain) routes, or it could be interpreted as the Roman numeral four (IV). Abbreviations for drug administration routes are best avoided and must be taken carefully in the context of each medication order or clarified when necessary.

Intravitreal. **Intravitreal,** or **intravitreous,** medications are administered by direct injection into the vitreous fluid of the eye. Many drugs do not enter the interior eye from the bloodstream, and often the only way to deliver medications inside the eye is to inject them intravitreally behind the lens of the eye. Antibiotics to treat sight-threatening eye infections and other medications that treat conditions that threaten eyesight are administered intravitreally. Ranibizumab (Lucentis) is an example of a medication administered by this route.

Intrathecal. **Intrathecal** is the route by which drugs are injected into the space around the spinal cord. This route may be used to deliver agents that treat infections or cancerous tumors of the central nervous system.

Intravesicular. The **intravesicular** route delivers drugs directly into the urinary bladder. This route is used to treat bladder infections or bladder cancer.

Intrauterine. The levonorgestrel intrauterine insert (Mirena) and Paragard intrauterine copper contraceptive are devices that deliver contraceptive medication or effect by the **intrauterine** (into the uterus) route. These devices are placed within the uterus and release medication into the uterine cavity. The medication is then absorbed into the bloodstream and prevents pregnancy.

Topical

The **topical** route usually refers to the application of medications to the skin or mucous membranes, although it also applies to other external parts of the body, such as fingernails and toenails (e.g., ciclopirox [Penlac] nail lacquer) and hair (e.g., permethrin [RID] shampoo). Medications administered topically include antibiotics, antiseptics, astringents, emollients, and corticosteroids. Topical medication dosage forms include creams, ointments, lotions, foams, sprays, and aerosols. In most cases, the skin or mucous membrane acts as a barrier to prevent the medication from entering the bloodstream. The medication then produces a local effect—its action is confined to the area in which it is applied or administered. As a result, drugs used for treating diseases of the skin and mucous membranes can be applied topically in higher concentrations than can drugs administered internally.

Some ointments and creams (e.g., topical corticosteroid ointments) are formulated to deliver a drug into the skin to treat a condition of the deeper skin layers. Sometimes creams and ointments are designed so that the drug diffuses through the skin into the bloodstream, making the drug available to the whole body to produce a systemic effect. Nitroglycerin ointment used to treat chest pain is one such medication.

In some cases, systemic absorption is not desired and may result in unwanted side effects. For example, when topical corticosteroids are absorbed systemically over prolonged periods of time, the patient can develop cataracts or glaucoma. Patients who use some types of eye drops (beta blockers) for glaucoma can experience slow heart rates if too much of the medication is absorbed systemically. Topical medications should not be applied to skin that is not intact (e.g., inflamed, irritated, or burned). Topical medications are more likely to penetrate into the bloodstream through non-intact, fragile, or thin skin. This may result in patients receiving higher than intended doses of medication and experiencing side effects as a consequence. Babies, young children, and the elderly are especially at risk.

Safety First To avoid systemic absorption, care must be taken when topical preparations are applied to large areas of the skin, when the medication concentration is high, or when the medicated skin surface is covered with an occlusive (barrier) material such as plastic bandages or diaper covers. Also, topical preparations should not be applied to non-intact, fragile, or thin skin.

Transdermal. The **transdermal,** or **percutaneous** [pur-kyoo-tay-nee-uhs], route of medication administration delivers drugs across, or through, the skin. Transdermal medications are applied to the skin, released from a vehicle, and absorbed continuously into the bloodstream, and consequently are delivered throughout the body. Adhesive patches are commonly used to deliver medications transdermally.

Ointments are sometimes used to deliver drugs percutaneously. Nitroglycerin ointment for chronic chest pain was often used in the past. Its use has been widely replaced by nitroglycerin transdermal patches, although the ointment may still be used to transition, or wean, patients from continuous nitroglycerin IV infusions to oral nitroglycerin medications.

PLO (pluronic lecithin organogel) gel is a vehicle used to deliver medication transdermally. The gel is formulated to allow penetration of medication into the deeper layers of the skin. Medications are added to the gel and are often customized to the needs of the patient. Commonly, nonsteroidal anti-inflammatory drugs for the treatment of painful skin conditions are added to PLO gel, but medications for other conditions (e.g., nausea or skin infections) may also be administered in this fashion.

Rectal. Drugs delivered by the rectal route are inserted through the anus into the rectum. Rectally administered drugs can be formulated as solids (suppositories), liquids or suspensions (enemas), and aerosol foams. Once the drug reaches the rectum, its activity may be limited to the lower gastrointestinal tract (a local effect), or the drug may be absorbed into the bloodstream and delivered to its site of action elsewhere in the body (a systemic effect). The rectal route is often used for children or other patients who are unable to take oral medications or when a local effect is desired (e.g., treatment of hemorrhoids).

Vaginal. Drugs can also be inserted into the vagina. Drugs delivered by the vaginal route may be in the form of a vaginal suppository (e.g., miconazole [Monistat-7] vaginal suppositories), tablet (e.g., nystatin vaginal tablets), cream (e.g., terconazole [Terazol 3]), ointment (tioconazole [Vagistat-1]), gel (e.g., nonoxynol [Ortho-Gynol Contraceptive]), or solution (e.g., Massengill Douche). A contraceptive ring, ethinylestradiol (NuvaRing), and a hormone-replacement ring, estradiol (Femring), are examples of vaginal rings, one of the newer vaginal drug delivery forms.

Drug effect may be limited to the vagina, as it is when vaginal medications are used to treat vaginal infections, or the drug may be absorbed into the bloodstream and delivered to another part of the body where the drug takes effect. Dinoprostone vaginal suppositories (Prostin E2), used to stimulate uterine contractions, is an example of a drug administered vaginally to produce systemic effects in another part of the body (the uterus).

Otic. The otic route is used to deliver drugs into the ear canal. Otic drugs can be formulated as solutions or suspensions. Local conditions of the ear, such as ear infections or excessive earwax, may be treated with otically administered drugs.

Safety First The term "aural" may also be used to refer to delivery of medications into the ear canal. However, even though the term aural (into the ear) is spelled differently than the term oral (by mouth), it is difficult to distinguish between the two when the two terms are heard. Use care when interpreting verbal orders for these routes of administration.

Ophthalmic. Drugs given via the ophthalmic route are administered onto the exterior surface of the eye. The ophthalmic route differs from the intravitreous route in that medications administered ophthalmically are applied only to the surface of the eye. They are not directly injected *into* the eye, like those administered intravitreously.

Ophthalmic medications are formulated as solutions, suspensions, gels, or ointments. Special medicated inserts (e.g., hydroxypropyl cellulose [Lacrisert]) placed in the pouch of the lower eyelid can also be used to deliver medications to treat conditions of the eye. The ophthalmic route is advantageous in that diseases of the eye, such as glaucoma and infections of the conjunctiva, can be treated without administering the drug systemically. As a result, medication can reach the intended site without exposing the patient to unnecessary side effects in other parts of the body.

Nasal. Drugs are administered into the nostrils by the nasal route. Solutions can be nasally administered as sprays or drops. This route enables conditions of the nose, such as nasal congestion or allergic rhinitis, to be treated without administering the drug systemically. Azelastin (Astelin) is an example of a nasal spray that treats nasal symptoms caused by allergies. Often, drugs given nasally act more quickly and with fewer side effects than those administered by another route, such as orally or intravenously, which introduces medication into the whole body. In other cases, drugs may be administered nasally to treat conditions not involving the nose (e.g., nicotine [Nicotrol NS] as an aid in smoking cessation).

Inhalation. Drugs can be inhaled through the mouth into the lungs. This route is used when a rapid drug effect is desired to treat lung conditions or when a local effect in the lungs is desired. The inhalation route is most often used to deliver medications for the treatment of asthma or COPD. Examples of inhaled drugs include the over-the-counter product epinephrine aerosol (Primatene Mist), the prescription drug albuterol (Proventil), and the nicotine (Nicotrol) inhaler, which is used to aid in smoking cessation.

Dosage Form versus Route of Administration

A particular medication dosage form often implies a specific administration route, and a particular route often implies a specific dosage form. For instance, the tablet dosage form is most often administered orally, although it is also used to administer drugs intravaginally. When the rectal route is used, the suppository is the dosage form commonly considered. However, suppositories are not the only dosage form used for the rectal route, because many medications are formulated as rectal foams or enemas.

Sometimes a dosage form intended for use via one route may be delivered through another route when other options or routes are impractical or infeasible. For example, oral morphine tablets may be administered rectally to terminally ill cancer patients who are unable to swallow and do not have intravenous access. Finally, as discussed previously, one term may be used to describe both a route and a dosage form—for example, the terms sublingual and buccal.

Safety First A pharmacist should always be consulted when a medication is being considered for administration via a route other than that for which it is intended. Some medications may not be suitable for use via non-intended routes. When a medication is used for conditions or administered via routes which the Food and Drug Administration (FDA) did not originally approve for the medication, its use is considered "off-label."

Many drugs are available in a number of dosage forms and may be delivered via a number of administration routes. In some cases, a condition may be treated by using two or more routes. For example, meningitis, an infection of the brain, may be treated with antibiotics administered intravenously or intraventricularly. Medication for glaucoma, a condition of the eye, may be administered directly into the eye with ophthalmic drops or systemically with oral capsules. Physicians and pharmacists select the most appropriate dosage form and route based on the patient's condition, need for immediate drug action, or availability of a drug in a particular dosage form or administration route.

Summary

Medications are available in many dosage forms and may be administered by a variety of routes. By carefully considering the desired effects of a medication, its potential undesired effects, and a patient's characteristics and situation, the best combination of dosage form and route of administration route is selected. This results in optimal use of the medication and guarantees that the patient will receive the maximal benefit with minimal side effects.

Self-Assessment Questions

1. Which of the following is the vehicle in an aqueous solution?
   a. ethyl alcohol
   b. water
   c. propylene glycol
   d. glycerin
2. For which of the following situations would a liquid medication dosage form be a better choice than a solid one?
   a. A patient has just had throat surgery and cannot easily swallow.
   b. A traveling salesman needs to take a medication on a regular basis.
   c. A patient is very sensitive to unpleasant tastes and refuses to take "bad-tasting" medicine.
   d. An elderly patient has a hand tremor.
3. The intravenous route of administration may be advantageous over the oral route for what reason?
   a. There is less chance of bacterial contamination in the bloodstream.
   b. The drug effects are easily reversed if too high a dose is given.
   c. Rapid IV administration of a drug may avoid adverse effects such as low blood pressure or feelings of warmth.
   d. The drug is available to immediately act in the body.
4. Medication administered by the intravenous route means that the medication is injected directly into
   a. a ventricle of the heart.
   b. an eye.
   c. a vein.
   d. a ventricle of the brain.
5. A parenteral route of medication administration is one that bypasses
   a. the gastrointestinal tract.
   b. the heart and circulatory system.
   c. the kidneys.
   d. the skin barrier.
6. Injection of a drug into a joint, such as the knee or elbow, is known as the ________ route of medication administration.
   a. intra-arterial
   b. intrapleural
   c. intra-articular
   d. intravesicular
7. Which of the following is NOT an advantage of oral liquid medication dosage forms?
   a. Oral liquid medication dosage forms usually are faster-acting than solid medication dosage forms.
   b. Oral liquid medication dosage forms may be easier to take for a patient who has difficulty swallowing than an oral solid medication dosage form.
   c. Oral liquid medication dosage forms may be used in cases where solid medication dosage forms are not practical to administer.
   d. Drug particles are present in oral liquid medications and come in contact with the taste buds of the tongue.
8. A local effect is one that occurs
   a. at a site distant from the point at which the medication enters the body.
   b. throughout the body.
   c. as a result of absorption of the medication into the body.
   d. in the area where the medication is applied or administered.
9. Which of the following statements about water-in-oil (W/O) emulsions is false?
   a. W/O emulsions are often used on unbroken skin.
   b. W/O emulsions spread more evenly than O/W emulsions because the natural oils on the skin readily mix with the external phase.
   c. W/O emulsions soften the skin better than O/W emulsions because they retain moisture and are not readily washed off with water.
   d. W/O emulsions are water-washable and do not stain clothing.
10. Drugs that are administered on the surface of the eye are given by the __________ route.
    a. otic
    b. ophthalmic
    c. oral
    d. aural

Part 2

Self-Assessment Answers

1. b. The term "aqueous" refers to water. Ethyl alcohol, glycerin, and propylene glycol are all examples of nonaqueous vehicles.
2. a. Liquids are a good option for patients who have difficulty swallowing oral solid medication dosage forms. Liquids mask tastes less effectively than other oral dosage forms. They may spill or leak, require a measuring device, or need refrigeration, so they are less convenient for travelers or for patients who may have difficulty pouring or measuring a fluid.
3. d. Drugs given via the IV route are immediately available to act in the body. The IV route is more easily contaminated by bacteria and less easily reversed. Rapid administration may be more likely to produce adverse effects, and slowing the infusion rate may avoid these effects.
4. c. "Intravenous" refers to administration into the vein. The ventricle of the heart (intracardiac), the eye (intravitreous), and the ventricle of the brain (intraventricular) are other routes of administration.
5. a. Parenteral means bypassing the "enteral" or gastrointestinal system.
6. c. "Intra-articular" refers to injection into a joint. Intra-arterial (into an artery), intrapleural (inside the sac surrounding the lungs, the pleura), and intravesicular (into the urinary bladder) are other routes of administration.
7. d. Particles of some drugs in liquids are able to come into contact with taste buds on the tongue. When this happens, some patients may experience an unpleasant taste or sensation on their tongues.
8. d. A local effect is confined to the area where the medication comes into contact with a part of the body. The other options describe a systemic effect.
9. d. Because water is emulsified within an oil base in W/O emulsions, they resist washing with water but do adhere to the skin and may stain clothing.
10. b. "Ophthalmic" refers to the eye. "Otic" and "aural" both refer to the ear, and oral administration is by mouth.

References

Allen LV, ed. *Pharmaceutical Dosage Forms and Drug Delivery Systems*. 8th ed. Baltimore, MD: Lippincott Williams & Wilkins; 2004.

University of the Sciences in Philadelphia. *Remington: The Science and Practice of Pharmacy.* 21st ed. Baltimore, MD: Lippincott Williams & Wilkins; 2006.

Part Three

Practice Basics

This section includes the chapters directly related to processing, preparing and dispensing prescriptions and medication orders. It also includes a chapter on Calculations and Medication Errors, which are essential for safe and accurate medication use.

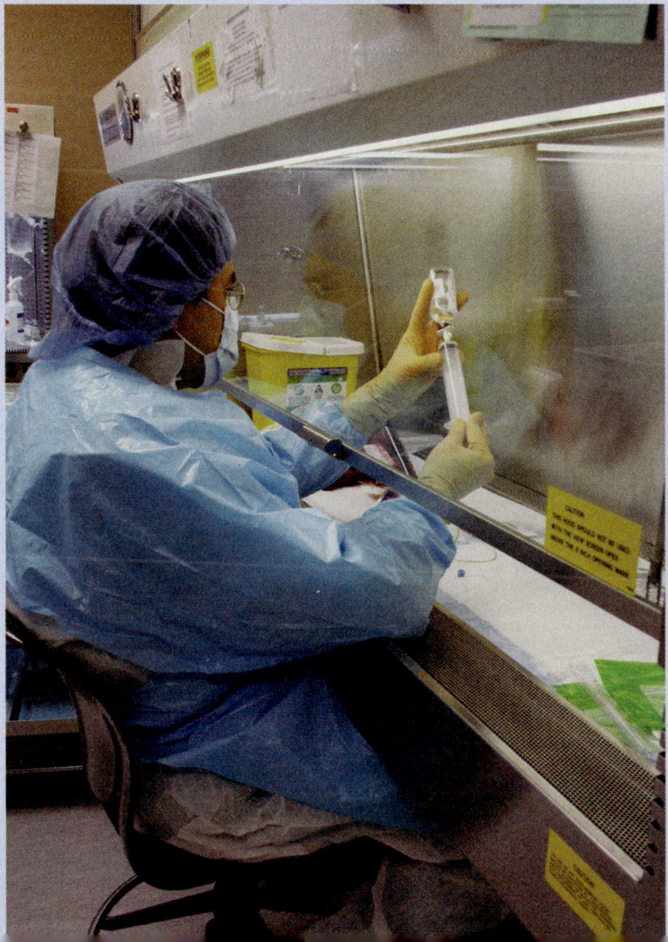

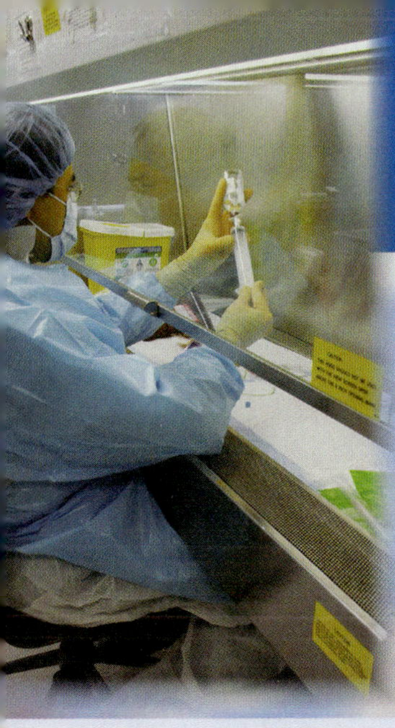

Chapter 13

Processing Medication Orders and Prescriptions

Christopher M. Kutza

Learning Outcomes

After completing this chapter you will be able to

- Identify the components of a complete prescription or medication order.
- Prioritize prescriptions and medication orders on the basis of pertinent criteria.
- Describe the necessary steps in processing a prescription or medication order.
- List the information that is typically contained in a patient profile.
- Identify the information that is necessary to make a medication label complete.

Key Terms

automated dispensing technology Electronic storage cabinets or robotics that secure medications and dispense them to nurses or other caregivers when needed.

auxiliary prescription label A label affixed to a drug product that alerts users to special handling or administration concerns.

centralized dispensing automation Technology that assists in the selection and dispensing of drug products that are located in a central location, such as the pharmacy, and that can include robotics and carousels that use bar code scanning to select and label drug products for patients.

computer physician order entry (CPOE) The entering of patient orders directly into a computer system.

decentralized automation system Drug distribution devices placed in patient care areas.

electronic medication administration record (eMAR) A component of the computerized patient medical record in which nurses and other healthcare providers document times and dates when a medication was administered to the patient.

medication administration record (MAR) A component of the paper patient medical record in which nurses and other healthcare providers document times and dates when a medication was administered to the patient.

medication order A written, electronic, telephone, or verbal request for a patient medication in an inpatient setting.

mnemonic A shorthand name for a drug product that facilitates faster computer data entry.

patient identification number A unique code number that identifies a given patient (for example, a medical record number) or a patient and specific admission date (for example, an account number).

patient profile A list of information about a patient, including name, identification number, date of birth, sex, height, weight, lab values, admitting and secondary diagnoses, room and bed number, names of admitting and consulting physicians, allergies, medication history, special considerations, and clinical comments.

primary prescription label A label, affixed to a dispensed drug product, that contains legally required information, including pharmacy name and address, patient name, prescriber name, drug name, directions for use, date dispensed, cautionary statements, sequential prescription number, initials or name of dispensing pharmacist, quantity dispensed, number of refills, expiration date, and lot number.

STAT Abbreviation of the Latin word *statim,* meaning immediately; commonly used on medication orders to indicate the need for the drug right away.

This chapter describes the pharmacy technician's role in evaluating and processing medication orders and prescriptions from the time they are received until the medications leave the pharmacy. The differences between the process in the inpatient and outpatient settings are described as well, although the reader should refer to the separate chapters on specific settings (in Part I of this textbook) to achieve a complete understanding of the topic.

Typically, the term **medication order** refers to a physician's written, electronic, telephone, or verbal request for a medication in an inpatient setting. This order is part of the patient's medical record. The term "prescription" refers to a medication order on a prescription blank that is transmitted in writing, verbally, or electronically to be filled in an outpatient or ambulatory care setting. Medication orders and prescriptions both represent means for the prescriber to give instructions to the dispenser of the medication (i.e., the pharmacy), the individuals who will be administering it (i.e., nurses), and/or the patients who will be taking it.

The specific roles fulfilled by technicians vary by practice site. This text assumes that technicians will perform all processes they may legally be allowed to perform, which requires a basic understanding of medication order processing activities. Actually performing these functions also requires specialized training in the procedures of the specific practice site, such as the use of the organization's computer system or manual record-keeping system.

Inpatient Pharmacies

The following section discusses processes and considerations for receiving and processing medication orders in an inpatient hospital setting.

Receiving Medication Orders

Medication orders come to the pharmacy in various ways. Figure 13-1 shows an example of a written **medication order**. Orders are hand-delivered to the pharmacy or one of its satellites or are sent via a mechanical method, such as fax transmission or pneumatic tube. Some institutions utilize technology that allows a scanned image of a written order to be transmitted to the pharmacy for processing (figure 13-2). Medication orders may also be entered directly into the computer system by the prescriber, which is commonly referred to as **computer physician order entry,** or **CPOE** (see section on CPOE later in this chapter for more information).

Orders may be telephoned to the pharmacy by either the prescriber or an intermediary, such as a nurse. Legal restrictions are placed on who may telephone in an order or a prescription and who may receive that information in the pharmacy, particularly when controlled substances are involved. Technicians should consult their employer's policies and procedures or their job descriptions to determine what restrictions apply in their particular practice setting. Many states require that prescriptions be phoned in by the prescriber or a licensed professional operating under the prescriber's authority. It is also common to require that a pharmacist or another licensed professional receive telephone prescriptions.

Upon receipt of a medication order, two steps should be taken. The first is to review the order for clarity and completeness. The second is to prioritize the order on the basis of a number of factors, including the time the

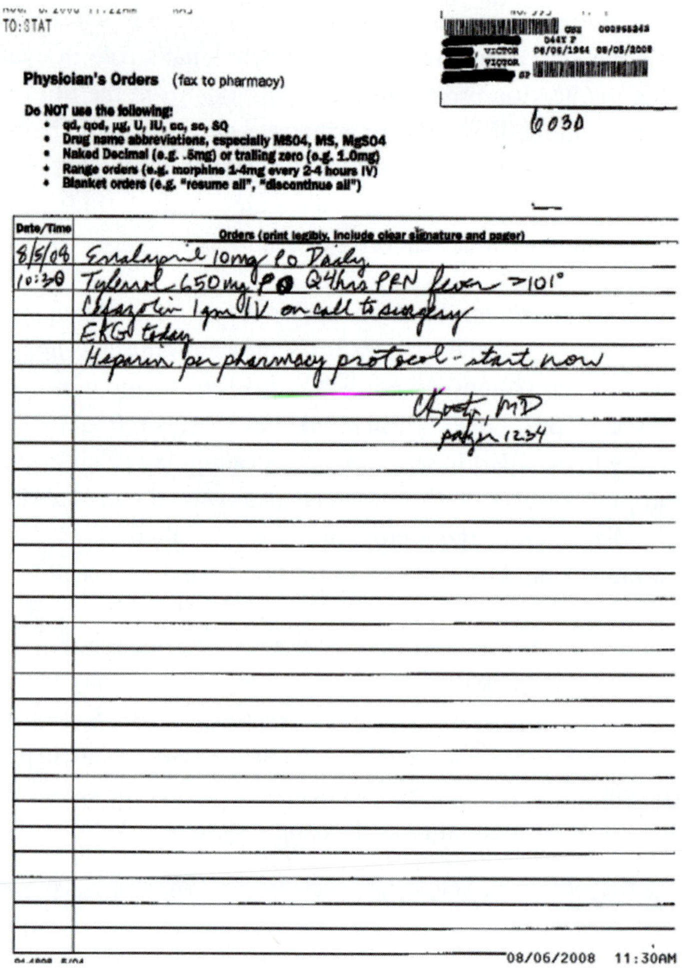
TO:STAT

[redacted] 044Y F
VICTOR 06/08/1964 08/05/2008

6030

Physician's Orders (fax to pharmacy)

Do NOT use the following:
- qd, qod, μg, U, IU, cc, sc, SQ
- Drug name abbreviations, especially MSO4, MS, MgSO4
- Naked Decimal (e.g. .5mg) or trailing zero (e.g. 1.0mg)
- Range orders (e.g. morphine 1-4mg every 2-4 hours IV)
- Blanket orders (e.g. "resume all", "discontinue all")

Date/Time	Orders (print legibly, include clear signature and pager)
8/5/08	Enalapril 10mg PO Daily
10:30	Tylenol 650mg PO Q4hrs PRN fever >101°
	Cefazolin 1gm IV on call to surgery
	EKG today
	Heparin per pharmacy protocol - start now
	[illegible], MD
	pager 1234

08/06/2008 11:30AM

Figure 13-1. Sample written inpatient medication order from a medication chart.

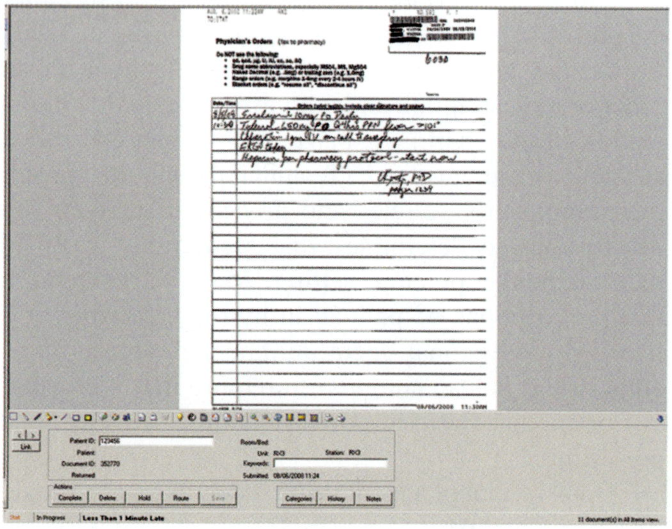

Figure 13-2. Sample image from order scanning technology.

medication is needed, the seriousness of the condition that is being treated, and the urgency of the other medication orders waiting to be processed.

Clarity and Completeness. When a new order is received, the first step is to ensure that it is clear and complete. Ideally, every medication order contains the following elements:

- Patient name, hospital identification number, and room/bed location
- Generic drug name (it is recommended that generic drug names be used, and many institutions have policies to this effect.)

- Brand drug name (if a specific product is required)
- Route of administration (with some orders, the site of administration should also be specified.)
- Dosage form
- Dose/strength
- Frequency and duration of administration (if duration is pertinent; may be open-ended)
- Rate and time of administration, if applicable
- Indication for use of the medication
- Other instructions for the person administering the medication, such as whether it should be given with food or on an empty stomach
- Prescriber's name/signature and credentials (some hospitals require a printed name, physician number, or pager number in addition to the signature, to assist with identification.)
- Signature and credentials of person writing the order, if other than prescriber
- Date and time of the order

Some of this information is required by state law or by policy. As shown in figure 13-1, however, not all of the elements are included in every order.

If information is missing—for example, the room number—the technician may be allowed to clarify the order without pharmacist intervention. However, most clarifications must involve the pharmacist. For example, the pharmacist may wish to discuss with the prescriber the choice of medication, the dose, or a potential drug interaction. When an order is deferred for clarification, it is important to make sure the other caregivers (e.g., the nurse waiting to administer the medication) are aware of any anticipated delays.

Prioritization. Once orders are deemed clear and complete, they must be prioritized so that the most urgent orders are filled first. Prioritizing orders means comparing the urgency of new orders with the urgency of all of the orders requiring attention. Prioritizing ensures that the most-needed orders will be processed first. Technicians can prioritize orders by evaluating the route, time of administration, type of drug, intended use of the drug, and patient-specific circumstances.

For example, an order for phenylephrine, a medication used intravenously to maintain blood pressure in critically ill patients, would usually receive priority over an order for an orally administered stool softener. Remember to think of patient needs first.

Rx for Success

Additional clues about urgency can be gleaned from the orders themselves. For example, when surgery or diagnostic procedure is indicated, such as in this order: "Give 1 gram cefazolin IVPB 30 minutes prior to incision," the technician can consult the operating room schedule to determine the priority of the order.

Some orders are designated as **STAT** (abbreviation of *statim,* Latin for *immediately*), which indicates an urgent need. A prescriber may also designate that a medication is to be started "now" or "ASAP" (as soon as possible), or simply state "start today" or "start this morning."

It is also necessary to consider whether a medication might already have been started prior to the pharmacy's receipt of the order—a first dose of an antibiotic administered in the emergency room prior to the patient's admission, for example. If no apparent urgency or specific time is denoted in the order, it may receive a lower priority. Most pharmacies designate a standard amount of time it should take to process and deliver an order. A typical turnaround time for filling an order in an institutional setting might be 15 minutes for a STAT order and 1 hour for a routine order.

If no specific designation about the urgency of a medication is given in the body of the order, technicians can use critical thinking skills to prioritize orders. Most of the decisions involved in prioritizing orders require some basic knowledge of the drugs and common sense. It is also helpful for technicians to be familiar with their hospital's specific policies regarding prioritization of orders. Some hospitals, for example, treat all orders from a particular unit—such as an intensive care unit—as urgent. Many hospitals have designated administration times for certain drugs, such as warfarin, that may alter prioritization of the order depending on the time the order is received. Policies vary by pharmacy, and technicians need to become familiar with the system of prioritization used at their institution.

✔ Medications ordered for the initial treatment of pain, fever, or nausea and vomiting are generally high priority because of the desire to relieve the patient's discomfort. A regularly scheduled vitamin, on the other hand, would be a lower priority.

Processing Medication Orders

After an order has been received, determined to be clear and complete, and prioritized, it is ready to be processed. Processing usually involves a computer, but some pharmacies still use a manual system (typewriters, pen and paper, profile cards, or notebooks). The discussion in this chapter focuses on computerized operations.

A number of steps are involved in processing an order. First, the patient must be positively identified to avoid dispensing medication to the wrong patient. Second, the order typically is compared against the patient's existing medication profile, or a new profile is created for the patient. Then, a number of order entry steps occur to update the patient's medication profile. These steps include such tasks as choosing the correct medication from the database, identifying the administration schedule, and entering any special instructions (later in this section, a step-by-step procedure walks the technician through the order entry process). Finally, the medication must be selected, prepared or compounded, checked, and dispensed for use.

Identifying the Patient. Identifying the patient entails comparing the patient identification on the medication order to the one in the patient profile system (i.e., the patient's computer record) to make sure they match. Although it may seem like a very elementary task, its importance cannot be overstated, and the technician must pay an appropriate level of attention to this detail—particularly when dealing with very common names.

In an institutional setting, **patient identification numbers** are generally used. Most commonly, patients are identified by two numbers: a unique medical record number that distinguishes patients from one another, and an account number that is specific to a transaction or set of transactions, such as an individual hospitalization. A patient's medical record number never changes, but account numbers change every time a patient is admitted to an institution. The account number may also be known by other names, such as a billing number, a financial number, or an admission number.

Technology Topics

Some institutions are now using bar codes or magnetic strips to facilitate accuracy in verifying patient identification. As more hospitals employ electronic charting, the use of bar-coded or magnetic strip patient identifiers will play a larger role.

In the meantime, many hospitals rely on a computer-generated adhesive label that is affixed to the documents or a printed name that is generated by an addressograph (a raised-letter registration card similar to a credit card).

When entering the order into the computer or other patient record, it is important to make sure the patient name matches the number and vice versa. It is easy to make errors when keying in numbers, and some patients may have the same or very similar names. Occasionally, orders get marked with the wrong patient name, and checking the profile may prevent this error from causing any harm to the patient.

✔Because of the possibility of an order being marked with the wrong patient name, it is vital to ensure that each order makes sense for the patient by checking the order against the patient profile.

For example, an order for oxytocin (a medication typically used to induce labor in pregnant women) placed for an elderly male patient would warrant an investigation by the pharmacist to determine if it was ordered for the wrong patient.

Creating, Maintaining, and Reviewing Patient Profiles. The pharmacy's **patient profile** is a fundamental tool that pharmacists use in reviewing orders. It is vital that pharmacists and technicians build and review patient profiles while they are processing medication orders. The following information is generally found in the hospital pharmacy's patient profile, although system capabilities may limit access to some components:

- Patient name and identification numbers
- Date of birth or age
- Sex
- Height and weight
- Lab values, such as serum creatinine
- Admitting and secondary diagnoses (including pregnancy and lactation status)
- Room and bed number
- Names of admitting and consulting physicians
- Allergies
- Medication history (current and discontinued medications; medications from a previous admission, if applicable)
- Special considerations (e.g., foreign language, disability)

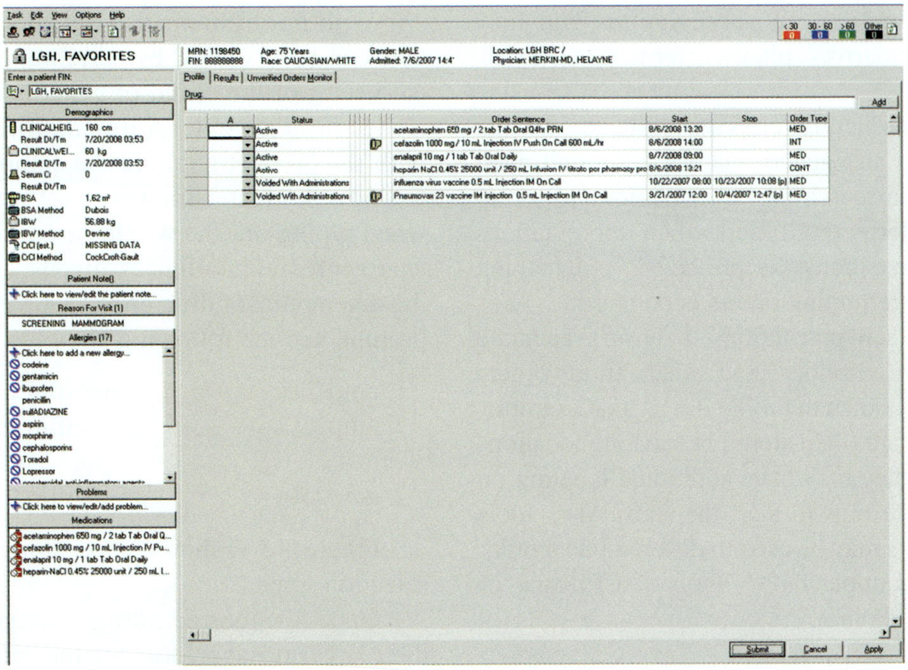

Figure 13-3. Sample patient profile.

- Clinical comments (e.g., therapeutic monitoring, counseling notes)

Figure 13-3 shows an example of a patient profile.

Before medication orders are entered into a patient's profile, the profile should be reviewed in relation to the changes indicated on the new orders. In some cases, information in the profile may raise questions about whether the patient should receive the medication as it is prescribed. For example, the patient may be allergic to the medication or may already be on a similar medication. In addition, the profile may contain information that changes how the order will be processed or prioritized. For example, a new order may simply represent a change in administration time that does not require any additional dispensing. A technician who suspects that the prescribed medication is inappropriate for the patient should consult the pharmacist or follow the pharmacy's standard procedure for order clarification.

Processing medication orders involves adding a medication to a patient's regimen or modifying or discontinuing a previously ordered medication. Computerized systems make processing orders faster and more accurate because patient profiles can be easily created or modified and medication labels quickly printed, all within a single step. In manual systems, two separate steps are needed: the patient's profile is modified, and the medication labels are typed or handwritten separately. Generally, for safety reasons, labels and medication administration records (MARs, discussed later in the chapter) are not produced until the medication order entry/transcription process has been completed and verified.

Order Entry Steps. This next section will describe the steps involved in entering a medication order into the pharmacy computer system.

Selecting the Drug Product. Once the order has been compared against the profile, the technician can proceed with selecting the drug product indicated on the medication order. It is recommended that prescribers order drug products by generic name instead of brand name. However, drug products are often prescribed by either or both names, which can result in confusion. Abbreviations, although best avoided, are also sometimes used in ordering medications. Certain abbreviations have been associated with contributing to medication errors because their meaning can be confusing. Therefore, many institutions have implemented lists of abbreviations that *cannot* be used when ordering medications. Some examples of unapproved abbreviations might include MSO4 for morphine sulfate or QD for daily. In these instances, the full word or drug name must be spelled out. For more information on abbreviations and how they can contribute to errors, please refer to Chapter 17, Medication Errors.

Selecting drug products requires a working knowledge of both brand names and generic names (although most computer systems can search for either name) and a sensible approach to interpreting orders when abbreviations are used. Patient safety must be protected, and making assumptions when interpreting orders is dangerous. Most pharmacies take special precautions to ensure accurate interpretation of prescriptions and medication orders involving look-alike and sound-alike drugs. For example, drugs that look alike are often stored in separate locations in the pharmacy, or they may have additional labeling on the product or storage bins to alert the staff. Also, tools such as tall man letters may be used to differentiate similar looking names (for example, buPROPion – busPIRone, or niCARdipine – NIFEdipine).

Safety First When in doubt about a drug name or an abbreviation, it is always best to have the pharmacist clarify the order with the prescriber, or with the person who wrote the order if it is a telephone order.

With most pharmacy computer systems, drug products can be reviewed by scrolling through an alphabetical listing of the brand or generic names or by entering a code or mnemonic. A **mnemonic** is a code, associated with the product name in the computer, that allows one to find a product using fewer keystrokes than is required when typing out the whole name. For example, to enter an order for ampicillin 250 mg, the technician might enter the mnemonic, or drug code, "amp250," at the drug name prompt, and the following choices would appear:

1. amp250c — ampicillin 250 mg capsule
2. amp250s — ampicillin 250 mg/5 mL oral suspension
3. amp250i — ampicillin 250 mg injection

Figure 13-4 shows an example of a drug product selection screen.

Once the correct drug and strength are located, the correct dosage form for the route of administration must be selected. If the order were for a 250 mg/5 mL suspension, the proper choice above would be number 2. Choosing the correct dosage form is not only important for the purposes of dispensing, but also, the dosage form often determines the type of label that prints from the

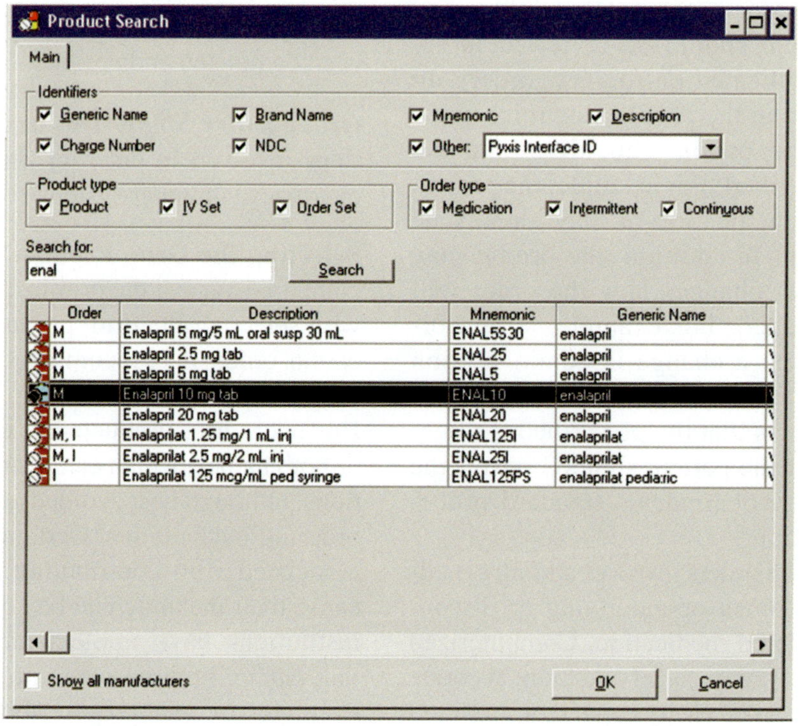

Figure 13-4. Sample drug product selection screen.

pharmacy computer system. For example, an IV label format is generally very different from a unit dose tablet label format, and it includes different information (such as an expiration date for IV products).

Multiple dosage forms of the drug may make sense for an order. For example, the order "ampicillin 250mg po q6h" could be entered using either the capsule, for someone who can swallow pills, or the suspension, for someone who may have trouble swallowing a pill. Patient and caregiver considerations must be taken into account when choosing the form of the drug to dispense. For example, when providing an oral medication, checking with the nurse or parent to determine if an older child would prefer to swallow tablets or take a liquid medication is a common practice. Providing liquid forms of oral medications when patients are receiving drugs through tubes (e.g., nasogastric tubes or gastric tubes) is another example of tailoring dispensing to the needs of patients and caregivers.

In many institutions, the technician may enter only those drugs approved for use in the institution (i.e., formulary drugs). Input from the pharmacist is required to process an order for a medication that is not on the institution's formulary (i.e., non-formulary drugs).

Many computer systems fire an alert if the operator attempts to enter medications that interact with preexisting orders, conflict with the patient's drug allergies, or represent therapeutic duplications. Many systems also check the dosage range and fire an alert if the operator enters a dose that exceeds the recommended dose for that patient. Although these alert systems help prevent errors, they are not always relevant to the patient's situation. Therefore, the technician should consult the pharmacist if an alert fires. The pharmacist may bypass the alert on the basis of his or her professional judgment or may call the prescriber to discuss the alert. Technicians should know and follow the procedure at their practice site regarding computer alerts.

In addition to choosing the correct drug product, some other related choices are included in this step. For example, if an IV medication is being entered, it might be necessary to choose the correct diluent into which the drug should be mixed. Most hospitals have standard diluents that are used for IV compounding, and in a computerized system the diluent will often automatically be specified with the drug.

Another decision is the choice of the correct package type and size, such as bulk or unit dose, 15-gram tube or 30-gram tube, and 100-mL bottle or 150-mL bottle.

Scheduling Medication Administration Times. The medication administration time can have an impact on drug efficacy and other treatment factors, such as diagnostic laboratory testing, and this impact can be important for some medications. The timing of gentamicin in relation to a laboratory test to measure the amount of drug circulating in the blood, for example, is important because it might affect the blood level result and subsequent dosing recommendation by the pharmacist or physician. Many drugs should be given at specific times in relation to meals for the best effect.

In institutions, standard medication administration times are generally set. These times are often defined by institutional policy or by a drug therapy protocol. Such policies and protocols may define times for common dosing frequencies. For example, daily = 0900 (9 a.m.), bid = 0900 and 1700 (5 p.m.), and every 8 hours = 0600 (6 a.m.), 1400 (2 p.m.), and 2200 (10 p.m.). A specific administration time may be specified for certain drugs; for example, warfarin may be administered at a set time each day (e.g., 1700) to allow enough time to review lab results from the morning and to make changes to the dose if necessary. Standardized schedules of drug administration are usually based on therapeutic issues, nursing and pharmacy efficiency, or coordination of services. Pharmacy, nursing, and the hospital's medical staff usually agree on standard administration schedules and protocols. Many pharmacies have a written document that staff can refer to when the appropriate administration time is unclear. These times are usually conveyed on the pharmacy's patient profile, on medication labels, and on the **medication administration record (MAR).** The MAR is the part of the patient's medical record in which the caregiver (generally the nurse) documents when medications ordered for a patient are administered. Pharmacy technicians should be aware of standardized medication administration times.

Standardized administration times usually appear as default entries associated with a particular drug or administration schedule that was selected in the computer during the order entry process. This means that if a "bid" administration schedule were entered for a particular drug, the computer would automatically assign its default administration times, which might be 0900 and 1700.

Default time schedules may differ on some specialized nursing units. For example, scheduling for "daily" may default to 0900; however, a physical rehabilitation unit might require daily administration to occur at 0800 so as not to interfere with physical therapy. During order

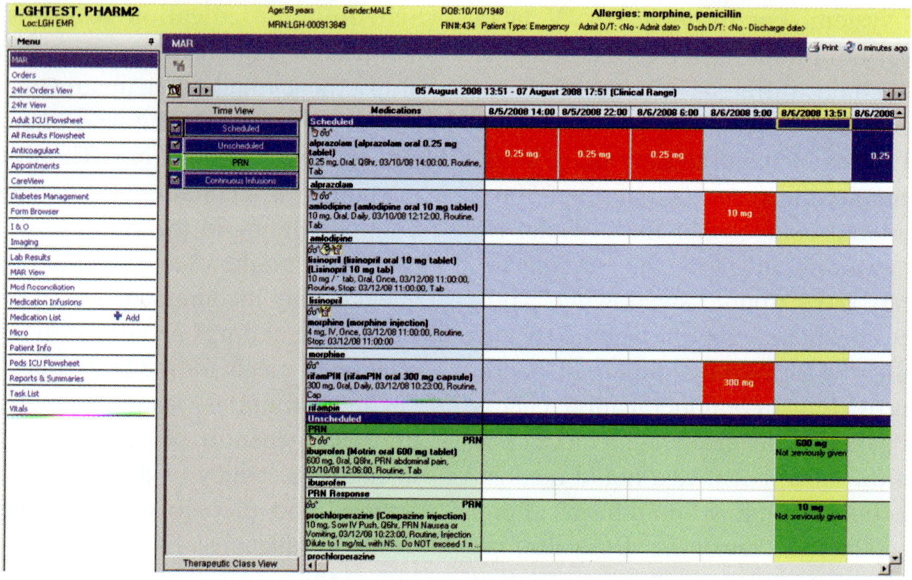

Figure 13–5. Sample electronic medication administration record (eMAR).

entry, the technician must be aware of such exceptions and change the default entries when necessary.

When scheduling medication administration times for a new medication, pharmacists also must consider other medications the patient is taking. For example, if a patient is taking both ciprofloxacin and calcium carbonate, there must be an adequate amount of time between the doses of each agent. If these medications are taken too close together, the calcium carbonate can reduce the amount of ciprofloxacin the patient absorbs. The resulting reduced absorption of ciprofloxacin could render therapy ineffective.

Another consideration is the day or days of the week that a medication is due. Medications are sometimes ordered to be given every other day, every three days, or once per week. In these cases, it is important to coordinate with the patient's home schedule if this is a continuation of home therapy. One must also be careful with every-other-day orders, to avoid advising the caregiver to give the medication on odd days or even days, because depending on the number of days in a month, "every other day" will change with respect to odd/even.

Special Instructions. The prescriber's directions for proper use of the medication must be conveyed clearly and accurately. In the institutional setting, the style used to convey the prescriber's directions is geared toward another healthcare professional at the bedside. Medical abbreviations tend to be used, and information may be provided in a kind of shorthand that might be difficult for a patient to interpret. As shown later in this chapter in the discussion of ambulatory care, the style is vastly different when the end user is a patient or family member.

In institutions, physicians' orders are input into the patient profile in the pharmacy information system. Then, this information is used to generate MARs for nursing documentation (figure 13-5), medication profiles and fill lists (for pharmacy use), and labels for medications to be issued to patient care areas (figure 13-6). Because only healthcare personnel will use this information, the directions for use may contain only the name of the medication, strength, dose and schedule, and administration

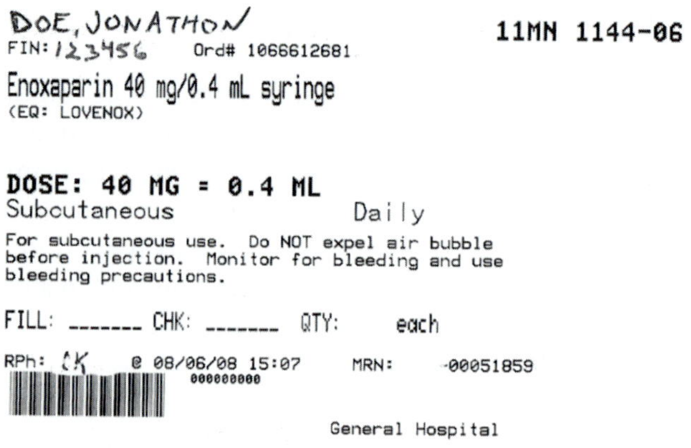

Figure 13–6. Sample medication label for inpatient use.

times, much of which may be written in medical terminology and Latin abbreviations.

It is important to note that MARs may be either paper or electronic. Electronic systems are more common and allow for efficient transfer and sharing of information among the physician, pharmacist, and bedside nurse. For example, in an electronic system, medications will appear on the **electronic medication administration record (eMAR)** the moment they are entered into the computer system. Also, healthcare providers can determine from the record exactly when a medication has been administered and by whom, simply by pulling it up on the computer. A traditional paper system would require going to the bedside or nursing unit to review the record.

Additional instructions for the nurses are often entered into the pharmacy information system for presentation on one of the many documents printed from the profile (or for the nurses' use in an electronic system) or simply as additional information for the pharmacists' use at a later time. These special instructions might include storage information, such as the need to refrigerate, or administration instructions, such as how fast to give an IV push injection. Another example would be physician-specified parameters for use, such as "hold if systolic blood pressure is less than 100 mm Hg" or "repeat in 1 hour if ineffective." These types of instructions would typically be displayed on the MAR and also on the medication label.

Many pharmacy systems also allow for notes between the pharmacist and the technician to be displayed only on a fill list or work list. These instructions might include something like "reconstitute with normal saline only."

Most systems include a field or location in the pharmacy patient profile system where pharmacists can note clinical comments. Such comments may include indications for use, incidents of adverse drug reactions, laboratory values, or any other information that may help the pharmacist provide pharmaceutical care. During the initial screening and evaluation of the drug order, for example, the pharmacy technician might notice in the clinical comments field that therapeutic monitoring may be needed or that recent monitoring parameters are outside normal limits. To ensure safe and effective drug therapy, the technician should alert the pharmacist to such situations as soon as possible.

The last step in the order entry process is generally an acceptance (also called verification or validation) function in which the pharmacist verifies that the order is correctly entered for the right patient and is clinically appropriate. Once this step is completed, the medication order is released for preparation and dispensing. This is generally the point at which labels and other documents are generated, although some systems allow printing prior to pharmacist validation.

Sample Inpatient Order Entry. Inpatient order entry usually proceeds as follows (see written order example in figure 13-1 and sample order entry screen in figure 13-7):

1. *Enter the patient's name or account number, and verify the patient.* To begin, key in the account number or the name. Compare the patient profile to the written medication order to verify that the patient represented on the screen is the one for whom the order was written.
2. *Compare the order to the patient profile in detail.* The order to be entered is "enalapril 10 mg PO daily." Check for general appropriateness of the order; it should make sense with regard to patient profile information, such as the patient's age, allergy profile, and drugs currently being taken. Note that the patient's allergies are sometimes listed on the physician's order form. It is useful to check this information against the patient's profile to make sure they agree.
3. *Enter the drug.* Go into the order entry mode, and type in the drug mnemonic or find the drug in an alphabetical listing. For example, typing "enal" might result in a short list of enalapril products to select from, whereas typing "enal10" (the mnemonic for enalapril 10-mg tablets, as in the example) might result in a match for the specific product. After the product has been selected, most systems check for drug interactions, therapeutic duplication, and drug allergies. At this point, department policy determines what action the technician should take if an alert occurs. Once interaction checks are cleared, the computer will show the drug on the screen, and order entry may proceed.
4. *Verify the dose.* Check the dose on the order against the drug product entered. Most computer systems have a field that allows for some modifications here. In the enalapril example, the drug product chosen was a 10-mg tablet, and the dose is 10 mg, so no adjustments are necessary. However, if entering the Tylenol (acetaminophen) order (see figure 13-1), the technician may find only a 325-mg tablet in the computer. Therefore, the dose field would have to be modified to two tablets, which equals 650 mg.

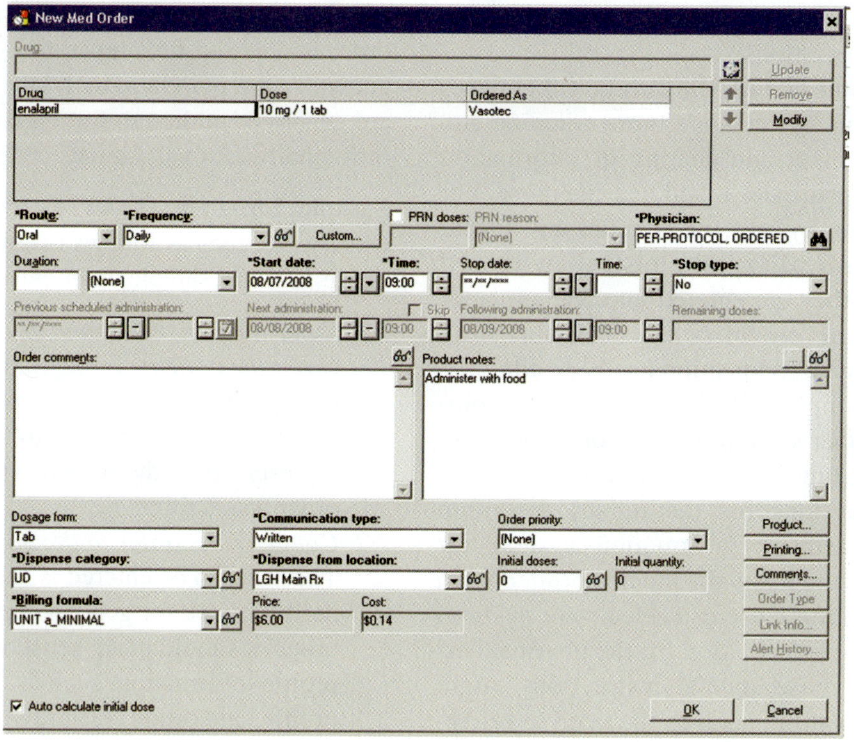

Figure 13–7. Sample inpatient medication computer order entry.

It is important to review all the available products and become familiar with available drug product dosages. For example, if a patient needs 100 mg of a drug and it comes in 10-, 25-, and 50-mg tablet strengths, it would be preferable to give the patient two 50-mg tablets rather than ten 10-mg tablets. Also, the technician should be aware that odd dosages may indicate a prescribing error. In the previous example, if the only available tablet strength were 10 mg, a 100-mg dose would be odd and should be verified by the pharmacist. For another example, if an ordered dose requires multiple vials or tablets or a small fraction of a tablet to prepare, it should be clarified with the pharmacist.

Safety First A good rule of thumb to follow to help determine if a dose might be too high or too low is that if the dose requires less than half of one, or more than two, dosage units (capsules, tablets, vials, etc.), double-check with the pharmacist before continuing. Often the dosage units designed by manufacturers are intended to be a single unit of use or very close to a typical dose.

5. *Enter the administration schedule.* Select the interval (e.g., daily) and the route of administration (e.g., orally, IV, etc).
6. *Enter any comments in the clinical comments field.* In the Tylenol example, "for fever > 101" should be entered as a comment.
7. *Verify the prescriber name.* Depending on the computer system, the accuracy of the prescriber name may need to be verified. Most systems default to the admitting or attending physician, but some allow or require changing to the actual prescriber, who may be the medical resident or a specialist.
8. *Fill and label the medication.* The correct product (e.g., enalapril 10 mg tablets) must be obtained and supplied in the correct quantity with proper labeling. In this case, one or two tablets might be sent in a traditional inpatient setting, depending on the time of day, the time the next dose was due, and the next scheduled filling time. This would vary dramatically, however, depending on the degree and type of automation. Whether dispensing occurs on a patient-specific basis or as part of a batch automated system fill, this is the final opportunity for the technician to check the medication

against the label, the fill list, or the order to ensure accuracy.

Filling, Labeling, and Checking Medications. Once the computer entry has been completed and labels have been generated, the medication order must be filled with the correct quantity of the right drug. Generally, enough doses are sent to provide medication to carry through to the next scheduled delivery time. For example, if the institution is using a 24-hour cart fill system, doses will be sent to account for all administration times up until the next cart delivery occurs. During this step, it is important to review the label carefully against the order and the product to make sure the correct product has been chosen. This is the final opportunity for the pharmacy to catch an error prior to dispensing to a patient care area.

The accuracy of the label should be checked before the medication order is filled. If an order is filled from an inaccurate label and the pharmacy system of checking fails, the wrong product could be dispensed and given to the patient.

When a label seems to indicate an error, the first step is to review the label against the order and profile. Using the example in figure 13-1, if the label indicated a 100-mg enalapril dose, and it were reviewed against the original order, it would be clear that an error was made when the order was entered. The label would be discarded, and the entry in the computer would have to be corrected. If, however, the original order did specify a 100-mg dose, the order should be brought to the attention of the pharmacist. The pharmacist can then evaluate the order and take action to get it corrected if necessary.

Finally, the medication order is filled and left for the pharmacist to check.

✔A pharmacist check is legally required in most cases, and must occur before any drug is dispensed to a patient care area.

Medication orders may need to be filed after they are filled. An advantage of using technology that allows viewing of written order images is that such systems automatically archive all of the orders that are received and allow users to search for specific orders if needed. Policies and legal requirements differ regarding how orders are filed and how long the files have to be maintained. Consult state and federal laws and your organization's policies with regard to these rules.

Special Considerations in Hospital Order Processing. This section will discuss the issues of charge processing as related to orders, pharmacist-performed dosing protocols, diagnostic preparation orders, computer physician order entry, and technology used to automate dispensing.

"Charge-Only" and "No-Charge" Entries. In some situations, order entry into the pharmacy computer system is done for record-keeping or billing purposes only. Technicians are often involved in these practices when charging patients for medications used from floor stock, for example. Most hospitals keep some inventory in floor stock (i.e., inventory stored in a controlled space in the patient care areas) for use as first doses, emergency doses, or convenience medications. When these drugs are used, the pharmacy is generally notified for the purposes of patient charging and floor stock replenishment.

Another situation is the dispensing of medication for which there is no charge but for which record-keeping is still required. An example would be investigational medications, which are often provided free of charge but still need to be accounted for.

A similar situation involves medications brought in from home to be used while a patient is in the hospital. Because they are the patient's property, there is typically no charge for the drugs. However, it is important for the medications to show up on the MAR and in the patient profile so that all caregivers are aware that the patient is receiving the medication and there is a legal record that the doses were administered.

Pharmacist Protocols. Many institutions have developed protocols in which the pharmacist is requested to dose and monitor certain medications. These protocols are used to assist the managing physician in the dosing and monitoring of some medications that require close laboratory monitoring, unique patient-specific doses, and/or small ranges of acceptable blood levels to maintain their therapeutic effect without resulting in toxicity. Examples of pharmacist protocols include heparin, warfarin, and aminoglycoside dosing and monitoring. The prescriber will submit a medication order requesting the specific protocol, which is then executed by the pharmacist. These orders should be given to the pharmacist for processing. Please refer to institution-specific policies and procedures for more details.

Diagnostic Preparation Orders. Many hospitals (as well as some retail pharmacies that are affiliated with a physician's office practice) dispense "preparations" (or preps) for diagnostic procedures. An example might be a colonoscopy prep that includes a large volume of laxative solution to be ingested over a period of several hours. Sometimes these orders are very vague (e.g., "routine prep for colonoscopy"), and the pharmacists and technicians are expected to follow a specific protocol for dispensing medications. These protocols are generally agreed upon by the individual hospital's medical staff and are recorded in policies for everyone's reference.

Computer Physician Order Entry. In many hospitals, instead of handwriting orders, physicians enter orders directly into the hospital's computer system. This is commonly referred to as computer physician order entry (CPOE). Figure 13-8 shows a sample list of pending computer physician order entry orders.

With CPOE, a pharmacist still reviews and verifies the order before the medication is dispensed. Advantages of CPOE include more complete orders, no errors caused by illegible handwriting, and quicker processing of orders since the additional time required to send a paper order to the pharmacy is eliminated. However, pharmacists and pharmacy technicians must be aware of potential hidden errors that can be made by the prescriber, such as choosing the wrong medication or patient from a list or entering orders into the wrong patient's electronic medical record. Because of such potential errors, it is still extremely important for the pharmacist to evaluate the appropriateness of all medication orders, whether they are written on an order sheet or entered via CPOE. When computer physician order entry is used, technicians may not be involved in the order entry process at all, but still fulfill many of the same dispensing roles.

Automated dispensing technology can have a profound effect on the filling, labeling, and checking functions performed in the pharmacy. This allows for electronic record-keeping and/or password-protected access to the medications. There are two basic approaches to automation: centralized dispensing automation in the pharmacy and decentralized automation at the point of care. The two approaches can be employed independently or combined.

> **TECHNOLOGY TOPICS**
>
> Automated dispensing technology is electronic storage cabinets or robotics that secure medications and dispense them to nurses or other caregivers when needed.

Centralized dispensing automation assists in the selection and dispensing of drug products that are located in a central location, such as the pharmacy. It

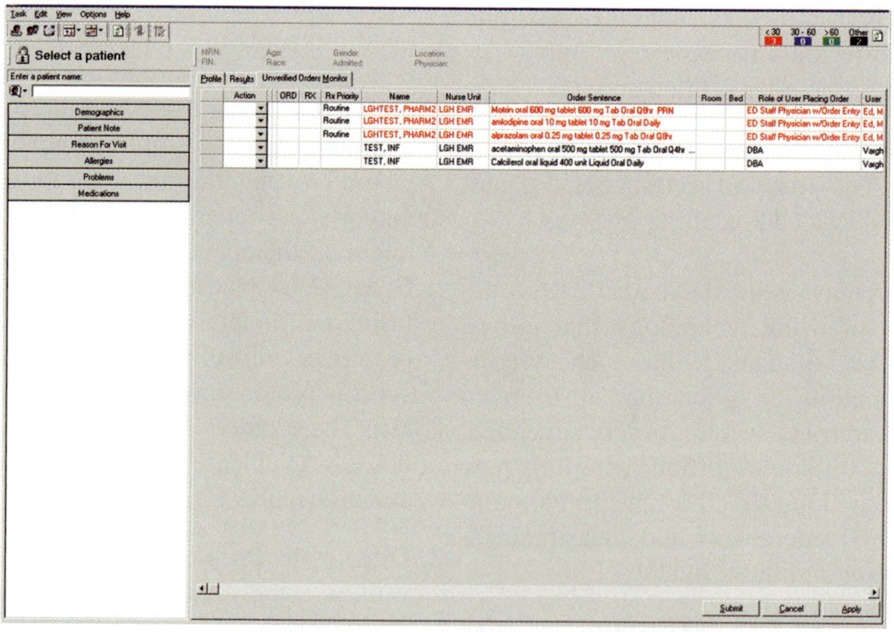

Figure 13-8. Sample list of pending computer physician order entry (CPOE) orders.

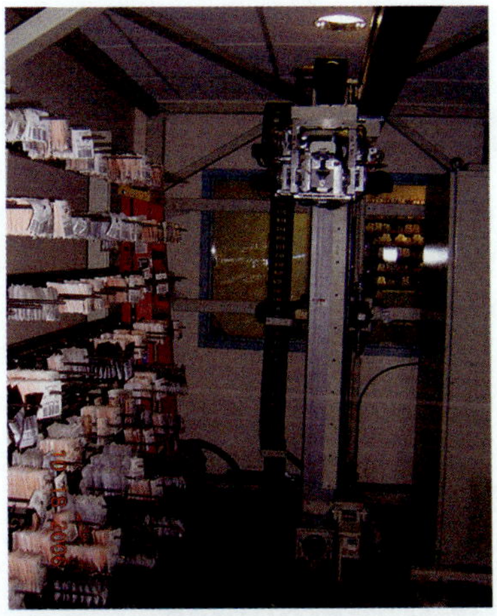

A.

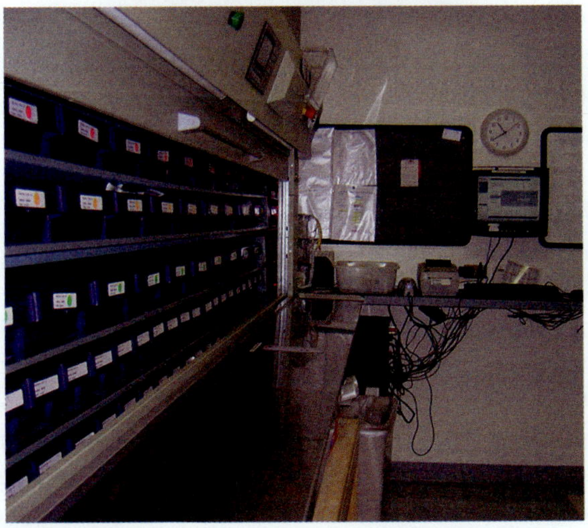

B.

Figure 13-9. Centralized dispensing automation A. Example of a dispensing robot B. Example of a dispensing carousel.

generally takes the form of robotics (figure 13-9A) or carousel systems (figure 13-9B). These systems use bar codes to identify medications accurately during filling. In a fully automated robotic example, the following steps might take place:

1. The technician scans a bulk container's bar code to fill a bulk bin in an automated packaging device. Because an error at this point in the process might result in many patients' getting incorrect medication, this is often a checkpoint for a pharmacist.
2. The technician packages the drug into robot-friendly containers, using a packaging device. Packages may include a hole at the top to fit on spindles on the robot and a bar code imprint for product identification.
3. The technician restocks the robot. This process is automated as well. The technician puts all individual containers to be stocked into the machine on a single spindle, and the robot reads the bar code on each package and places the drug in the correct location.
4. When an order is entered into the pharmacy's computer system for a medication that is stocked in the robot, the information is communicated to the robot, and the correct drug and quantity are pulled for the specific patient—again, by using the bar code to match the drug order to the correct product.
5. The technician removes each patient's drugs from the machine and distributes them to the patient care area by whatever distribution method is used. Routine quality assurance (QA) checks are often used to ensure that the robot is consistently dispensing doses accurately. Because of the inherent accuracy of these systems, a routine check of all dispensed drugs from a robot is not typical. State law may determine the amount of double-checking by a pharmacist that is required.
6. A batch fill of patient medications is generally scheduled at some point during the day. When this happens, the robot does a complete 24-hour fill of medications by patient and unit. Again, a random checking procedure may occur at this point.

In **decentralized automation systems,** distribution devices are placed in patient care areas. These devices may be used for only floor stock distribution and narcotic control or for the majority of drug distribution in a facility. When used for the majority of drug distribution, point-of-care automation makes distribution more of a batch system. In a traditional (non-automated) system—as has been described—most of the dispensing is "on demand," which means an order comes to the pharmacy by some means and is entered and filled at that time. When decentralized automation is used, orders are entered upon receipt, but the drugs are already "distributed" to the automation devices. A fully implemented decentralized system would work something like this:

1. An order is received in the pharmacy and is entered into the pharmacy computer system.
2. Once order entry is completed, a computer interface sends the information to the automation device, effectively "releasing" the medication for use for a specific patient.

3. The nurse goes to the machine and keys in the patient's name and the drug name, and the appropriate location in the device "unlocks" so that the medication can be removed.
4. For continuing medications (e.g., a tid medication), the nurse goes back to the device at designated times (standard administration times) throughout the day and removes the medication for administration to the patient.
5. When it is time to restock the machine, the technician prints a batch restock report that is filled by a technician and then checked by a pharmacist. The technician then makes a delivery to each unit and restocks the medications into the machines. Some devices allow for bar code verification of the medication to ensure that the correct medication goes to the correct bin (see figure 13-10).

These types of automation allow for the safer dispensing of medications. The use of bar code technology makes dispensing more accurate, since the opportunity for human error is minimized. However, errors can still occur. This generally results from the end user bypassing the bar code technology or not using it properly.

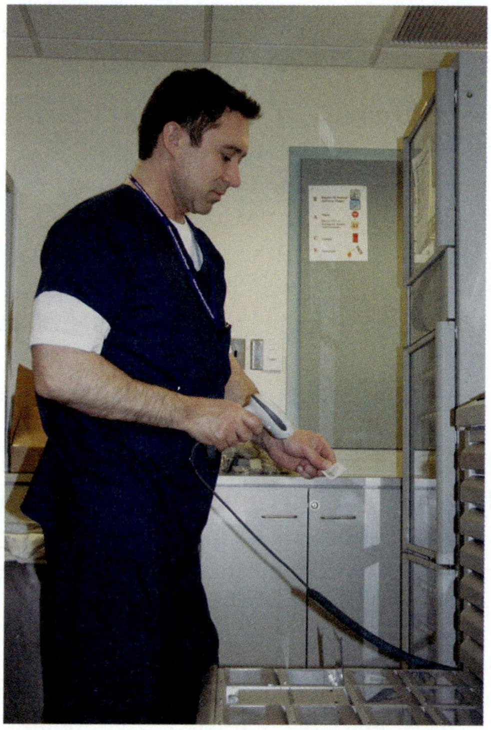

Figure 13-10. Example of a technician restocking an automated dispensing device, using bar code verification of the medication.

Both types of automation allow for some efficiencies as well. For example, with point-of-care automation, medication orders must still be filled, but by moving that function to a batch report, all of the orders for all of the patients on a particular floor can be filled at the same time, and the filling can be scheduled at a time that is convenient for the pharmacy instead of on demand at the convenience of the nurse. Centralized automation makes the filling process more efficient by automating the filling act itself. The machine does the filling—no more walking around the pharmacy to pull inventory from different locations.

Outpatient Pharmacies

The following section discusses processes and considerations for receiving and processing prescriptions in an outpatient pharmacy setting.

Receiving Prescriptions

Traditionally, prescriptions are presented to outpatient pharmacies in person after having been written by the prescribing physician on a prescription blank. It is now possible, however, for prescriptions to come into the pharmacy by a number of other means. Many pharmacies accept refill requests over the phone via a pharmacy Web site. As in the inpatient setting, there are regulatory restrictions on who can receive a telephone order, and the technician should refer to state laws for specific information.

Other means of communication include facsimile and electronic transmission. These methods are also regulated, with state-by-state variations, especially as related to electronic signatures and prescribing of controlled substances. Many pharmacies accept refill requests over the Internet through a pharmacy Web site or over the phone, either a person or using an automated system. Eventually, patients may use these Web sites routinely to log in to their own accounts to view a refill history, print an insurance receipt, or access drug information online.

Obtaining payer information is an important step in receiving a prescription in the outpatient setting. This information is used for a number of purposes, including establishing the primary payer for the prescription, the patient's portion of the reimbursement (copayment), and, in some cases, the drug formulary. Most prescriptions are now electronically filed with a third-party payer at the time they are entered into the pharmacy information system; this is called electronic claims adjudication. If the information is not available when the prescription is received, it may be held until the patient is present. This is generally an issue only the first time a pharmacy fills a prescription for a patient, because the information typically becomes a part of the patient's profile.

However a prescription comes in to the pharmacy, a technician is often the first person to handle it. The initial treatment, as in an inpatient pharmacy, must include screening for completeness and clarity. Then the order is prioritized for processing.

Clarity and Completeness. Reviewing a prescription for clarity and completeness is similar in the outpatient and inpatient settings. The following prescription elements are *typically* present (please refer to individual state laws and regulations to determine what elements are required in your area):

- Patient name
- Patient home address
- Date the prescription was written
- Drug name, strength, and dose to be administered
- Directions for use, including route of administration, frequency, and duration of use as applicable (some durations are open-ended)
- Quantity to be dispensed
- Number of refills to be allowed
- Substitution authority or refusal
- Signature and credentials of the prescriber and DEA number if required
- Prescriber's name, address, and phone number
- Reason for use, or indication (not required, but recommended)

An example of an outpatient prescription is presented in figure 13-11.

In an outpatient practice, some special clarity and completeness issues must be considered. When the prescriber uses "Dispense as Written" (or "DAW") on the prescription blank, the brand name drug written on the prescription must be dispensed. In some states, the phrase used is "Do Not Substitute" (or DNS). In this case, substituting the generic equivalent is not allowed. Depending on state law, pharmacy policy, or both, some prescription blanks come preprinted with areas the prescriber can use to designate either "DAW" or "generic substitution acceptable." In some practice settings, the prescriber must write "DAW," and preprinted prescription blanks are not recognized as official.

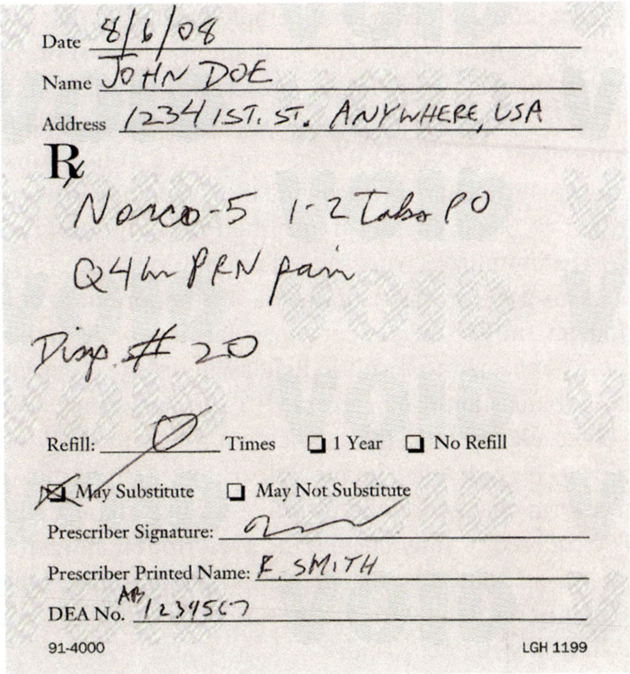
Date 8/6/08
Name JOHN DOE
Address 1234 1ST. ST. ANYWHERE, USA
℞
Norco-5 1-2 Tabs PO
Q4hr PRN pain
Disp. #20
Refill: Ø Times ❑ 1 Year ❑ No Refill
☒ May Substitute ❑ May Not Substitute
Prescriber Signature:
Prescriber Printed Name: F. SMITH
DEA No. AB 1234567
91-4000 LGH 1199

Figure 13-11. Sample outpatient prescription.

Another outpatient issue is prescription forgeries. Screening prescriptions, particularly those for controlled substances, for potential forgeries should be part of the technician's routine. Some prescription forgeries may be fairly easy to identify, such as erasure or overwriting of the strength or dispensing quantity of the drug (e.g., changing a 3 to an 8). Some forgeries are much more subtle and may involve, for example, theft of preprinted prescription pads and legitimate-looking prescriptions. Forged prescriptions may also be telephoned in to the pharmacy. Forgeries are not typically a concern for inpatient pharmacies because of their much more controlled environment.

Rx for Success

Technicians should screen prescriptions for anything that looks unusual, such as a dispense quantity in excess of normal quantities or an unrecognizable signature. Any suspicious prescription should be *discreetly* presented to the pharmacist for further evaluation. A telephoned prescription that is suspected of "forgery" should be validated with the prescriber.

Checking for clarity and completeness includes considering legibility problems and interpreting abbreviations. If there is any doubt, the prescribing physician must be contacted by the pharmacist for clarification. Making assumptions in either of these instances compromises patient safety. There is a growing movement toward typewritten or electronically transmitted prescriptions in an effort to minimize errors related to poor legibility.

As is true for inpatient orders, it is important to communicate fully to the patient when clarification or another issue is expected to result in a delay in order processing. The patient should be informed if the prescriber needs to be contacted or if the medication is not in stock and needs to be ordered. The prescriber may wish to make a short-term change in therapy while waiting for a product to be ordered or may change the prescription altogether. The patient should be made aware if the problem cannot be readily resolved with the prescriber, resulting in a delay in filling the prescription.

Prioritization. Prioritization of prescription processing in an outpatient pharmacy is generally an issue of customer service. Although some outpatient pharmacies may experience the equivalent of the inpatient STAT order, most outpatient pharmacy prioritization is based on the customer's needs. In general, prescriptions are filled in the order in which they are presented to the pharmacy, and many pharmacies use some type of "take-a-number" system. Some common-sense judgment does apply, however. For example, regardless of the order in which they were presented, prescriptions for customers who are waiting are generally filled before prescriptions to be mailed the next day.

Processing Prescriptions

Prescription processing involves many of the same steps as medication order processing in the inpatient setting. There are some differences, however, which are covered in the following sections.

Identifying the Patient. Patient identification in the outpatient pharmacy is an important step that helps ensure that prescriptions are filled for and dispensed to the correct patients. Proper attention needs to be paid to similar or identical names, to make sure the medication is entered in the right patient's profile. Another important concern at this stage is to ensure that there is no forgery and that individuals obtaining controlled substances are lawfully entitled to do so.

Most outpatient pharmacies use some type of patient identification system—often a numeric identifier that is unique to the patient, such as an account number. These systems are used to ensure accurate identification of patients for profiling and billing purposes.

Creating, Maintaining, and Reviewing Patient Profiles. Patient profiles are just as important in outpatient sites as they are in inpatient pharmacies. There are legal requirements for profiling, just as there are for hospital pharmacies. More importantly, however, patient profiles serve as a basis for providing patient care. The pharmacist is an integral participant in outpatient healthcare. The pharmacist is often the first provider to interact with a patient who is ill and intends to self-medicate, and also the last professional to interact with a patient who has been prescribed medication prior to implementation of the treatment plan. The pharmacist has a tremendous opportunity and responsibility to help patients use their medications safely and effectively. Patient profiles are an important tool in supporting that care.

A number of pieces of information are typically collected in the patient profile—some according to law (which varies from state to state) and some for efficiency and convenience purposes for both the pharmacy and the patient. They include the following:

- Patient's name and identification number
- Age or date of birth
- Home address and telephone numbers where patient can be reached
- Allergies
- Principal diagnoses
- Primary healthcare providers
- Third-party payer(s) and other billing information
- Over-the-counter medications and herbal supplements used by the patient
- Prescription and refill history
- Patient preferences (e.g., child-resistant packaging waiver or prefers prescriptions to be mailed)

Maintaining patient profiles is a function that technicians commonly perform in the outpatient setting. For this reason, technicians must be aware of the types of information that should be obtained from the patient to create and update the profile, and should bring any profile issues to the attention of the pharmacist. For example, the technician should notify the pharmacist if a medication is a duplication of something the patient has already been taking. As is true of the inpatient setting, outpatient pharmacy computers generally screen for many potential medication problems at the time of order entry. These alerts should be given to the pharmacist for follow-up according to the pharmacy's policies.

Prescription Entry into the Computer. Selecting the appropriate drug product is the first step in the order entry process, once the patient's profile is located or created. Most outpatient computer systems, like inpatient systems, allow the operator to choose a drug product by typing in a mnemonic or by accessing an alphabetical listing. It may also be possible to access the drug by National Drug Code (NDC) number.

Selecting the correct drug is not just a matter of choosing the correct product by name. It is also important to choose the correct strength and package size to match the NDC number with the product dispensed, especially when generic products are used. Accuracy ensures correct billing in addition to correct dispensing and is important in regulatory compliance and in protecting the pharmacy against accusations of fraud.

Keying in a mnemonic will generally result in a short list of options, from which the correct drug is then chosen. At this step it is important to pick the correct dose, dosage form, and, in the case of a bulk item, package size.

A variety of information must be entered into the computer at this point, and systems differ as to the order in which they are entered. Required elements include the following:

- Prescriber's name, address, & telephone number
- Directions for use
- Fill quantity
- Initials of the pharmacist checking the prescription
- Number of refills authorized

Once this information is entered into the computer, the technician accepts the prescription and, if applicable, the prescription entry is electronically submitted to the patient's insurance carrier for adjudication. Drug formularies were mentioned earlier in relation to choosing drug products in an institutional setting. Outpatient dispensing may be governed by numerous formularies, because each third-party payer has the option of identifying a formulary for its patients. Unfortunately, identification of a non-formulary medication does not generally happen until this step in the process. If a product is not covered by a patient's insurance, it is important to bring this fact to the pharmacist's attention so that the pharmacist can discuss the issue with the patient. Because non-formulary costs may be prohibitive for some patients, many will ask the pharmacist to contact the prescriber to determine if a formulary product might be an option.

Filling, Labeling, and Checking Prescriptions. The prescription entry process typically generates a label (figure 13-12) and may also produce additional documents, such as the patient's insurance receipt, a mailing label, and a drug information sheet for the patient. At this point, the technician fills the prescription and labels the container.

The following components must generally appear on the **primary prescription label,** whether typed or computer-generated (information may vary by state):

- Patient's name
- Date the prescription is being filled (or refilled)
- Prescriber's name
- Sequential prescription number
- Name and strength or concentration of the drug (including manufacturer, if filled generically)
- Quantity dispensed
- Directions for use
- Number of refills remaining (or associated refill period)
- Expiration date
- Physical description of the medication, if required by state law

GENERAL DRUG STORE
PHONE: 123-456-7891 ANYWHERE, USA AB 1234567
PT. John Doe — Prescription #1234
DR. Robert Smith — DATE 8/6/2008
Take 1-2 tablets by mouth every 4 hours as needed for pain.
Hydrocodone 5mg/Acetaminophen 325mg #20 CMK RPh
MFG Lot # ______
REFILLABLE 0 TIMES BEFORE ____
Caution: Federal law prohibits the transfer of this drug to any person other than the patient for whom it was prescribed

Figure 13-12. Sample outpatient prescription label.

Figure 13-13

BRAND NAME(S): Vicodin, Vicodin ES, Lortab 7.5/500, Lortab 10/500, Lortab 5/500, Lorcet Plus, Lorcet 10/650, Maxidone, Zydone, Xodol, Lortab 2.5/500, Anexsia, Vanacet, Co-Gesic, VicodinHP

GENERIC NAME: Hydrocodone/Acetaminophen (hye-droe-KOE-done) (a-seet-a-MIN-oh-fen)

DO NOT USE THIS MEDICINE if you have had an allergic reaction to acetaminophen (Tylenol®), to hydrocodone, or to other narcotic medicines (such as Darvon®, Percocet®, Percodan®).

COMMON USES: This medicine treats moderate to moderately severe pain. This medicine contains a narcotic pain reliever.

HOW TO USE THIS MEDICINE: Follow the directions for using this medicine provided by your doctor. TAKE THIS MEDICINE with food or milk if it upsets your stomach. Do not take more medicine or take it more often than your doctor tells you to. **It is not safe to use more than 4 grams (4,000 milligrams) of acetaminophen in one day (24 hours).** Measure the **oral liquid** with a marked measuring spoon or medicine cup. IF YOU MISS A DOSE OF THIS MEDICINE, take it as soon as possible. If it is almost time for your next dose, wait until then to take the medicine and skip the missed dose. Do not take 2 doses at once.

STORE THIS MEDICINE at room temperature in a closed container, away from heat, moisture, and direct light. Do not freeze. Ask your pharmacist, doctor, or health caregiver about the best way to dispose of any leftover medicine after you have finished your treatment. You will also need to throw away old medicine after the expiration date has passed. Keep all medicine away from children and never share your medicine with anyone.

CAUTIONS: MAKE SURE YOUR DOCTOR KNOWS if you are pregnant or breastfeeding, or if you have lung disease, liver disease, kidney disease, problems with urination, underactive thyroid, Addison's disease, prostate problems, a stomach disorder, or a history of head injury or brain tumor. This medicine may be habit-forming. If you feel that the medicine is not working as well, **do not take more than your prescribed dose**. Call your doctor for instructions. Make sure any doctor or dentist who treats you knows that you are using this medicine. Acetaminophen may affect the results of certain laboratory tests. This medicine may make you dizzy or drowsy. Avoid drinking, using machines, or doing anything else that could be dangerous if you are not alert.

POSSIBLE SIDE EFFECTS: SIDE EFFECTS include anxiety, mood changes, constipation, mild skin rash or itching. If they are bothersome, check with your doctor. CHECK WITH YOUR DOCTOR **AS SOON AS POSSIBLE** if you notice allergic reactions: itching or hives, swelling in face or hands, swelling or tingling in mouth or throat, tightness in chest, trouble breathing extreme weakness, shallow breathing, slow heartbeat, sweating, cold or clammy skin lightheadedness or fainting nausea, vomiting, loss of appetite, pain in the upper stomach problems with urination unusual bleeding or bruising yellow skin or eyes, dark-colored urine or pale stools. If you notice less severe side effects not listed above, tell your doctor.

BEFORE YOU BEGIN TAKING ANY NEW MEDICINE, **prescription, over-the-counter drug, vitamin, or herbal product check with your doctor or pharmacist for possible drug interactions.** Make sure your doctor knows if you are using an MAO inhibitor (Eldepryl®, Marplan®, Nardil®, Parnate®), medicine for depression (such as amitriptyline, imipramine, Norpramin®, Vivactil®), or any medicines that may make you sleepy (such as sleeping pills, cold and allergy medicine, other narcotic pain relievers, or sedatives). Do not drink alcohol while you are using this medicine. Acetaminophen can damage your liver and drinking alcohol can increase this risk. **If you regularly drink 3 or more alcoholic drinks every day, do not take acetaminophen without asking your doctor.** Many combination medicines contain acetaminophen, including products with brand names such as Alka-Seltzer Plus®, Comtrex®, Drixoral®, Excedrin Migraine®, Midol®, Sinutab®, Sudafed®, Theraflu®, and Vanquish®. Carefully check the labels of all other medicines you are using to be sure they do not contain acetaminophen.

The information in this monograph is not intended to cover all possible uses, directions, precautions, drug interactions, or adverse effects. This information is generalized and is not intended as specific medical advice. If you have questions about the medicines you are taking or would like more information, check with your doctor, pharmacist, or nurse

Figure 13-13. Sample drug information sheet to be given to the patient at the time of dispensing.

Labeling includes more than just the primary prescription label. The inpatient section of the chapter noted that labeling for inpatient use is often abbreviated or in a form of shorthand. For home use, however, this is not acceptable. Beyond the directions on the prescription label itself, auxiliary information is often included in the form of special labels affixed to the container or written drug information leaflets for patients to read at home (figure 13-13).

Of primary importance is that the instructions for use be presented very clearly on the label or within the **auxiliary prescription label,** a label affixed to a drug product that alerts users to special handling or administration concerns. This information also is commonly shared verbally with the patient at the time of dispensing. Instructions for use must include at least the following:

- Administration directions (e.g., "Take," "Insert," "Apply")
- Number of units constituting one dose and the dosage form (e.g., two tablets)
- Route of administration (e.g., "by mouth" or "vaginally")

- How frequently or at what time (e.g., "twice daily," "daily at 9 a.m.")
- Length of time to continue, if applicable (e.g., "for 10 days," "until finished")
- Indication, or purpose, if applicable (e.g., "for pain" or "for blood pressure")

At the time of dispensing, it is important to ensure that the patient fully understands how to use the medication. This is an appropriate time to consider language barriers, such as illiteracy or a non-English primary language. Many pharmacies now have interpreters available if they serve a large non-English-speaking population, and some pharmacies translate prescription labels and offer educational materials in languages other than English. Please refer to Chapter 8, Communication & Teamwork, for more information on this topic.

The pharmacist generally counsels the patient about the correct use and side effects of the medication.

Sample Outpatient Prescription Process. This section highlights how the outpatient order entry process differs from the inpatient order entry process (refer to the prescription in figure 13-11).

1. *Enter the patient's medical record number or name, and verify the patient* (same as for inpatients). On the basis of the prescription or by questioning the patient directly, verify that the rest of the patient information (address, date of birth, allergies, insurance information, etc.) is correct.
2. *Enter or verify existing third-party billing information.* Accurate third-party billing information is essential. Often, drug product choices must coincide with the payer's formulary for the patient's medication to be covered. If third-party payer information is incorrect, the patient may have significant out-of-pocket expenses or may choose not to use the medication because of the expense.
3. *Compare the order to the patient profile in detail* (same as for inpatients).
4. *Enter the drug* (same as for inpatients).
5. *Enter the label direction mnemonic.* This step will encompass steps 4 and 5 of the inpatient process. Remember, outpatient directions must be in a language the patient can understand so they must go beyond giving a milligram dose and scheduled time to take the medication. The dosing mnemonic for the Norco prescription might be t1-2poq4hp, which consists of encoded characters for all of the major elements of the directions ("sig" text): *t* = take *1-2* = one to two tablets, *po* = by mouth, *q* = every, *4* = four, *h* = hours, *p* = as needed.
6. *Enter comments.* Comments, such as "to control blood pressure," are added to the label and the medication profile at this point.
7. *Enter the prescriber's name.* Depending on the computer system, the technician might enter the full name, a mnemonic, or a numeric code.
8. *Enter the amount to dispense and the refill information.* In the example, the amount dispensed is 30, and no refills are authorized.
9. *Fill and label the prescription.* The correct medication must be chosen, the fill quantity counted and packaged, and the appropriate labeling applied. As in the inpatient setting, this is the final opportunity for the technician to ensure the accuracy of the process by checking the chosen product against the original order—not just against the label.

Summary

As a member of the healthcare team, the technician provides considerable assistance in operations of the pharmacy. The technician's ability to evaluate and assist in processing orders and prescriptions adds another measure of safety and efficiency to the system and is an opportunity for the technician to contribute significantly to the welfare of patients, whether inpatient or outpatient.

Self-Assessment Questions

1. Anyone who has worked in a pharmacy for a minimum of 1 year may receive a telephone prescription from a physician.
   a. True
   b. False
2. Generally, the first step when a prescription is received is a review of the prescription for completeness and accuracy, and the second is to prioritize the prescription in relation to the other work to be done.
   a. True
   b. False
3. An outpatient pharmacy generally has a single formulary that is used for all patients, regardless of the third-party payer.
   a. True
   b. False
4. Which of the following pieces of information should be on a prescription in an outpatient pharmacy and is also required on a medication order for a hospitalized patient?
   a. patient's address
   b. prescriber's address and telephone number
   c. refill information
   d. patient's name
5. What does "dispense as written" on a prescription mean?
   a. The brand name product ordered by the prescriber must be used to fill the prescription.
   b. Generic substitution is prohibited, but an alternative brand name product may be used if the one ordered is not available.
   c. Generic substitution may occur, but only if the patient insists on it.
   d. The brand name drug can be substituted with a generic, if available.
6. Any suspicious prescription should be brought to the attention of the pharmacist because it may be a forgery.
   a. True
   b. False
7. Considerations in determining an inpatient or outpatient order's priority include all of the following *except*
   a. the type of medication prescribed and what it is used to treat.
   b. the type of patient identification used.
   c. the patient's or caregiver's expectation for the time of delivery.
   d. specific instructions from the prescriber as to the delivery time.
8. A typical "turnaround time" for a STAT order in a hospital is 15 minutes.
   a. True
   b. False
9. Patient identification is not a concern in an outpatient pharmacy, because the technician has no control over who actually takes the medication.
   a. True
   b. False
10. Once a bar-coded account number system is instituted in an organization, less attention needs to be paid to patient identification because these systems are basically foolproof.
    a. True
    b. False
11. A thorough review of a well-kept patient profile in an outpatient pharmacy will generally allow the technician to identify all of the following *except*
    a. existing orders for the same medication.
    b. allergies that may indicate that the medication should not be used.
    c. a disability, such as blindness, that requires special attention.
    d. how the patient will pay for the amount the insurance company does not pay (i.e., the copay).

Self-Assessment Questions

12. Common screening options during a pharmacy- or nursing-operated computerized order entry process in a hospital include all of the following *except*
    a. therapeutic duplication.
    b. price range checking.
    c. allergy screening.
    d. dose range checking.
    e. drug interactions with existing orders.
13. Medication administration times are generally standardized within hospitals.
    a. True
    b. False
14. In the outpatient setting, appropriate medication administration times must be discussed with the patient or family member to ensure optimal benefit.
    a. True
    b. False
15. In the case of a prescription with complex directions, such as "tid for 3 days, bid for 3 days, qd for 3 days, and dc," it is acceptable to use the Latin abbreviations on the label as long as they are carefully explained to the patient.
    a. True
    b. False
16. Which of the following statements about prescription labeling is *false*?
    a. Some prescriptions require labeling beyond what will fit on the label itself.
    b. Auxiliary labels are often used to clarify or elaborate on directions for use.
    c. If the patient is in a hurry, it is acceptable to dispense the prescription without an affixed label as long as you talk to the patient about how to use the medication and he or she understands.
    d. Most states have specific requirements about what information must be included in prescription labeling.
17. Which of the following best incorporates all recommended components of label directions for outpatient use?
    a. Take one tablet by mouth three times daily.
    b. Take one tablet three times daily.
    c. Take one tablet by mouth three times daily for 10 days.
    d. Take one tablet by mouth three times daily for 10 days as needed for pain.
18. Inpatient pharmacies may become more efficient by implementing decentralized dispensing automation, thereby moving more of the filling functions to batch runs.
    a. True
    b. False
19. Which of the following is *not* true of hospital pharmacy dispensing automation?
    a. Dispensing automation may be centralized in the pharmacy or decentralized at the point of care.
    b. Decentralized automation is superior to centralized automation.
    c. Both centralized and decentralized automation make dispensing more efficient.
    d. Some institutions combine both centralized and decentralized automation to incorporate advantages of both systems.
20. When a filling label seems to indicate an error, which of the following would be an appropriate *initial* action for the technician?
    a. Alert the pharmacist that an error has been made.
    b. Check the label against the original order to determine if an error was made.
    c. Call the physician to clarify the order.
    d. Call the nursing unit (institutional setting) or notify the patient (outpatient setting) that an error was made on the prescription order and that delays will result.

Self-Assessment Answers

1. b. State laws vary in their requirements for telephone prescriptions, particularly when controlled substances are involved. In many states, only a pharmacist is allowed to receive telephone prescriptions.
2. a. An initial review of the prescription for completeness and accuracy will identify problems and facilitate their efficient resolution. Prioritization will help to ensure that the most urgent work is done first.
3. b. An outpatient pharmacy generally does not have a single formulary, as a hospital pharmacy might, but must conform to the various formularies of all the different third-party payers its customers use.
4. d. All of the listed pieces of information would appear on an outpatient prescription. The only one that would be seen on an inpatient order is the patient's name. Several other pieces of information would appear on inpatient orders but not outpatient prescriptions—most commonly a room and bed location for the patient and an admission number or account number of some type.
5. a. A "dispense as written" order must be filled with the brand listed by the prescriber.
6. a. Prescription pads can be lost or stolen and then used in attempts to obtain controlled drugs. It is also possible for forged prescriptions to be called in to the pharmacy. Although telephone forgeries may be more difficult to spot than written forgeries, the technician should consider anything unusual in a phone order as potentially indicating an attempt to obtain medications illegally. These calls should be directed to the pharmacist.
7. b. The type of identification offered or placed on the order does not influence priority.
8. a. STAT is derived from the Latin word *statim,* meaning immediately. Most hospitals have a designated time limit on these orders, typically 15 minutes.
9. b. Although the person picking up the prescription may not be the one who will ultimately be using it, patient identification is still an important function. The technician must always make sure prescriptions are filled for the correct patient and that the pharmacy's dispensing records are correct.
10. b. No identification system is completely free from potential error. Patient identification is one of the most important steps in the order processing sequence.
11. d. The patient profile should contain a full range of patient information, including patient demographics, such as date of birth, allergies, medical conditions, and disabilities, as well as a complete list of currently prescribed medications. Although it would typically contain information regarding the type of insurance coverage the patient has and the amount of any required deductible or copay, how the patient chooses to meet that requirement would not usually be indicated.
12. b. There is no screening for prices of drugs, although price information may be available. Some outpatient systems may offer price information for generic equivalents.
13. a. The majority of administration times are standardized in a hospital setting. However, there may be exceptions to such a policy, such as in pediatric or neonatal units, which might have specialized administration schedules that differ from other units.
14. a. Because there are fewer controls on medication administration in the outpatient setting, scheduling should be discussed with the patient or a family member to make sure the instructions are clear and the patient will not have difficulty using the medication as intended.
15. b. Latin abbreviations should never be used on labeling for home use. Although patients may fully understand the directions when they leave the pharmacy, they may forget by the time they get home. If detailed instructions do not fit on the prescription label itself, it would be appropriate to give the patient a separate piece of paper with instructions written in plain English.
16. c. There are legal requirements for labeling that must be met, including a label affixed to the prescription itself.

17. d. Six pieces of information are recommended for inclusion in outpatient labeling: (1) the administration directions, (2) the number and type (dosage form) of units constituting one dose, (3) the route of administration, (4) the frequency of administration, (5) the duration of therapy, and (6) the indication or purpose.
18. a. One way of improving efficiency through automation is to decentralize the inventory into automated dispensing machines. This allows more of the work to be completed on a batch basis as opposed to "on-demand" filling in response to a physician's order.
19. b. Both centralized and decentralized automation offer efficiencies, although at different points in the dispensing system. They represent different choices, but one is not inherently superior to the other. The choice of which system to use is a matter of organizational fit and determining which system best achieves the organization's objectives.
20. b. Checking the label against the original order is a good initial step because the error may have been a simple keystroke error in the computer, which could be easily corrected, eliminating the need for many of the other options listed.

Resources

To help you fully understand what is expected of you by your employer and how to comply with your state's applicable laws, it is strongly recommended that you read the following:

1. Your employer's policy and procedure manual and orientation materials regarding receiving and processing orders, filling and labeling medication orders, using the computer system, preventing errors, standard administration times, delivery expectations and turnaround time, and duties of the technician involved in dispensing functions.
2. Rules and Regulations for the Administration of the Pharmacy Practice Act for the state in which you are employed. These may generally be obtained from the regulating body in the state.

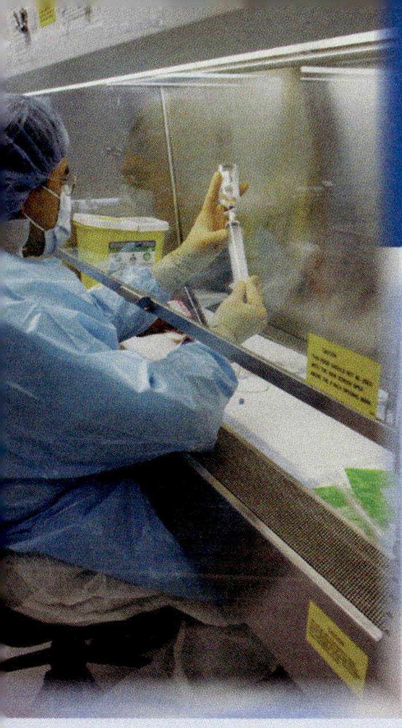

Chapter 14

Pharmacy Calculations

Susan P. Bruce

ASHP acknowledges Mary B. McHugh's work as a contributing editor on this chapter.

Learning Outcomes

After completing this chapter, you will be able to

- Explain why it is important to follow a standardized approach when using math in pharmacy.
- Convert between fractions, decimals, and percentages.
- Convert between different systems of measurement.
- Perform and check key pharmacy calculations, including the calculations needed to interpret prescriptions and those involving patient-specific information.

Key Terms

alligation method A way to help determine how many parts of each strength should be mixed together to prepare the desired strength.

apothecary system A system of measurement, originally developed in Greece for use by physicians and pharmacists but now largely replaced by the metric system, including the grain and the dram, the most common apothecary measures seen today.

avoirdupois system A French system of mass that includes ounces and pounds; the system of mass most commonly utilized in the United States.

body mass index (BMI) A measure of body fat based on height and weight, used to determine if a patient is underweight, of normal weight, overweight, or obese.

body surface area (BSA) The total surface area of the body, taking the patient's weight and height into account and expressed in m^2.

days supply The amount of medication dispensed for a specified time period.

denominator The bottom number of a fraction, representing the total number of parts.

fraction A part of a whole number, used to express quantities less than one or quantities between two whole numbers.

household system A system of measurement commonly used in cooking, including the teaspoon, the tablespoon, and the cup.

ideal body weight (IBW) An estimate of how much a patient should weigh based on his or her height and gender; expressed in kg.

metric system The most widely used and accepted system of measurement in the world; based on multiples of ten.

numerator The top number of a fraction, representing the number of parts present.

proportion A combination of two ratios with the same units; a statement of equality between two ratios.

ratio A representation of the relationship between two items. For example, when calculating a dose, a ratio can be used to show the number of milligrams in the dose per one kilogram of patient weight (mg/kg).

ratio strengths A ratio expressed as 1:something, where the units are g per mL. The concentrations of weak solutions, such as 1:1000 or 1:10,000 epinephrine, are sometimes expressed this way.

Pharmacy technicians and pharmacists in many settings use pharmacy calculations every day to determine, for example, the correct dose of a medication for a patient, the correct amount of ingredients to include in a compounded product, or the amount of medication a patient should receive. It is important to develop a systematic approach to solving pharmacy calculations that is reliable and consistent, with built-in checks along the way to ensure accuracy. Although it may seem as though completing a calculation two or three times is too time-consuming, it is time well spent when considering the potential for patient harm. Double-checking pharmacy calculations can lead to identification of abnormal doses, requests for early refills, incorrect quantities, or even incorrect medications. This chapter outlines the steps necessary to perform essential calculations and provides opportunities to apply the information to patient-specific scenarios.

Math Concepts

Most pharmacy calculations involve basic math. Numerals or numbers in different forms commonly appear on prescriptions and medication orders. Each of these basic math concepts is reviewed below.

Review of Basic Math

A numeral is a symbol, letter, or group of symbols or letters that represents a number. Common numerals in pharmacy calculations are Arabic numerals (e.g., 0, 1, 2) and Roman numerals (e.g., ss, I, V, X). Roman numerals are used in pharmacy only to designate a quantity on a prescription. Common Roman numerals in pharmacy include:

ss = 1/2	L or l = 50
I or i = 1	C or c = 100
V or v = 5	M or m = 1000
X or x = 10	

When presented with a Roman numeral, it is important to pay attention to the order of the symbols. First, identify the largest Roman numeral. If more than one numeral of the same quantity is present, then add them together. Second, locate the smaller numerals. If the smaller numerals are to the right of the largest numeral(s), the quantity of the small numerals is added to the largest numeral. If the smaller numerals are to the left of the largest numeral(s), the quantity of the smaller numerals is subtracted from the largest numeral(s).

Example: XXI = 10 + 10 + 1 = 21
Example: XIX = 10 + 10 – 1 = 19

Self-Assessment 14-1

Note: Answers to self-assessment questions can be found at the end of the chapter.

Convert Roman numerals to Arabic numerals:

a. iv
b. iii
c. xvi
d. MCX
e. cxx

A number is a numeral or a group of numerals. Examples of numbers are whole numbers (0, 1, 2), fractions (1/4, 2/3, 7/8), mixed numbers (1 1/4, 2 2/3, 10 1/2), and decimals (0.5, 1.5, 2.25).

Fractions

A **fraction** represents a part of a whole number. It is used to express quantities less than one or quantities between two whole numbers. A fraction is written as two whole numbers separated by a division line, for example, $^3/_4$. The number on top, or the **numerator,** represents the number of parts present. The number on the bottom, or the **denominator,** represents the total number of parts. Considering the simple fraction 3/4, 3 is the numerator and 4 is the denominator. Compound fractions or mixed numbers contain a whole number in addition to the fraction, such as 1 1/4. This can also be written as 1 + 1/4.

Fractions may be used in a variety of situations in pharmacy. For example, commonly used IV fluids include 1/2 NS (one-half normal saline) or 1/4 NS (one-quarter normal saline). Fractions appear when the prescriber intends to prescribe less than one unit of measure. For example, 3/4 teaspoon may be the prescribed volume of a medication dose for a child.

Safety First Fractions may lead to medication errors if someone mistakes the / for a 1. When using fractions, it is important to write clearly to avoid misinterpretation.

To simplify, or reduce, a fraction, find the greatest number that can divide into the numerator and denominator evenly. If you are not sure, begin with small numbers like 2 or 3. In the following example, both the numerator and denominator are divisible by 2. Fractions are usually represented in their simplest form.

Example: Simplify the fraction 66/100.

66	divided by 2	⇒	33
100	divided by 2	⇒	50

This fraction cannot be reduced further because no single number can be divided into both 33 and 50 evenly.

It is important to understand how to add, subtract, multiply, and divide fractions.

Adding Fractions

There are 3 simple steps to remember:

1. Make sure all the fractions have common denominators. The easiest way to do this is to enlarge the fraction by either multiplying both parts of the fraction by the denominator of the other or by using the lowest (or least) common denominator.

   Example A: 3/4 + 2/3
   3/4 * 3/3 = 9/12
   2/3 * 4/4 = 8/12
   In this case, the least common denominator is 12, since both denominators are divisible by 4.

   Example B: 3/4 + 1/2
   1/2 * 2/2 = 2/4
2. Add the numerators.
   A: 9/12 + 8/12 = 17/12
   B: 3/4 + 2/4 = 5/4
3. Reduce to the simplest fraction or mixed number.
   A: 17/12 = 1 5/12
   B: 5/4 = 1 1/4

Subtracting Fractions

The steps are similar to the steps followed for addition:

1. Make sure all fractions have common denominators.

   Example: 1 7/8 – 1/2
   In this example, the compound fraction, 1 7/8, needs to be converted to a simple fraction before we can find the common denominator. Remember, 1 7/8 is the same as 1 + 7/8, which is the same as writing 8/8 + 7/8, and 8/8 + 7/8 = 15/8. The number 2 goes into 8 evenly, so the common denominator of 1/2 and 15/8 is 8.
   1/2 * 4/4 = 4/8
2. Subtract the numerators.
   15/8 – 4/8 = 11/8
3. Simplify the fraction.
   Because the numerator is greater than the denominator, we can simplify by removing the part of the numerator that is equivalent to the value of the denominator to equal one whole number, and continue doing this until the remaining numerator is less than the denominator. In this example, subtract 8 from the numerator to represent one whole number.
   11/8 = 1 3/8

Multiplication

When multiplying fractions, it is not necessary to convert to common denominators. Steps to multiply fractions:

1. Multiply the numerators.

   Example: 9/10 * 4/5
   9 * 4 = 36
2. Multiply the denominators.
   10 * 5 = 50
3. Express your answer as a fraction.
   9/10 * 4/5 = 36/50
4. Simplify the fraction. In this example, both the numerator and denominator are divisible by 2.
   36 divided by 2 = 18
   50 divided by 2 = 25
   Final answer = 18/25

Division

When dividing fractions, it is not necessary to convert to common denominators. Steps to divide fractions:

1. Convert the second fraction (divisor) to its reciprocal; that is, trade the places of the numerator and the denominator.

   Example: 2/3 ÷ 1/3
   1/3 is converted to 3/1.
2. Multiply the first fraction by the second fraction's reciprocal.
   2/3 * 3/1 = 6/3
3. Simplify the fraction.
   $$\frac{6 \text{ divided by } 3}{3 \text{ divided by } 3} = \frac{2}{1}$$
   Final answer = 2

Self-Assessment 14-2

1. $\frac{1}{2} + \frac{3}{4} =$
2. $\frac{7}{8} - \frac{1}{9} =$
3. $\frac{4}{5} \times \frac{3}{20} =$
4. $\frac{9}{10} + \frac{2}{5} =$

Decimals

Because fractions can be challenging to work with, some individuals prefer to convert them to decimals. Like fractions, decimals are also used to represent quantities less than one or quantities between two whole numbers. For example, 0.5 teaspoon means one-half of a teaspoon. Numbers to the left of the decimal point represent whole numbers, and numbers to the right of the decimal point represent quantities less than one (figure 14-1).

Medication errors can occur when decimals are used incorrectly or misinterpreted. Sloppy handwriting, stray pen marks, and poor quality faxed copies can lead to misinterpretation. Decimal point errors can lead to medication underdoses or overdoses. To avoid errors, healthcare professionals should follow a standardized approach to documenting decimals.

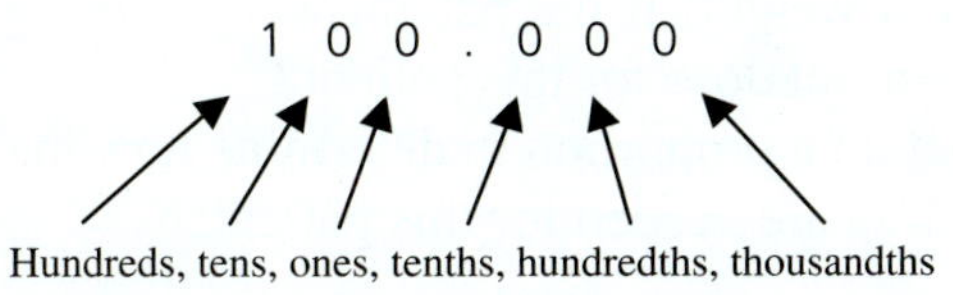

Figure 14-1. Numbers to the left of the decimal point represent whole numbers, and numbers to the right of the decimal point represent quantities less than 1.

First, decimals should only be used when absolutely necessary. For example, five milligrams should be written as 5 mg, not 5.0 mg; the decimal point and *trailing zero* are not necessary. Use of a trailing zero in this example could cause the quantity to be misinterpreted as 50 mg. Second, only zeros serving as placeholders should be included after the decimal. For example, if you wish to write seven and five hundredths, it should be written as 7.05, with no zeros following the last significant digit (in this case, the 5). Third, a decimal point should not appear without a number before it. If you wish to write one-half milligram, it should be written as 0.5 mg, not .5 mg. This is referred to as proper use of a *leading zero.* Failure to use a leading zero in this example could lead someone to mistakenly read the quantity as 5 mg rather than 0.5 mg. Also, notice that there are no zeros following the 5, the last significant digit.

Part 3

Safety First To prevent errors, remember to "always lead, never trail." Use a leading zero when writing decimals that are less than 1 (e.g., 0.5 mg), and never use a trailing zero (e.g., 5.0 mg).

Pharmacy technicians need to know how to convert fractions to decimals. Using a calculator, divide the numerator by the denominator to obtain a decimal. If a whole number is present, that number is placed to the left of the decimal. For example, when converting 1 2/3 to a decimal, first place the 1 to the left of the decimal. Then divide the 2 by 3 to determine the numbers to the right of the decimal.

Example:
1 2/3 → place 1 to the left of the decimal: 1.xx
To determine the numbers to the right of the decimal, divide: 2/3 = 0.6667
Final answer = 1.6667

In most pharmacy calculations, decimals are rounded to tenths (most common), hundredths, or thousandths, depending on the situation. To round a number to hundredths, look at the number in the thousandths place. If it is 5 or larger, then you increase the hundredths value by 1. If the number in the thousandths place is less than 5, the number in the hundredths place stays the same. In either case, the number in the thousandths place is then dropped.

In the example above, if rounding to hundredths, the final answer is 1.67.

With respect to rounding, pharmacy numbers must be measureable and practical. For example, one would never see a dose of 4.324 mL of a medication. Depending

Table 14–1. Examples of Rounding

Number to be rounded	Round to tenths (look at the hundredths place)	Round to hundredths (look at the thousandths place)	Round to thousandths (look at the ten-thousandths place)
1.515151	1.5	1.52	1.515
0.22222222	0.2	0.22	0.222
100.444445	100.4	100.44	100.444
4.56959	4.6	4.57	4.570 or 4.57

on the medication, most milliliter (mL) measurements are rounded to the closest mL or tenth of a mL. Likewise, one would never see 4.1 teaspoons (which would typically be converted to mL anyway), 6.1 tablets, or 4.1 days. Table 14-1 includes examples of rounding.

Self-Assessment 14-3

Convert the fractions to decimals, and round to the nearest hundredth:

a. 3/4 =
b. 2/5 =
c. 6/8 =
d. 9/16 =
e. 4/5 =
f. 2 3/8 =
g. 1/100 =
h. 7/8 =
i. 1 15/16 =
j. 3 7/8 =

To convert back to a fraction, write the decimal as the fraction you would say when you read the decimal. For example, 0.5 is read as "five tenths," so write the fraction as = 5/10 Then simplify the fraction—in this case, to 1/2.

Percentages

Percentages are a blend of fractions and decimals. Because percentage means "per 100," percentages can be converted to fractions by placing them over 100.

Example:

$$78\% = \frac{78}{100}$$

Percentages also convert simply to decimals. Just remove the % sign and move the decimal point two places to the left.

Example:

$$78\% = 0.78$$

Self-Assessment 14-4

Express each percentage as a fraction and as a decimal.

	Percentage	Fraction	Decimal
a.	8%	$\frac{8}{100} = \frac{2}{25}$	0.08
b.	67%		
c.	14%		
d.	92%		
e.	56.92%		
f.	0.05%		

Ratios and Proportions

A **ratio** shows the relationship between two items. For example, when calculating a dose, a ratio can be used to show the number of milligrams in the dose required for each kilogram of patient weight, which is written as mg/kg and read as "milligrams per kilogram." Two ratios with the same units can be combined to create a **proportion,** or a statement of equality between two ratios. Write the units next to each number and double check that the units are lined up correctly (the same units appear on top of the equation and the same units appear on the bottom of the equation). If the units are mismatched, convert to matching units before solving.

✔When solving proportions, it is critically important to make sure the equation is set up correctly before you solve for the unknown variable (x in the following examples).

Example:

The standard dose of a medication is 4 mg per kg of patient weight. If the patient weighs 70 kg, what is the correct dose for this patient?

Set up a proportion to determine how many mg of the drug are needed for this patient:

$$\frac{4\,\text{mg}}{1\,\text{kg}} = \frac{x\,\text{mg}}{70\,\text{kg}}$$

x represents the unknown value (in this case, the number of mg of drug in the dose) that you will find when you solve this problem. It takes two steps to solve for x:

Step 1: Cross-multiply.

$$\frac{4\text{ mg}}{1\text{ kg}} \times \frac{x\text{ mg}}{70\text{ kg}}$$

$$4\text{ mg} * 70\text{ kg} = 1\text{ kg} * x\text{ mg}$$

Step 2: Divide both sides of the equation by 1 kg to isolate the unknown, x, on one side of the equation. Then you can solve for x.

$$\frac{4\text{ mg} * 70\text{ kg}}{1\text{ kg}} = \frac{1\text{ kg} * x\text{ mg}}{1\text{ kg}}$$

The kg units in the numerator and denominator cancel each other out, and any amount divided by one is equal to that amount.

$$\frac{4\text{ mg} * 70\,\cancel{\text{kg}}}{\cancel{1\text{kg}}} = \frac{\cancel{1\text{kg}} * x\text{ mg}}{\cancel{1\text{kg}}}$$

Therefore the equation becomes:

$4\text{ mg} * 70 = x\text{ mg}$

$x = 280\text{ mg}$

Example:

Diphenhydramine 12.5 mg / 5 mL contains 12.5 mg per 5 mL. How many mg of diphenhydramine are in 10 mL of the solution?

Set up a proportion and solve for x.

$$\frac{12.5\text{ mg}}{5\text{ mL}} = \frac{x\text{ mg}}{10\text{ mL}}$$

$$12.5\text{ mg} * 10\text{ mL} = x\text{ mg} * 5\text{ mL}$$

$$x = \frac{12.5\text{ mg} * 10\text{ mL}}{5\text{ mL}}$$

$$x = 25\text{ mg}$$

Self-Assessment 14-5

1. A solution of morphine sulfate contains 10 mg of active drug per 5 mL of solution. How many mg of drug are found in 30 mL of drug solution?
2. A suspension of sucralfate contains 1g of active drug per 10 mL of solution. How many mL are needed to obtain a dose of 575 mg for a child?
3. The usual dose of cefazolin for a child is 40 mg/kg. How many mg are needed for a 22-pound patient?
4. When cefuroxime powder for suspension is reconstituted, the final concentration is 125 mg/5 mL. How many mL of the solution are needed to obtain a 50-mg dose?

Systems of Measurement

Multiple systems of measurement are used in pharmacy. The most common system is the metric system, also known as the international system of units (SI). Pharmacy technicians and pharmacists need to know how to convert from this system to the apothecary, avoirdupois, and household systems.

Metric System (International System of Units)

The **metric system** is the most widely used and accepted system of measurement in the world. It is based on multiples of ten. The standard units used in healthcare are:

- meter (distance)
- liter (volume)
- gram (mass)

The relationship among these units is: 1 mL of water occupies 1 cubic centimeter and weighs 1 gram.

There are prefixes that can be added to these standard measures to indicate a unit's relationship to the standard unit. For example, "milli" means one thousandth; 1 milliliter is 1/1000 of a liter. Table 14-2 lists the common prefixes relevant to healthcare.

Oral solid medications are usually expressed in mg or g. Liquid medications are usually expressed in mL or L. If a dose or volume is not available commercially, the correct amount must be compounded or measured. Doing so may require converting between units of the metric system.

Safety First When filling medication orders, it is critically important that the technician pays careful attention to the units to prevent medication errors and potential patient harm.

In the metric system, each move of the decimal to the left or to the right in the number represents an increase or decrease in the magnitude of the unit. As long as you know the order of prefixes and the magnitude each represents,

Table 14-2. Commonly Used Metric Units and Prefixes, with Correct Abbreviations

Relationship to standard unit	1/1,000,000 micro (mc)*	1/1000 milli (m)	1/100 centi (c)	Standard Unit	1000 kilo (k)
Weight	microgram (mcg)	milligram (mg)		**gram (g)**	kilogram (kg)
Volume		milliliter (mL)		**liter (L)**	
Distance		millimeter (mm)	centimeter (cm)	**meter (m)**	kilometer (km)

*Note that μ has been used as an abbreviation for micro, but this is an unsafe symbol because it can be confused with an "m." The correct abbreviation for micro is mc.

you can easily convert from one metric unit to another. The stem of the unit represents the type of measure. If you are converting to the left in Table 14-2, move the decimal to the right; your number will get bigger and your unit will get smaller. If you are converting to the right in the table, move the decimal to the left; your number will get smaller and your unit will get bigger. For example:

0.004 kg = 4 grams = 4000 mg

✔A kilogram is 1000 times as big as a gram. A gram is 1000 times as big as a milligram. A milligram is 1000 times as big as a microgram.

Example: sodium bicarbonate 650 mg tablets
1 tablet = 0.65 g = 650 mg = 650,000 mcg

Self-Assessment 14-6
Convert to the requested units:

a. 42 mg = ___ g	b. 26 km = ___ m	c. 2 m = ___ mm
d. 84 L = ___ mL	e. 13.6 m = ___ mm	f. 0.4 L = ___ mL
g. 56 m = ___ cm	h. 43 kg = ___ g	i. 98.2 cm = ___ mm
j. 54 mg = ___ mcg	k. 96 mL = ___ L	l. 5.2 m = ___ cm
m. 0.87 mm = ___ m	n. 43.2 g = ___ kg	o. 32.5 mcg = ___ mg

Apothecary System

The **apothecary system** was originally developed in Greece for use by physicians and pharmacists. This system has historical significance for the profession of pharmacy, but it has largely been replaced by the metric system. The Joint Commission (TJC) recommends that healthcare providers avoid using apothecary units because they are largely unfamiliar and often confused with metric units. There has been a decrease in the use of the apothecary system in hospitals, but apothecary units are still used in community pharmacy.

The most common apothecary measures appearing today are the grain and the dram. One grain represents approximately 60 milligrams for most medications (e.g., thyroid, phenobarbital). However, 1 grain of aspirin is 65 mg, so 5 grains is 325 mg and 10 grains is 650 mg. One dram is used to represent 5 mL or 1 teaspoon. Drams rarely appear on prescriptions but are still used to describe the capacity of prescription vials.

Avoirdupois System

The **avoirdupois system** is a French system of mass that includes ounces and pounds. In the United States, this is the system of mass commonly utilized, in which 1 pound equals 16 ounces. Assume this conversion when performing pharmacy calculations unless otherwise stated.

Household System

The **household system** may be familiar to people who like to cook. Prescribers frequently refer to teaspoons or tablespoons when writing prescriptions. It is a good practice to dispense a dosing spoon or oral syringe with both metric and household system units for liquid medications. The patient or the patient's caregiver should be instructed on how to interpret the units of measure on the spoon or oral syringe.

Converting Between Systems of Measurement

When preparing a prescription or medication order, it is important to know how to convert from one system of measurement to another. Table 14-3 is a summary of helpful conversions. Some of these conversions are not exact—the numbers have been rounded to make them more convenient.

Table 14–3. Common Conversions

Converting Measures of Length		
Metric		**Household**
2.54 cm	=	1 inch

Converting Measures of Mass		
Metric		**Avoirdupois**
1 kg	=	2.2 pounds (lb)
454 g	=	1 lb
28.4 g (usually rounded to 30 g)	=	1 ounce (oz)

Converting Measures of Volume		
Metric		**Household**
5 mL	=	1 teaspoon (tsp)
15 mL	=	1 tablespoon (T)
30 mL	=	1 fluid ounce (fl oz)
473 mL (usually rounded to 480 mL)	=	1 pint

Converting Within the Household System		
1 cup	=	8 fluid ounces
2 cups	=	1 pint
2 pints	=	1 quart
4 quarts	=	1 gallon

Converting Temperature		
Metric		**Household System**
degrees Celsius	=	degrees Fahrenheit

Formula for converting Fahrenheit temperature (T_F) to Celsius temperature (T_c):

$$T_C = \frac{5}{9} * (T_F - 32)$$

Formula for converting Celsius temperature (T_c) to Fahrenheit temperature (T_F):

$$T_F = \frac{9}{5} * (T_C + 32)$$

Example: Convert 35.4 degrees Celsius to Fahrenheit.

$$T_F = \frac{9}{5} * (35.4 + 32)$$

$$T_F = 95.72\ °F$$

Converting Time

It is important to know how to convert between the 12-hour and 24-hour clocks, since many institutions refer to medication administration by the 24-hour clock. The 24-hour clock, also known as military time, does not include a.m. or p.m. to designate hours of the day and does not use a colon to separate hours and minutes. Instead, the number represents the number of hours and minutes since midnight and ranges from 0 to 2359. (Example: 2130 = 9:30 p.m.)

Example: Convert 4:15 p.m. to the 24-hour clock.
12 + 4 = 16 hours
4:15 p.m. = 1615 in the 24-hour clock

It is good practice for individuals to work within the system with which they are most comfortable, to minimize error. Most practitioners prefer to work within the metric system because there are fewer conversions to remember. Instead of memorizing all conversions from one system of measurement to another, remember the key conversions listed and then use conversions within each system.

Using the proportion method, you can convert from household to metric units.

Example:
How many mL in 2.5 teaspoons?

Set up a proportion, starting with the conversion you know.

$$\frac{5\text{ mL}}{1\text{ tsp}} = \frac{x\text{ mL}}{2.5\text{ tsp}}$$

To solve for *x*, use the two-step process of cross-multiplying and dividing to isolate *x:*

$$5\text{ mL} * 2.5\text{ tsp} = 1\text{ tsp} * x\text{ mL}$$

$$\frac{5\text{ mL} * 2.5\text{ tsp}}{1\text{ tsp}} = \frac{1\text{ tsp} * x\text{ mL}}{1\text{ tsp}}$$

$$5\text{ mL}*2.5 = x\text{ mL}$$
$$x = 12.5\text{ mL}$$

The following practice problems will help to ensure you are competent with conversions.

Self-Assessment 14-7

Convert between systems of measure and round to the nearest tenth of a unit:

a. 3 in = ___ cm	b. 4 T = ___ mL
c. 36.2 g = ___ lb	d. 324 lb = ___ kg
e. 972 g = ___ oz	f. 386 mL = ___ tsp
g. 473 mL = ___ fl oz	h. 3.2 qt = ___ mL

Patient-Specific Calculations

As science progresses, we are learning more about medications and how they work in the body. Researchers are also discovering how medications target specific sites and how their safety or efficacy may differ from one patient to the next. Some medications may be administered at a common dose across all patient types, while doses of other medications must be calculated based on factors specific to the individual patient to be safe and effective. Three examples of patient-specific calculations that may influence drug dosing include body surface area, ideal body weight, and body mass index. While some of the calculations may be confusing or cumbersome, such as body surface area, nomograms—graphical representation of the key variables in the calculation—are available to use and may provide a quick and easy way to determine the result.

Body Surface Area

Calculating the dose of a medication may first require determining a value that is specific to the patient. **Body surface area (BSA)** is a value that takes the patient's weight and height into account and is expressed as m^2. For example, a man weighing 150 lb (68.2 kg) and standing 5'10" (177.8 cm) tall has a BSA of 1.8 m^2.

BSA values are frequently used to calculate doses of chemotherapeutic agents. There are several similar equations that are used, such as the Mosteller formula, which is:

$$\text{BSA}(\text{m}^2) = \sqrt{\frac{([\text{height(cm)} * \text{weight(kg)}])}{3600}}$$

Find out which equation is preferred at your institution by asking your pharmacist. Hospital computer systems will usually calculate the BSA value. Because this is a complex equation prone to error when performed manually, it is wise to count on the computer system, but it is helpful to understand how the calculation is performed.

Ideal Body Weight

Ideal body weight (IBW) is an estimate of how much a patient should weigh, based on his or her height and gender. IBW is expressed as kg. The formulas for determining IBW are:

IBW (kg) for males = 50 kg + 2.3(inches over 5')
IBW (kg) for females = 45.5 kg + 2.3(inches over 5')

Example:
Calculate the IBW for a 72-year-old male who is 6'2" tall.

$$\text{IBW (kg)} = 50 \text{ kg} + 2.3(14)$$
$$\text{IBW} = 82.2 \text{ kg}$$

Example:
Calculate the IBW for a 52-year-old female who is 5'9" tall.

$$\text{IBW (kg)} = 45.5 \text{ kg} + 2.3(9)$$
$$\text{IBW} = 66.2 \text{ kg}$$

Self-Assessment 14-8

Determine the IBW, to the nearest pound, for the patients below:

a. Male Wt: 230 lb Ht: 6'2"	b. Female Wt: 306 lb Ht: 5'11"
c. Female Wt: 266 lb Ht: 5'7"	d. Male Wt: 284 lb Ht: 5'6"
e. Female Wt: 320 lb Ht: 6'5"	f. Male Wt: 145 lb Ht: 5'2"

Body Mass Index

Body mass index (BMI) is a measure of body fat based on height and weight. This value is used to determine if a patient is underweight, of normal weight, overweight, or obese. The BMI is not generally used in medication calculations, but it may be mentioned in the pharmacy and in the literature. BMI is calculated by using this formula:

$$\text{BMI}\left(\frac{\text{kg}}{\text{m}^2}\right) = \frac{\text{weight (kg)}}{[\text{height (m)}]^2}$$

Key Pharmacy Calculations

Dosage Calculations

Certain medications require patient-specific dosing. Depending on the medication, BSA-based or weight-based dosing may be employed. For example, pediatric dosing is frequently determined by the weight of the child.

Example: If diphenhydramine syrup is dosed 5 mg/kg per day and the child weighs 43 lb, how many mg should the child receive in one day?

First, convert all necessary values to the appropriate units.

$$\frac{2.2\,\text{lb}}{1\,\text{kg}} = \frac{43\,\text{lb}}{x\,\text{kg}}$$

$$x\,\text{kg} = \frac{43}{2.2} = 19.5\,\text{kg}$$

Second, set up a proportion with the available information, and solve for *x*.

$$\frac{5\,\text{mg}}{1\,\text{kg}} = \frac{x\,\text{mg}}{19.5\,\text{kg}}$$

$$x\text{ mg} = 5\text{ mg} * 19.5 = 97.5\text{ mg}$$

Self-Assessment 14-9

1. The pediatric dose of phenytoin suspension (125 mg/5 mL) is 5 mg/kg/day in 2 or 3 equally divided doses. The patient is a 10-year-old boy who weighs 96 lb and stands 4’3” tall.
   a. What is the total daily dose of phenytoin for this patient?
   b. If the patient receives a dose twice daily, how many mL of suspension should be administered for each dose?
2. HumaLog Mix 75/25 contains 75% long-acting insulin and 25% short-acting insulin.
   a. How many units of long-acting insulin and short-acting insulin are found in 63 units of HumaLog Mix?
   b. If the initial dose of HumaLog Mix is 0.3 units/kg/day, how many units of long-acting and short-acting insulin will a 42-year-old female weighing 212 lb receive per day?
   c. If an insulin pen contains 3 mL (100 units/mL), how many days until the pen is empty?
3. You receive a medication order for diphenhydramine 25 mg IV. Diphenhydramine injection (50 mg/mL) is available in a 10-mL vial.
   a. How many mL of diphenhydramine solution are needed to prepare this injection?
   b. How many 25-mg doses can be prepared from one vial?

Days Supply

Part of the dispensing process is to ensure that a patient receives a sufficient quantity of the medication to last for the desired duration. To determine the **days supply,** evaluate the dosing regimen to determine how much medication per dose, then how many times the dose is given each day, and then for how many days the medication will be given.

Part 3

Example:
Metoprolol tartrate 50 mg po twice daily for 30 days (25-mg tablets available)

1. The dose is 50 mg, which will require 2 of the 25-mg tablets. The dose is given twice daily, which will require 2 tablets * 2 = 4 tablets per day.
2. The medication regimen will last 30 days, so 4 tablets per day * 30 days = 120 tablets.

Calculating the quantity needed of an oral medication is fairly straightforward, but calculating topical products may be a bit more challenging. For eye drops, the drops per mL may vary, depending on the viscosity of the drops.

Example:
Betaxolol ophthalmic solution 2 drops in each eye twice daily for 10 days

A 5-mL dropper bottle is available; assume 1 mL = 20 drops for this ophthalmic solution, which is a common estimate for many ophthalmic solutions.

1. The patient will take 4 drops twice daily, for a total of 8 drops per day.
2. The patient will use 8 drops per day for 10 days, for a total of 80 drops.
3. Set up a proportion to determine mL needed per day.

$$\frac{8\text{ drops per day}}{x\text{ mL per day}} = \frac{20\text{ drops}}{1\text{ mL}}$$

$$20 * x\text{ mL} = 8 * 1\text{ mL}$$
$$x = 0.4\text{ mL per day}$$

The patient is taking the medication for 10 days, so 0.4 mL/day * 10 days = 4 mL total volume needed to fill the prescription.

4. Determine if the available product will provide a sufficient quantity of medication. Since the total volume of the dropper vial is 5 mL and this prescription calls for 4 mL, one unit would be dispensed to fill the prescription. It is acceptable for the patient to receive slightly more volume than the calculated amount in case he or she has difficulty applying the drops and accidentally misses applying the medication in the eyes.

Self-Assessment 14-10

1. Atorvastatin (Lipitor) 40 mg tablets, 1/2 tab po daily. Dispense 30 tabs. How many days supply?
2. Omeprazole 2 mg/ml suspension, 1 mL PO BID. Disp 120 mL. This suspension has a 30-day shelf life. How many mL should be dispensed now, and how many mL will be available as a refill?
3. Testosterone 5 mg/mL gel; apply 1 mL to skin BID. Disp 30 day supply. How many mL should be dispensed?
4. Cyclosporine 2% 1 drop in each eye x 10 days (assume 1 mL = 20 drops). How many mL should be dispensed?
5. Methimazole 5 mg/mL suspension; 2.5 mg PO BID, Disp 90 mL. How many days supply?
6. Methotrexate 25 mg/mL injection 1 mL IM every week. Dispense 8 mL. How many days supply?
7. Prednisone 20 mg/mL give 1 mL PO daily x 5 days, then 0.5 mL PO daily x 5 days, then 0.5 mL PO every other day thereafter. Dispense 10 mL. How many days supply?

Concentration and Dilution

Some pharmacy mixtures are created by adding two solids together. When this occurs, the percentage strength is measured in weight in weight (w/w) or grams of drug/100 grams of mixture. This measurement is mainly used when compounding ointments and creams. When mixtures are created by adding two liquids together, the percentage strength is measured in volume in volume (v/v) or mL of drug/100mL of mixture. When mixtures are created by adding a solid to a liquid, the percentage strength is measured in weight in volume (w/v) or grams of drug per 100mL of mixture.

Standard solutions are used for IV administration, which are usually w/v mixtures. Table 14-4 represents some of the more common solutions, but there are many more.

To determine how much dextrose is in 1 liter of D5W, which is a weight (dextrose) in volume (water) type of mixture (w/v), set up a proportion starting with the concentration you know and then solve for *x*.

The first step is to make sure you have matching units in the numerators and denominators. Since D5W means 5% dextrose in water, it is expressed as 5 g/100 mL. Starting with 5 g/100 mL, determine how many grams of dextrose are in 1 liter by converting 1 liter to mL so that the denominator units are mL on both sides of the equation. Then set up the equation and solve for *x*.

$$\frac{5\,\text{g}}{100\,\text{mL}} = \frac{x\,\text{g}}{1000\,\text{mL}}$$

$$x\,\text{g} = \frac{5\,\text{g} * 1000}{100} = 50\,\text{g}$$

This method of determining amounts of drug in solution may be used for any mixtures expressed as percents.

Table 14-4. Standard IV Solutions

Solution	Also Known As	Also Written As	Contains
NS	normal saline	0.9% NaCl (sodium chloride)	0.9 g NaCl in 100 mL water
1/2NS	half normal saline	0.45% NaCl	0.45 g NaCl in 100 mL water
1/4NS	quarter normal saline	0.225% NaCL	0.225 g NaCl in 100 mL water
D5W	dextrose 5% in water	5% dextrose in water	5 g dextrose in 100 mL water
D10W	dextrose 10% in water	10% dextrose in water	10 g dextrose in 100 mL water
D5NS	dextrose 5% in normal saline	5% dextrose in 0.9% NaCl	5 g dextrose and 0.9 g NaCl in 100 mL water

Self-Assessment 14-11

1. In 250mL of D5W, how many grams of dextrose are there?
2. In 1 liter of D5NS,
   a. how many grams of dextrose are there?
   b. how many grams of sodium chloride are there?
3. How many grams of sodium chloride are in 5mL of a 23.4% solution?
4. How many grams of amino acids are in 500mL of a 10% amino acid solution?

Some medications are available in units per mL. Examples include insulin, heparin, and aqueous penicillin. Using the proportion method, you can determine what volume of medication is needed, starting with the available concentration.

Safety First When writing units, never use the abbreviation "u" for unit. It may be mistaken for a zero or the number 4 and cause an overdose.

Example:
How many mL of aqueous penicillin 500,000 units/mL are needed for a 5-million-unit dose?

Set up the proportion equation, beginning with the available strength and the unknown. Solve for *x*, using the two-step process of cross-multiplying and dividing:

$$\frac{500,000\,\text{units}}{1\,\text{mL}} = \frac{5,000,000\,\text{units}}{x\,\text{mL}}$$

$$500,000 \text{ units} * x \text{ mL} = 5,000,000 \text{ units} * 1 \text{ mL}$$

$$x\,\text{mL} = \frac{5,000,000}{500,000} = 10\,\text{mL}$$

Self-Assessment 14-12

1. How many mL of heparin 10,000 units/mL are needed for a 2000-unit dose?
2. How many mL of regular insulin 100 units/mL are needed for a 30-unit dose?

Frequently, the exact concentration of a product necessary to fill a prescription is not available. Through the concentration and dilution processes, a solution can be made more potent or less potent. In these cases, calculations are required to determine the appropriate proportions of one or more concentrations needed to fill the prescription. Many times, the medication is available in a concentrated stock solution, in which case a specified amount of the stock solution is added to a diluent to prepare the final product.

Example:
A medication order is received for the drug gentamicin 120 mg in 100 mL of normal saline. Gentamicin is available as a 40 mg/mL stock solution. How many mL of the stock solution are needed to prepare one dose?

First, set up a proportion, beginning with the strength of the stock solution. Make sure the units are consistent.

$$\frac{40\,\text{mg}}{1\,\text{mL}} = \frac{120\,\text{mg}}{x\,\text{mL}}$$

Use the two-step process of cross-multiplying and then dividing to isolate and solve for the unknown *x*.

$$x \text{ mL} * 40 \text{ mg} = 120 \text{ mg} * 1 \text{ mL}$$

$$x\,\text{mL} = \frac{120}{40} = 3\,\text{mL}$$

Draw up 3 mL of gentamicin 40 mg/mL and add this amount to a 100-mL minibag of NS to obtain 120 mg of gentamicin in 100 mL of NS.

When working with electrolytes (e.g., potassium, calcium, or magnesium), you will encounter milliequivalents (mEq). A milliequivalent is a measure of mass that takes into account the molecular weight (MW) and ionic charge, or valence, of an electrolyte. Vials containing electrolytes express concentrations in both mEq and mg.

Calculations involving milliequivalents are similar to calculations using units or milligrams as units of measure. Be sure to always check to see that you are using matching units in your equations.

Example:
Potassium acetate is available in a concentration of 40 mEq/20 mL. If you need to give a dose of 5 mEq of potassium IV, how much potassium do you need?

Start with the given concentration of potassium and set up an equation to determine the volume of the needed potassium:

$$\frac{40\,\text{mEq}}{20\,\text{mL}} = \frac{5\,\text{mEq}}{x\,\text{mL}}$$

This equation can be simplified to:

$$\frac{2\,\text{mEq}}{1\,\text{mL}} = \frac{5\,\text{mEq}}{x\,\text{mL}}$$

Cross-multiply:

$$2\ \text{mEq} * x\ \text{mL} = 1\ \text{mL} * 5\ \text{mEq}$$

Divide both sides of the equation by 2 mEq to isolate *x*.

$$\frac{2\,\text{mEq} * x\,\text{mL}}{2\,\text{mEq}} = \frac{1\,\text{mL} * 5\,\text{mEq}}{2\,\text{mEq}}$$

When you divide both sides of the equation by 2 mEq, the mEq units cancel out, and you are left with this equation:

$$x\,\text{mL} = \frac{5\,\text{mL}}{2}$$

$$x\ \text{mL} = 2.5\ \text{mL}$$

2.5 mL of potassium concentrate will deliver 5 mEq of potassium.

The concentrations of very weak solutions are sometimes expressed as **ratio strengths.** Ratio strengths are usually expressed as 1:something, where the units are g per mL. For example, epinephrine is available in concentrations of 1:1000 and 1:10,000. This type of expression has caused medication errors, especially for medications ordered in mL, because 1000 and 10,000 look alike and people have assumed that only one concentration is available. It is recommended that the more concentrated version (1:1000) be clearly labeled, stating that the concentration requires dilution prior to administration.

To solve a problem utilizing a medication that is labeled by ratio strength, first convert the ratio to a standard fraction.

Example:

A medication order is for 1 mg of epinephrine. You have a vial of epinephrine 1:10,000. What volume of medication is needed for a dose of 1 mg?

Start your equation with the ratio you have been given:

1:10,000 means 1 gram in 10,000mL, or

$$\frac{1\,\text{g}}{10{,}000\,\text{mL}}$$

Since you need to find the volume in mL for 1 mg, you need to convert units. Remember that 1 g=1000 mg, so you can replace 1 g with 1000 mg and set up your equation:

$$\frac{1\,\text{g}}{10{,}000\,\text{mL}} = \frac{1000\,\text{mg}}{10{,}000\,\text{mL}}$$

$$\frac{1000\,\text{mg}}{10{,}000\,\text{mL}} = \frac{1\,\text{mg}}{x\,\text{mL}}$$

Cross-multiply and divide to get:

$$x\,\text{mL} = \frac{10{,}000\,\text{mL} * 1\,\text{mg}}{1000\,\text{mg}} = 10\,\text{mL}$$

10 mL of this solution (epinephrine 1:10,000) contains 1 mg of epinephrine.

Self-Assessment 14-13

1. A medication order is received for digoxin 0.5 mg po daily. Available is a digoxin 50 mcg/mL solution. How many doses of the medication are available in a 60-mL bottle of the stock solution?
2. The dose of vancomycin is 15mg/kg in 250 ml of D5W. The patient weighs 50 kg. How many mL of a 100 mg/mL solution are needed to prepare the dose?
3. A medication order is received for a child for dexamethasone 0.15 mg/kg/day divided into 2 doses. The patient weighs 11 kg. Dexamethasone solution for injection is available as 4 mg/mL concentration.
   a. You are asked to prepare 4 mL of a pediatric dilution of dexamethasone (final concentration 100 mcg/mL) from the commercially available solution. How much of the dexamethasone solution is needed to prepare the pediatric dilution? How much sterile water for injection is needed to prepare the pediatric dilution?
   b. How many mL of the dexamethasone pediatric dilution are needed to prepare one dose of the dexamethasone for this patient?
4. How many grams of pure coal tar should be added to prepare a prescription for 5% coal tar in ointment base with a total weight of 60 g?
5. How many mL of a commercially available phenobarbital 130 mg/mL solution are needed to prepare 1 L of a 10 mg/mL pediatric solution? How many mL of sterile water are needed to prepare the pediatric solution?

This column is %.	This column is %.	This column is PARTS.
High concentration →	→	(Desired concentration) – (low concentration) = number of parts of high concentration needed
Low concentration	Desired concentration	
→	→	(High concentration) – (desired concentration) = number of parts of low concentration needed
		Total parts (add numbers of parts from above)

Figure 14–2. Alligation method. This method helps to determine how many parts of each strength should be mixed together to prepare the desired strength.

6. How many mL of potassium 40 mEq/20 mL are needed to provide 10 mEq of potassium?
7. How many mL of epinephrine 1:1000 are needed to deliver 1 mg?

Alligation Method. At times, the desired concentration of a product is not readily available, but concentrations above and below the desired concentration are available. The **alligation method** will help to determine how many parts of each strength should be mixed together to prepare the desired strength. The easiest way to visualize an alligation is to set up a tic-tac-toe board, as shown in figure 14-2. The contents of the cells in the right-hand column are added to determine the total number of parts.

> **Example:** You have an order for 550 mL of a 25% solution. You have a 45% solution and a 10% solution available. How many mL of the 45% solution will you need to mix with the 10% solution to prepare the amount of 25% solution that you need? Figure 14-3 shows use of the alligation method to solve this problem.

If we mix 15 parts of the 45% concentration with 20 parts of the 10% concentration, we will get a 25% solution. To determine what volume of each concentration is needed to make 550 mL of 25% solution, set up a proportion representing one of the two concentrations you will be using. If you start with the high concentration (45%), you know that this represents 15 of the 35 parts. Therefore the equation will start with that information:

$$\frac{15\,\text{parts}}{35\,\text{parts}} = \frac{x\,\text{mL}}{550\,\text{mL}}$$

Use the two-step process of cross-multiplying and dividing to isolate *x:*

$$x\,\text{mL} = \frac{15 * 550\,\text{mL}}{35} = 235.7\,\text{mL of the 45\% solution}$$

%	%	PARTS
45%		15 parts of high concentration
	25%	
10%		20 parts of high concentration
		35 parts total (550 mL)

Figure 14–3. Example of using the alligation method.

Knowing that the total is 550 mL, you can subtract the amount of the 45% (235.7mL) from the total to calculate the amount of the 10% solution needed.

$$550 \text{ mL} - 235.7 \text{ mL} = 314.3 \text{ mL of } 10\% \text{ solution needed}$$

It is helpful to double-check your work and calculate it both ways.

Remember, if the product does not contain active ingredient, its concentration is 0%. Similarly, if the product is pure active ingredient, its concentration is 100%.

Another method to solve similar problems uses the equation below:

$$C_1V_1 = C_2V_2$$

C represents concentration, *V* represents volume, and the subscript numbers represent two different solutions.

Example: You have an order for 5 mL of a 70% ethanol solution. You only have 98% ethanol. How many mL of the 98% solution will you add to sterile water to make 5 mL of the 70% ethanol solution?

$$C_1V_1 = C_2V_2$$

$$98\%_{\text{conc of 98\% soln}} X_{\text{volume needed of 98\% soln}} = 70\%_{\text{conc of 70\% soln}} 5_{\text{volume desired of 70\% soln}}$$

$$98x = 70 * 5$$

$$x = \frac{70 * 5}{98} = 3.6 \text{ mL}$$

So you would add 3.6 mL of the 98% solution to 1.4 mL of sterile water to make 5 mL of the 70% solution.

Self-Assessment 14-14

1. How many grams of pure hydrocortisone powder are needed to prepare 45 grams of a 3% w/w ointment if you mix the powder with a 0.5% hydrocortisone ointment? (Note: pure hydrocortisone powder is considered 100%.)
2. How many mL of water should be added to 1 liter of normal saline (0.9% NaCl) to reduce the concentration to 0.45% w/v?
3. How many grams of salicylic acid powder are needed to prepare 60 grams of a 2.5% w/w ointment if you have 100 g of a 1% w/w ointment available to you?

Specific Gravity

Specific gravity is a number unique to each substance. It is the ratio of the weight of the compound to the weight of the same amount of water. For example, the specific gravity of milk is 1.035 and the specific gravity of ethanol is 0.787. In other words, milk is denser than water and ethanol is less dense than water. Knowing the specific gravity of a substance is helpful when converting between weight and volume. Generally, units do not appear with specific gravity. In pharmacy calculations, specific gravity and density are used interchangeably; therefore, we can use the following formula:

$$\text{specific gravity} = \frac{\text{weight (g)}}{\text{volume (mL)}}$$

✔The specific gravity of water is 1, so 1 mL of water weighs 1 gram.

Example:
What is the weight of 473 mL of coal tar if the specific gravity is 0.84?

To answer this question, start with the known specific gravity of 0.84, which means 0.84 g/mL, and set up this proportion:

$$\frac{0.84 \text{ g}}{1 \text{ mL}} = \frac{x \text{ g}}{473 \text{ mL}}$$

Solve for *x:*

$$x \text{ g} = 0.84 * 473 = 397.3 \text{ g}$$

Self-Assessment 14-15

1. What is the volume of a sorbitol solution that weighs 2.6 kg if the specific gravity is 1.3?

Chemotherapy Calculations

Accurate pharmacy calculations are critically important in the oncology setting, where medications administered to patients are extremely potent and can cause patient harm or death if miscalculations occur. A system of checks and rechecks is in place in most institutions that compound chemotherapy, to ensure accurate calculations and medication preparation prior to patient administration.

Example: A medication order is received for amifostine 200 mg/m² over 3 minutes once daily 15–30 minutes prior to radiation therapy. The patient is a 79-year-old man weighing 157 lb and standing 6' tall. He has a BSA of 1.9 m². What is the dose of amifostine for this patient?

The easiest way to solve this problem is to set up a proportion:

$$\frac{200\,\text{mg}}{\text{m}^2} = \frac{x\,\text{mg}}{1.9\,\text{m}^2}$$

$$x\,\text{mg} = \frac{200 * 1.9}{1} = 380\,\text{mg}$$

Self-Assessment 14-16

1. Medication orders are received for irinotecan 125 mg/m² IV in 250 mL D5W over 90 minutes, followed by a leucovorin 20 mg/m² IV bolus, followed by a 5-fluorouracil 500 mg/m² IV bolus. The patient is a 56-year-old man weighing 187 lb and standing 5'11" tall. He has a BSA of 2.06 m².
   a. What is the dose of irinotecan for this patient?
   b. What is the dose of leucovorin for this patient?
   c. What is the dose of 5-fluorouracil for this patient?
2. Medication orders are received for doxorubicin 60 mg/m² IV push, cyclophosphamide 600 mg/m² in NS over 30 minutes, paclitaxel 80 mg/m² in 250 mL NS over 1 hour, and trastuzumab 4 mg/kg IV in 250 mL NS over 90 minutes. The patient is a 42-year-old female weighing 146 lb and standing 5'7" tall. Her BSA is 1.77 m².
   a. What is the dose of doxorubicin for this patient?
   b. What is the dose of cyclophosphamide for this patient?
   c. What is the dose of paclitaxel for this patient?
   d. What is the dose of trastuzumab for this patient?

IV Flow Rate

When working in an institutional setting or home care, it is important to know how to perform calculations related to intravenous medications. This includes calculating the rate at which a medication should be infused. Use the math concepts practiced above to find the necessary information.

Example:
How many mL per minute will a patient receive if a 500 mL solution is infused over 2 hours?

To solve this problem, set up a proportion:

$$\frac{500\,\text{mL}}{120\,\text{min}} = \frac{x\,\text{mL}}{1\,\text{min}}$$

$$500\text{ mL} * 1\text{ min} = 120\text{ min} * x\text{ mL}$$

$$x = \frac{500}{120} = 4.2\text{ mL/min}$$

Therefore, the rate is 4.2 mL per minute.

Example: How many drops per minute will a patient receive if a 250-mL solution is infused over 1 hour and the infusion set delivers 10 drops/mL?

First set up a proportion to determine the mL per minute.

$$\frac{250\,\text{mL}}{60\,\text{min}} = \frac{x\,\text{mL}}{1\,\text{min}}$$

$$250\text{ mL} * 1\text{ min} = 60\text{ min} * x\text{ mL}$$

$$x = \frac{250}{60} = 4.2\text{ mL/min}$$

Now determine how many drops this would be by setting up a second proportion:

$$\frac{10\,\text{drops}}{1\,\text{mL}} = \frac{x\,\text{drops}}{4.2\,\text{mL}}$$

$$x\text{ drops} = 10 * 4.2 = 42\text{ drops per minute}$$

Self-Assessment 14-17

1. The dose of vancomycin is 15 mg/kg and should be infused at no more than 10 mg/min or for a total of 60 minutes (whichever is longer). The patient weighs 226 lb. A 50 mg/mL stock solution of vancomycin is available to you.
   a. Calculate the dose of vancomycin.
   b. Determine how many mL of solution are needed to prepare each dose.
   c. Determine the duration of infusion in minutes.
2. A medication order is received for aminophylline 6 mg/kg IV. The rate of infusion should not exceed 25 mg/minute. The aminophylline stock solution for injection is available as a 20-mL vial in a concentration of 25 mg/mL. The patient is a 72 year old female who stands 5'6" tall and weighs 174 lb.
   a. What is the dose of aminophylline?

b. How many mL of the stock solution are needed to prepare the dose?
c. How many minutes will it take to infuse the aminophylline?

3. A medication order is received for gentamicin 3 mg/kg/day administered in 3 equal doses every 8 hours. Each dose should be placed in 50 mL of normal saline. The patient weighs 198 lb. Gentamicin (40 mg/mL) 2-mL vials are available.
   a. Determine the mg per dose of gentamicin.
   b. How many mL of gentamicin solution are needed to prepare each dose?
   c. If the dose is administered over 30 minutes, how many mL per minute will the patient receive?
4. An order is received for amiodarone 150 mg in 100 mL D5W infused over 10 minutes. A 3-mL vial (50 mg/mL) of amiodarone solution is available to prepare the infusion.
   a. How many mL of amiodarone solution are needed to prepare one dose?
   b. At what rate (mL/min) should the medication be infused?
   c. If the administration set delivers 15 drops/mL, how many drops per minute will this patient receive?
5. An order is received for piperacillin/tazobactam (Zosyn) 3.375 g IV every 6 hours in 100 mL of NS infused over 1 hour. A bulk vial contains 40.5 g of piperacillin/tazobactam.
   a. If 152 mL of diluent is added to the bulk vial to create a total volume of 180 mL, how many mL are needed to prepare one dose of piperacillin/tazobactam?
   b. How many doses of piperacillin/tazobactam can be prepared from one bulk vial?
   c. If 3.375 g of piperacillin/tazobactam contains 3000 mg of piperacillin, how many g of piperacillin will the patient receive per day?
   d. How many mL/min will the patient receive during each infusion?

Summary

Accurately performing pharmacy calculations is an essential skill for a pharmacy technician. No matter how busy your day is in the pharmacy, take your time to complete the necessary calculations and double-check your work. If you are unsure of your result, ask another technician or your pharmacist for assistance. Reducing and avoiding medication errors is worth the extra time.

Self-Assessment Answers

Self-Assessment 14-1

a. 4
b. 3
c. 16
d. 1110
e. 120

Self-Assessment 14-2

1. $\frac{1}{2}+\frac{3}{4}=\frac{2}{4}+\frac{3}{4}=\frac{5}{4}=1\frac{1}{4}$

To add fractions, you must first find the common denominator. Then add the numerators. The denominators remain the same. Finally, change to a proper fraction.

2. $\frac{7}{8}-\frac{1}{9}=\frac{63}{72}-\frac{8}{72}=\frac{55}{72}$

To subtract fractions, find the common denominator first. Then subtract the numerators. The denominators remain the same. This fraction cannot be reduced any further.

3. $\frac{4}{5}*\frac{3}{20}=\frac{4*3}{5*20}=\frac{12}{100}=\frac{3}{25}$

To multiply fractions, multiply the numerators together and multiply the denominators together. Simplify the fraction.

4. $\frac{9}{10}\div\frac{2}{5}=\frac{9}{10}*\frac{5}{2}=\frac{45}{20}=\frac{9}{4}=2\frac{1}{4}$

To divide fractions, invert the divisor (second fraction) and then multiply. In this case, the answer could be simplified (from 45/20 to 9/4) and changed to a proper fraction (from 9/4 to 2 1/4).

Self-Assessment 14-3

a. 0.75
b. 0.4
c. 0.75
d. 0.56
e. 0.8
f. 2.38
g. 0.01
h. 0.88
i. 1.94
j. 3.88

Self-Assessment 14-4

	Percentage	Fraction	Decimal
a.	8%	$\frac{8}{100}=\frac{2}{25}$	0.08
b.	67%	$\frac{67}{100}$	0.67
c.	14%	$\frac{14}{100}=\frac{7}{50}$	0.14
d.	92%	$\frac{92}{100}=\frac{23}{25}$	0.92
e.	56.92%	$\frac{5692}{10000}=\frac{1423}{2500}$	0.5692
f.	0.05%	$\frac{0.05}{100}=\frac{1}{2000}$	0.0005

Self-Assessment 14-5

1. $\frac{10\text{ mg}}{5\text{ mL}}=\frac{x\text{ mg}}{30\text{ mL}}$

   x mg * 5 mL = 10 mg * 30 mL

   $x\text{ mg}=\frac{10*30}{5}=60\text{ mg}$

2. First, convert 1g to mg so that the units match:
   1 g = 1000 mg
   Then determine the number of mL to obtain the dose of 575 mg:

   $\frac{1000\text{ mg}}{10\text{ mL}}=\frac{575\text{ mg}}{x\text{ mL}}$

   1000 mg * x mL = 575 mg * 10 mL

   $x\text{ mL}=\frac{575*10}{1000}=5.75\text{ mL}$

   Remember that values must be measurable. In this example, the dose should be rounded to 6 mL, because this medication is available as a thick suspension and it would be difficult to measure it in tenths of a mL.

3. First determine how many kg this 22-pound patient weighs, using this equation:

   1 kg = 2.2 lb
   $\frac{1\text{ kg}}{2.2\text{ lb}}=\frac{x\text{ kg}}{22\text{ lb}}$

   x kg * 2.2 lb = 1 kg * 22 lb

   $x\text{ kg}=\frac{22}{2.2}=10\text{ kg}$

   Then determine the correct dose:

   $\frac{40\text{ mg}}{1\text{ kg}}=\frac{x\text{ mg}}{10\text{ kg}}$

   x mg = 40 * 10 = 400 mg

4. $\frac{125\text{ mg}}{5\text{ mL}}=\frac{50\text{ mg}}{x\text{ mL}}$

   $x\text{ mL}=\frac{5*50}{125}=2\text{ mL}$

Self-Assessment 14-6

a. $\frac{1000\text{ mg}}{1\text{ g}}=\frac{42\text{ mg}}{x\text{ g}}$

   $x\text{ g}=\frac{42}{1000}=0.042\text{ g}$

b. $\frac{1000\text{ m}}{1\text{ km}}=\frac{x\text{ m}}{26\text{ km}}$
   x m = 1000 * 26 = 26,000 m

c. $\frac{1000\text{ mm}}{1\text{ m}}=\frac{x\text{ mm}}{2\text{ m}}$
   x m = 2 * 1000 = 2000 mm

d. $\frac{1000\text{ mL}}{1\text{ L}}=\frac{x\text{ mL}}{84\text{ L}}$
   x mL = 1000 * 84 = 84,000 mL

e. $\frac{1000\text{ mm}}{1\text{ m}}=\frac{x\text{ mm}}{13.6\text{ m}}$
   x mm = 1000 * 13.6 = 13,600 mm

f. $\frac{1000\text{ mL}}{1\text{ L}}=\frac{x\text{ mL}}{0.4\text{ L}}$
   x mL = 1000 * 0.4 = 400 mL

g. $\frac{100\text{ cm}}{1\text{ m}}=\frac{x\text{ cm}}{56\text{ m}}$
   x cm = 100 * 56 = 5600 cm

h. $\frac{1000\text{ g}}{1\text{ kg}}=\frac{x\text{ g}}{43\text{ kg}}$
   x g = 1000 * 43 = 43,000 g

i. $\frac{10\text{ mm}}{1\text{ cm}}=\frac{x\text{ mm}}{98.2\text{ cm}}$
   x mm = 10 * 98.2 = 982 mm

j. $\frac{1000\,\text{mcg}}{1\,\text{mg}} = \frac{x\,\text{mcg}}{54\,\text{mg}}$

x mcg = 1000 * 54 = 54,000 mcg

k. $\frac{1\,\text{L}}{1000\,\text{mL}} = \frac{x\,\text{L}}{96\,\text{mL}}$

x L = 96 ÷ 1000 = 0.096 L

l. $\frac{100\,\text{cm}}{1\,\text{m}} - \frac{x\,\text{cm}}{5.2\,\text{m}}$

x cm = 100 * 5.2 = 520 cm

m. $\frac{1\,\text{m}}{1000\,\text{mm}} = \frac{x\,\text{m}}{0.87\,\text{mm}}$

x m = 0.87 ÷ 1000 = 0.00087 m

n. $\frac{1\,\text{kg}}{1000\,\text{g}} = \frac{x\,\text{kg}}{43.2\,\text{g}}$

x kg = 43.2 ÷ 1000 = 0.0432 kg

o. $\frac{1\,\text{mg}}{1000\,\text{mcg}} = \frac{x\,\text{mg}}{32.5\,\text{mcg}}$

x mg = 32.5 ÷ 1000 = 0.0325 mg

Self-Assessment 14-7

a. $\frac{2.54\,\text{cm}}{1\,\text{in}} = \frac{x\,\text{cm}}{3\,\text{in}}$

x cm = 3 * 2.54 = 7.62 cm = 7.6 cm

b. $\frac{15\,\text{mL}}{1\,\text{T}} = \frac{x\,\text{mL}}{4\,\text{T}}$

x mL = 15 * 4 = 60 mL

c. $\frac{2.2\,\text{lb}}{1000\,\text{g}} = \frac{x\,\text{lb}}{36.2\,\text{g}}$

$x\,\text{lb} = \frac{2.2 * 36.2}{1000} = 0.\,07964\,\text{lb} = 0.1\,\text{lb}$

d. $\frac{2.2\,\text{lb}}{1\,\text{kg}} = \frac{324\,\text{lb}}{x\,\text{kg}}$

$x\,\text{kg} = \frac{324}{2.2} = 147.2727\,\text{kg} = 147.3\,\text{kg}$

e. $\frac{28.4\,\text{g}}{1\,\text{oz}} = \frac{972\,\text{g}}{x\,\text{oz}}$

$x\,\text{oz} = \frac{972}{28.4} = 34.225\,\text{oz} = 34.2\,\text{oz}$

f. $\frac{5\,\text{mL}}{1\,\text{tsp}} = \frac{386\,\text{mL}}{x\,\text{tsp}}$

$x\,\text{tsp} = \frac{386}{5} = 77.2\,\text{tsp}$

g. $\frac{30\,\text{mL}}{1\,\text{fl oz}} = \frac{473\,\text{mL}}{x\,\text{fl oz}}$

$x\,\text{fl oz} = \frac{473}{30} = 15.7666\,\text{fl oz} = 15.8\,\text{fl oz}$

h. $\frac{473\,\text{mL}}{1\,\text{pt}} = \frac{x\,\text{mL}}{2\,\text{pt}}$

x mL = 2 * 473 mL = 946 mL

$\frac{946\,\text{mL}}{1\,\text{qt}} = \frac{x\,\text{mL}}{3.2\,\text{qt}}$

x mL = 946 * 3.2 = 3027.2 mL

Self-Assessment 14-8

Use these formulas:
IBW (kg) for males = 50 kg + 2.3(inches over 5')
IBW (kg) for females = 45.5 kg + 2.3(inches over 5')

a. A male who is 6'2" should ideally weigh 50 kg + 2.3(14) = 82.2 kg = 181 lb.
b. A female who is 5'11" should ideally weigh 45.5 kg + 2.3(11) = 70.8 kg = 156 lb.
c. A female who is 5'7" should ideally weigh 45.5 kg + 2.3(7) = 61.6 kg = 136 lb.
d. A male who is 5'6" should ideally weigh 50 kg + 2.3(6) = 63.8 kg = 140 lb.
e. A female who is 6'5" should ideally weigh 45.5 kg + 2.3(17) = 84.6 kg = 186 lb.
f. A male who is 5'2" should ideally weigh 50 kg + 2.3(2) = 54.6 kg = 120 lb.

Self-Assessment 14-9

1.

a. First convert the weight to kg. Then calculate the total daily dose:

$\frac{96\,\text{lb}}{x\,\text{kg}} = \frac{2.2\,\text{lb}}{1\,\text{kg}}$ x kg * 2.2 lb = 1 kg * 96 lb $x = \frac{96}{2.2} = 44\,\text{kg}$

$\frac{5\,\text{mg}}{\text{kg}} = \frac{x\,\text{mg}}{44\,\text{kg}}$

x = 5 * 44 = 220 mg phenytoin per day

b. First calculate the amount (mg) per dose, and then calculate the volume (mL) per dose:

$$\frac{220\text{ mg}}{2\text{ doses per day}} = 110\text{ mg per dose}$$

$$\frac{125\,\text{mg}}{5\,\text{mL}} = \frac{110\,\text{mg}}{x\,\text{mL}}$$

$125\text{ mg} * x\text{ mL} = 110\text{ mg} * 5\text{ mL}$

$$x = \frac{110*5}{125} = 4.4\text{ mL}$$

2.

a. $\frac{75}{100} = \frac{x\,\text{units}}{63\,\text{units}}$

$$x = \frac{75*63}{100} = 47.25\text{ units of long-acting insulin}$$

63 units – 47.25 units = 15.75 units short-acting insulin

You can check this answer by determining if 15.75 is 25% of 63.

b. 212 lb = 96.36 kg rounded to 96 kg

$$\frac{0.3\,\text{units}}{\text{kg}} - \frac{x\,\text{units}}{96\,\text{kg}}$$

x units = 28.8 units

75% of this is long-acting insulin, so $\frac{75}{100} = \frac{x\,\text{units}}{28.8\,\text{units}}$

$$x = \frac{28.8*75}{100}$$

$x = 21.6$ units are long-acting and the rest (28.8 – 21.6 = 7.2 units) are short-acting insulin.

a. $\frac{28.8\,\text{units}}{1\,\text{day}} = \frac{300\,\text{units}}{x\,\text{days}}$

$$x\,\text{days} = \frac{300\,\text{units}}{28.8\,\text{units}}$$

$x = 10.42$ days

So 1 insulin pen will last approximately 10 days.

3.

a. $\frac{50\,\text{mg}}{1\,\text{mL}} = \frac{25\,\text{mg}}{x\,\text{mL}}$

$$x = \frac{50\,\text{mg}}{25\,\text{mg}} = 0.5\,\text{mL}$$

b. $\frac{0.5\,\text{mL}}{1\,\text{dose}} = \frac{10\,\text{mL}}{x\,\text{doses}}$

$$x\,\text{doses} = \frac{10\,\text{mL}}{0.5\,\text{mL}} = 20\,\text{doses}$$

Self-Assessment 14-10

1. $\frac{0.5\text{ tab}}{\text{day}} = \frac{30\text{ tabs}}{x\text{ days}}$

   $x = 60$ days

2. 1 mL PO BID means 1 mL by mouth twice daily. First determine how many mL are needed for a 30-day supply.

   $\frac{2\text{ mL}}{\text{day}} = \frac{x\text{ mL}}{30\text{ days}}$

   $x = 60$ mL

   Dispense 60 mL for a 30-day supply and one 60-mL refill for a total of 120mL.

3. 1 mL to skin BID means apply 1 mL to skin twice per day. The patient will be using 2 mL per day, so for 30 days, the patient will need 60 mL.
4. 1 drop in each eye daily means 2 drops per day.

   $\frac{2\text{ drops}}{\text{day}} = \frac{x\text{ drops}}{10\text{ days}}$

   $x = 20$ drops

   If there are 20 drops per mL, then 1 mL is needed to fill this prescription. Consider overfilling, because sometimes drops are wasted if the eye is missed on application attempts.

5. 2.5 mg PO BID means 2.5 mg by mouth twice daily. The patient will be taking 2.5 mg twice per day, or 5 mg per day. Since the concentration of the medication is 5 mg/mL and you need 5 mg (1 mL) per day, 90 mL will last 90 days.
6. If 1 mL per week will be given and there are 8 mL in the vial, this med should last 8 weeks, or 56 days.
7. The patient will use 5 mL total in the first 5 days and 2.5 mL the second 5 days for a total of 7.5 mL in 10 days. 10 mL – 7.5 mL = 2.5 mL left after 10 days. 2.5 mL divided by 0.5 mL = 5 doses left. 5 * 2 (every other day) = 10 more days. 10 + 10 = 20 days supply.

Self-Assessment 14-11

1. $\frac{5\,\text{g}}{100\,\text{mL}} = \frac{x\,\text{g}}{250\,\text{mL}}$

   $x\,\text{g} = \frac{5*250}{100} = 12.5\,\text{g}$ of dextrose in 250 mL

2.

a. $\frac{5\,g}{100\,ml} = \frac{x\,g}{1000\,ml}$

$$x\,g = \frac{5 * 1000}{100} = 50\,g$$

b. $\frac{0.9\,g}{100\,mL} = \frac{x\,g}{1000\,mL}$

$$x\,g = \frac{0.9 * 1000}{100\,mL} = 9\,g$$

3. $\frac{23.4\,g}{100\,mL} = \frac{x\,g}{5\,mL}$

$$x\,g = \frac{23.4 * 5}{100} = 1.17\,g$$

4. $\frac{10\,g}{100\,mL} = \frac{x\,g}{500\,mL}$

$$x\,g = \frac{10 * 500}{100} = 50\,g$$

Self-Assessment 14-12

1. $\frac{10000\,units}{1\,mL} = \frac{2000\,units}{x\,mL}$

$$x\,mL = \frac{2000}{10000} = 0.2\,mL$$

2. $\frac{100\,units}{1\,mL} = \frac{30\,units}{x\,mL}$

$$x\,mL = \frac{30}{100} = 0.3\,mL$$

In this case it is appropriate to leave the value as it is, without rounding to a whole number. This amount of insulin is measurable; insulin syringes can deliver very accurate small doses.

Self-Assessment 14-13

1. First, determine how many mL are needed per dose. In this case, this also represents the amount needed per day since the patient is taking the medication once daily. Pay careful attention to the units—the order was written for 0.5 mg daily, which equals 500 mcg daily.

$$\frac{50\,mcg}{1\,mL} = \frac{500\,mcg}{x\,mL}$$

$$x\,mL = \frac{500}{50} = 10\,mL$$

10 mL of the solution would be used for one dose of the medication. 60 mL of the solution will provide 6 doses, or 6 days' worth of medication.

2. First determine the correct dose for the 50-kg patient:

$$\frac{15\,mg}{kg} = \frac{x\,mg}{50\,kg}$$

$x = 15 * 50 = 750$ mg

Next, determine how many mL you would need of the 100 mg/mL solution.

$$\frac{100\,mg}{mL} = \frac{750\,mg}{x\,mL}$$

$x = 7.5$ mL

3.

a. First prepare the pediatric dilution. Determine how many mcg of dexamethasone are needed to prepare the dilution. Remember, the commercially available solution is available as 4 mg/mL, so convert mcg to mg (0.4 mg).

$$\frac{x\,mcg}{4\,mL} = \frac{100\,mcg}{1\,mL}$$

x mcg = 100 * 4 = 400 mcg = 0.4 mg

Next, determine how many mL of the commercially available solution are needed to equal 0.4 mg.

$$\frac{4\,mg}{1\,mL} = \frac{0.4\,mg}{x\,mL}$$

x mL = 0.4 ÷ 4 = 0.1 mL

If the final volume is to be 4 mL, and you need 0.1 mL of the dexamethasone solution, then 3.9 mL of sterile water is needed to prepare 4 mL of the pediatric dilution.

b. First, determine the dose:

$$\frac{0.15\,mg/day}{1\,kg} = \frac{x\,mg}{11\,kg}$$

$x = 1.65$ mg/day

$$\frac{1.65\,mg}{1\,day} * \frac{1\,day}{2\,doses} = 0.825\,mg/doses$$

Next determine the volume of medication for this dose:

$$\frac{0.1\,mg}{1\,mL} = \frac{0.825\,mg}{x\,mL}$$

$x = 8.25$ mL

4. This mixture is a w/w type. Both ingredients are weighed. Determine what 5% of 60 g is.

$$\frac{5\,\text{g}}{100\,\text{g}} = \frac{x\,\text{g}}{60\,\text{g}}$$

$x = 3$ g

You will need 3 g of pure coal tar for this mixture.

5. First, determine how many mg of phenobarbital are needed in the pediatric dilution.

$$\frac{10\,\text{mg}}{1\,\text{mL}} = \frac{x\,\text{mg}}{1000\,\text{mL}}$$

$x = 10000$ mg

Second, determine how many mL of the commercially available solution are needed to prepare the dilution.

$$\frac{130\,\text{mg}}{1\,\text{mL}} = \frac{10{,}000\,\text{mg}}{x\,\text{mL}}$$

$x = 76.9$ mL phenobarbital solution needed

To determine the amount of sterile water needed, subtract the volume of phenobarbital solution from the total volume:

1000 mL – 76.9 mL = 923.1 mL sterile water needed

6. $$\frac{40\,\text{mEq}}{20\,\text{mL}} = \frac{10\,\text{mEq}}{x\,\text{mL}}$$

$x = 5$ mL

7. 1 g is equal to 1000 mg.

$$\frac{1\,\text{g}}{1000\,\text{mL}} = \frac{1000\,\text{mg}}{1000\,\text{mL}}$$

$$\frac{1000\,\text{mg}}{1000\,\text{mL}} = \frac{1\,\text{mg}}{x\,\text{mL}}$$

$x = 1$ mL

Self-Assessment 14-14

1.

%	%	PARTS
100%		2.5 parts
	3%	
0.5%		97 parts
		99.5 total parts

100 – 3 = 97, so there are 97 parts of the 0.5% cream.

3 – 0.5 = 2.5, so there are 2.5 parts of the 100% powder.

97 parts + 2.5 parts = 99.5 parts

Now you know that if you were making 99.5 parts of this cream, 97 parts would be the 0.5% cream and 2.5 parts would be 100% HC powder. Knowing this, you can set up a proportion to calculate how much of each you need for 45 grams of cream.

$$\frac{97}{99.5} = \frac{x}{45\,\text{g}}$$

$x = \dfrac{97 * 45}{99.5} = 43.869$ g rounded to 44 g of the 0.5% cream

If the total is 45 grams, and 44 grams are 0.5% cream, you can subtract and calculate what is left, which must be the pure hydrocortisone powder.

45 – 44 = 1 g of pure hydrocortisone powder.

2. Note: Water is considered 0%.

%	%	PARTS
0.9%		0.45 parts
	0.45%	
0 %		0.45 parts
		0.9 total parts

You will need 0.45 parts each of water and normal saline to make 0.9 total parts. No matter how much 0.45% half-normal saline you are making, you will always mix water and normal saline in equal amounts. Therefore, the answer to this question is that you add 1 liter of water to 1 liter of normal saline to make 2 liters of half-normal saline (0.45%NS).

3.

%	%	PARTS
100%		1.5 parts
	2.5%	
1%		97.5 parts
		99 total parts

Of a total of 99 parts, 97.5 parts are the 1% ointment.

$$\frac{97.5\,\text{parts}}{99\,\text{parts}} = \frac{x\,\text{g}}{60\,\text{g}}$$

$x = \dfrac{97.5 * 60}{99} = 59.09$ g of the 1% ointment rounded to 59.1g

60 – 59.1 = 0.9 g of the salicylic acid powder

Self-Assessment 14-15

1. Remember that specific gravity is in terms of weight and volume.

$$\text{specific gravity} = \frac{\text{weight (g)}}{\text{volume (mL)}}$$

Plug the known quantities into the formula and solve for x. Be sure to convert to the appropriate units:

$$1.3 = \frac{2600\text{ g}}{x\text{ mL}}$$

$$x\text{ mL} = \frac{2600}{1.3} = 2000\text{ mL}$$

Self-Assessment 14-16

1.

a. $\frac{125\text{ mg}}{\text{m}^2} = \frac{x\text{ mg}}{2.06\text{ m}^2}$

$125\text{ mg} * 2.06\text{ m}^2 = \text{m}^2 * x\text{ mg}$

$\frac{125\text{ mg} * 2.06\text{m}^2}{\text{m}^2} = \frac{\text{m}^2 * x\text{ mg}}{\text{m}^2}$

$x\text{ mg} = 125\text{ mg} * 2.06 = 257.5\text{ mg}$

b. $\frac{20\text{ mg}}{\text{m}^2} = \frac{x\text{ mg}}{2.06\text{ m}^2}$

$x = 20 * 2.06\text{ mg} = 41.2\text{ mg}$

c. $\frac{500\text{ mg}}{\text{m}^2} = \frac{x\text{ mg}}{2.06\text{ m}^2}$

$x = 500\text{ mg} * 2.06 = 1030\text{ mg}$

2.

a. $\frac{60\text{ mg}}{\text{m}^2} = \frac{x\text{ mg}}{1.77\text{ m}^2}$

$x = 60\text{ mg} * 1.77 = 106.2\text{ mg}$

b. $\frac{600\text{ mg}}{\text{m}^2} = \frac{x\text{ mg}}{1.77\text{ m}^2}$

$x = 600\text{ mg} * 1.77 = 1062\text{ mg}$

c. $\frac{80\text{ mg}}{\text{m}^2} = \frac{x\text{ mg}}{1.77\text{ m}^2}$

$x = 80\text{ mg} * 1.77 = 141.6\text{ mg}$

d. First convert weight in pounds to kg: 146/2.2 = 66.4 kg

$\frac{4\text{ mg}}{\text{kg}} = \frac{x\text{ mg}}{66.4\text{ kg}}$

$x = 4\text{ mg} * 66.4 = 265.6\text{ mg}$

Self-Assessment 14-17

1.

a. The patient weighs 226 lb, which is equal to 102.7 kg (226/2.2 = 102.7)

$\frac{15\text{ mg}}{\text{kg}} = \frac{x\text{ mg}}{102.7\text{ kg}}$

$x = 102.7 * 15\text{ mg} = 1540.5\text{ mg}$, rounded to 1540 mg

b. $\frac{50\text{ mg}}{\text{mL}} = \frac{1540\text{ mg}}{x\text{ mL}}$

$x = \frac{1540}{50} = 30.8\text{ mL}$

c. $\frac{10\text{ mg}}{1\text{ min}} = \frac{1540\text{ mg}}{x\text{ min}}$

$x = \frac{1540}{10} = 154\text{ min}$

Since the instructions are to infuse for 60 min or at 10 mg/min, whichever is longer, and since 154 min is more than 60 min, the correct infusion time is 154 min.

2.

a. 174 lb ÷ 2.2 lb/kg = 79 kg

$\frac{6\text{ mg}}{\text{kg}} = \frac{x\text{ mg}}{79\text{ kg}}$

$x = 474\text{ mg}$

b. $\frac{25\text{ mg}}{1\text{ mL}} = \frac{474\text{ mg}}{x\text{ mL}}$

$x = 19\text{ mL}$

c. $\frac{474\text{ mg}}{x\text{ min}} = \frac{25\text{ mg}}{1\text{ min}}$

$x = 19$ minutes

3.

a. 198 lb ÷ 2.2 lb/kg = 90 kg

$\frac{3\text{mg}}{\text{kg}} = \frac{x\text{ mg}}{90\text{ kg}}$

$x = 270\text{ mg}$

This is the dose per day. Each dose would be 90 mg (270 mg ÷ 3).

b. $\frac{40\text{ mg}}{\text{mL}} = \frac{90\text{ mg}}{x\text{ mL}}$

$x = 2.25\text{ mL}$

c. $\frac{50\text{ mL}}{30\text{ min}} = \frac{x\text{ mL}}{1\text{ min}}$

$x = 1.7$ mL per minute

4.

a. $\frac{50\,mg}{1\,mL} = \frac{150\,mg}{x\,mL}$

$x = 3$ mL

b. Note: use 100 mL for calculation.

100 mL / 10 min = 10 mL/min

c. $\frac{15\,drops}{1\,mL} = \frac{x\,drops}{10\,mL}$

$x = 150$ drops

5.

a. $\frac{40.5\,g}{180\,mL} = \frac{3.375\,g}{x\,mL}$

$x = \frac{3.375 * 180}{40.5} = 15\,mL$

b. $\frac{15\,mL}{1\,dose} = \frac{180\,mL}{x\,dose}$

$x = 12$ doses

c. Every 6 hours is 4 doses per day, so 4 * 3000 mg = 12,000 mg = 12 g.

d. 100 mL of NS and 15 mL of piperacillin/tazobactam will be infused each hour.
115 mL/60 min = 1.9 mL/min

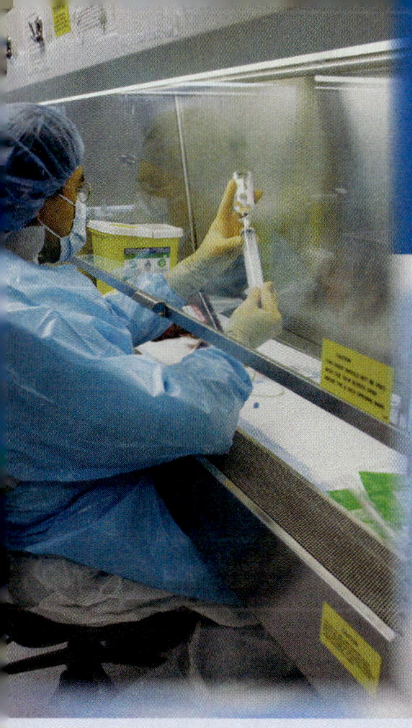

Chapter 15

Nonsterile Compounding and Repackaging

John F. Falkenholm, Jane E. Krause

Learning Outcomes

After completing this chapter, you will be able to

- Define compounding.
- Describe the steps involved in the compounding process.
- Describe the equipment commonly used when compounding preparations.
- Identify the types of preparations commonly compounded.
- Explain the concept of and reasons for repackaging medications.
- Explain the importance of record keeping for compounding and repackaging.

Key Terms

active ingredient Ingredient in the compounded preparation that is responsible for the therapeutic or pharmaceutical action of the medication.

batch record (or batch log) The compounding record for a batch, usually filed by lot number.

batch repackaging The periodic repackaging of large quantities of medications in unit-dose or single-unit packages.

beyond-use labeling A date that is given to a medication noting when it should no longer be used, also referred to as the expiration date.

blister packages Often called "bubble packs." Composed of a plastic bubble that forms a cavity for the medication. The package is then sealed with a backing material that also acts as a label.

compounding Usually takes place in a pharmacy and includes the preparation, mixing, packaging, and labeling of a small quantity of a drug based on a practitioner's prescription or medication order for a specific patient.

compounding environment Includes the facilities (i.e., compounding area) and equipment in the pharmacy.

compounding record The log or record of an actual compounded preparation or batch that was prepared.

extemporaneous repackaging Repackaging quantities of medications that will be used within a short period of time.

formulation record An individual record (like a recipe) for a preparation. It includes a listing of the ingredients, compounding equipment, and instructions for preparing the compound. A formulation record may also be referred to as a formula or master formula.

geometric dilution Compounding technique used to ensure the uniform mixing when there is a wide discrepancy in amounts of individual ingredients. The preparer starts with the smallest ingredient amount and mixes it with an equal amount (estimated by sight) of the next smallest ingredient amount and continues adding and doubling the size until all ingredients are integrated.

graduates Compounding equipment used to measure the volume of liquid ingredients; generally glass or plastic cylinders and conicals.

inactive ingredient An ingredient that is necessary to prepare the formulation, but is not intended to cause a pharmacologic response. Inactive ingredients may also be referred to as inert ingredients, added ingredients or substances, or excipients, and include, for example, colorants, flavorants, sweeteners, and wetting agents.

levigation A compounding method of incorporating a solid (i.e., powder) into an ointment. A small amount of a levigating agent is added to the powder to form a paste, which is then incorporated into the ointment.

manufacturing Typically occurs in licensed manufacturing facilities and includes the production, conversion, and/or processing of a drug, generally in bulk quantities and without a prescription or medication order.

master formula Also known as a formulation record.

nonsterile compounding Compounds prepared in a pharmacy that do not require strict aseptic technique and include preparations such as oral and topical medications.

peristaltic pumps Pumps with a series of roller wheels that press against tubing to force a volume of liquid down the length of the tubing.

prescription compounding A medication individualized for a specific patient that requires the mixing of ingredients in a pharmacy and is based on a prescription or drug order.

stability Defined in USP-NF as the extent to which a preparation retains, within specified limits and throughout its period of storage and use, the same properties and characteristics that it possessed at the time of compounding.

sterile compounding Compounds prepared in a pharmacy using strict aseptic technique including preparations such as injections, ophthalmic solutions, and irrigation solutions.

trituration The act of mixing powders or crushing tablets using a mortar and pestle (i.e., solid is rubbed with mortar and pestle) until a state of fine, evenly sized particles is achieved.

unit-dose package A non-reusable container designed to hold a quantity of drug to be administered as a single dose.

unit-of-use packaging Characterized by a vial, an envelope, or a plastic bag containing several doses of the same medication.

volumetric pumps Pumps that allow the user to preset a volume to be dispensed into a container on the basis of the draw back setting.

As the benefits of individualized drug therapy have been recognized over the past few decades, prescription compounding has experienced renewed popularity. It is estimated that 30 million compounded prescriptions are prepared each year, which comprises 1% of all dispensed prescriptions.[1] Several thousand pharmacies have thriving practices in human and veterinary compounding; in fact, some are compounding-only pharmacies. Providing individualized patient care through compounding offers a unique clinical experience through the patient-physician-pharmacist triad.

When commercial medications are available but not in the packaging best suited to the needs of the patient or staff, repackaging offers a convenient, cost-effective method of providing medications to the patient. The role of technicians in the preparation of nonsterile compounds and repackaging medications is very important.

✔ While pharmacists evaluate patient needs, counsel patients, interact with other health care professionals, and perform other clinically oriented activities, technicians perform much of the actual dosage form preparation through compounding and repackaging medications.

Overview of Prescription Compounding

Prescription compounding allows the prescriber and the pharmacist to meet the unique needs of a patient. For example, a physician may determine that a patient requires a medication in a strength or dosage form that is not commercially available. Compounding is often associated with several specialty practice areas, including veterinary medicine, dermatology, hormone replacement therapy, pain management, hospice, and home care.

It is important to differentiate between compounding and manufacturing. **Compounding** involves the preparation, mixing, packaging, and labeling of a small quantity of a drug based on a practitioner's prescription or medication order for a specific patient. This is contrasted with **manufacturing,** which is the production, conversion, and/or processing of a drug, generally in bulk quantities and without a prescription or medication order. In other words, compounding a preparation for a specific patient usually takes place in a pharmacy, whereas manufacturing products in bulk typically occurs in licensed manufacturing facilities.

It is also necessary to understand that **sterile compounding** is different from **nonsterile compounding**. Sterile compounds must be prepared using strict aseptic technique and include preparations such as injections, ophthalmic solutions, and irrigation solutions. Sterile compounding is explained in Chapter 16, Aseptic Technique, Sterile Compounding, and IV Admixture Programs. This chapter focuses on nonsterile compounding, which includes preparations such as oral and topical medications. The topics of pharmacy calculations (Chapter 14) and processing medication orders and prescriptions (Chapter 13) are also important to understand in relation to compounding.

USP-NF Chapter 795

The *United States Pharmacopeia and The National Formulary* (USP-NF) offers guidelines and an enforceable set of standards describing procedures and requirements for compounding in Chapter 795 (Pharmaceutical Compounding–Nonsterile Preparations).[2] The intent of the USP is to protect both patients and pharmacists.

Once a technician's knowledge and proficiency have been demonstrated and documented, they are allowed to participate in the compounding process. The pharmacist is responsible for the finished product and quality assurance in all aspects of the compounding process. The intent and emphasis of USP Chapter 795 is summarized here in relation to nonsterile compounding.

Rx for Success

All technicians involved in compounding must be properly trained, knowledgeable about USP Chapter 795 (Pharmaceutical Compounding–Nonsterile Preparations), and proficient with pharmaceutical calculations.

Compounding Environment

The **compounding environment** includes the facilities (i.e., compounding area) and equipment. The compounding area should have adequate space for the orderly placement and storage of equipment and support materials. Controlled temperature and lighting are needed for chemicals and finished medications. The area must be kept clean for sanitary reasons and to prevent cross-contamination. A sink with hot and cold running water is essential for hand washing and equipment cleaning. Compounding equipment must be appropriate in design and size for its intended purpose and must always be cleaned immediately after use. Equipment must be properly maintained and calibrated.

✔ Some pharmacies compound both sterile and nonsterile preparations. In these pharmacies, the compounding area for sterile preparations is separate and distinct from the area used for compounding nonsterile preparations.

Stability of Compounded Preparations

Stability is defined in USP-NF as "the extent to which a preparation retains, within specified limits, and throughout its period of storage and use, the same properties and characteristics that it possessed at the time of compounding."[2] Primary packaging of the finished medication is of utmost importance. The choice of the proper container is guided by the physical and chemical characteristics of the finished medication. Whether the medication is light sensitive or binds to the container are examples of considerations in maximizing stability. **Beyond-use labeling** (i.e., the preparation is labeled with a beyond-use date) should be included on all medications. The beyond-use date is the date after which a preparation is not to be used and is calculated from the date it was compounded. Things to consider for determining beyond-use dates include whether the medication is aqueous (water-based) or nonaqueous, the expiration dates of the ingredients used, the storage temperature, and the references documenting the stability of the finished medication. Expiration dates apply to manufactured products.

Ingredient Selection

Sources of ingredients vary widely. USP or National Formulary (NF) chemicals are the preferred chemicals for compounding. Other sources may be used, but the pharmacist is responsible for ensuring that the chemical meets purity and safety standards. Manufactured medications (prescription and nonprescription drugs) are another acceptable source of ingredients. Any drug that is withdrawn from the market by the FDA should not be used.

Compounded Preparations

Preparations should contain at least 90%, but not more than 110%, of the labeled active ingredient, unless more restrictive guidelines apply. Compounding guidelines in USP-NF specifically address the following dosage forms: capsules, powders, lozenges, tablets, emulsions, solutions, suspensions, suppositories, creams, topical gels, ointments, and pastes.

Compounding Process

The goal of the compounding process is to "minimize error and maximize the prescriber's intent."[2] Depending upon state laws and regulations, technicians who are trained in preparing compounded prescriptions may be involved in the steps listed in this section.

✔ As stated in USP Chapter 795, the compounding process includes several steps and for quality assurance, it is suggested that the steps be accomplished in an orderly and methodical manner.

Prior to the technician compounding the preparation, the pharmacist clinically evaluates the appropriateness of the prescription or drug order in terms of safety and intended use for the patient. In addition, as these steps are reviewed, it is important to understand that only one preparation should be compounded at one time in the compounding area to avoid errors and cross-contamination.

1. **Calculate the amount of ingredients needed for the preparation.**
2. **Identify equipment needed to compound the preparation.** Compounding equipment is discussed later in this chapter.
3. **Wash hands and wear proper attire.** Clean clothing with a clean laboratory jacket is considered proper attire for most nonsterile compounding. It may, however, be necessary to wear head covering, safety glasses, gloves, mask, gown, and foot covers if the ingredient(s) in the compound are considered potentially hazardous. An example of compounding attire is shown in figure 15-1. These precautions are for the safety and protection of the individual preparing the compound. Procedures for working with an ingredient can be found in the Material Safety Data Sheet (MSDS), which are forms readily accessible to all employees in the pharmacy (electronically or in hardcopy) for each drug substance in the compound. Pharmacists are responsible for instructing technicians on how to retrieve and interpret needed information from the MSDS.
4. **Clean the compounding area and needed equipment.**
5. **Collect all materials and ingredients needed.**
6. **Compound the preparation following a formulation record (file of individually compounded preparations) or prescription and according to the art and science of pharmacy.** Compounding procedures are discussed later in this chapter.

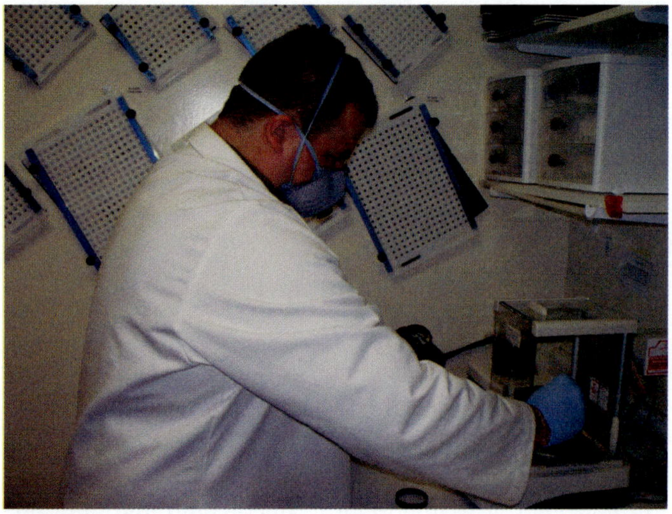

Figure 15-1. An example of compounding attire (laboratory jacket, gloves, and mask).

7. **Document name on the compounding record/log.** In addition to the name of the technician preparing the compound, the compounding record also includes the name, strength, and amount of preparation, formulation record reference, lot numbers of ingredients, name of the pharmacist checking the compound, date of preparation, prescription number (or other assigned identification number), and beyond use date.
8. **Label the final preparation appropriately.** The label should include the name of the preparation, strength, dosage form, quantity, beyond-use date, initials of the pharmacist checking the preparation, storage requirements, and any other statements or information that may be required by law.
9. **Properly clean and store all equipment.**

The pharmacist is responsible for checking the final preparation for weight variation, proper mixing, odor, color, consistency, and pH as appropriate. In addition, the pharmacist is responsible for signing and dating the prescription or drug order documenting and ensuring quality.

Rx for Success

The pharmacist reviews each step in the compounding process and is responsible for accuracy, quality, completeness, and final checks prior to dispensing the prescription to the patient.

Compounding Records and Documents

Each step of the compounding process should be documented. USP Chapter 795 requires pharmacies to maintain a **formulation record,** also known as the **master formula,** and a **compounding record** for each compounded preparation. The formulation record is an individual record (like a recipe) that is stored in a file with other formulas. These are usually filed alphabetically, so it is easy to find the desired formula. This record includes a listing of the ingredients, compounding equipment, and instructions for preparing the formula.

✔ The goal of documentation is for quality purposes, to allow another individual to reproduce the same formulation at a later date, and to trace each ingredient in the compound, if necessary.

The compounding record is the log (or record) of an actual compounded preparation (i.e., based on an individual prescription or drug order) or batch being prepared (i.e., for compounds prepared in anticipation of orders). It includes manufacturer and lot numbers of chemicals used, the date of preparation, an internal identification number (commonly called a lot number), a beyond-use date, the names of the individuals who prepared and verified the preparation, and any other pertinent information regarding the preparation. The compounding record for a batch (**batch record**) is usually filed by lot number, whereas the compounding record for an individual prescription or drug order is a chronological list of preparations made. Depending upon state laws and regulations, the formulation and compounding records may be maintained as paper copies or electronically in the pharmacy.

Rx for Success

Always remember that accurate and complete documentation is essential in all aspects and areas of pharmacy.

Quality Control

Quality control is the final check on the preparation to ensure its safety and quality. The pharmacist must evaluate the finished preparation both physically and by reviewing the compounding procedure to be certain the preparation is accurate. Discrepancies should be noted and evaluated to determine if the preparation is acceptable.

Patient Counseling

Patient counseling is important with all medications, including compounded formulations. The patient should be counseled by the pharmacist on the correct use, storage, beyond-use date, and evidence of instability in the compounded medication.

Inactive Ingredients

In addition to the **active, or therapeutic, ingredient(s)**, compounded medications may contain a number of inactive, or nontherapeutic, ingredients. **Inactive ingredients** are needed to prepare the formulation, but are not intended to cause a pharmacologic response. Inactive ingredients are also referred to as inert ingredients, added ingredients or substances, or excipients.

Examples of categories of inactive ingredients used in compounded prescriptions include diluents or fillers, binders, colorants, lubricants, flavorants, sweeteners, suspending agents, emulsifying agents or surfactants, coating agents, preservatives, perfumes, acidifying agents, alkalizing agents, vehicles, and wetting agents. Although they do not cause pharmacologic activity, inactive ingredients are a necessary part of the product, and the specific chemicals used as excipients must be named in the formula.

Compounding Equipment and Procedures

The compounding equipment found in a pharmacy depends upon the type and scope of compounding performed. The most common types of equipment are those used to weigh and measure ingredients in the preparation. An electronic or class A torsion balance is used to weigh solids (i.e., powders, crystals) needed for the compound (figure 15-2 A and B). The surface on which the balance rests must be stable and solid. It is essential that technicians develop a proficient and accurate technique when using balances. Powder papers or weigh boats are used to hold the solid being weighed and help to keep the balance pans clean and free of corrosion. Brass weight sets are used with class A torsion balances.

✔ The balance must be maintained and calibrated regularly.

Graduates (i.e., glass or plastic cylinders and conicals) are used to measure the volume of liquid ingredients. Various sizes of graduates (e.g., 5 mL, 10 mL, 25 mL, 100 mL, 250 mL, etc.) are used when compounding (figure 15-3). It is recommended to use the smallest graduate that will hold the volume to be measured. In addition, it is important to measure the volume of liquid accurately by placing the graduate on a stable surface (i.e., counter top of work area) and read the measurement at the bottom of the meniscus. The meniscus is the natural curvature of the surface of the liquid and it is lower in the middle than at the edges. The bottom of the meniscus should be read at eye level. Do not look down or up at the bottom of the meniscus as this will yield an inaccurate reading (figure 15-4). In terms of graduates, the cylinder shaped graduates usually yield more accurate readings. Conical shaped graduates are often used when mixing

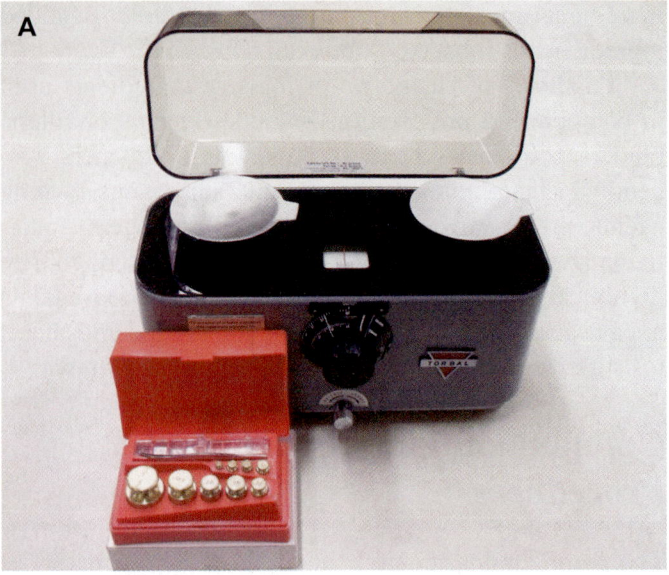

Figure 15–2A. Class A torsion balance and weight set.

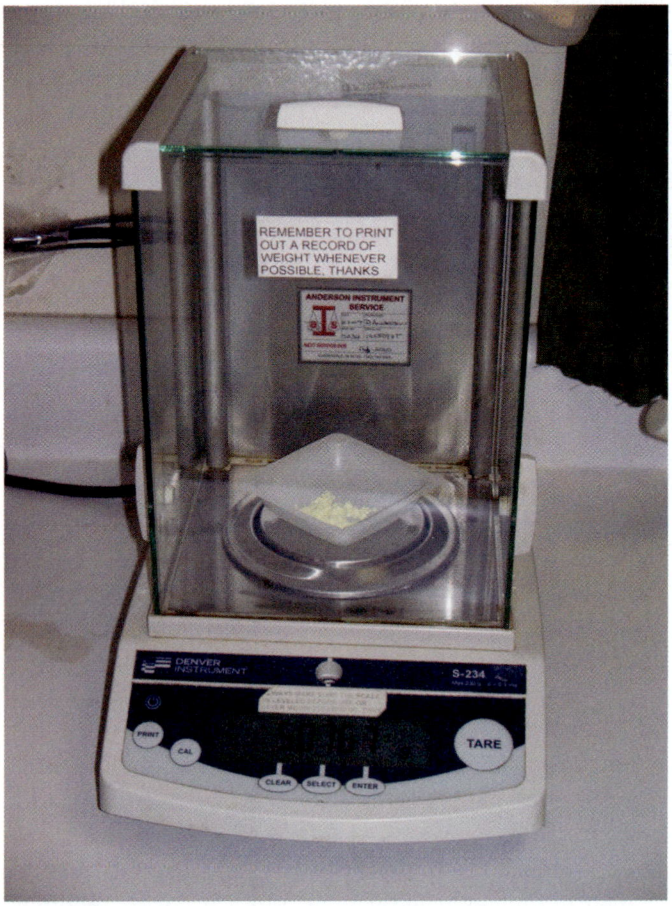

Figure 15–2B. Electronic balance with weigh boat.

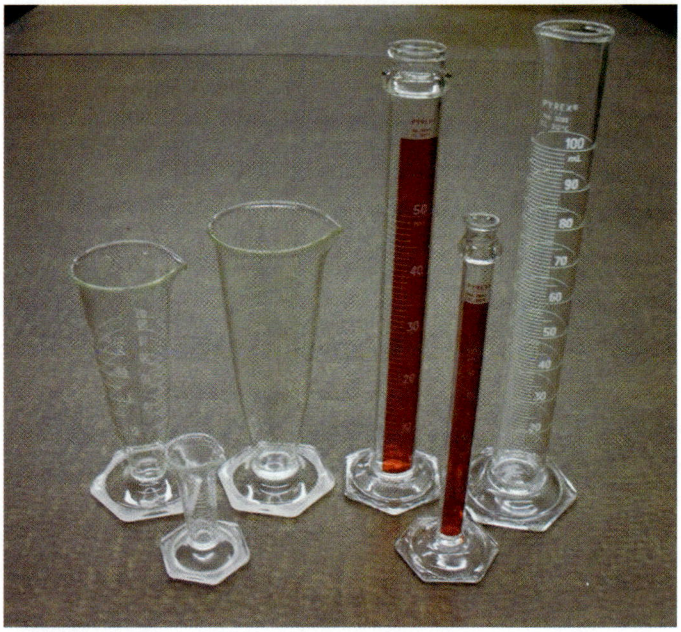

Figure 15–3. Graduates (conicals and cylinders).

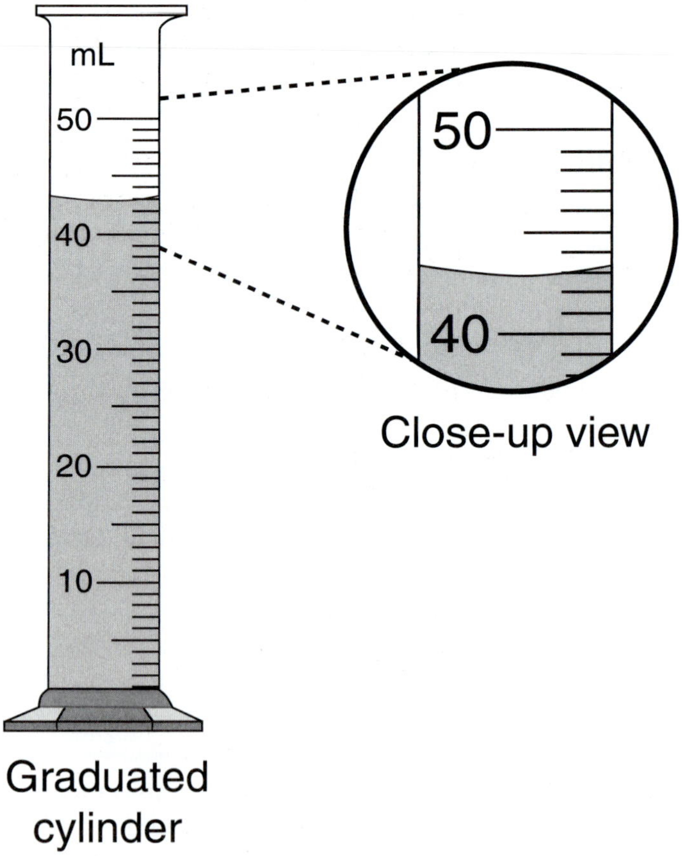

Figure 15–4. Measuring using a graduated cylinder. Read the bottom of the meniscus at eye level.

liquids. The likelihood of error in accurately reading the bottom of the meniscus in a conical graduate increases as the sides flare. Pipets and calibrated syringes are used to accurately measure very small volumes of liquids.

Rx for Success

As part of quality assurance, it is essential to develop correct and accurate technique with all compounding equipment.

Mortars and pestles (figure 15-5 A, B, and C) are used to crush, grind, and blend various medicinal ingredients. Mixing powders or crushing tablets is achieved by moving the pestle in a circular motion in the mortar (i.e., solid is rubbed with mortar and pestle) until a state of fine, evenly sized particles is achieved. This is termed **trituration.** It is necessary to reduce particle size and blend the ingredients into a homogenous mixture to ensure accurate dosing. Mortars are available in a variety of materials (e.g., glass, porcelain, Wedgewood) and sizes (e.g., 2 oz, 4 oz, 8 oz, etc). Glass mortars are preferable when mixing liquids or preparing solutions, suspensions, or lotions. Glass mortars are also non-staining and therefore should be used when adding flavoring oils and coloring. Wedgewood mortars have a rough interior surface and are ideal for intense grinding and trituration to reduce particle size. Wedgewood mortars stain easily and are porous; therefore, extra care must be taken when cleaning Wedgewood to ensure that all particles are removed to avoid cross contamination. Porcelain mortars are also very durable and are often used for blending powders and reducing particle size. Porcelain mortars have a glazed interior surface that is less porous than Wedgewood.

An ointment slab (also called a pill tile) is a square glass tile that is used for preparing and mixing creams and ointments. Similarly, many facilities use ointment paper (e.g., pads of 12" × 12" disposable parchment paper) instead of an ointment slab because of convenience in reducing clean-up time (figure 15-6 A and B). The ingredients are placed on the ointment slab/paper and blended with a spatula (plastic or stainless) by moving the spatula in a "figure eight" motion. Before incorporating a powder into the ointment, a paste is first formed by adding a small amount (sufficient to form a paste) of an appropriate levigating agent (e.g., mineral oil). Particle size is then reduced by rubbing the paste on the ointment

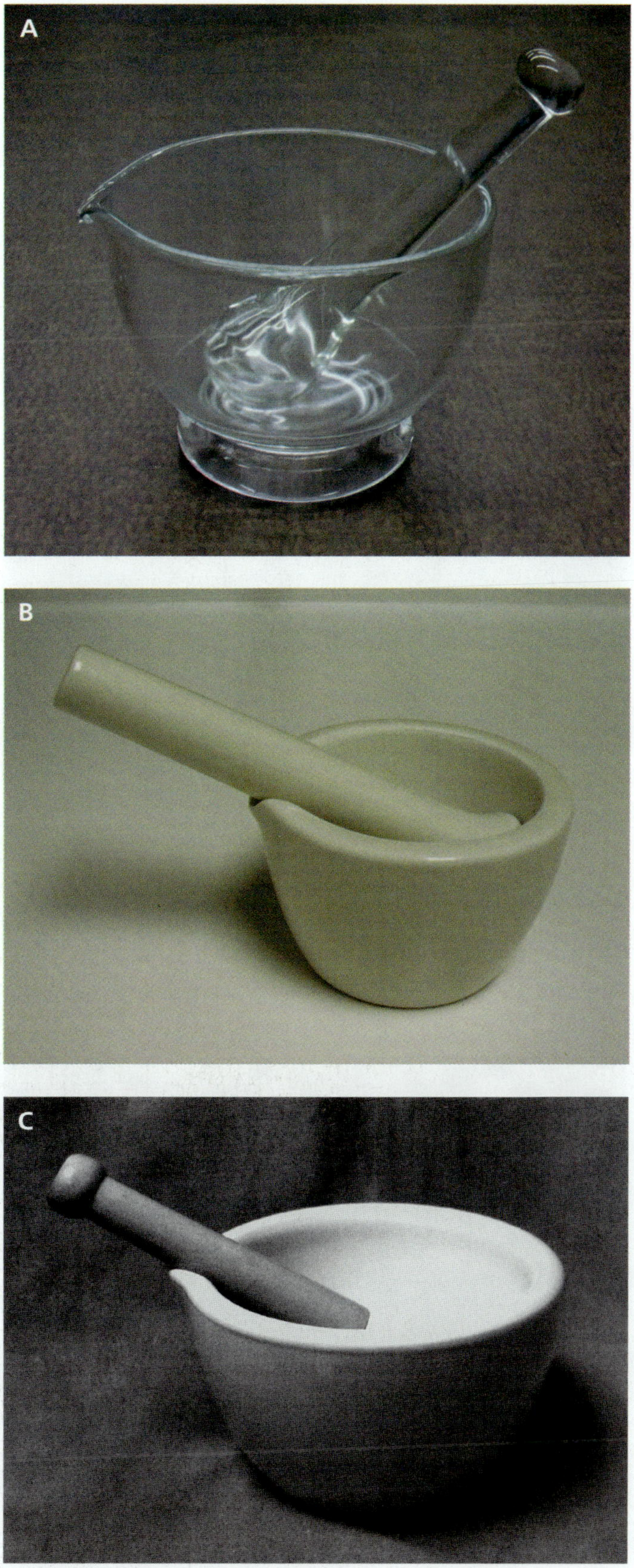

Figure 15-5 Mortar and pestles.

slab/paper using a spatula. This method of incorporating a solid into the ointment is termed **levigation**. The levigating agent used is based on its compatibility in the final preparation.

A variety of sizes and types of spatulas should be available in a compounding area. Smaller spatulas (i.e., blades four or six inches long) are suggested when working with dry chemicals. Larger spatulas (i.e., blades eight inches long) are recommended when working with large quantities of ointments or creams. Plastic spatulas should be used when working with chemicals that may react with stainless steel.

Electronic mortars and pestles are often used for the preparation of ointments and creams. The chemicals in the preparation can be conveniently weighed, mixed, and dispensed in the same ointment jar (figure 15-7). In addi-

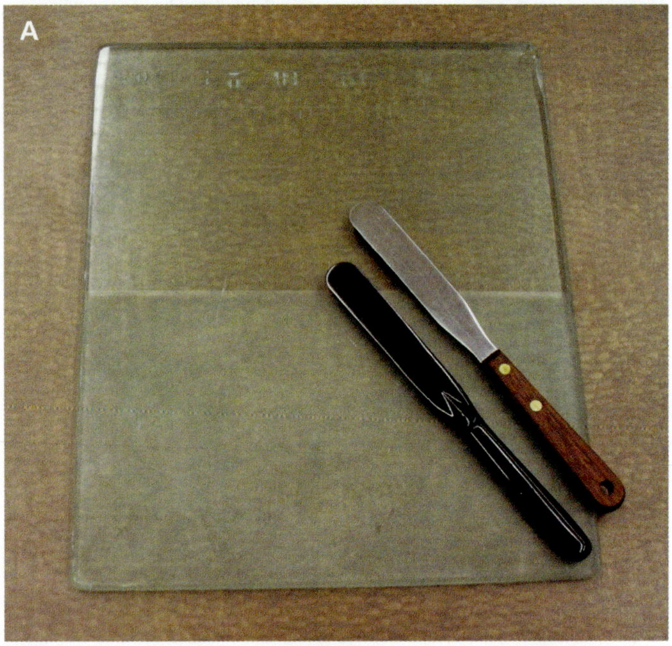

Figure 15-6A Ointment slab and spatulas.

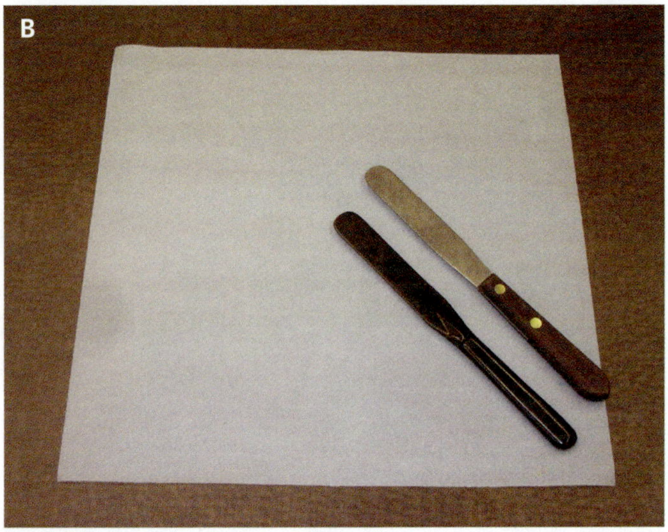

Figure 15-6B Ointment tablet.

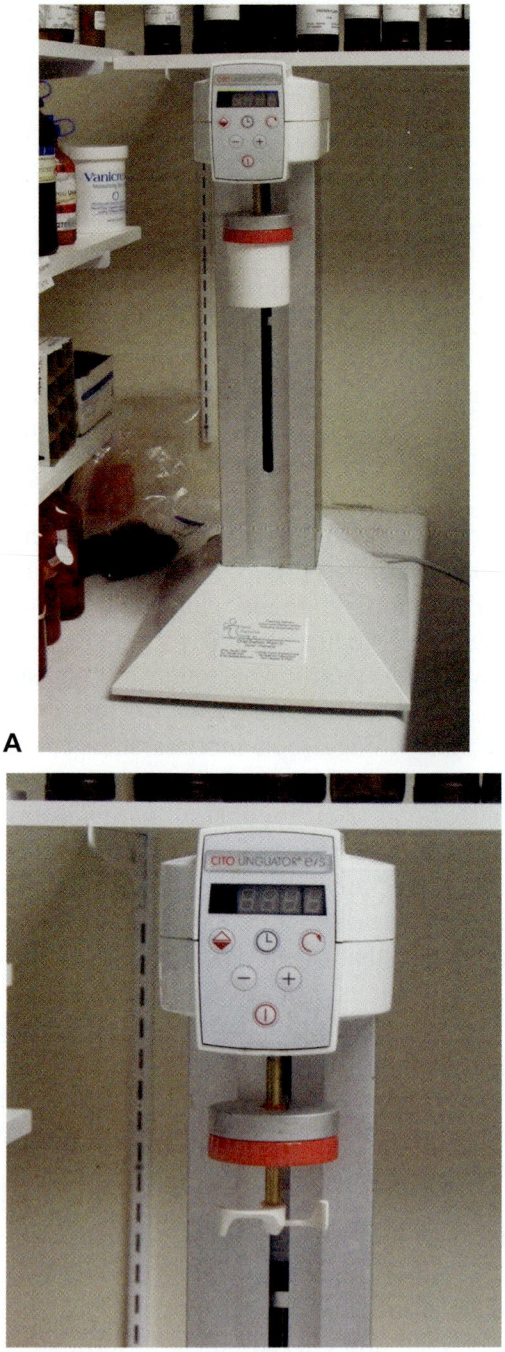

Figure 15-7. Electronic mortar and pestle (often used for preparing creams and ointments).

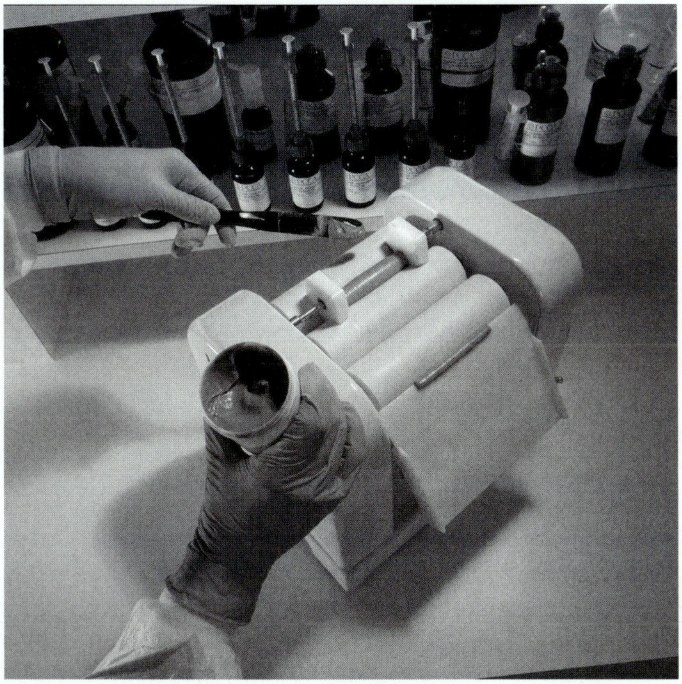

Figure 15-8. Ointment mill.

tion, ointment mills are commonly found in compounding pharmacies (figure 15-8). Most have three rollers with small, adjustable spaces between the rollers. When preparations pass through the rollers, particle size is reduced.

Geometric dilution is a technique that is used to ensure the uniform mixing of various amounts of different ingredients. This process is used when there is a wide discrepancy in amounts of individual ingredients. To mix ingredients using geometric dilution, the technician starts with the smallest ingredient amount and mixes it with an equal amount (estimated by sight) of the next smallest ingredient amount. This process then continues (adding and doubling the size) until all ingredients are integrated.

Other useful equipment and supplies include funnels and filter paper. Filtration refers to the process of separating solid particles from a liquid. Filtering a liquid preparation will help obtain a clear product (i.e., will brighten the appearance) and remove any impurities or minute particles. In the process, the liquid (called the filtrate) is passed through a barrier (commercially available filter paper). Mechanical filtering machines may be available in more advanced compounding pharmacies that cut the filtration time down extensively.

Depending on the needs of the pharmacy, other general compounding equipment may include beakers, hot plates, refrigerator with freezer, stirring rods, stir plates with magnetic stir bars, strainers, and molds (e.g., suppository, troche). Examples of more advanced compounding equipment found in some pharmacies include blenders, capsule filling equipment, mixers, and motorized stirrers.

Rx for Success

Although the pharmacist is responsible for overseeing that the compounding equipment is continually checked and maintained for accuracy and quality, the technician plays an important part in this process. This documentation is referred to as equipment maintenance records.

Commonly Compounded Preparations

Types of commonly compounded preparations include ointments, creams, solutions, suspensions, suppositories, lozenges/troches, capsules, and other preparations. Generally, the prescriber will indicate a specific dosage form that is to be compounded, such as an oral solution, topical cream, or a rectal suppository. The prescriber, however, sometimes depends upon the clinical knowledge of the pharmacist to decide on an appropriate dosage form for a preparation.

Ointments and Creams

Ointments and creams are generally applied topically, but other routes of administration (e.g., rectal and vaginal) may also be appropriate based on the prescription. Usually, an active ingredient is incorporated into a commercially prepared base (e.g., petrolatum-based products, emollient creams, vanishing creams). The choice of base depends on the type of condition being treated and the route of administration.

When mixing the active ingredient into the base, the preparation may be prepared manually using an ointment slab and spatula, or mechanically using a mixer or an electronic mortar and pestle. Some examples of medications incorporated into ointments and creams include corticosteroids, antifungals, antibiotics, and hormones. Ointments and creams are generally dispensed in an ointment jar. Depending on the preparation, however, the prescription may also be dispensed in a tube, syringe, or applicator.

Dermatology Clinic
West Lafayette, Indiana
555-2317

Patient: John Wilson | Age: 61
Address: 1958 Washington Street | Date: today

Rx

Coal Tar Solution		10%
Hydrocortisone 1% Cream		10%
Loprox 1% Cream		50%
Eurax Cream	qs	60 g

Sig: apply as directed to affected areas TID

Dispense as Written

Jessica Smith, M.D
May Substitute

Refill: 2 times

Figure 15–9. Example of a prescription for a compounded cream preparation.

It is important that the patient is counseled by the pharmacist on the correct way to use or apply the preparation. Prescriptions for compounded preparations generally look different from prescriptions for commercially available medications. An example of a compounded prescription for a cream preparation is shown in figure 15-9.

Solutions and Suspensions

Solutions and suspensions are both liquid preparations and are generally administered orally. These preparations may be prepared for other routes of administration, however, such as topical, rectal, or vaginal application. Solutions and suspensions are generally easy to compound and offer wide flexibility of dosing. Dosing can be individualized to the patient by varying the concentration of the medication.

Solutions contain one or more drug ingredients that once mixed result in a homogenous or single phase and therefore contain no visible undissolved particles. In most pharmaceutical preparations, solutions result from a drug that is a solid that dissolves in the liquid. This is contrasted to suspensions. Suspensions contain two phases: the insoluble solid particles (active ingredient) and a liquid. The insoluble particles will eventually settle in the bottom of a bottle of a compounded prescription. Suspending agents are added in the compounding process that allow the insoluble particles to re-suspend uniformly upon shaking. This explains why it is important for patients to shake a suspension until no powder remains on the bottom of the container before using.

Suspensions are generally prepared by levigating the insoluble powder to a smooth paste in the mortar with an appropriate wetting agent. A small amount of vehicle is then added to the mortar to make the preparation pourable into a graduate or calibrated dispensing bottle. This process is repeated in order to transfer all of the medication from the mortar.

Most vehicles used in the preparation of solutions and suspensions are water based, but oil-based vehicles may be used as well. Flavoring and sweetening the preparations is almost always necessary. A wide variety of sweeteners,

Oncology Clinic
West Lafayette, Indiana
555-1212

Patient: Mary Jones | Age: 56
Address: 1315 West Main Street | Date: today

Rx

Mary's Magic Mouthwash
Hydrocortisone Powder 240 mg
Tetracycline 6 gm (use capsules)
Nystatin Suspension 240 ml (100,000 U/ml)
Benadryl Elixir QS 720 ml

Sig: 10 ml tid (pc) and hs. Swish & spit.

Dispense as Written

Paul Hunt, MD
May Substitute

Refill: 5 times

Figure 15–10. Example of a prescription for a compounded suspension.

including sucrose, aspartame, and saccharin are available. Flavors range from traditional grape, raspberry, cherry, and chocolate to newer flavors such as piña colada, green apple, and bubble gum. Some flavorings are available in both water- and oil-soluble forms. For veterinary use, flavors include fish, chicken, beef, and liver.

Whenever possible, it is preferable to obtain the pure chemical to compound the solution or suspension. When the pure chemical is unavailable, tablets or capsules may be used to compound the medication. An example of a compounded prescription for a suspension preparation is shown in figure 15-10.

Suppositories

Suppositories are a solid dosage form used to administer medication rectally or vaginally. Suppositories are most commonly used to deliver medications such as analgesics, hormones, anti-nausea agents, laxatives, and vaginal anti-infectives. Once inserted, the suppository melts or dissolves, allowing the release of the active ingredient in the body cavity. Because of this, suppositories must remain a solid at room temperature, but melt at body temperature. This is accomplished through the use of special bases (i.e., cocoa butter or polyethylene glycol) in the compounding of the suppositories.

To prepare suppositories, the base material is first melted by placing it in a beaker on a hot plate with a magnetic stirring rod. After the base is melted, the active ingredient(s) are added to the base with rapid stirring and mixed thoroughly. In addition, a suspending agent (i.e., silica gel powder) may be added to the mixture to minimize settling of the active ingredients while the suppository hardens. The material is then poured into the clean and dry molds (generally disposable plastic molds are used) by starting at one end of the mold and slowly filling each cavity (figure 15-11). The suppositories are allowed to solidify at room temperature and are then refrigerated.

Suppository molds are available in a variety of sizes and the size used is dependent upon the amount of active ingredient in each suppository. Adult rectal suppositories generally weigh about 2 grams and are about 1–1.5 inches in length. Infant suppositories weigh

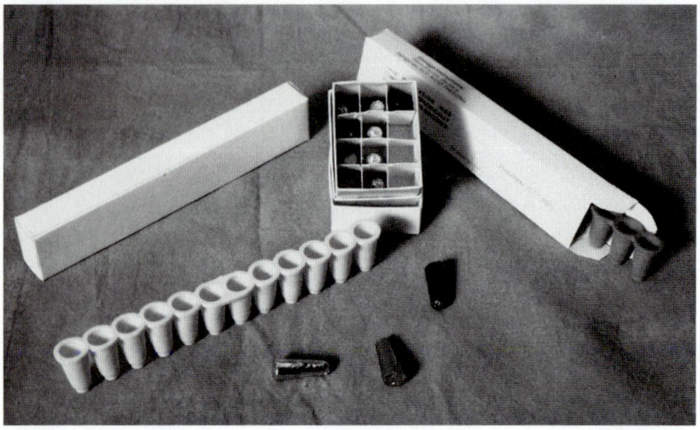

Figure 15-11. Suppositories and molds.

about one-half that of adult rectal suppositories.[3] When preparing suppositories it is important to calculate a 10% overage of materials to allow for the inevitable loss of material during the preparation process.

Lozenges/Troches

Lozenges and troches (also known as pastilles) are small, medicated squares that can be soft or hard. Lozenges and troches are intended to dissolve slowly between the cheek and gum and allow for the medication(s) to be absorbed through the oral mucosa. This medication form is useful for pediatric and geriatric patients who may be unable to swallow solid oral dosage forms.

The molds are commonly plastic and contain twenty-four or thirty separate molds. After the base is melted, the active ingredient(s), flavoring(s), and inactive ingredients are added. The mixture is then poured into the mold and allowed to cool and solidify. Similarly, molds are also available to make lollipops.

Safety First It is important that children do not mistake lozenges, troches, or lollipop dosage forms for candy.

Capsules

Pharmacists who specialize in compounding may prepare a wide variety of capsules. In the past, capsules were packed by hand, but most pharmacists specializing in compounding now use a capsule-filling machine. Powders are commonly mixed in a mortar, zippered plastic bag (to prevent spills), or specialized blender. After the capsules are loaded into the machine, the lids or capsule tops are removed, the capsules drop even with the plate, the powder is distributed into the capsules, and the lids

A

B

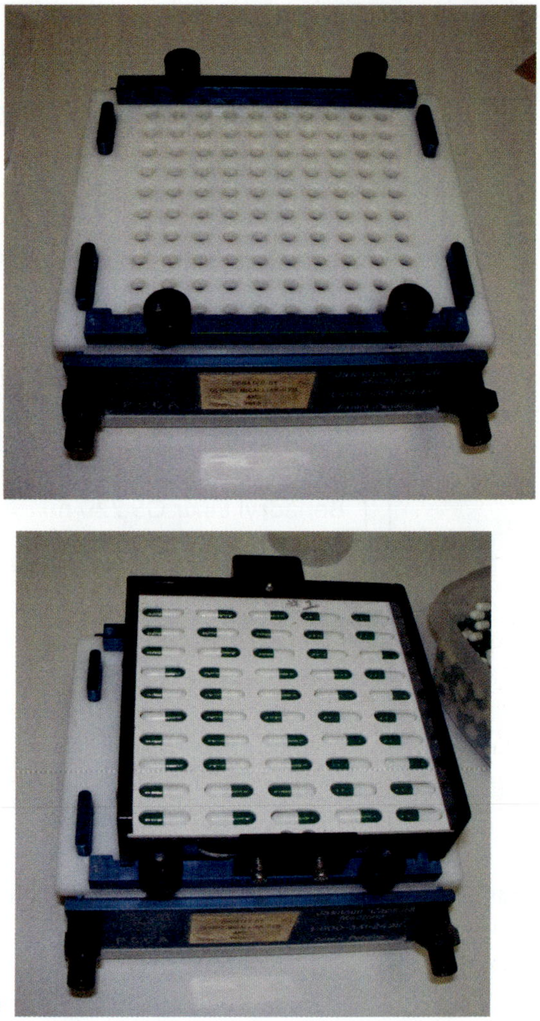

Figure 15-12. Capsule machine and loader.

or tops are replaced (figure 15-12). Many capsules can be filled in a short time using this method.

Numerous capsule sizes and colors are available (figure 15-13), depending upon the amount of powder to be placed in each capsule. For human use, eight sizes of gelatin capsules are used, ranging from the smallest (No. 5) to the largest (No. 000).[3] Note that the smaller the capsule number, the larger its capacity for holding the capsule powders. For compounding purposes, the capsule size used for a preparation should be slightly larger than that needed to hold the powders necessary for the preparation of each capsule.

Additional Compounded Preparations

In addition to the types of commonly compounded preparations just described, additional examples of compounded preparations include powders, granules, emulsions, gels, and tablets. Powders are mixtures of very fine, dry

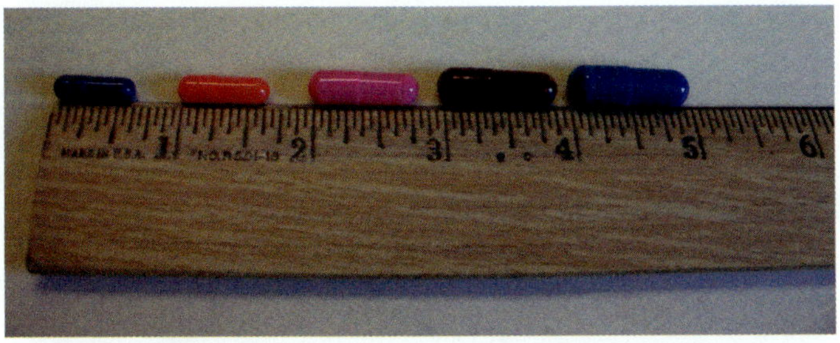

Figure 15–13. Capsules in various sizes and colors.

active and inactive ingredients that can be used for topical or internal preparations. Granules are dosage forms that consist of particles of larger size and are formed when powders are moistened and passed through a screen. Emulsions are generally a mixture of two liquids (i.e., oil and water) that are immiscible, or incapable of being mixed. An emulsifying agent (i.e., acacia) is added to the preparation to bring the two liquids together. Emulsion preparations may be prepared for external or internal use. Gels are semi-solid systems consisting of suspensions that can be administered through many different routes of administration. Tablet presses are used to compound individual tablets by compression. A mixture of the active and inactive powders are weighed and placed in the press, the handle is lowered and tablets are prepared.

Repackaging

As pharmaceutical manufacturers prepare, package, and distribute most prescribed medications, the role of the pharmacy has expanded from formulator, compounder, and packager to include repackager of commercially available products. Pharmacies repackage medications from bulk containers into patient-specific containers, including unit-of-use, single-unit, and unit-dose packaging.

Unit-of-Use Packaging

Unit-of-use packaging is characterized by a vial, an envelope, or a plastic bag containing several doses of the same medication. Most unit-of-use packages contain enough medication for the entire treatment period (e.g., ten days of an antibiotic). In an outpatient setting, this is usually a one-month supply for chronic medications. Before dispensing, a pharmacy label with the patient's name and administration directions is affixed to the package. Unit-of-use packaging is suitable for inpatient and outpatient dispensing. Medications can be packaged this way in advance of their request, which is sometimes referred to as pre-packaging.

As the benefits of unit-of-use packaging became known, further modifications gave rise to the unit-dose concept. A **unit-dose package** is a non-reusable container designed to hold a quantity of drug to be administered as a single dose. The package may contain one unit or multiple units, depending on the dose ordered. The benefits of unit-dose packaging include improved patient safety, reduced waste, more accurate patient charges, ability to use automated dispensing machines, and improved control of medications.

Single-Unit Packaging

Single-unit packaging contains one unit of a dosage form. Examples include one tablet or capsule, or one teaspoonful (5 mL) of an oral liquid.

Part 3

Safety First If the actual dose for the patient is more (e.g., 2 tablets) or less (e.g., 1/2 tablet) than the single-unit package, a notation should be made or a "check dose" sticker can be applied to remind the nurse or caregiver to double check the dose.

Unit-Dose Packaging

The unit-dose or single-dose package is often confused with the single-unit package. The important difference is that the unit-dose package contains one dose of the drug for a given patient. For example, a unit-dose package contains two tablets when a given patient's dose is two tablets, whereas a single-unit package contains only one tablet, regardless of the dose ordered.

The availability of single-unit and unit-dose packages from manufacturers has somewhat reduced the need for pharmacy personnel to repackage. Repackaging, however, is still performed because not all medications are available in unit-dose packages. Most oral liquid medications for pediatric patients and a number of less commonly prescribed oral solids are not available in unit-dose forms. Also, it is usually more expensive to purchase drugs already in unit-dose form than in bulk form. The cost of repackaging will depend on several factors, including what equipment is used, the repackaging materials, the number of doses being repackaged, and labor. Typical costs associated with repackaging average \$0.05–\$0.35 per dose. In addition to costs, facilities need to consider the size of the final product and the types of dispensing equipment when deciding on whether to buy in unit dose or to repackage from bulk.

Extemporaneous Versus Batch Repackaging

Extemporaneous repackaging is repackaging quantities of medications that will be used within a short period of time. Extemporaneous repackaging is done on an as-needed basis. The quantities repackaged are based on the anticipated immediate need. Usually these medications have limited or unknown stability, or are prescribed infrequently. Extemporaneous repackaging is also known as "just-in-time" packaging.

Batch repackaging is the periodic repackaging of large quantities of medications in unit-dose or single-unit packages. Batch repackaging is done for medications that have extended stability and are prescribed more frequently. Since the packages are prepared in advance of when they are needed, batch repackaging is sometimes called pre-packaging. Batch repackaging is also thought to save time, materials, and money when compared to extemporaneous repackaging.

Containers and Repackaging Materials

Repackaging materials and the package itself must protect the drug from harmful external elements, such as light, heat, moisture, air, and (in the case of sterile products) microbial contaminants. The material must not deteriorate during the shelf life of the drug. Packages should be lightweight and made of materials that do not interact with the dosage form. Repackaging materials should not absorb, be absorbed by, or chemically interact with the drug. Materials that are recyclable or biodegradable are preferred over those that are not.

Packages should be constructed so they do not deteriorate with normal handling. They should be easy to open and use, and should not require any additional training or experience to use. Packages should allow for the contents to be inspected by the person administering the medication unless the pharmaceutical properties of the drug preclude its being exposed to light.

USP defines containers and closures on the basis of the degree to which the contents are protected (table 15-1).[2]

Table 15-1. Degrees of Protection of Containers and Closures

Degree of Protection	Description
Light-resistant containers	■ Protects the drug from the effects of incident light by virtue of specific properties of which they are composed, including any coating applied ■ If protection from light is required, a clear and colorless or a translucent container may be made light-resistant by means of an opaque enclosure
Well-closed containers	■ Protects the contents from extraneous solids and from loss of the drug under ordinary handling, shipment, storage, and distribution conditions
Tightly-sealed containers	■ Protects their contents from contamination by extraneous liquids, solids, or vapors; from loss of the drug; and from effervescence, deliquescence, or evaporation under ordinary handling, shipment, storage, and distribution conditions
Hermetic containers	■ Are impervious to air or any other gas under ordinary or customary conditions of handling, shipment, storage, and distribution

Repackaging Equipment

Repackaging equipment can be manual, semi-automated, or fully automated. These systems are reviewed as they pertain to repackaging of oral solids and oral liquids. Manual systems introduce more variability into the final package quality. More repackaging systems are available for oral solids than for any other dosage form, because most doses dispensed in institutions are oral solids.

Oral Solid Systems

Oral solids can be packaged in blister packages or in pouch packages and they can be manual or automated systems.

Blister Packaging Systems **Blister packages** (often called bubble packs) are composed of an opaque and non-reflective backing that is typically used for printing or labeling. The backing, generally composed of paper or a paper-foil laminate, is easy to peel from the blister portion of the package. Backing that is made entirely of paper can range in thickness from light (about the thickness of construction paper) to heavy (about the thickness of light cardboard).

The blister portion is composed of a flat-bottomed dome or bubble of transparent plastic. Blister packages are more rigid than pouch packages and therefore may protect the contents better, but they do not lend themselves to the automated repackaging systems found in institutional practice. Automated blister packaging is generally confined to the pharmaceutical industry, but blister packages are used with some manually operated repackaging programs in institutional practice.

Pouch Packaging Systems Pouch packages have one or both sides composed of an opaque, non-reflective surface intended for printing. This surface is generally a paper-foil laminate. The opposite side of the pouch can be made of the same paper-foil laminate, a paper-foil-polyethylene laminate, or transparent polyethylene-coated cellophane. The pouch package is probably the most common type of packaging used for batch repackaging. The pouch package lends itself to relatively inexpensive automated machinery applications in institutional practice.

Manual Systems Manually operated oral solid repackaging systems use either pouch packages or blister packages. Both pouch packages and blister packages use either heat sealing or adhesive sealing. Manual pouch repackaging systems use clear or light-resistant plastic bags (usually PVC). The tablet or capsule is dropped into the bag, and the bag opening is sealed with an adhesive or zipper mechanism. Manual pouch systems can also be heat sealed by a hot knife blade, which seals the end of the plastic bag and provides a better seal than adhesive. A label is typed directly on the package before the product is added or on a regular stock label and affixed to the package after it is sealed. This system is generally reserved for extemporaneous packaging.

Manual blister repackaging systems use a plastic blister package made of clear PVC or a laminate of PVC and low-density polyethylene plastic. The blisters or bubbles come in various sizes, depending on the type and size of the product being repackaged. The blisters can be filled on a tabletop or placed in specially designed holders to cradle the package (figure 15-14). The blisters are filled with the drug, and then a paper, paper-foil, or vinyl-paper-foil backing is attached to the blister by removing a protective covering from an adhesive strip on the backing material and applying pressure to the blister and backing material. Some blister packages are then heat sealed in a heat seal press, which resembles a waffle iron. The heat seal applies heat and pressure to the backing material, while the blisters remain protected by the well-like device that holds them.

Automated Systems Automated oral solid repackaging systems, or unit-dose strip packaging machines, can be semi-automated or fully automated. They all produce

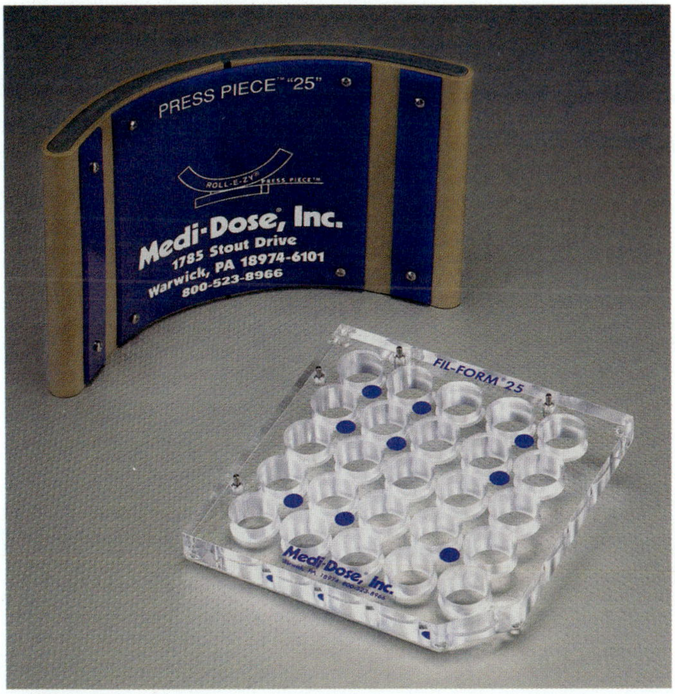

Figure 15–14. Blister holder and press. (Courtesy of Medi-Dose®, Inc./EPS®, Inc.)

a pouch package made of two polyethylene-paper-foil laminates or a polyethylene-paper-foil laminate and a polyethylene-cellulose laminate.

TECHNOLOGY TOPICS

Automated repackaging machines can package 60 to 120 doses of a single drug per minute. Automated repackaging machines are often used for batch repackaging so larger quantities can be done more efficiently.

To prevent contamination of oral solid packaging equipment, only non-penicillin and non-hazardous drugs should be repackaged using one of these machines.

Safety First

Penicillin-containing medications and hazardous medications should not be placed in automated repackagers to prevent cross-contamination. Traces of these medications in the repackaging equipment could lead to severe allergic reactions or harmful effects.

In semi-automated systems, tablets or capsules are manually fed into a wheel that drops the dose into a pouch formed by two heated wheels or a heated press and then package is sealed. A serrated knife blade that perforates or cuts the strip of pouches as it passes out of the machine separates individual packages. The labeling information is printed on the paper laminate by a computer-generated printing system that interfaces with the packaging machine. The printing process occurs before the dose is dropped into the pouch. A device can be attached to the top of the strip-packaging machine to eliminate the need for an operator to feed tablets and capsules into the wheel.

Newer fully automated repackaging systems have canisters that are calibrated for one specific National Drug Code (NDC) number or product and can hold up to 500 different oral solid products. The National Drug Code is a unique three-segment number that is used to identify a specific drug product.

✔ In an automated repackaging system that uses drug-specific, calibrated canisters, each canister can *only* be used for the specific medication and manufacturer that the canister was calibrated for.

These machines are controlled by computers that "tell" the machine when to drop pills into a package prior to the package getting sealed. These machines produce a strip of packages that is perforated between each dose that comes out the front or side of the machine (figure 15-15). They can produce a few different sizes of packages depending on the machine and can produce packages with one or more pills in the same package.

The advantages and disadvantages of placing multiple medications in the same pouch vary depending on the setting in which they are used. In the hospital setting where doses are typically dispensed for a twenty-four hour period or removed from an automated dispensing machine, it is more cost effective to package pills individually. This allows for crediting and reuse of doses that are not used by the patient. In an outpatient or long-term care environment, having all of the medications that are due at a particular time in the same pouch has multiple benefits. This system would make it easier for patients to know if they had taken all of the medications that were due at a particular time. This could also lead to improved adherence to drug regimens and lessen the possibility of taking a second dose if they were unsure as to whether they had already taken the dose. Disadvantages to placing multiple medications in the same pouch include not being able to reuse doses and having to re-dispense pouches when there is a change in the medication regimen.

Figure 15–15. Examples of output from an automated oral solid repackaging machine.

Oral Liquid Systems

Oral liquids can be packaged with manual, semi-automated, and automated systems.

Manual Systems Manual repackaging systems for oral liquids can be divided into those that use a glass or plastic vial as the reservoir for the liquid medication and those that use a glass or plastic syringe. Manual repackaging systems that require vials have several different closure systems: screw cap vials, vials with permanently affixed tops and small fill holes for medication that a plastic ball fits into to prevent liquid from escaping from the container, and vials that require the addition of a cap that must be crimped (figure 15-16 A, B, and C). An operator uses syringes, burettes, pipettes, or graduates to measure and transfer the liquid into the vial.

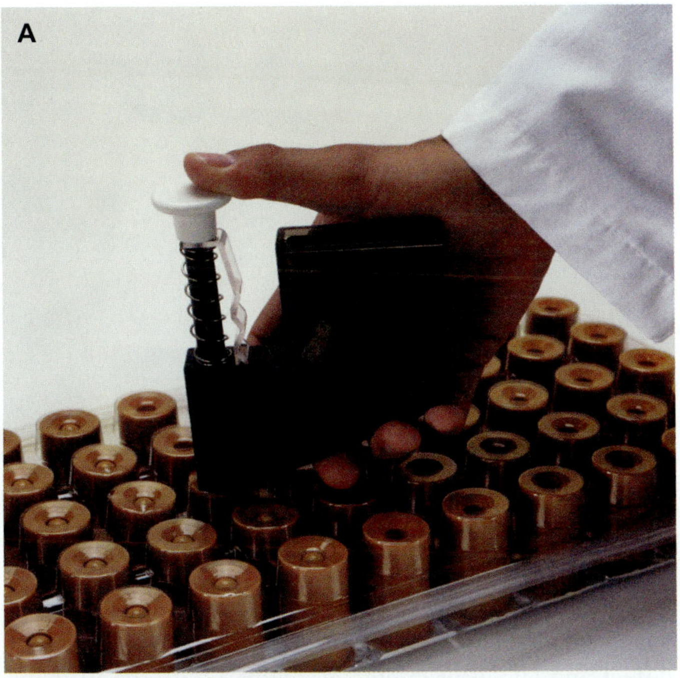

Figure 15-16A. Kwik-Vial™ containers. (Courtesy of Baxa Corporation.)

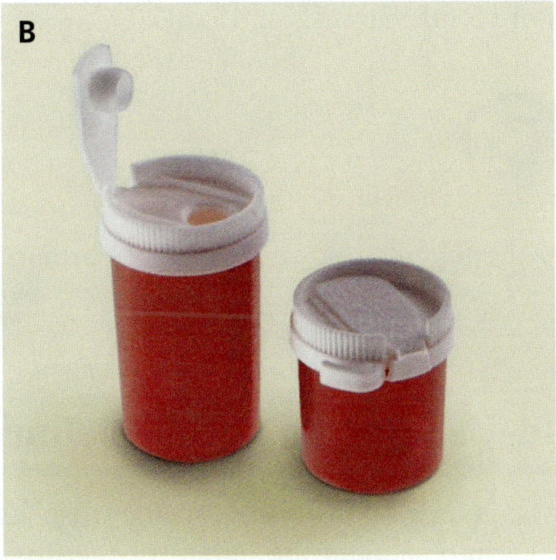

Figure 15-16B. Tamper-Tuf™ containers. (Courtesy of © Bectin, Dickinson and Company.)

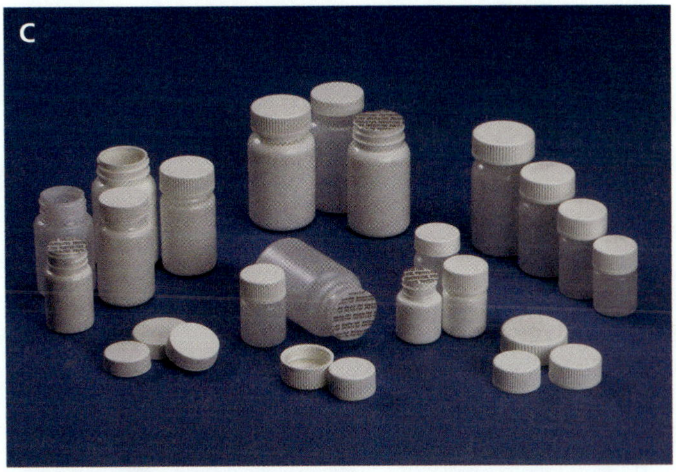

Figure 15-16C. TampAlerT containers. (Courtesy of Midi-Dose® Inc./EPS®, Inc.)

Manual systems for repackaging oral liquids into syringes use one of two methods of repackaging. The first method relies on the operator transferring the liquid to a suitable vessel (such as a beaker) and withdrawing the liquid into the syringe. An ordinary oral syringe can be used for this process if the number of dosage units is relatively small. Many pharmacies use a reusable glass or disposable plastic Cornwall-type syringe (often referred to as a magic syringe or a spring-loaded syringe) to speed the filling process. The Cornwall syringe method also offers greater reliability in fill volume because the syringe is preset with the appropriate volume to dispense. Another method is where the operator attaches a specially designed cap or cork to the bulk bottle that allows a syringe to be introduced into the cap; the contents are then withdrawn via the syringe by inverting the bottle (figure 15-17). Oral syringes are similar to injectable syringes, except they are not sterile, and a hypodermic needle cannot be connected to the syringe, which prevents the injection of oral products parenterally.

Safety First Caregivers who use the oral syringe system should be cautioned to ensure that the syringe caps are kept out of reach of small children to prevent the children from accidentally swallowing a cap. These caps should not be placed on syringes intended for outpatient use.

Semi-Automated Systems Semi-automated systems are manual systems that use some piece of automated equipment as part of the filling or sealing process. Semi-automated filling pumps are either volumetric or peristaltic in design and can be used with oral syringes or vials.

Volumetric pumps operate on the same principle as the Cornwall syringes. The volume to be dispensed into the container is preset on the basis of the draw back setting and the type of reservoir selected for the pump.

Peristaltic pumps get their name from the form of pumping action they employ in delivering fluid. Peristaltic

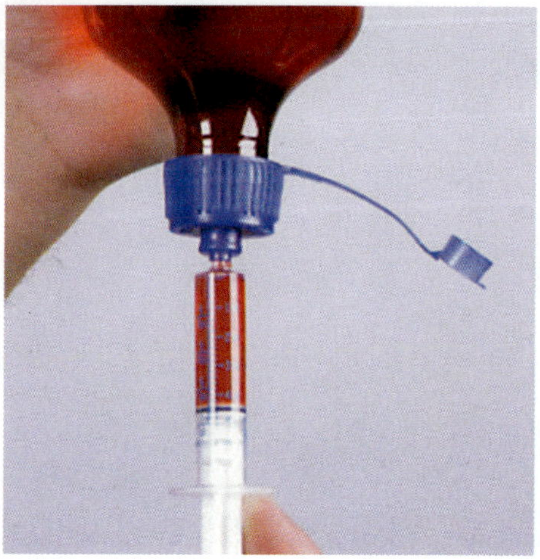

Figure 15-17. Adapta-Cap™ bottle adapter. (Courtesy of Baxa Corporation.)

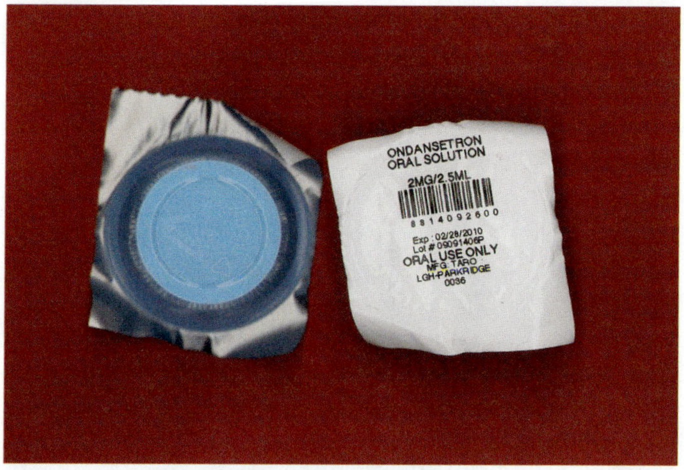

Figure 15-18. Example of output from an automated oral liquid repackaging machine.

action is created by a series of roller wheels being pulled across a length of tubing. As each wheel passes over the tubing, the tubing is crimped, and a small volume of fluid is forced down the tubing. Peristaltic pumps offer some advantages over volumetric pumps, including a faster rate of delivery for larger volumes (10 mL and above) and the ability to deliver viscous liquids.

When many units need to be produced, a peristaltic pump usually requires frequent recalibration. Volumetric pumps need less recalibrating than peristaltic pumps and are more accurate and reliable for delivering fluid volumes of less than 10 mL.

Like most mechanical devices, these pumps offer several convenience factors. Most pumps display the volume of fluid being dispensed and the number of dispensing cycles (number of units filled), allow fill cycle times to be set automatically with rest periods established between each fill, and are equipped with alarms to alert the operator to an empty container. Pumps also are furnished with foot pedal actuators that allow the operator to control the delivery and rest cycle of the fill.

Automated Systems Plastic cups are used as the fluid reservoir and the sealing system is a PVC-paper-foil overseal. The overseal acts as the label stock, and the labeling is printed directly on the seal as the machine fills and seals the product in much the same way as automated oral solid packaging machines. A peristaltic pump delivers a predetermined amount of fluid into each cup as the cups pass by the filling orifice. The overseal is attached by applying heat and pressure until a strong bond is made between the cup and the PVC-paper-foil seal. The individual finished packages are separated when the machine cuts the over seal paper between cups (figure 15-18). Machines are equipped with a variety of sensors that detect and signal problems associated with the fill cups, sealing foil, printing tape, and general machine failure. These machines, capable of producing twenty to thirty-two units per minute, are used in packaging liquids with volumes of 15 mL, 30 mL, or 45 mL.

TECHNOLOGY TOPICS

Automated liquid repackaging machines are available that fill, seal, and label medications.

Beyond-Use Dating and Labeling

Labeling is the responsibility of the dispenser, who should take into account the nature of the drug repackaged, the characteristics of the containers, and the storage conditions to which the medication may be subjected in order to determine a beyond-use date for the label. USP offers standards for determining an appropriate expiration date in the absence of published stability data, "For nonsterile solid and liquid dosage forms that are packaged in single-unit and unit-dose containers, the beyond-use date shall be one year from the date packaged or the expiration date on the manufacturer's container, whichever is earlier."[2]

Considerable technical advances have occurred in the area of labeling, partly as a result of using computers in institutional practice. In particular, personal computers have greatly improved the quality and efficiency of the label production process. Current federal labeling requirements are described in the *ASHP Technical Assistance Bulletin on Single Unit and Unit Dose Packages of Drugs*.[5] The technical bulletin states that the nonproprietary name (generic name), proprietary name (brand name) if appropriate, dosage form, strength, amount delivered in package, notes (such as storage conditions, preparation or administration instructions), expiration date, and control number or lot number should appear on the package. Inclusion of a barcode on repackaged items is highly recommended and is necessary to facilitate bedside barcode scanning in hospitals.

TECHNOLOGY TOPICS

Most computerized packaging machines include the ability to include a bar code to identify the medication in the package.

Some labels are applied manually to the finished product. Newer semi-automated and automated repackaging machines have printers built in so the label can be printed on the package prior to the dosage form being inserted.

Record Keeping

Standards of practice and government regulations require maintaining accurate and complete records of the repackaging process. Accurate records help in managing inventory and monitoring the efficiency of the repackaging process. Such records can provide a focal point for a quality assurance program and maximize the technician's role in repackaging.

Most repackaging record keeping systems are now computerized and individual state laws and regulations will dictate what needs to be kept, whether records may be maintained as paper or electronic records, and how long records must be maintained.

Quality Control

A well-defined quality control program is essential to ensure the continuous production of high-quality repackaged medications. Quality control of repackaging involves written procedures, formal training of the operators of the equipment, maintenance of equipment, checkpoints during the process, and end product testing.[6]

Because several technicians and pharmacists may deal with many products when repackaging medications, strict adherence to the principles of good manufacturing practices (GMP) is essential to quality control. GMP refers to guidelines for various aspects of production that would affect the quality of the final product and include the following:

- Manufacturing/repackaging processes are clearly defined and controlled.
- Instructions and procedures are written in clear and unambiguous language.
- Documentation of personnel training.
- Records are kept that show that the procedures were followed.
- Storage and distribution of the final product minimizes negative effects to the quality.
- A system for recalling any batch of product.

Written Procedures

Technicians should be familiar with the pharmacy's procedures for repackaging. Most procedures will include expectations regarding cleanliness; labeling format; assignment of beyond-use dates; container size in relation to the size or volume of the drug being repackaged; operational procedures for the setup, operation, and cleanup of equipment; the type and detail of records; and quality assurance and testing procedures. Because procedures are usually reviewed and updated annually, it is a good idea to continually review the procedures to make sure your knowledge is up to date.

Personnel Training and Competency

Formal training programs are important because they promote consistency and standardization. Over time, training programs can pay for themselves by preventing the loss of medication, supplies, and personnel time associated with improper repackaging. Training can extend the life of equipment by teaching proper operating procedures, cleaning and maintenance, and adjustment and repair of malfunctioning machinery. Teaching aids, such as programmed texts and video presentations, are available through professional organizations.

Maintenance of Equipment

Most equipment that is used in the repackaging process requires maintenance. Some maintenance will be part of the daily operation of the equipment and some can be done on a set schedule. Refer to the instructions that came with the equipment to see what needs to be done every time the equipment is used and what can be done less often. Regularly scheduled preventive maintenance can extend the life of equipment, which decreases overhead in the repackaging operation.

✔ Preventive maintenance reduces equipment failures and ensures that equipment is operating to the manufacturer's specifications.

Checkpoints

Checkpoints are the steps in the repackaging process that are crucial to ensuring a high-quality package. It is important to double-check each step. Checkpoints may include the following:

1. Double-checking to ensure that the drug and dosage form being repackaged are the ones that are supposed to be repackaged. It is also important to ensure that the bulk product has not expired and has a long enough remaining shelf life to warrant repackaging.
2. Double-checking the fill volumes to ensure that the amount of liquid delivered is proper for the dose and the container selected.
3. Double-checking any calculations.
4. Double-checking the information (e.g., spelling) on a label or computer screen to ensure that the label is complete and accurate.

End-Product Testing

End-product testing is the type of quality control most industries practice. End-product testing requires sampling the final product and determining whether it meets all of the standards it met before being repackaged. Examples of end-product testing include testing a sterile product for sterility and testing a package of a solid or liquid oral dosage for moisture impermeability. The uniformity and potency of a product can be tested by a number of chemical analyses. End-product testing is not generally performed for basic repackaging processes, but it may be used more commonly in institutional practice to validate certain types of sterile compounding. End product testing of repackaged oral liquids may include validating that the package delivers the specified volume of medication.

Summary

Compounding offers a unique clinical experience in meeting patient needs. Patients benefit from the customized medication and the care of the pharmacist in meeting their needs with dosage forms, routes of administration, or strengths of medication not commercially available. The demand for compounded medications is increasing as more pharmacies offer this service. With the superb technical support provided by compounding support services, compounding pharmacists and technicians offer a new level of patient care. When commercial medications are available but not in the packaging best suited to the needs of the patient or staff, repackaging offers a convenient, cost-effective method of providing medications to the patient.

Self-Assessment Questions

1. When preparing compounded preparations, what should the preparer *avoid*?
   a. having food or beverages in the preparation area
   b. using a mask to prevent inhalation of chemical powders
   c. using gloves to protect hands from chemical contact
   d. using hazardous chemicals
2. Examples of nonsterile compounded preparations include all of the following *except:*
   a. emulsions
   b. injections
   c. suppositories
   d. troches
3. Technicians are allowed to be involved in the nonsterile compounding process (as regulated by state law) once knowledge has been demonstrated regarding all of the following *except*:
   a. pharmacy calculations
   b. the compounding process
   c. USP-NF Chapter 795
   d. USP-NF Chapter 797
4. Compounded preparations could include all of the following *except*:
   a. medications produced by a manufacturer
   b. prescription for a dermatologic preparation
   c. prescription for a preparation discontinued by the manufacturer
   d. prescription for a veterinary preparation
5. Which of the following statements about inactive ingredients is *false*?
   a. Flavoring agents are an example of an inactive ingredient.
   b. Inactive ingredients are also referred to as therapeutic agents.
   c. Inactive ingredients should not interfere with the absorption of the active ingredient(s) in the preparation.
   d. Suspending agents are examples of inactive ingredients.
6. When choosing repackaging materials, what should one refer to?
   a. USP standards
   b. Food and Drug Administration standards
   c. State pharmacy board standards
   d. Local health department standards
7. Dispensing units of repackaged medications would *not* commonly include which of the following?
   a. Unit-of-use packaging
   b. Single-dose packaging
   c. Single-unit packaging
   d. Reusable containers
8. Repackaging records
   a. may be destroyed when the medication supply has been dispensed
   b. may be useful for quality control purposes
   c. are not used to evaluate whether or not the medication was correctly packaged
   d. are not useful for monitoring inventory and the efficiency of the repackaging process
9. Considerations for repackaging materials include
   a. the day of the week to repackage
   b. the type of packaging material and medication to be repackaged
   c. the sensitivity of the repackaging person to light
   d. the time of day when repackaging

Self-Assessment Answers

1. a. Food or beverages can contaminate the preparation(s) and also can be contaminated by the chemicals in the compounding area.
2. b. Injections are made using aseptic or sterile technique.
3. d. These are the standards for sterile compounding. The other choices are all expectations for technicians involved in nonsterile compounding.
4. a. Compounding, by definition, is not manufacturing.
5. b. Active ingredients (not inactive) are also referred to as therapeutic agents.
6. a. USP standards are the published standards for repackaging.
7. d. Reusable containers would be difficult to use due to sanitary reasons.
8. b. Knowing details from repackaging records can be useful in many quality control areas, such as knowing expiration dates and the person who did the repackaging.
9. b. The repackaged medication may have stability needs, such as light sensitivity, to be met by the materials.

Resources

It is important for pharmacies to have adequate availability of resources on compounding. This may include books, journals, Web sites, telephone access to compounding centers, etc. Examples of suggested compounding resources include the following:

Extemporaneous Formulations (ASHP)
PCCA: Professional Compounding Centers of America (http://www.pccarx.com)
Pediatric Drug Formulations
Pharmaceutical Dosage Forms and Drug Delivery Systems
Remington: The Science and Practice of Pharmacy
Secundum Artem (http://www.paddocklabs.com)
Trissel's Stability of Compounded Formulations

References

1. Galston SK, U.S. Food and Drug Administration. Federal and State Role in Pharmacy Compounding and Reconstitution: Exploring the right mix to protect patients. Statement to the Senate Committee on Health, Education, Labor, and Pensions 10/23/03. Available at: http://www.fda.gov/NewsEvents/Testimony/ucm115010.htm. Accessed May 5, 2010.
2. USPC. *The United States Pharmacopeia*, 32nd rev., and the *National Formulary*, 27th ed. Rockville, MD: The United States Pharmacopeial Convention; 2009.
3. Allen Jr. LV. *The Art, Science, and Technology of Pharmaceutical Compounding.* 15th ed. Washington, DC: American Pharmacists Association; 2008.
4. Lippincott, Williams & Wilkins. *Remington: The Science and Practice of Pharmacy.* 20th ed. Philadelphia, PA: University of the Sciences; 2000.
5. American Society of Hospital Pharmacists. ASHP technical assistance bulletin on single unit and unit dose packages of drugs. *Am J Hosp Pharm.* 1985;42:378–379.
6. American Society of Hospital Pharmacists. ASHP technical assistance bulletin on repackaging oral solids and liquids in single unit and unit dose packages. *Am J Hosp Pharm.* 1983;40:451–452.

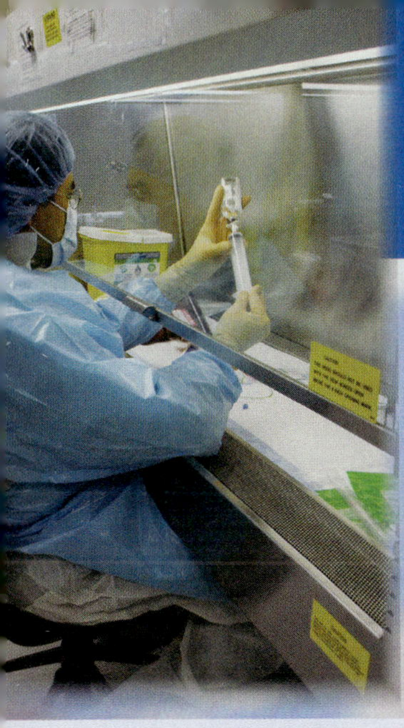

Chapter 16

Aseptic Technique, Sterile Compounding, and IV Admixture Programs

Scott M. Mark, Thomas E. Kirschling

Learning Outcomes

After completing this chapter, you will be able to

- Describe the basics of intravenous drug therapy.
- Describe the key elements of working in laminar airflow workbenches.
- List the common types of contamination that may occur when working in a laminar flow hood and describe how to minimize the risks of these types of contamination.
- Perform basic manipulations needed to prepare a sterile product by using aseptic technique.
- Describe the risks of handling cytotoxic and hazardous drugs.
- List the steps in drug preparation and handling that are unique to cytotoxic and hazardous drugs.
- List the typical ingredients of a total parenteral nutrition solution.
- Describe the manual and automated means of preparing total parenteral nutrition solutions.
- Describe the benefits of having a formal intravenous admixture program.
- Describe how USP 797 has impacted the preparation of sterile products.

Key Terms

aseptic technique The technique and procedures designed to prevent contamination of drugs, packaging, equipment, or supplies by microorganisms during preparation.

biological safety cabinet A vertical laminar airflow workbench (LAFW) used for the preparation of hazardous medications that confines airflow within the hood.

coring Introducing particulate matter in the form of a plastic or rubber "core" or plug into a sterile fluid through the process of penetrating the outer seal of a vial or bag with a needle.

free-flow protection A feature that prevents "free-flow" of medication or fluid, which can lead to unintentional overdoses.

HEPA filter A high-efficiency particulate air (HEPA) filter that removes 99.97% of all air particles 0.3 micrometers or larger. It is composed of pleats of filter medium separated by rigid sheets of corrugated paper or aluminum foil that direct the flow of air forced through the filter in a uniform parallel flow.

laminar airflow workbench (LAFW) A work area (hood) where parenteral products are compounded. Twice-filtered laminar layers of aseptic air continuously sweep the work area inside the hood to prevent the entry of contaminated room air. There are two common types of laminar flow workbenches, horizontal flow and vertical flow.

large volume parenteral (LVP) IV solutions greater than 100 mL in volume. LVPs are usually solutions of dilute dextrose and/or sodium chloride with or without drug additives. They are usually given as continuous infusions, but they may be used for intermittent infusions as well.

total parenteral nutrition (TPN) Also known as hyperalimentation, refers to the IV administration of nutrients needed to sustain life.

small volume parenteral (SVP) Also called an IV piggyback (IVPB). Any IV solution with a total volume of less than or equal to 100 mL.

Aseptic technique, along with its application to different dispensing and administration systems and dosage types, is the primary focus of this chapter. Potential risks of parenteral therapy are addressed in the next section in order to emphasize the importance of using proper techniques and appropriate caution when preparing these products. Nurses are often referred to as the primary caregivers involved in administering the products described in this chapter; however, in some hospitals or home care settings, the primary caregiver may be another health care professional, the patient, or the patient's family members. The training and skill of the caregiver or caregivers should be taken into consideration when products are prepared and dispensed because this may influence the intravenous (IV) delivery system chosen for the patient.

The purpose of this chapter is to help the pharmacy technician develop a basic understanding of sterile products and the methods used to prepare them. This chapter should be mastered in sequence with the rest of the *Manual for Pharmacy Technicians,* especially chapters that have related information, including Chapter 4, Hospital Pharmacy Practice, Chapter 5, Home Care Pharmacy Practice, Chapter 13, Processing Medication Orders and Prescriptions, and Chapter 14, Pharmacy Calculations.

Many small hospitals prepare and administer hundreds of sterile products daily; larger hospitals may prepare thousands. As such, pharmacy technicians play an important role in the preparation of sterile products. In addition, many patients now receive intravenous drug therapy in the home. It is important that correct procedures are followed when preparing intravenous drug therapy to ensure that the final product is safe and effective. For example, a structured intravenous admixture program is needed to ensure the stability, sterility, and appropriate labeling of intravenous products. Technicians and pharmacists work as a team in the IV preparation environment, each with their own role and expertise, to ensure that the patient receives the right drug in the right amount, concentration, and dosage form.

Drugs are given parenterally if patients cannot take oral medications; if they have difficulty absorbing oral medications (i.e., absorptive capacity is limited); if a more rapid onset of action is desired (as in an emergency situation); or if the drug is not available in a suitable oral dosage form. Though the parenteral route of drug administration offers many advantages, it also has some unique preparation requirements to ensure that patients are not harmed.

Because the drug or solution is being injected directly into the body, it bypasses the body's barriers to infection.[1] Therefore, it is extremely important that the solution be sterile; that is, it must be free from bacteria or other living organisms. If a drug or solution that is contaminated with bacteria is inadvertently injected into a patient, the patient can suffer fatal adverse effects. Aseptic technique is the term used for all procedures and techniques utilized to keep a sterile product from becoming contaminated with live bacteria or other microorganisms.

Parenteral Drug Administration

Medications can be administered to patients in numerous ways. Medications not given to patients through the digestive tract (enterally) are referred to as parenterally administered. These can include intravenous (IV), intramuscular (IM), intrathecal (IT), epidural, intraarticular, intraarterial, intraocular, intraperitoneal, and subcutaneous (SQ, SC, SubQ) routes of administration. IV solutions are commonly administered to patients as a means of replacing body fluids and as a vehicle for introducing drugs into the body. Medications are not beneficial to the patient until they reach the blood and are distributed to the body. Medications given via IV are introduced directly into the blood and therefore have the most rapid onset of action. This has many benefits over oral medications, which have to be absorbed from the gastrointestinal tract, or IM medications, which have to be absorbed from the muscle mass. Intravenous medications are also beneficial in that they can be given to patients who are unconscious, uncooperative, nauseated, vomiting, or otherwise unable to take medications orally. Direct administration of IV medications into the blood also provides a predictable rate of administration. Some medications, however, are simply not suitable for IV administration due to their instability or adsorptive properties. Disadvantages of IV medications include the risk of infection, pain on injection, and immediate effect of the medication in the event of an error.

Special training is required for all personnel who prepare and administer sterile intravenous solutions. Basic aseptic technique should be used when handling parenteral dosage forms, as well as irrigations and ophthalmics (see Chapter 10, Medication Dosage Forms and Routes of Administration). Much of this chapter will address the intravenous route of administration because it is the most common route through which parenteral doses are administered in health systems today.

Risks of Intravenous Therapy

Intravenous therapy offers a rapid, direct means of administering many life-saving drugs and fluids. A high percentage of IV therapy is administered without any problems, but there are some risks. Many of the issues addressed in this training manual are aimed at teaching proper technique and therefore minimizing the potential for risks associated with these medications. What follows are some reported complications of IV therapy that may increase the risk to patients.[3]

Infection. Infections can result if a product contaminated with microorganisms or pathogens is infused into a patient. Because the IV route bypasses the body's normal barrier system, microorganisms reach the bloodstream directly. These may be introduced into products during preparation, administration, production, or through improper storage. The rate of infection or sepsis due to a contaminated infusion has steadily decreased because health care practitioners and product manufacturers have implemented training, good manufacturing practices (GMPs), and quality assurance programs. Despite these efforts, human touch contamination (improper product handling) continues to be the most common source of IV-related contamination.

Air embolus. The incidence of an air embolus is low because many solutions are administered using infusion pumps equipped with an alarm that sounds when air is in the IV line. These are called air-in-line alarms. Solutions infused by gravity do not need alarms because the infusion automatically stops when there is no more fluid for gravity to push through the IV line. Even when a bag runs dry, large amounts of air are not infused. In adults, it takes 15–20 mL of air given quickly to result in harm, which may include shortness of breath, chest pain, blood pressure and heart rate changes, and even death. Infants and pediatric patients are adversely affected by much lower amounts of air.[3] Air-eliminating filters are available on some IV sets, which also stop air bubbles and add another measure of safety.

Bleeding. Bleeding may or may not be caused by intravenous therapy. When the IV catheter is removed, bleeding may occur around the catheter site. Also, if the patient has a condition that results in prolonged bleeding time or takes an anticoagulant medication, extra care and caution should be used, especially when removing the catheter.

Allergic reaction. When a patient has an allergic reaction to a substance given parenterally, the reaction is usually more severe than if the same substance were given by another route (e.g., orally, topically, or rectally). One reason for this is that substances given parenterally cannot be retrieved like substances given by other routes. For example, substances administered topically can often be washed off, those given orally can be retrieved by inducing vomiting or by pumping the stomach, and those substances given rectally can be flushed out using an enema. When a drug that has a higher likelihood of causing allergic reactions (e.g., penicillin) is given intravenously, the patient should be monitored closely. If the likelihood of an allergic reaction is especially high and there is no alternative therapy allowing for risk mitigation, a test dose (a small amount of the drug that is often called a challenge) may be given to see how the patient reacts before administering the full dose of the medication.

Incompatibilities. Some drugs are incompatible with other drugs, containers, or solutions. If an incompatibility exists, the drug may precipitate, be inactivated, or adhere to the container. These outcomes are undesirable and may be difficult to detect with the naked eye. A visual inspection of the final product should always be performed to observe any cloudiness or signs of irregularity. Solutions with known or detectable incompatibilities should not be administered to patients.

Extravasation. Extravasation occurs when the IV catheter punctures and exits the vein under the skin, causing drugs to infuse or infiltrate into the tissue. Extravasation may happen when the catheter is being inserted or after it is in place if the extremity with the IV catheter is moved or flexed too much. Using a stiff arm board to prevent excessive movement near the catheter site may help maintain regular flow and prevent extravasation and infiltration. Extravasation and infiltration can be painful and usually requires that the IV be restarted in a different location. Some drugs, such as certain chemotherapy agents, may cause severe tissue damage if they infiltrate the tissue. Although there are medications that can alleviate some of the effects of the drug and hot or cold compresses can stop progression and reduce swelling, in some cases the tissue damage is severe enough to require surgery or can result in the loss of the limb.

Particulate Matter. Particulate matter refers to unwanted particles present in parenteral products. Particulate matter that is injected into the bloodstream can cause adverse effects to the patient. Some examples of particulate matter are glass fragments, hair, lint or cotton fibers, cardboard fragments, undissolved drug particles, and fragments of rubber stoppers, known as cores. Improvements in manufacturing processes have greatly reduced the presence of particulates in commercially available products. Similar care must be taken in the pharmacy so that particulate matter is not introduced into products.

Safety First When using glass ampules, filters are required to prevent glass fragments from entering the compounded sterile product. All products should be visually inspected for particulate matter before dispensing.

Some institutions may additionally use inline filters to help minimize the amount of particulate that reaches the patient, especially in situations where medications need to be prepared in emergency situations outside the controlled environment of a pharmacy.

Pyrogens. Pyrogens, the by-products or remnants of bacteria, can cause reactions (e.g., fever and chills) if injected in large enough amounts. Since a pyrogen can be present even after a solution has been sterilized, great care must be taken to ensure that these substances are not present in quantities that would harm the patient via filtration when appropriate. If the pyrogen is smaller than the filter being used, however, it may be introduced into the bloodstream.

Phlebitis. Phlebitis, or irritation of the vein, may be caused by the IV catheter, the drug itself due to its chemical properties or its concentration, the location of the IV site, the rate of administration, or the presence of particulate matter. The patient usually feels pain or discomfort along the path of the vein, which is often severe. Red streaking can also occur. If phlebitis is caused by a particular drug, it may be helpful to further dilute the drug, give it more slowly, or give it via an IV catheter placed in a larger vein with a higher, faster-moving volume of blood.

Types of IV Administration

Medications can be administered intravenously through several different systems or processes. While they are commonly larger volume solutions, they may not be in the case of pediatric doses. Infusions can be given either continuously or intermittently. While continuous infusions of IV fluids or medications are given over extended periods of time (often twenty-four hours or more), intermittent infusions of medications are given over a short period of time, such as over 15 minutes up to several hours. In most IV solutions, one or more drugs are added to the IV solution to prepare the final sterile product. The drug is referred to as the additive and the final product is referred to as the admixture.

✔ An IV injection is generally a small volume of solution administered directly from a syringe into the vein. When given over a short period of time, it is referred to as IV push. Solutions in IV bags or bottles that are administered over a longer period of time are known as IV infusions.

IV Containers

Large Volume Parenterals **(LVPs). Large volume parenterals** are defined as IV solutions greater than 100 mL in volume. LVPs are usually solutions of dilute dextrose and/or sodium chloride with or without drug additives. These are usually given as continuous infusions, but they may be used for intermittent infusions as well. These preparations may be used in their commercially available form or may have drug additives added in the pharmacy.

Small Volume Parenterals or "Piggyback" Systems. A common method of preparing drugs is adding the drug solution to a **small volume parenteral** or piggyback (any IV solution less than or equal to 100 mL) and labeling it. The nurse simply attaches tubing to the piggyback and connects this secondary IV set to the

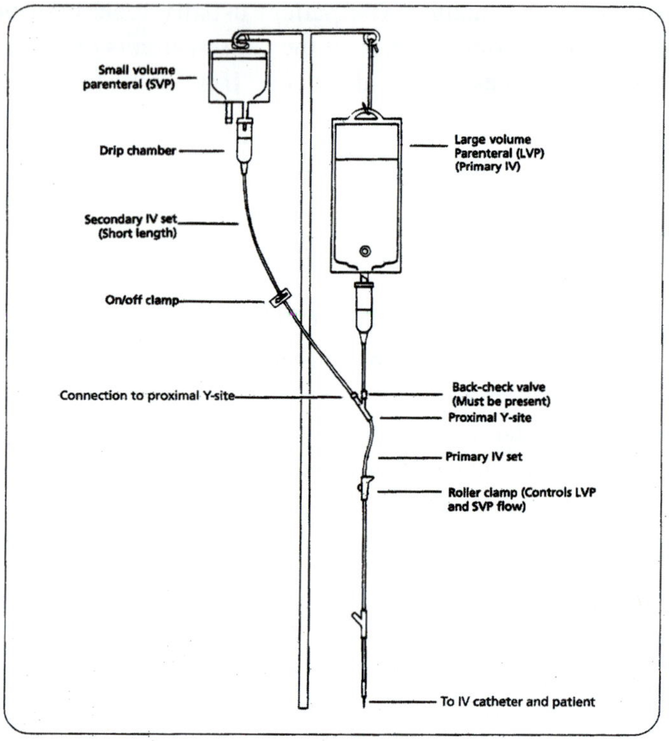

Figure 16–1. A small volume parenteral, or piggyback setup. Note that the piggyback hangs higher than the primary IV.

primary IV set at the proximal Y-site (figure 16–1). Piggybacking offers the benefits of flexibility and ease of administration.

The piggyback is placed higher than the primary IV (usually an LVP) so that gravity causes the drug solution to run into the patient's vein before the primary fluid. The back-check valve at the proximal Y-site closes while the piggyback is being administered, thus preventing the piggyback solution from entering the primary IV. Once the piggyback solution has infused, the primary IV resumes flowing. There are a number of systems that are variations of the basic piggyback concept.

Many drugs and doses for piggyback administration are available in premixed form. If premixed products are not stable for long periods of time at room temperature, they are often sold frozen, and thawed by the pharmacy shortly (hours or days) before being administered. Adding drugs to these solutions is generally not recommended, and most containers do not have an injection port. These solutions are administered and handled by the nurse in the same manner as other piggyback setups.

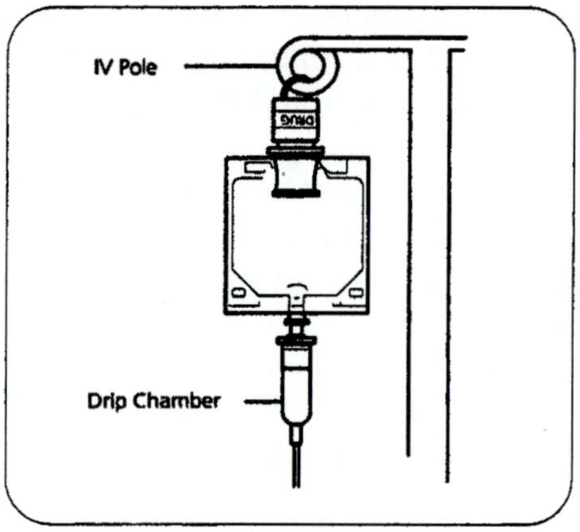

Figure 16–2. The ADD-Vantage® system setup is shown here. Note the special port at the top of the bag, which holds the medication vial.

Add-Vantage®. The Add-Vantage® system (figure 16–2) uses a specially designed bag and vial that contains drug for reconstitution. The vial is screwed into a special receptacle on the top of the bag. To reconstitute the drug, the vial's stopper is removed by manipulations done on the outside of the bag and the stopper remains in the bag. The IV solution then flows from the bag into the vial and dissolves and/or dilutes the drug. The bag is inverted several times to mix the drug and the IV solution. The bag is then administered to the patient in a fashion similar to the traditional piggyback setup.

The act of screwing the vial onto the bag receptacle should be performed in a laminar airflow workbench (LAFW) unless meeting criteria of Immediate-Use preparations as defined by USP. The actual vial top and receptacle are sterile and shielded by a protective cover until used. The pharmacy technician removes the cover at the time the vial is screwed on.

The bag's expiration date is usually thirty days after the date the vial is attached. The bag's expiration date changes to the drug expiration date when the stopper is pulled and the drug is mixed, or activated. For this reason, the stopper is usually left intact by the pharmacy and is pulled by the nurse just prior to administering the dose. This way, changes in the medication order do not result in wasted doses.

Vial Spike Systems. The Add-a-Vial®, AddEase®, Vial Mate, and Mini-Bag Plus® systems are similar in concept to the Add-Vantage® system. The drug-containing vial is attached to the bag in the pharmacy but is not activated or mixed until just before administration. The Add-a-Vial® system uses a vial adapter. The adapter has a spike at

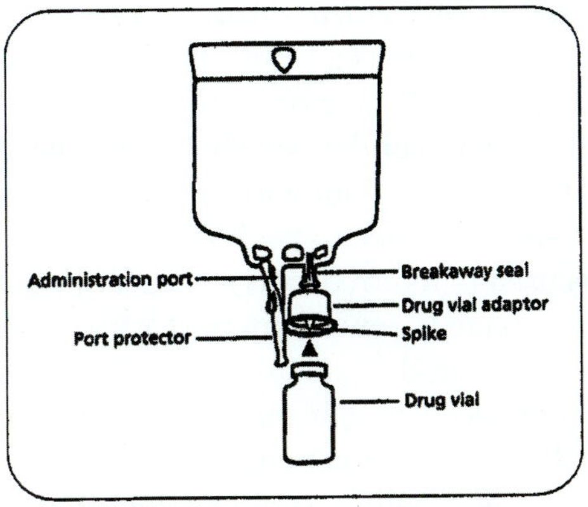

Figure 16–3. The Mini-Bag Plus® system has a special manufacturer's bag equipped with a drug vial adapter. The adapter is pushed down on the vial and snapped into place. The Add-a-Vial® system operates on a similar principle except the drug vial adapter is separate from the bag and is spiked on both ends. It is attached to the drug vial first, then assembled with the bag. With both systems, the assembled product is sent to the nursing unit, where, just prior to administration, the breakaway seal is broken and the solution is mixed with the drug.

each end; one is inserted into the drug vial and the other is inserted into the injection port of the bag. The Mini-Bag Plus® system (figure 16–3) uses a special container that has a vial adapter and a breakaway seal. The pharmacy is responsible for attaching the drug-containing vial to the bag.

The Add-a-Vial® spike that is inserted into the bag is snapped off or the Mini-Bag Plus® breakaway seal is broken just before administration, allowing solution from the bag to enter the drug vial and be mixed. The system does not require special vials because the adapters are designed to fit commonly used vial sizes. Add-a-Vial® can be used with various manufacturers' bags. Mini-Bag Plus® requires that the manufacturer's bag be used because the drug vial adapter is attached. With each of these systems, it is important to ensure that the product is activated to ensure that the patient receives the dose of medication.

Flexible Plastic Bags. Flexible plastic bags made of polyvinyl chloride (PVC) are used frequently. They are easier to store, are less breakable than glass bottles, and eliminate the need to vent the container when removing fluid.

PVC bags are available in several sizes and contain a variety of solutions. They are packaged in plastic overwrap designed to limit fluid loss. The protective overwrap should not be removed from a PVC bag until it is ready to be used. To minimize air turbulence in the critical area, position the injection port of a PVC bag, which is covered by an outside tip diaphragm, toward the HEPA filter when preparing an IV admixture.

✔ Various PVC bags will require a revision of the expiration date once the overwrap is removed. Review the product package insert for proper dating of IV bags once removed from their overwrap.

To add a drug to a PVC bag, swab the injection port, then insert a needle into the injection port and inject the appropriate volume of drug fluid. Use a needle at least one inch long because the injection port of the PVC bag has two diaphragms that must be pierced (figure 16–4). The outside diaphragm is the outside latex tip; the inside diaphragm, which is plastic, is about 3/8 inch inside the injection portal. Note that individual manufacturer's products may differ in appearance, but the design concept is the same.

Glass Containers. To add a drug to a glass infusion container, first remove the protective cap from the IV

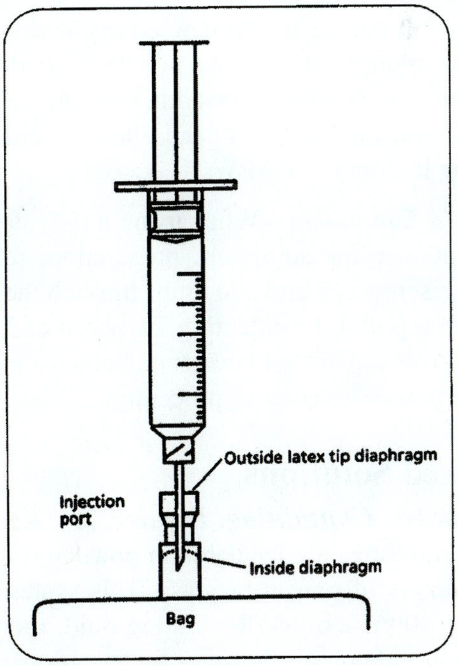

Figure 16–4. A syringe penetrating the injection port of a PVC bag. The needle must be long enough to penetrate the inside diaphragm. (Note: figure is not drawn to scale.)

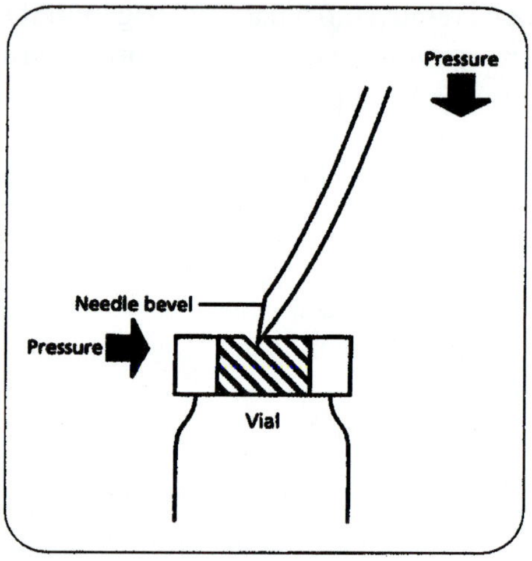

Figure 16–5. A non-coring technique of piercing a vial with a needle. Note that the needle is held on an angle—the bevel tip will pierce the vial first. As downward pressure is applied, there is a slight bend in the needle, and the bevel heel will enter through the opening made by the bevel tip.

bottle. Swab the rubber stopper with alcohol, let it dry, and then inject the drug fluid. To insert needles through rubber stoppers, use a non-coring technique (figure 16–5). After injecting the drug into the IV bottle, remove the bottle vacuum by removing the syringe needle used to inject the drug fluid and prepare a new empty syringe. Reattach the needle to the new empty syringe and remove the plunger. Insert the needle with the syringe barrel into the bottle. After admixing, place a protective seal over the stopper of the glass container before removing it from the LAFW.

Semi-rigid Containers—When using a polyolefin, semi-rigid container for admixture preparation, remove the protective screw cap and add drugs through the designated injection portal. Disinfecting the portal and replacing the protective cap are not necessary, but most pharmacies swab the port as a matter of procedure.

Premixed Solutions

Bags/Bottles Containing Powder for Reconstitution. Some drugs are available in powdered form in final containers of plastic or glass. This system requires that 20 to 100 mL of sterile diluting fluid, such as 0.9% sodium chloride or sterile water for injection, are added to the bottle to reconstitute the drug. Once reconstituted and labeled by the pharmacy, these products are administered via piggyback systems.

Basic Continuous Intravenous Therapy. In the basic setup, the IV fluid is a large-volume parenteral (LVP) that is hung on an IV pole or other device approximately 36 inches higher than the patient's bed or head. This allows the flow of IV solution to be maintained by gravity (figure 16–6).[2] Attached to the LVP is a set of sterile tubing that is usually referred to as a primary IV set. The primary IV set extends down from the LVP to a catheter that has been placed in the patient's vein. IV solution setups may differ between patients due to the infusion device or the special needs of the patient.

The LVP is usually a simple solution of dilute dextrose, sodium chloride, or both. It may contain additives, such as potassium, if the patient's clinical condition

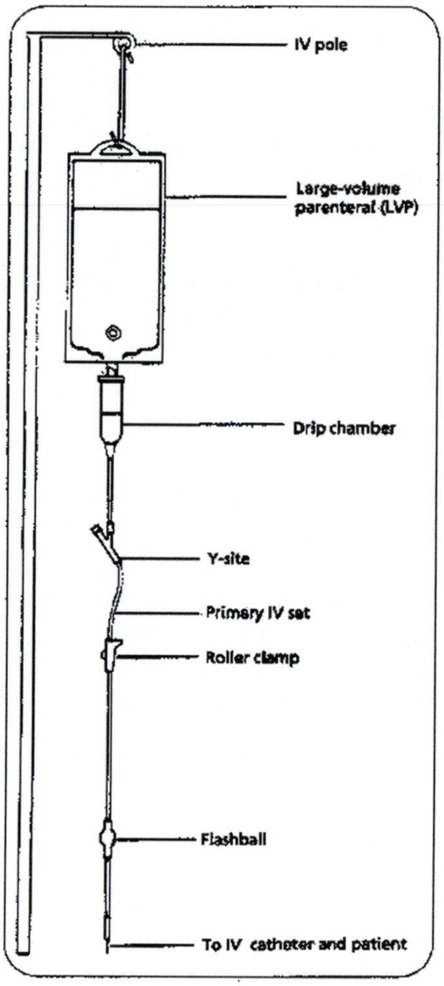

Figure 16–6. A LVP hanging on an IV pole, showing the primary IV set, including drip chamber, Y-site and flashball injection sites, and roller clamp, which can be used to control the flow of fluid.

warrants it. The solution is infused continuously to keep blood from clotting in the catheter and plugging it up. The fluid is also used to deliver drugs and to help prevent or reverse dehydration.

Administration Systems for Parenteral Products

Patients receiving IV therapy usually have a basic IV setup that includes a LVP solution, or they have a catheter specifically designed for periodic injections (heparin lock, butterfly, etc.). Based on this, IV drug administration systems are typically classified as either continuous infusions or intermittent injections.

Continuous Infusions

Some drugs are administered as a continuous infusion because they are more effective and less toxic than when given intermittently. Continuous infusions include basic fluid and electrolyte therapy, blood products, and drugs that require tight administration control to minimize adverse effects.

Intermittent Injections

Intermittent injection systems are used to administer medications that work better when infused at defined time intervals rather than when infused continuously. The reason may be that periodic administration of the drug increases efficacy or reduces toxicity. Examples of drugs commonly given intermittently are antibiotics and drugs used to treat or prevent gastrointestinal ulcers (e.g., proton pump inhibitors, such as pantoprazole).

Several types of systems are available for intermittent injections. Each system has advantages and disadvantages related to cost, flexibility, waste, and so on. This section addresses how to prepare products for use with each system. Institutional policies dictate specific labeling, expiration dating, and storage conditions, and so they are not addressed here.

Commercially Available Pre-Mixed Admixtures

LVPs with additives manufactured in standard concentrations are stable in solution for longer periods of time than those compounded in the pharmacy and are available in a variety of sizes (250 mL, 500 mL, 1000 mL) and containers (glass or plastic) depending on the product and its use. Examples include lidocaine, potassium, nitroglycerin, dopamine, and aminophylline. Ready-to-use products are advantageous because they reduce handling by the pharmacy and therefore, the potential for contamination. In some cases, these agents are used for emergency situations and may be stocked in the patient care area for immediate access. Standard concentrations of IV medications can decrease potential medication errors in compounding and administration.

Pharmacy Prepared Admixtures

Some solutions are made in the pharmacy to meet the specific needs of patients. Solutions are prepared in different volumes (100 mL, 250 mL, 500 mL, or 1000 mL) and different containers (glass, plastic, bag, bottle or syringe), depending on the drug and its intended use. The preparation of admixtures in the pharmacy should follow the techniques described in the section of this chapter titled "Aseptic Preparation of Parenteral Products."

Syringe Systems

The most common drug delivery systems that use syringes are syringe pumps, volume control chambers, gravity feed, and intravenous push systems. Syringe systems require that the pharmacy fill syringes with drugs and label them. Drug stability in syringes may differ from the stability of the same drug in other dosage forms because of concentration differences.

Syringe Pumps

Syringes can be used to administer drugs by means of a specially designed syringe pump and tubing set. The pump is adjusted to administer the desired volume from the syringe over a given period of time. Pumps are either operated by a battery or a compressed spring. Pumps are available to administer a single dose per setup or a supply at pre-programmed intervals. Many of these setups require a special small-bore tubing set that determines the rate at which the drug is administered. One important pharmacy implication is that doses must be sent from the pharmacy in standard syringe sizes and concentrations. This procedure allows doses to be administered to patients more safely because many syringe pumps are pre-programmed to deliver volumes that are based on standard concentrations.

Electronic Infusion Devices and "Smart Pumps"

Electronic infusion devices, typically categorized as either pumps or controllers, are used to increase the precision and accuracy of administration primarily of IV bags and syringes. Electronic infusion devices are usually used in fluid restricted patients or when the IV solution contains a drug that must be administered at a precise rate that cannot be ensured by using the gravity method.

The term "smart pumps" is used to refer to pumps designed to alert the user to an infusion setting that does not match a facility's drug administration guidelines. The medication's infusion parameters, such as dose, dosing unit (mcg/kg/min, units/hr, etc.), rate, or concentration can be safely chosen with notification for doses that fall outside the recommended range. Smart pumps also allow for updates to be sent to the pumps and pump log data to be sent to the information system via two-way communication over the hospital network. Most significantly, all smart pumps are designed to prevent unintentional overdoses of medication or fluid, referred to as **free-flow protection.**

Volume Control Chambers (Buretrol or Volutrol)

Syringes can be used to administer drugs through a volume control, or volumetric chamber (figure 16–7). The drug is injected through a port on top of the chamber and solution is added from the primary LVP. With this system, minimal amounts of fluid can be given per dose, a method that may be beneficial in fluid-restricted or pediatric patients. This setup allows for controlled administration of fluids, since the nurse can clamp off the solution after the volume in the chamber has infused. Since multiple drugs might be in the chamber at the same time, potential for incompatibilities and unpredictable rates of administration exist. For this reason, it is important that each medication be followed by an IV flush, usually with normal saline. A disadvantage to this system is the increased potential for infection because multiple manipulations may occur.

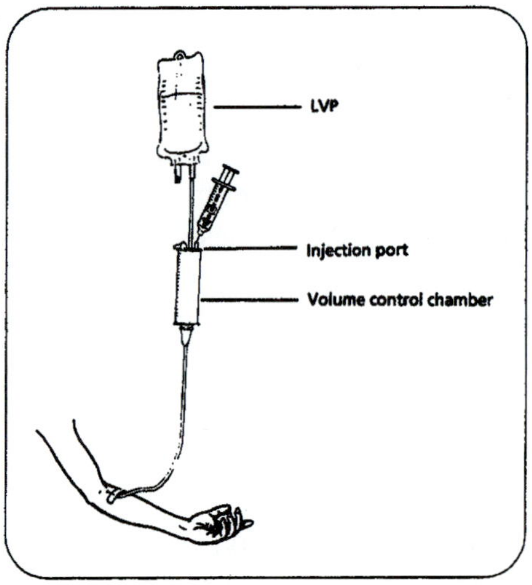

Figure 16–7. A volume control setup.

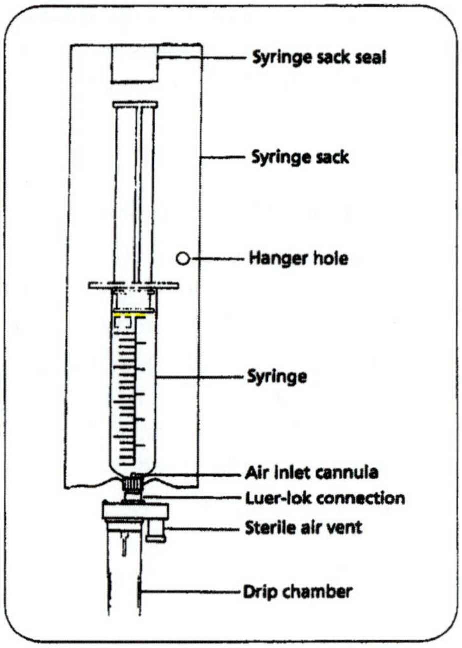

Figure 16–8. A gravity-feed syringe.

Gravity Feed

Syringes can be used to administer drugs directly by gravity if a specially designed tubing set is used (figure 16–8). The set has an air vent through which air enters the syringe as fluid is pulled out by gravity. The syringe is prepared in the pharmacy, labeled, and sent to the nurse for administration. The system is relatively inexpensive and requires no other special equipment.

Intravenous Push

Drugs given by IV push are injected directly into the IV tubing and pushed into the patient quickly (figure 16–9). With this method, the drug is injected into an injection port, a Y-site on the IV tubing, or an injection flashball. The primary IV set is usually clamped off just above the injection port so that the drug is delivered to the patient directly, resulting in the rapid onset of the drug's effects.

This system is used in emergencies as well as more routine situations. Disadvantages of the IV push method are that it is difficult to control the rate of drug delivery

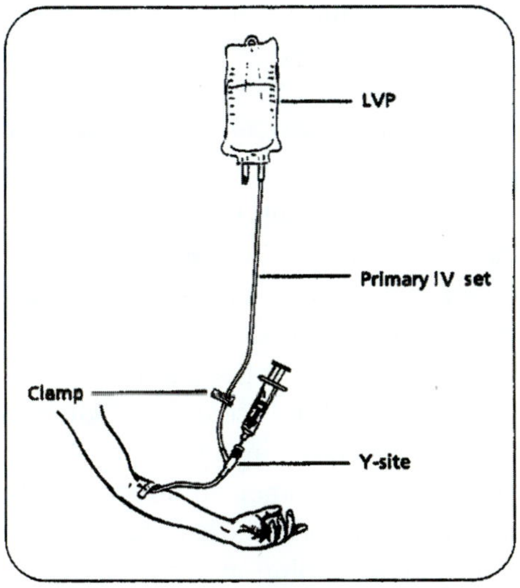

Figure 16–9. IV push setup using a Y-site.

with a syringe, and many drugs cause the patient to experience adverse effects when given too quickly.

Patient Controlled Analgesia

A method of drug administration used for injectable pain medications is patient controlled analgesia or PCA, which is very effective in managing pain. Two advantages of PCAs are that they eliminate the need for painful intramuscular injections and they give patients more control over managing their pain. The goal of PCA therapy is to relieve pain as soon as the patient recognizes a need for it. It may also reduce nursing time associated with the administration of pain medications. Patients are sometimes given a basal (or constant rate) of drug and have the ability to supplement this with a bolus or immediate dose of medication as needed.

PCA is usually administered by using either a stationary or a portable pump that infuses analgesics directly into an IV line. The pump releases a programmed amount of the pain medication into the IV tubing when the patient pushes a button. The pump is programmed to release an amount of pain medication that is specific for the patient's weight and condition. The pump is also programmed to limit how often the patient may push the button and receive pain medication. For example, the pump may be programmed to allow a patient to receive a maximum of 1 mg of morphine sulfate every fifteen minutes. When the patient pushes the button, the pump injects 1 mg. If the patient pushes the button again in ten minutes, the pump does not release drug. If the patient pushes the button at least five minutes later (fifteen minutes since the last injection), the pump again administers 1 mg. This is referred to as a fifteen-minute lockout period.

PCA preparations may be commercially available or be prepared in the pharmacy. Preparation of these products involves the same techniques as other parenteral products. They differ from most other products in two regards. First, if the patient does not have other means of pain control, there may be an urgency to initiate therapy. Much of this urgency can be avoided with preplanning among the physician, the nurse, and the pharmacy. Second, these doses usually contain enough medication to last at least eight hours and often up to twenty-four hours or more. The result is usually a very large amount of narcotic in one container, necessitating awareness of security issues in order to prevent diversion or theft. PCA solutions may sometimes be administered subcutaneously. As with IV infusions, PCAs should never be administered without an infusion pump to protect against inadvertent overdose.

Part 3

IV Locking Boxes—For infusions containing controlled substances, it is common for the final product to be hung in an IV locking box. This is a plastic box that encases the IV to prevent potential drug diversion (figure 16–10.)

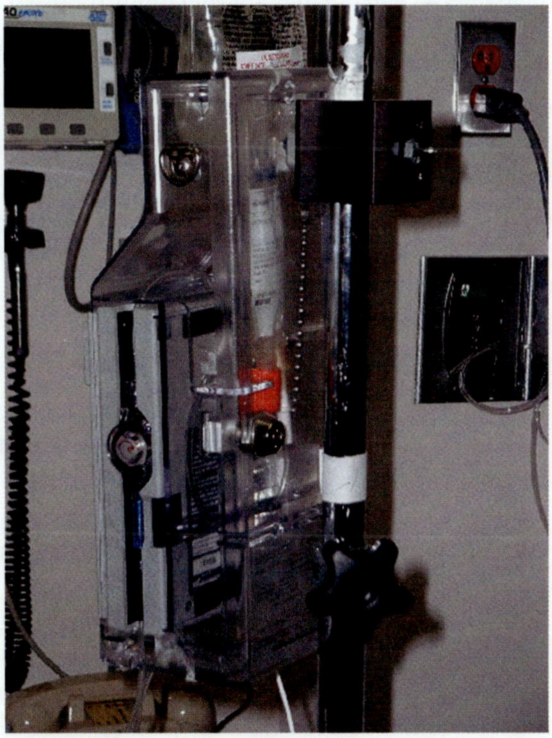

Figure 16–10. IV Lock Box.

Unique Infusion Devices and Containers

The delivery systems described thus far meet the needs of typical hospitalized patients. A number of new types of infusion devices and containers have been developed in the past twenty years to meet patient needs not met by traditional systems. Many of these products are designed to deliver drugs through a compact system that allows the patient to receive home infusion therapy. The system may be drug- or therapy-specific, such as an implanted pump with a drug reservoir for continuous low-dose chemotherapy administration. This type of system is surgically placed under the skin and the catheter is inserted in a vein. It has a built-in power source and space for the drug solution, so that the patient does not need to carry a pump, start a new IV periodically, or need any other supplies related to the IV therapy. The downside is that it requires surgery and can only be used for drug therapies administered in very small amounts over long periods of time.

Another type of system uses an elastomeric infusion device (EID) that acts as its own pump, not requiring gravity or an electronic infusion device. These systems are similar in concept to a water balloon inside a plastic bottle. The balloon is filled with drug solution, and the pressure of the container forces it through the tubing, eliminating the need for a separate pump. These systems, whether used for hospitalized patients or home care patients, present unique challenges in filling technique, drug stability, and administration methods. Personnel preparing drugs for use in these types of devices should become familiar with the devices themselves in order to prevent errors and complications. Some of the EIDs commercially available are the Intermate® and the Homepump Eclipse® Infusions systems. Each device is labeled with a flow rate in mL/hour. The duration of the infusion is dependent on the volume of the drug solution. The concentration of drug solution may determine the volume needed.

Administration Sets

Primary IV Set. The primary IV set attached to the LVP can be one of several varieties, but the IV sets that flow by the force of gravity have several common features. The tubing has a drip chamber that is used to estimate the administration rate by counting drops as they fall through the chamber. Drip chambers are typically classified as macrodrip or minidrip based on the size of the drop that is formed in the drip chamber. Each set of tubing is labeled according to the number of drops it produces from one milliliter of solution. This number is used to determine how many drops should fall in a minute for the desired volume of milliliters per hour. Macro-drip sets deliver ten to twenty drops per milliliter and minidrip sets deliver sixty drops per milliliter, which offers precision necessary for pediatric patients.

The rate of flow through the tubing is set by use of a roller clamp rate-controlling device or an electronic infusion device. The roller clamp crimps the IV tubing as it is adjusted to control the flow of fluid. Electronic infusion devices, typically categorized as either pumps or controllers, are used to increase the precision and accuracy of administration.

The tubing may have injection ports, either Y-sites or flashballs. Drugs or other solutions can be injected through the injection ports so that they may be administered with the main IV solution. The systems used to give drugs through this means vary in setup.

Secondary IV Sets. Drugs that are routinely given through the same basic IV setup are usually attached to a "secondary IV set" that is connected to the primary set.

Venous Access Devices

Peripheral Venous Catheters are inserted into a peripheral vein (a vein of the arm, leg, hand, foot, or scalp) or a central vein (existing in the chest near the heart). Where the catheter is inserted depends, in part, on the contents of the IV solution. Peripheral insertion is more common than central insertion. With peripheral catheters, there are limitations on what can be infused and at what rate. The central catheter is more complicated and riskier to insert and maintain, but has fewer restrictions with respect to concentration of drug, rate of administration, and time the venous access can remain in place.

There are several types of peripheral catheters. The most common is plastic, because it is flexible and can bend as the vein flexes or moves and is therefore the most comfortable for the patient. Another type is a steel needle with a short end of tubing. This type is commonly referred to as a scalp vein or butterfly because of its appearance. This type of catheter may be left in the patient's vein even without a running IV if it is periodically flushed (rinsed) with a solution to prevent it from being blocked by blood clots. It is usually used in patients that require IV therapy but are otherwise able to eat and drink, do not require supplemental fluids, and may even be ambulatory.

Central catheters can be temporary, meaning they are only used for days or weeks (such as during a hospital stay), or permanent, which can be used for months or years (such as with home care patients or cancer patients who require frequent infusions). Temporary central catheters are inserted by the physician via a minor surgical procedure in the patient's room. This involves a small incision and insertion of the catheter into a vein near the heart. Permanent placement of central catheters also involves minor surgery but must be done in an operating room. The central catheter gives direct access into a vein that has a high flow of blood. Therefore, solutions that might be irritating or damaging to peripheral blood vessels, which have a lower blood flow, are given centrally.

Two commonly used permanent catheters are the Hickman® and the Broviac®. Each of these are tunnel catheters, which remain outside the body to provide readily available access for patients receiving multiple injections. Port-a-cath® catheters are another form of central injection port that is located beneath the skin. Another type of catheter that offers some of the benefits of both central and peripheral catheters is called a peripherally inserted central catheter (PICC). The PICC line, as its name implies, is inserted peripherally, but it is a long flexible catheter that is threaded through the venous system and its tip ends near the heart, where there is a high volume of blood flow. Caution needs to be exercised when manipulating all catheters because they can become a source of infection and can become seeded or colonized with bacteria.

Heparin Lock. Heparin locks are used to maintain catheter access to a vein without having to run a continuous drip to keep the vein patent or unobstructed. Heparin locks have an IV catheter or needle on one end and a resealable rubber diaphragm at the other end. The main purpose is to provide a port through which medications can be administered intermittently. The concentration of heparin used in heparin locks is usually 10 units/mL or 100 units/mL (figure 16–11).

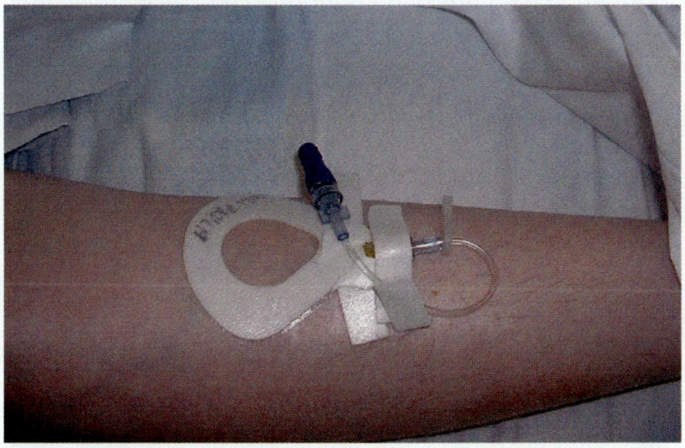

Figure 16–11. Heparin Lock.

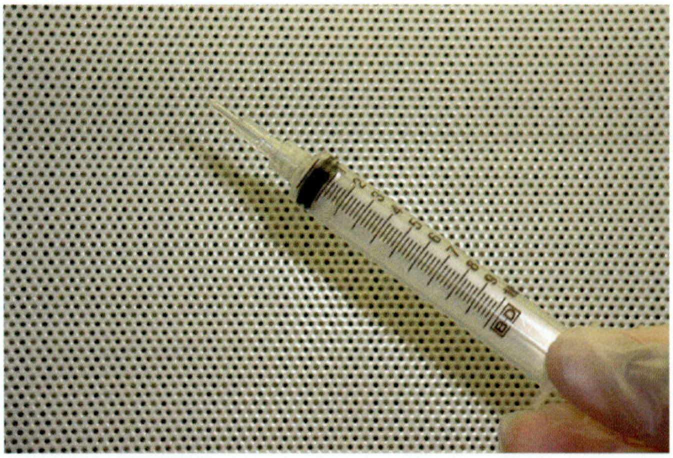

Figure 16–12. Syringe with cannula.

Part 3

Needleless Systems. Needleless systems are becoming a cost-effective alternative to traditional needle systems. They reduce the risks of needle sticks and subsequently the potential risk of disease transmission to healthcare workers who regularly draw blood or administer medications to patients. Needleless systems are required by law in some states and some health care systems. Needleless systems contain specially designed components, which may include a cannula or positive pressure cap that may be directly connected to a syringe tip and a needleless injection site. Cannulas functions like a needle but contain a blunt tip. The injection site must have the ability to accept the cannula (figure 16–12).

Final Filters. Final filters are inline filters located in the tubing used for drug administration. Final filters can be used to remove particles that may be present in the IV solution but are not visible to the naked eye. These particles, while small, can be harmful to patients if they become trapped in small capillaries or accumulate in the body. Final filters should be used with drugs that have a risk of particulate matter or crystals in the final solution, such as with phenytoin or mannitol.

Aseptic Preparation of Parenteral Products

As the use of parenteral therapy continues to expand, the need for well-controlled admixture preparation has also grown. Recognizing this need, many pharmacy departments have devoted increased resources to programs that ensure the aseptic preparation of sterile products. The main elements of these programs are[4,5]

- Development and maintenance of good aseptic technique in the personnel who prepare and administer sterile products
- Development and maintenance of a sterile compounding area, complete with sterilized equipment and supplies
- Development and maintenance of the skills needed to properly use a **laminar airflow workbench (LAFW)** or laminar airflow hood

Aseptic Technique

Aseptic technique is a means of manipulating sterile products without compromising their sterility. Proper use of a LAFW and strict aseptic technique are the most important factors in preventing the contamination of sterile products. Thorough training in the proper use of the LAFW and strict aseptic technique, followed by the development of conscientious work habits, is of utmost importance to any sterile products program.

Sterile Compounding Area (i.e., Clean Room)

Compounded sterile products must be free of living microorganisms, pyrogens, and visible particles. Room air typically contains thousands of suspended particles per cubic foot, most of which are too small to be seen with the naked eye. These include contaminants such as dust, pollen, smoke, and bacteria. Reducing the number of particles in the air improves the environment in which sterile products are prepared. This can be done by following several practices to maintain the sterile compounding area.

Compounding area counters, easily cleanable work surfaces, and floors should be cleaned daily while walls, ceilings, and storage shelving should be cleaned monthly at a minimum.[6] Segregated compounding areas must be separate from normal pharmacy operations, nonessential equipment, and other materials that produce particles. For example, the introduction of cardboard into the clean room environment should be avoided. Traffic flow into the sterile compounding area should be minimized. Trash should be removed frequently and regularly. Care should be taken to take the trash cans outside of the IV room before pulling the trash or otherwise removing it from the container. This will minimize the creation of particulate matter or the risk of spills in the IV room. Other, more sophisticated aspects of clean room design include special filtration or treatment systems for incoming air (figure 16–13), ultraviolet irradiation, air-lock entry portals, sticky mats to remove particulate matter from shoes, and positive room air pressure to reduce contaminant entry from adjacent rooms or hallways. Clean rooms are often adjoined by an anteroom that is used for non-aseptic activities related to the clean room operations, such as order processing, gowning, and handling of stock.

Figure 16–13. Ceiling HEPA filter.

Sterile products should be prepared in ISO Class 5 environments, which contain no more than 100 particles per cubic foot that are 0.5 micron or larger in size. LAFWs are frequently used to achieve an ISO Class 5 environment.

Laminar Airflow Workbenches

The underlying principle of LAFWs is that twice-filtered laminar layers of aseptic air continuously sweep the work area inside the hood to prevent the entry of contaminated room air. There are two common types of laminar flow workbenches, horizontal flow and vertical flow.

Horizontal LAFW. LAFWs that sweep filtered air from the back of the hood to the front are called horizontal LAFWs (figure 16–13). Horizontal flow workbenches use an electrical blower to draw contaminated room air through a prefilter. The prefilter, which is similar to a furnace filter, only removes gross contaminants and should be cleaned or replaced on a regular basis. The prefiltered air is then pressurized in a plenum to ensure that a consistent distribution of airflow is presented to the final filtering apparatus. The final filter constitutes the entire back portion of the hood's work area. This **high efficiency particulate air**, or **HEPA filter**, removes 99.97% of particles that are 0.3 micron or larger, thereby eliminating airborne microorganisms, which are usually 0.5 microns or larger.

Vertical LAFW. Laminar flow workbenches with a vertical flow of filtered air are also available. In vertical LAFWs, HEPA filtered air emerges from the top and passes downward through the work area (figure 16–14). Because exposure to antineoplastic (anticancer) drugs may be harmful, they should only be prepared in vertical LAFWs so that the risk of exposure to airborne drug particulates is minimized. The types of vertical LAFW used for the preparation of antineoplastics confine airflow within the hood and are referred to as biological safety cabinets (BSCs). BSCs and the preparation of antineoplastics and cytotoxic medications are covered later in this chapter.

The critical principle of using LAFWs is that nothing should interrupt the flow of air between the HEPA filter and the sterile object. The space between the HEPA filter and the sterile object is known as the critical area. The introduction of a foreign object between a sterile object and the HEPA filter increases wind turbulence in the critical area and contaminants from the foreign object may be carried onto the sterile work surface and thereby contaminate the injection port, needle, or syringe. This is referred to as downstream contamination.

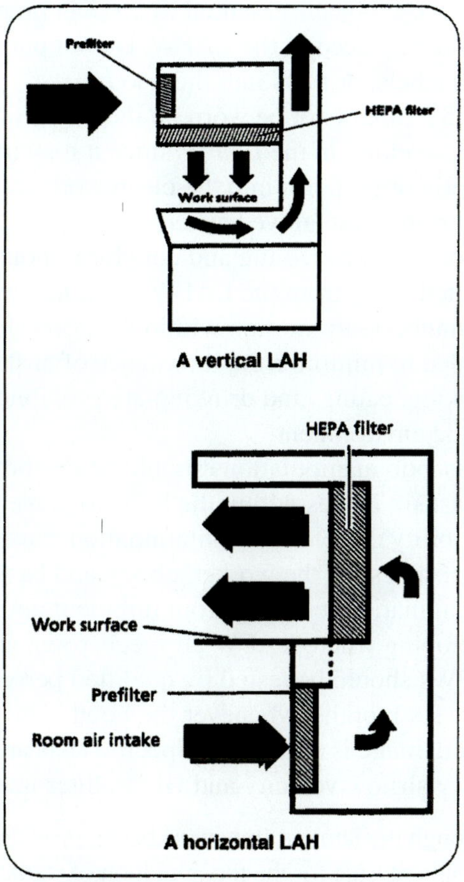

Figure 16–14. Horizontal and vertical laminar flow hoods with the basic components labeled.

Safety First To maintain sterility, nothing should pass behind a sterile object in a horizontal flow workbench or above a sterile object in a vertical flow workbench, including the technician's hands.

Part 3

All materials placed within the laminar flow workbench disturb the patterned flow of air blowing from the HEPA filter. This zone of turbulence created behind an object could potentially extend outside the hood, pulling or allowing contaminated room air into the aseptic working area (figure 16–15). When laminar airflow is moving on all sides of an object, the zone of turbulence extends approximately three times the diameter of that object. When laminar airflow is not accessible to an object on all sides (for example, when placed adjacent to a vertical wall), a zone of turbulence is created that may extend six times the diameter of the object. For these reasons, the hands should be positioned so that airflow in the critical area between the HEPA filter and sterile objects is not blocked.

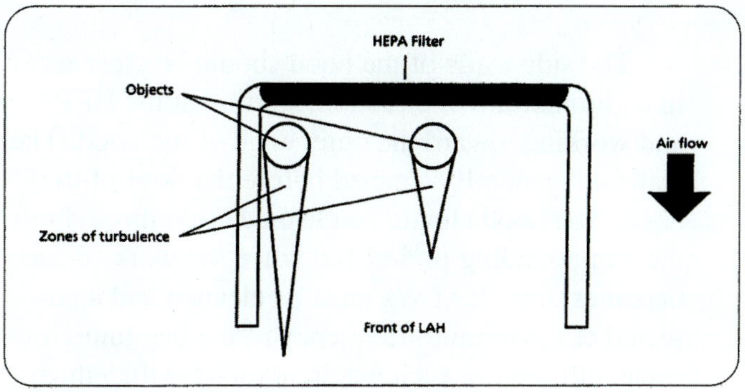

Figure 16–15. Examples of zones of turbulence created behind objects in a horizontal LAFW. Notice that the zone of turbulence of the object on the left is greater due to the object's proximity to the side of the hood, and has extended outside of the LAFW. (Note: figure is not drawn to scale.)

✔ It is advisable to work with objects at least six inches from the sides and front edge of the hood without blocking air vents, so that unobstructed airflow is maintained between the HEPA filter and sterile objects.

The following are general principles for operating LAFWs properly:

- A LAFW should be positioned away from excess traffic, doors, air vents, or anything that could produce air currents capable of introducing contaminants into the hood.
- If it is turned off, nonfiltered, nonsterile air will occupy the LAFW work area. Therefore, when it is turned back on, it should be allowed to run for fifteen to thirty minutes before it is used. Manufacturer recommendations should be consulted for each given hood. This allows the LAFW to blow the non-sterile air out of the LAFW work area. Then the LAFW can be cleaned for use.
- Before use, all interior working surfaces of the laminar flow workbench should be cleaned with 70% isopropyl alcohol or other appropriate disinfecting agent and a clean, lint-free cloth.

Safety First Cleaning should be performed from the HEPA filter beginning in the rear of the hood in a side-to-side motion *parallel to that surface's contact with the HEPA*, moving gradually away from the point of contact in overlapping strokes. Cleaning should never be done with a motion that carries contaminants from the outer edge back toward the HEPA.

The side walls of the hood should be cleaned in an up-and-down direction, starting at the HEPA and working toward the outer edge of the hood. The walls are generally cleaned before the floor of the hood. The hood should be cleaned often throughout the compounding period and when the work surface becomes dirty. LAFWs must be cleaned and disinfected at a minimum frequency of the beginning of each shift, before each batch, not longer than thirty minutes following the previous surface disinfection when ongoing compounding activities are occurring, after spills, and when surface contamination is known or suspected.[6] Some materials are not soluble in alcohol and may initially require the use of water in order to be removed. After the water is applied and wiped off, the surface should be cleaned with alcohol. In addition, spray bottles of alcohol should not be used in the hood because they do not allow for the physical action of cleaning the hood, they can accidentally damage the HEPA filter, and they do not ensure that alcohol is applied to all areas of the surface to be cleaned. Once applied, alcohol should also be allowed to air dry because this will increase its effectiveness as a disinfectant.

✔ In addition, Plexiglas sides, found on some types of laminar flow workbenches, should be cleaned with warm, soapy water rather than alcohol because the alcohol will dry out the Plexiglas and cause it to become cloudy and possibly cracked.

- Nothing should be permitted to come in contact with the HEPA filter. This includes cleaning solution, aspirate or drug spray from syringes, or glass from ampules. Ampules should not be opened directly toward the filter.
- Only those objects essential to product preparation should be placed in the LAFW. Do not put paper, pens, labels, or trays into the hood.
- Jewelry should not be worn on the hands or wrists when working in the LAFW since it may introduce bacteria or particles into the clean work area or compromise the glove barrier.
- Actions such as talking and coughing should be directed away from the LAFW working area and any unnecessary motion within the hood should be avoided to minimize the turbulence of airflow.
- Smoking, eating, and drinking are prohibited in the aseptic environment.
- All aseptic manipulations should be performed at least six inches within the hood to prevent the possibility of potential contamination caused by the closeness of the worker's body and backwash contamination resulting from turbulent air patterns developing where LAFW air meets room air.
- LAFWs should be tested by qualified personnel every six months, whenever the hood is moved, or if filter damage is suspected. Specific tests are used to certify airflow velocity and HEPA filter integrity.

Although the laminar flow workbench provides an aseptic environment, safe for the manipulation of sterile products, it is essential that strict aseptic technique be used in conjunction with proper hood operation. It is important to remember that the use of the LAFW alone, without the observance of aseptic technique, cannot ensure product sterility.

Personal Attire

The first component of good aseptic technique is proper personal attire. Compounding personnel should remove personal outer garments, all cosmetics, and all hand, wrist, and other visible jewelry or piercings before entering the ante room or segregated compounding area. Clean room attire should include dedicated shoes or shoe covers, head and facial hair covers, and face masks/eye shields applied in this order to help reduce particulate or bacterial contamination. After hand washing as described below, clean garments, which are relatively particulate free, should be worn when preparing sterile products. Clean room attire will depend on institutional policies and often are related to the type of product being prepared. Many facilities provide clean scrub suits or gowns for this purpose. Scrub suits should not be worn home to ensure that no contaminants are transported home and that the process of cleaning the clothing does not introduce lint onto the low-lint clothing. In addition, suits should be covered up when leaving the pharmacy to minimize the contamination from areas such as the cafeteria.

Handwashing

Touching sterile products while compounding is the most common source of contamination of pharmacy-prepared sterile products. Since the fingers harbor countless bacterial contaminants, proper hand washing is extremely important. Every entry into a sterile product area should include scrubbing your hands, nails, wrists, and forearms to elbows thoroughly for at least 30 seconds with a brush, warm water, and appropriate bactericidal soap before performing aseptic manipulations. Dry hands completely using either lint-free disposable towels or an electronic hand dryer.

Gloving

After appropriate hand washing is complete and attire is put on, antiseptic hand cleansing should be performed using a waterless, alcohol-based, surgical hand scrub just prior to the last item worn before compounding begins—sterile gloves. Sterile gloves are only sterile until they touch something unsterile or until they are torn and allow bacteria from the hands to enter the work area. For example, if it becomes necessary to scratch or touch the face while wearing gloves, they will need to be changed. For these reasons, always wash your bare hands thoroughly, as noted above, before unwrapping and putting on the gloves. Occasionally workers develop allergies to latex as a result of repeated use of latex gloves. As a result, many institutions have now turned to using only non-latex gloves.

Equipment and Supplies

In addition to hand washing and gloving, another important factor in aseptic preparation of sterile products is the correct use of appropriate sterile equipment and supplies, including syringes and needles.

Syringes. Syringes are made of either glass or plastic. Most drugs are more stable in glass, so glass syringes are most often used when medication is to be stored in the syringe for an extended period of time. Some medications may react with the plastics in the syringe, which would alter the potency or stability of the final product. Disposable plastic syringes are most frequently used in preparing sterile products because they are inexpensive, durable, and only in contact with substances for a short time. This minimizes the potential for incompatibility with the plastic itself.

Syringes are composed of a barrel and plunger (figure 16–16). The plunger, which fits inside the barrel, has a flat disk or lip at one end and a rubber piston at the other. The top collar of the barrel prevents the syringe from slipping during manipulation; the tip is where the needle attaches. To maintain sterility of the product, do not touch the syringe tip or the plunger. Many syringes have a locking mechanism at the tip such as the Luer-lock, which secures the needle within a threaded ring. Some syringes, such as slip-tip syringes, do not have a locking mechanism. In this case, friction holds the needle on the syringe.

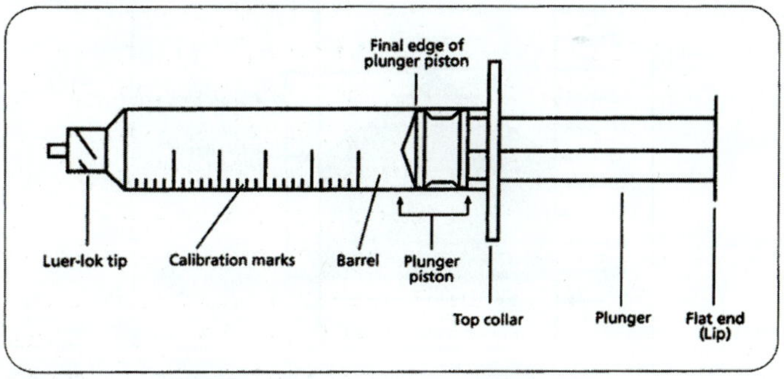

Figure 16–16. A syringe with the basic components labeled.

Syringes are available in numerous sizes ranging from 0.3 to 60 mL. Calibration marks on syringes represent different increments of capacity, depending on the size of the syringe. Usually, the larger the syringe capacity, the larger the interval between calibration lines. For example, each line on the 10 mL syringes represents 0.2 mL, but on a 30 mL syringe, each line represents 1 mL.

To maximize accuracy, the smallest syringe that can hold a desired amount of solution should be used. Syringes are accurate to one-half of the smallest increment marking on the barrel. For example, a 10 mL syringe with 0.2 mL markings is accurate to 0.1 mL and can be used to measure 3.1 mL accurately. A 30 mL syringe with 1 mL markings; however, is only accurate to 0.5 mL and should not be used to measure a volume of 3.1 mL.

Rx for Success

Ideally, the volume of solution should only take up 1/2 to 2/3 of the syringe capacity. This avoids inadvertent touch contamination caused when the syringe plunger is pulled all the way back.

When measuring with a syringe, line up the final edge (closest to the tip of the syringe) of the plunger piston, which comes in contact with the syringe barrel, to the calibration mark on the barrel that corresponds to the volume desired (figure 16–17).

Syringes are sent from the manufacturer assembled and individually packaged in paper overwrap or plastic covers. The sterility of the contents is guaranteed as long as the outer package remains intact. Therefore, packages should be inspected, and any that are damaged should be discarded. The syringe package should be opened within the laminar flow workbench in order to maintain sterility. The wrapper should be peeled apart and not ripped or torn. To minimize particulate contamination, do not lay discarded packaging or unopened syringes on the LAFW work surface.

Syringes may come from the manufacturer with a needle attached or with a protective cover over the syringe tip. The syringe tip protector should be left in place until it is time to attach the needle. For attaching needles to Luer-lock-type syringes, a quarter-turn is usually sufficient to secure the needle to the syringe.

Needles. Like syringes, needles are commercially available in many sizes. Two numbers, gauge and length, describe the needle size. The gauge of the needle corresponds to the diameter of its bore, which is the diameter of the inside of the shaft. The larger the gauge, the smaller the needle bore. For example, the smallest needles have a gauge of 27, while the largest needles have a gauge of 13. The length of a needle shaft is measured in inches and usually ranges from 3/8 to 3 1/2 inches.

The components of a simple needle are the shaft and the hub (figure 16–18). The hub attaches the needle to the syringe and is often color-coded to correspond to a specific gauge. The tip of the needle shaft is slanted to form a point. The slant is called the bevel, and the point is called the bevel tip. The opposite end of the slant is termed the bevel heel.

Needles are sent from the manufacturer individually packaged in paper and plastic overwrap with a protective cover or needle guard over the needle shaft. This guarantees

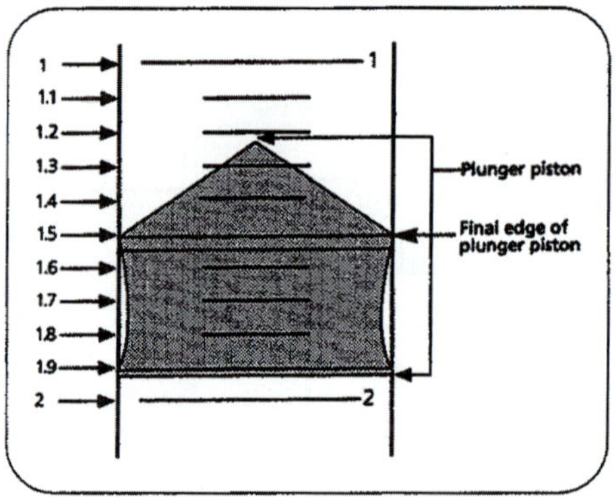

Figure 16–17. A close-up of a syringe showing how to measure 1.5 mL. Note that the final edge of the plunger piston is used to make the measurement.

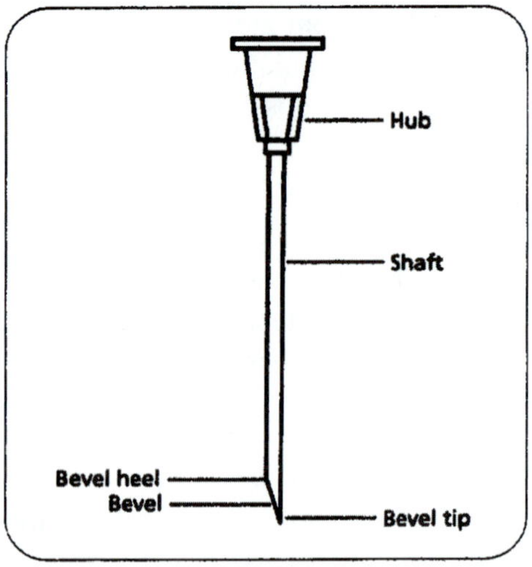

Figure 16–18. A needle with the basic components labeled.

the sterility as long as the package remains intact. Therefore, packages that are damaged should be discarded.

No part of the needle itself should be touched. Needles should be manipulated by their over-wrap and protective covers only. The protective cover should be left in place until the needle and/or syringe are ready to be used. A needle shaft is usually metal and is lubricated with a sterile silicone coating so that latex vial tops can be penetrated smoothly and easily. For this reason, needles should never be swabbed with alcohol.

Some needles are designed for special purposes and therefore have unique characteristics. For example, needles designed for batch filling have built-in vents (vented needles) to avoid the need to release pressure that might form in the vial. Another example is needles with built-in filters. These are intended for use with products requiring frequent filtering, such as drugs removed from a glass ampule.

✔ When dealing with small volumes, it is important to account for the volume of solution left in the shaft and hub of the needle, an area referred to as the dead space. As much as 0.3 mL may be present in the dead space of the needle, which could represent a significant amount of the dose for a pediatric patient.

When drawing up solutions using a needle, this volume remains in the dead space of the needle. Thus, when removing the needle and replacing it with a cannula, this volume is discarded and the patient does not receive the correct amount. It may be necessary to dilute the product to increase the volume or provide overfill in the syringe to account for this. Consult your institution's policies and procedures for guidance.

Drug Additive Containers

Injectable medication additives may be supplied in an ampule, vial, or prefilled syringe. Each requires a different technique to withdraw medication and place it in the final dosage form.

Vials. Medication vials are glass or plastic containers with a rubber stopper secured to the top, usually by an aluminum cover. Vials differ from ampules in that they are used to hold both powders and liquids. The rubber stopper is usually protected by a flip-top plastic cap or aluminum cover.

Protective covers do not guarantee sterility of the rubber stopper. Therefore, before the stopper is penetrated, it must be swabbed with 70% isopropyl alcohol and allowed to dry. The correct swabbing technique is to make several firm strokes in the same direction over the rubber closure, always using a clean swab. Swabbing helps achieve sterility in two ways: first, the alcohol acts as a disinfecting agent, and second, the physical act of swabbing in one direction removes particles.

When piercing vials with needles, avoid **coring** the rubber stopper with the needle. A core is carved out of the rubber stopper when the bevel tip and the bevel heel do not penetrate the stopper at the same point.

✔ To prevent core formation, hold the needle in a bevel-up position. Pierce the stopper with the bevel tip and then press downward and toward the bevel as the needle is inserted.

Vials are closed-system containers, since air or fluid cannot pass freely in or out of them. In most cases, air pressure inside the vial is similar to that of room air. In order to prevent the formation of a vacuum inside the vial (less pressure inside the vial than room air), the pressure should be normalized by first injecting a volume of air equal to the volume of fluid that is going to be withdrawn into the vial. This step should not be done with drugs that produce gas when they are reconstituted, such as ceftazidime, or with cytotoxic medications.

If the drug within a vial is in powdered form, it has to be reconstituted. Inject the desired volume of sterile diluting solution (the diluent), such as sterile water for injection, into the vial containing the powdered drug. An equal volume of air must be removed in order to prevent a positive pressure from developing inside the vial. This is particularly important when dealing with medications that can be harmful if aspirated (sprayed) into the air. Allow the air to flow into the syringe before removing the needle from the vial, or use a vented needle, which allows displaced air to escape the vial through a vent in the needle. Care must be taken to ensure that the drug is completely dissolved before proceeding. Usually, gentle shaking adequately dissolves the drug contents. There are some agents that can't be shaken because shaking will degrade the active ingredient in, for example, many biologic products. As always, if the user is not familiar with preparation methods for the product, the package insert and/or a supervisor should be consulted.

Vials with drugs in solution are classified as either multiple-dose (also called multi-dose or multiple-use) or single-dose. Multiple-dose vials contain a small amount of a preservative agent that is added to retard the growth of bacteria or other organisms that may inadvertently contaminate a product. The presence of these substances does not make the solution self-sterilizing, and the use of strict aseptic technique is still required. Preservatives are included in both bacteriostatic water for injection and in any multiple-dose product. Common substances used as preservatives include benzyl alcohol, parabens, phenol, and benzalkonium chloride. These substances are typically added by the manufacturer in small quantities that are not harmful when the product is dosed appropriately. Therefore, if a preparation calls for large amounts of drug solution that contains a preservative or a diluent with a preservative, the pharmacist should be consulted to verify that the total amount of preservative to be administered will not be toxic. Due to their toxicity, solutions with preservatives should not be used for epidural or intrathecal dosage forms and should only be used with caution in pediatric or neonatal preparations.

Rx for Success

Even if the drug *dose* is appropriate, the *number of doses* has to be considered. Diluents without preservatives are often used when just one dose is to be given in a short period of time, such as an IM injection in a physician's office or a piggyback given in the emergency room. If repeated doses are needed, a diluent with preservatives should be used.

Single-dose vials have no preservative and are intended to be used one time only. Once a vial is entered with a needle, whether in a patient care area or a LAFW, it should be discarded. It is best to consult your institution's policies with respect to handling single-dose vials.

Ampules. Ampules are composed entirely of glass and, once broken (i.e., opened), become open-system containers. Since air or fluid may now pass freely in and out of the container (no vacuum effect), it is not necessary to replace the volume of fluid to be withdrawn with air.

Before an ampule is opened, any solution visible in the top portion (head) should be moved to the bottom (body) by swirling the ampule in an upright position, tapping the ampule with one's finger, or inverting the ampule and then quickly swinging it into an upright position (figure 16–19).

To open an ampule, the head must be broken from the body of the ampule. To make the break properly, the ampule neck should be cleansed with an alcohol swab, which should be left in place. This swab can prevent accidental cuts to the fingers as well as shattering of glass particles and aerosolized drug. The head of the ampule should be

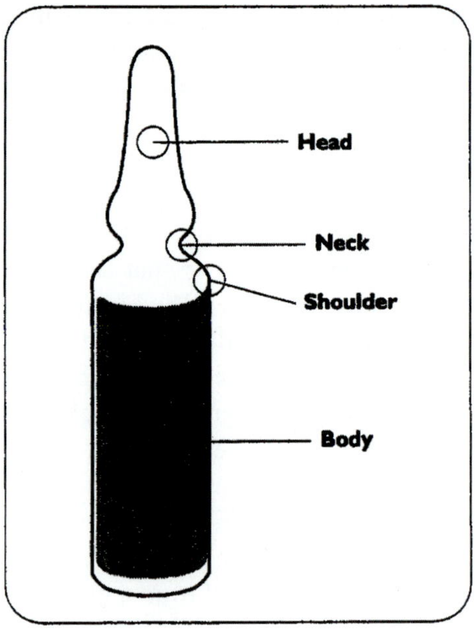

Figure 16–19. An ampule with the basic components labeled.

held between the thumb and index finger of one hand, and the body should be held with the thumb and index finger of the other hand. Pressure should be exerted on both thumbs, pushing away from oneself in a quick motion to snap open the ampule. Ampules should not be opened toward the HEPA filter of the laminar flow workbench or toward other sterile products within the hood. Extreme pressure may result in crushing of the head between the thumb and index finger. Therefore, if the ampule does not open easily, it should be rotated so that pressure on the neck is at a different point. Some ampules are scored or have designated pressure points to facilitate opening. Reusable plastic openers are available in various sizes to open ampules. They provide greater protection but must be kept clean.

✔ To withdraw medication from an ampule, the ampule should be tilted, and the needle should be placed bevel-downward in the corner space (or shoulder) near the opening.

Surface tension should keep the solution from spilling out of the tilted ampule. The syringe plunger is then pulled back to withdraw the solution.

The use of a filter needle (e.g. a needle with a 5-micron filter in the hub) keeps glass or paint chips that may have fallen into the solution from being drawn into the syringe. To withdraw the solution, either use a filter needle and change to a regular needle before expelling the contents, or start with a regular needle and change to a filter needle before expelling the contents. Either way, the filter needle must not be used for both withdrawing from the ampule and expelling from the syringe because doing so would nullify the filtering effect. Usually, the medication is withdrawn from the ampule with a regular needle, and then the needle is changed to a filter needle before pushing the drug out of the syringe. If the syringe is used as a final container for dispensing, a filter needle should be used to withdraw the solution. Some medications, such as those available as injectable suspensions, should not be filtered because active ingredients would also be filtered out in the process. In that case, the medication is withdrawn from the ampule using a regular needle. Most injectable suspensions are given intramuscularly, not intravenously.

Another device that can be used for withdrawing solutions from an ampule is the filter straw. The filter straw differs from the filter needle in that it is made out of plastic tubing rather than metal and it is longer, making it easier to reach the bottom of an ampule. It also reduces the risk of needlesticks during the manipulation, since it does not have a sharp tip. Once the solution is withdrawn with a filter straw, however, a regular needle must be attached to the syringe to inject the solution into its final container. Enough excess drug should be pulled from the straw into the syringe to refill the dead space of the needle.

Prefilled Syringes. Manufacturers produce a number of products that are packaged in ready-to-inject syringes. Drugs commonly given IM, IV, or subcutaneously are packaged this way to make them convenient for administration. It is also done if the drug is commonly used in emergency situations because a prefilled syringe saves time. Prefilled syringes often have calibrations on the syringe barrel and are labeled with the concentration and total volume. These products may be used in the pharmacy to prepare sterile products but are more likely to be kept in patient care areas.

Preparation of Intravenous Admixtures

The usual process for preparing an admixture is that an order is received in the pharmacy and reviewed by the pharmacist. If the order is deemed reasonable and appropriate, the pharmacist will input the information into the pharmacy records (usually by entering it into a pharmacy computer system) to document the preparation and generate a label. The pharmacist then assigns the preparation of the product to support personnel. The following sequence describes the common steps technicians follow to prepare intravenous admixtures. However, keep in mind that the final IV admixture may be prepared in a variety of containers, including flexible plastic bags, glass bottles, and semirigid plastic containers.

Before compounding, perform the necessary calculations, assemble all materials and visually inspect vials, ampules, and IV solution containers for signs of cloudiness, particulate matter, cracks and punctures, expiration dates, and anything else that may indicate that the product is defective. It is also important to ensure that an appropriate supply of all materials is available to complete the tasks. First, clean the hood and then only place materials that are necessary to prepare the product in the LAFW.

Next, disinfect all injection surfaces and allow them to dry. Withdraw and measure the drug fluid from its container, using the syringe size closest to the volume to be withdrawn. To obtain as accurate a measurement as possible, remove air bubbles from the syringe by first pulling back slightly on the plunger to draw any fluid trapped in the needle into the syringe barrel; then tap the barrel to move the air bubbles up to the tip, and slightly depress the plunger to expel the air. The syringe must be held in an upright position (tip up) during this maneuver.

Disposal of Supplies. Syringes and uncapped needles should be discarded according to institutional policy. In some institutions, they are discarded in puncture-resistant, sealable containers called sharps containers. If the pharmacist needs the syringe to verify the amount of drug added to the admixture, institutions may allow needles used in compounding to be recapped for removal and disposal. When a syringe is used to verify the amount of drug added, the plunger is drawn back to the calibration mark to indicate the amount of drug added. Then the syringe and the drug vial are placed next to the completed and labeled product for the pharmacist to verify. It should be noted that recapping needles is generally considered to be an unsafe practice. Most institutions have policies against recapping needles, as required by OSHA and the CDC, to decrease the risk of needlestick injuries with contaminated needles. Contaminated, uncapped needles and syringes must be disposed of in puncture-resistant containers. If recapping of needles is required, a one-handed scoop method should be used. For worker safety, two-handed recapping is never an acceptable practice for contaminated needles.

Luer Tips. When the final product being dispensed is not intended for injection (such as for inhalation), a Luer tip may be placed on it to maintain sterility. These are either attached by friction or threaded grooves (a Luer

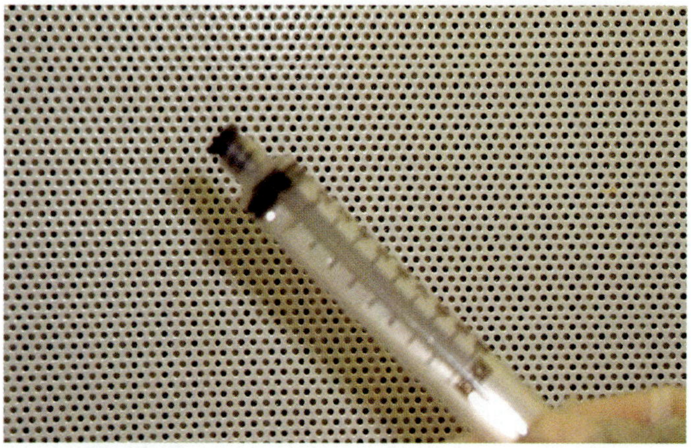

Figure 16–20. Luer Tip.

Lock). Luer tips are also used on syringes prepared for use with needleless systems (figure 16–20).

Seals and Closures. Once a port has been penetrated with a needle, it will need to be properly sealed to reduce the risk of contamination from bacteria. The most common seals used are IV additive seals, which are placed over the sterile port of a vial or a final product. (figure 16–21). They are made from aluminum and have a sterile pad in the center that maintains contact with the port to ensure the sterility. Other closures include tamperproof caps that are placed on bottles or IV bags to prevent tampering. Tamperproof caps are commonly used on IV preparations containing controlled substances to discourage drug diversion once the product has left the pharmacy. Injection ports on IV bags are often sealed with metallic adhesive seals in the LAFW after an admixture is made.

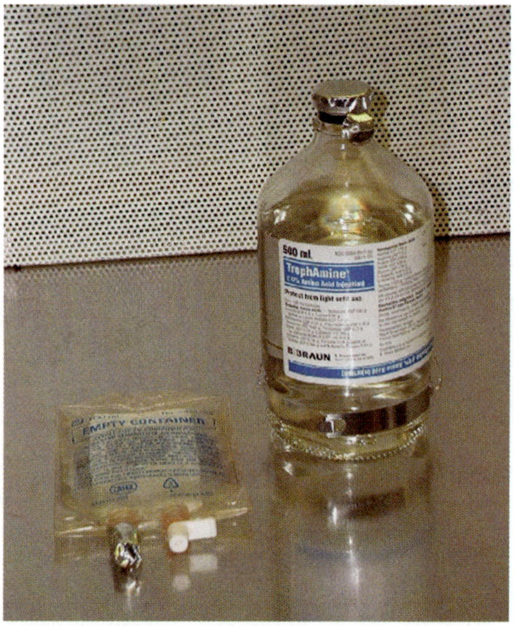

Figure 16–21. IV additive seals.

Automated Compounding Sterile Product Filling Equipment

Although hospitals and regulatory agencies have strict guidelines that must be followed, including rigorous training and competencies, the technical complexity of sterile product preparation lends itself to inconsistency among employees. Additionally, compounded sterile products create potentially challenging situations for pharmacists to verify product preparation accuracy. Automation can eliminate sources of preparation errors inherent to human factors; this technology ensures proper handling and accurate, sterile preparation of the IV product. Enclosed IV preparation environments that utilize robotics to prepare, label, and dispense IV syringes, SVPs and LVPs ready for dispensing are becoming more common, given these considerations (figures 16–22 and 16–23).

TECHNOLOGY TOPICS

Automation incorporates tools to mitigate math errors, including an algorithm to mathematically scale fluid transfers to match the requested order. For example, if a vial's fluid volume, concentration, and, if applicable, the vial's reconstitution information (fluid and volume) is entered into the system, it can automatically scale the fluid transfers to accommodate the range of doses defined. This means that generic rules for a medication are defined and the automation can then handle a dose range without needing information specific to the requested dose.

Stated another way, the automation does not need to be taught each step value over the range. Auditing tools are often provided to allow a pharmacist to review and confirm the calculated values for the ranges. Systems should and typically do allow for specific handling of drug levels

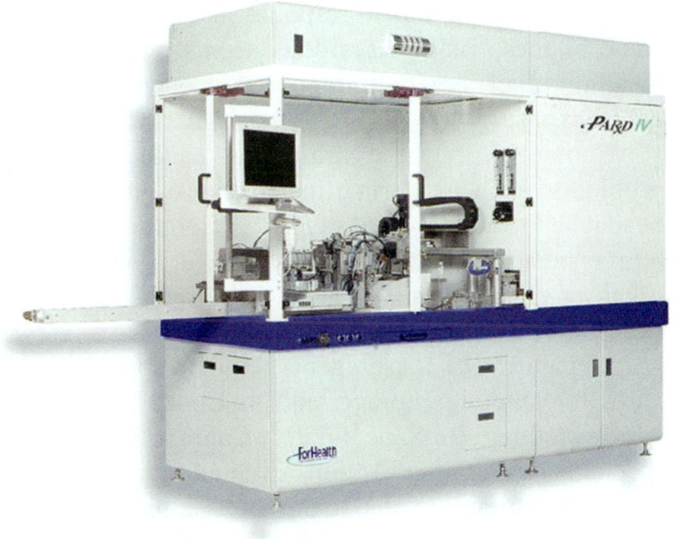

Figure 16–22. Automated syringe filling cabinet.

sort the order for production (if desired). A queue of requests determines what vials, syringes, and IV bags are required by the automation to fulfill the requests. The automation then pulls from a selection of drug vials that are pre-loaded into the cabinet, using bar-code verification. The vial is disinfected, reconstituted, in some cases shaken or rolled, and the appropriate amount of final product is removed and labeled for dispensing. Tracking mechanisms capture NDC codes and provide a complete audit trail.

In addition to the varied speed of preparation between platforms, the time required to clean these units may take between twenty to sixty minutes daily and will vary among systems. Internal complexity contains various surface topographies that require physical contact for cleaning. Also, automation that utilizes loading trays needs to be cleaned during the daily set up.

that do not scale in this manner or to create mixes where a dispensed product requires more than one drug.

Most often, items prepared in this type of environment are produced in high volumes and are repetitive in nature. Batch orders can be entered directly into the system's user interface. Alternatively, the automated compounded sterile product filling cabinets may receive data from the pharmacy information system, instructing it to prepare the appropriate patient specific doses. Operators can review the drug orders, set priorities, and

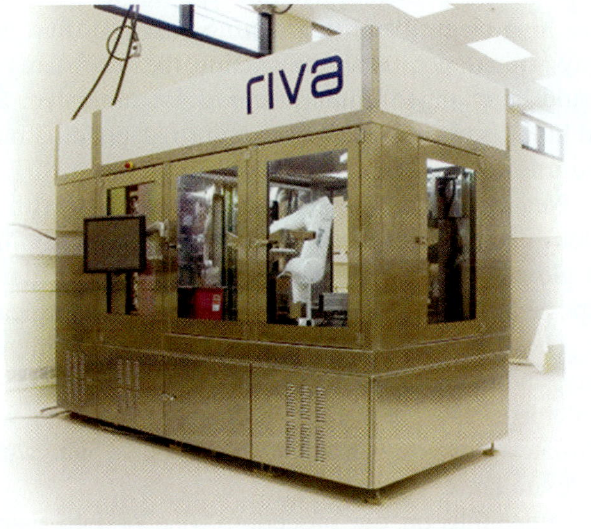

Figure 16–23. Automated IV syringe, SVP and LVP filling cabinet.

Labeling

Once an IV admixture or other sterile product is compounded, it should be properly labeled with the following information:

1. Patient name, identification number and room number (if applicable)
2. Bottle or bag sequence number, when appropriate
3. Name and amount of drug(s) added
4. Name and volume of admixture solution
5. Approximate final total volume of the admixture, when applicable
6. Prescribed flow rate (in milliliters per hour)
7. Date and time of scheduled administration
8. Date and time of preparation
9. Expiration date
10. Initials of person who prepared and person who checked the IV admixture
11. Auxiliary labeling—supplemental instructions and precautions

Many labels also now contain a bar code that contains information regarding the medication, the patient, and the anticipated administration. These are generated by the pharmacy computer to reduce the frequency of medication administration errors (figure 16–24).

After the drug is properly labeled, a final inspection of the admixture for cores and particulates is performed. All drug and IV solution containers used in preparing the admixture should be checked by the pharmacist to

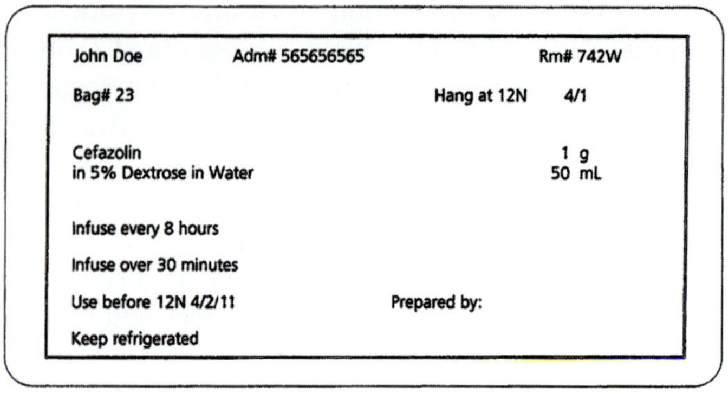
John Doe Adm# 565656565 Rm# 742W
Bag# 23 Hang at 12N 4/1
Cefazolin 1 g
in 5% Dextrose in Water 50 mL
Infuse every 8 hours
Infuse over 30 minutes
Use before 12N 4/2/11 Prepared by:
Keep refrigerated

Figure 16–24. A sample IV label.

verify that the technician added the proper amount of the correct drug to the correct IV solution. The label and final sterile product must be validated by a registered pharmacist against the order for accuracy and completeness before dispensing it for patient use.

Each product should also include an expiration date beyond which it should not be used. This might include a time twenty-four hours after preparation so that unused preparations are returned for potential reuse, or it might reflect the actual time that the product is considered stable. Typically, drugs are considered stable as long as they are within 10% of their labeled potency. In addition to stability, sterility concerns also factor into the assignment of expiration times. The pharmacist should assign the expiration time. Methods for assigning those times for both standard and non-standard preparations should be reflected in policies and procedures and substantiated by references, published literature, or reasonable professional judgment.

Preparation and Handling of Cytotoxic and Hazardous Drugs

Some medications can be hazardous to those who touch or inhale them. Because hazardous drugs initially involved drugs used to treat cancer, the terms antineoplastic and chemotherapeutic were used to describe them. The term cytotoxic, or cell killer, was later used to refer to any agent that may be genotoxic (a substance that may cause cancer or mutation by damaging DNA), oncogenic (causing, inducing, or being suitable for development of neoplasm), mutagenic (promoting mutation), teratogenic (producing malformed neonates), vesicant (an agent that produces a blister), or hazardous in any way. Exposure to antineoplastics, as well as immunosuppressants, antiviral agents, and biological response modifiers, may pose some of these risks. Hazardous agents require special handling procedures to minimize the potential for accidental exposure.

Contact with these drugs can cause immediate problems, such as dermatitis, dizziness, nausea, and headache.[7] Studies also suggest that repeated long-term exposure to small amounts of the drugs may cause organ or chromosome damage, impaired fertility, and even cancer.[7]

Preparation of these agents requires special procedures for labeling, storage, and transport. Use of protective clothing, Biological Safety Cabinets (BSCs), and special handling of spills and waste are also important. Special techniques related to the actual administration of these products to patients are not covered in this chapter. Additional information is available from ASHP in the form of a *Technical Assistance Bulletin on Handling of Cytotoxic and Hazardous Drugs.*[7]

Protective Apparel

There is no substitute for good technique, but protective apparel is another fundamental element in protecting personnel who handle or prepare hazardous drugs. Protective garments such as disposable coveralls or gowns, gloves, and shoe and hair covers may be used to shield personnel from exposure.

Most procedures require the use of disposable coveralls or a solid front gown. These garments should be made of low-permeability, lint-free fabric. They must have long sleeves and tight-fitting elastic or knit cuffs. They should not be worn outside the work area and should be changed immediately if contaminated. Shoe and hair covers may also be required, depending on the institution's policies.

Wearing gloves is essential when working with hazardous drugs. Wash hands thoroughly before putting on the gloves and after removing them. Use good quality, disposable, powder-free latex gloves, such as surgical latex. These gloves are preferred because of their fit, elasticity, and tactile sensation. If only powdered gloves are available, wash powder off before beginning to work. Non-latex gloves are also available for those who with an allergy to latex.

Depending on the procedure, one or two pairs of gloves may be required. If two pairs are needed, tuck one pair under the cuffs of the gown and place the second pair over the cuff. If an outer glove becomes contaminated, change it immediately. Change both the inner and the outer gloves immediately if the outer glove becomes torn, punctured, or heavily contaminated. If only one pair is worn, tuck the glove under or over the gown cuff so that the skin is not exposed.

Every work area in which hazardous drugs are prepared should have an eyewash fountain or sink and appropriate first aid equipment. If skin or eye contact occurs, follow established first aid procedures, obtain medical attention without delay, and document the injury.

Biological Safety Cabinets

One of the most important pieces of equipment for handling hazardous drugs safely is the **biological safety cabinet (BSC).** A BSC is a type of vertical LAFW that is designed to protect workers from exposure as well as to help maintain product sterility during preparation. BSCs must meet standards set by the National Sanitation Foundation (NSF Standard 49).

Do not use horizontal LAFWs to prepare hazardous drugs. They blow contaminants directly at the preparer. If possible, prepare sterile hazardous drugs in a Class II BSC. The front air barrier of the BSC protects the handler from contact with hazardous drug dusts and aerosols that are generated in the work zone. Room air is pulled into the front intake grill and filtered through a HEPA filter. The air then passes vertically, that is, downward, through the work zone. The air that has passed through the work zone goes through front intake and rear exhaust grilles, passes through a separate HEPA filter, and is recirculated through the work zone or exhausted to the outside. Placing objects on or near the front intake or rear exhaust grilles may obstruct the airflow and reduce the effectiveness of the cabinet.

There are several types of Class II BSCs. Type A BSCs pump about 30% of the air out the hood exhaust after it passes through a HEPA filter (figure 16–25). This air is then circulated to the room or exhausted to the outside, depending on how the hood is vented. Be sure not to block airflow from the exhaust filters. Type B BSCs send air from the work zone through a HEPA filter and then to the outside of the building through an auxiliary exhaust system (figure 16–26). Type B BSCs offer greater protection because filtered air is sent outside the building, and they have a faster inward flow of air. It is preferable to have the BSC exhausted directly to the outside through dedicated venting rather than venting into the general hospital circulation.

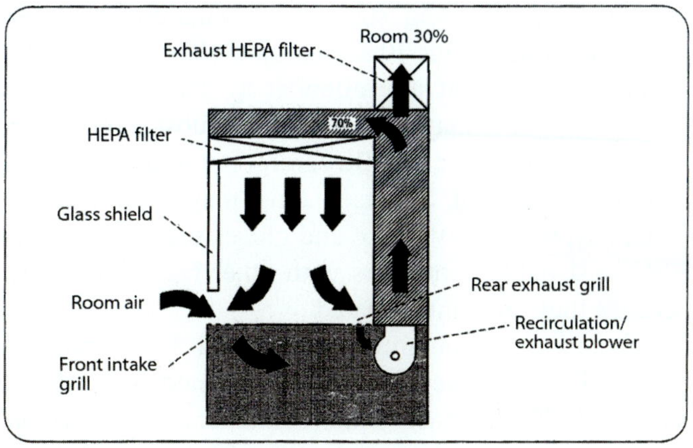

Figure 16–25. Class II Type A biological safety cabinet.

BSCs must be operated continuously, twenty-four hours per day, and they should be inspected and certified by qualified personnel every six months. Follow the manufacturer's recommendations for proper operation and maintenance, particularly replacement of HEPA filters.

Clean and disinfect the BSC regularly. Clean the work surface, back, and side walls with water or a cleaner recommended by the cabinet manufacturer. Do not use aerosol cleaners; they could damage the HEPA filters and cabinet and could allow contaminants to escape.

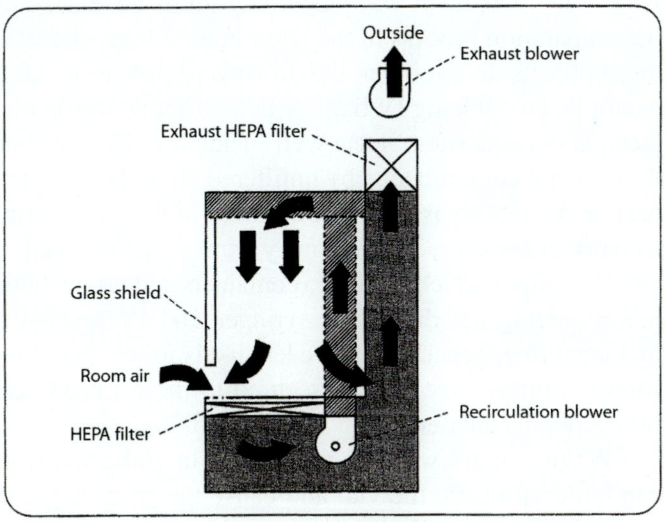

Figure 16–26. Class II Type B biological safety cabinet.

Before performing sterile manipulations, disinfect the work surface with 70% isopropyl alcohol or another suitable disinfectant and allow it to dry. Alcohol is a disinfectant and may remove some substances in the hood that water does not. Be careful not to use excessive amounts of alcohol, because vapors may build up in the BSC. Dispose of any gauze and gloves used to clean the BSC in sealable containers with other hazardous waste because they are contaminated.

Extensive decontamination should be performed, preferably on a weekly basis and immediately after a large spill. The cleaner, water containers, protective apparel, and cleaning materials all must be handled and discarded as contaminated waste. Refer to the facility's procedure on hood maintenance for specific cleaning procedures and schedules.

Preparing Hazardous Drugs

Before technicians handle a cytotoxic or other hazardous drug, they must demonstrate proper manipulative technique and use of protective equipment and materials.

Before preparing sterile hazardous drugs in a BSC, wash your hands and put on a gown and one or two pairs of latex gloves. Disinfect the work surface with alcohol. Place yourself so the front shield protects your eyes and face. Some institutions place a plastic-backed liner on the work surface. Though this liner may introduce particles into the work zone, it will absorb any small spills.

Assemble sufficient materials for the entire preparation process so you will not have to leave and re-enter the work zone. Disinfect and place only items necessary to the preparation process in the work zone. Make sure that these objects do not block the downward flow of air; for example, do not hang IV bags or bottles above sterile objects. Handle sterile objects well inside the BSC so that they are not contaminated by unfiltered air at the front air barrier. Air quality is lowest at the sides of the work zone, so work at least three inches away from each side wall.

If possible, attach IV sets to containers and prime them before adding the drug. Use syringes and IV sets with locking fittings because they are less likely to separate than friction fittings. Needles are secured to these Luer-Lock fittings with a quarter turn.

When you are working with drugs in vials, pressure can build up inside the vial and cause the drug to spray out around the needle. Maintain a slight negative pressure inside the vial to prevent this. Too much negative pressure, however, can cause leakage from the needle when it is withdrawn from the vial. Another way of preventing pressure buildup is to use a chemotherapy dispensing pin. This disposable device is attached at one end to the Luer-Lock fitting of the syringe, and a pin on the opposite end is inserted into the drug vial. The device also has a venting unit that allows for constant pressure equalization, therefore eliminating any problems due to pressure imbalances. Many pharmacies use needleless systems when preparing chemotherapy to reduce the risk of needlestick injuries.

When reconstituting a drug in a vial, use a syringe that can hold twice as much diluent as you will be drawing into the syringe barrel. This ensures that the plunger will not be pulled out of the barrel when the diluent is being drawn into the syringe. After drawing the diluent into a syringe, insert the needle into the vial top and draw the plunger back to draw air into the syringe to create a slight negative pressure inside the vial. Inject small amounts of diluent slowly and draw equal volumes of air out of the vial. Keep the needle in the vial and swirl the contents carefully until they dissolve completely. With the vial inverted, gradually withdraw the proper amount of drug solution while exchanging equal volumes of air for drug solution. Excess drug should remain in the vial. With the vial in the upright position, draw a small amount of air from the vial into the needle and hub. Then withdraw the needle from the vial.

If there is a need to transfer a hazardous drug to an IV bag, be careful not to puncture the bag. Wipe the IV container and set with moist gauze and put a warning label on the IV bag. Place the IV in a sealable bag so any leakage will be contained.

When withdrawing cytotoxic or hazardous drugs from an ampule, gently tap the contents down from the neck and top portion. Spray or wipe the ampule neck with alcohol. Attach a 5-micron filter needle or filter straw to a syringe that is large enough to hold the ampule's contents. The syringe should not be more than 1/2 to 2/3 full. Draw the fluid through the filter needle and clear it from the needle and hub. Exchange the filter needle for a regular needle of similar gauge and length. Eject any air and excess drug into a sterile vial, leaving the desired volume in the syringe. Be careful not to create aerosols. You may then transfer the drug to an IV bag or bottle. If the dose is to be dispensed in the syringe, draw back the plunger to clear fluid from the needle and hub. Replace the needle with a locking cap. Wipe the syringe with moistened gauze and label it appropriately. In some institutions, it is the responsibility of the pharmacy to prime the line with the chemotherapeutic agent. Additional precautions will need to be taken if this is the case.

To properly prime the line, obtain the proper IV tubing and the IV bag being prepared. Then unwrap the tubing inside the BSC. Close the tubing flow by using the roller clamp, remove the tubing tip, and place it aside. Insert the tubing spike (located above the fluid chamber) into the IV bag and slowly roll open the roller clamp, allowing IV fluid to flow through the tubing. Follow the fluid until the IV fluid reaches the end of the tubing. Allow a few drops of fluid to exit the tubing and then close the roller clamp as well as the on/off clamp and replace the tubing tip. Proper priming should have minimal to no air bubbles in the tubing. Proper manipulation of the roller clamp will ensure minimal bubbles. Priming the IV bag should be done prior to preparing any chemotherapy IV bags.

Good technique does not end with drug preparation. There are special requirements for waste disposal and cleanup. Put any glass fragments and needles in a puncture- and leak-resistant container. Do not clip the needles before disposal. Place all other materials in sealable plastic bags along with the outer pair of gloves. Seal all waste containers before removing them from the BSC and dispose of them in designated, labeled containers for chemotherapy disposal. Next, remove and dispose of the gown and, last, the inner pair of gloves. When removing the gloves, be careful not to touch the fingertips of the gloves to the skin or the inside of the gloves. Finally, wash your hands.

Labeling, Storage, and Transport

Safe and effective labeling, storage, and transportation practices are essential to prevent accidental exposure to hazardous drugs. Following the appropriate guidelines with respect to these processes should begin the moment hazardous drugs enter the facility. Hazardous drugs should be identified by distinctive labels indicating that the product requires special handling (figure 16–27). Attach the labels to drug packages and their storage shelves, bins, and areas. All areas where hazardous drugs are stored should be marked clearly as containing hazardous drugs. Access to these areas should be limited to authorized personnel who have been trained in handling hazardous drugs.

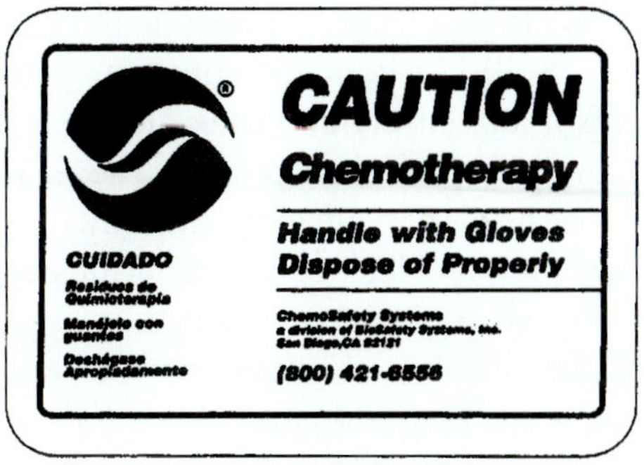

Figure 16–27. Example of a suitable warning label for cytotoxic and hazardous drugs.

Part 3

Storage equipment should be designed to minimize breakage. For example, shelves should have front barriers and carts should have rims. Hazardous drugs should be kept at eye level or lower and stored in bins. Refrigerated hazardous drugs should be stored in bins that are separated from non-hazardous drugs.

Transporting hazardous drugs requires special precautions to prevent container leakage or breakage. For example, pneumatic tube systems cause mechanical stress to containers and should never be used for transporting hazardous drugs. Carts used to transport hazardous materials should have rims to prevent the containers from falling off the cart and breaking. Hazardous drug containers must be securely capped or sealed and properly packaged to protect against leakage or breakage during transport. If leakage or breakage occurs, follow procedures described later in this section.

Waste Disposal and Spill Cleanup

Review your institution's policies and procedures for identifying, containing, collecting, segregating, and disposing of hazardous waste. Hazardous waste should be disposed of in separate containers. Regular trash should not be placed in hazardous waste containers. Handle the outside of hazardous waste containers only with uncontaminated gloves.

If you handle hazardous drugs, you should be familiar with the techniques and procedures for handling spills. In the event of a hazardous drug spill, you should use a spill kit, and the cleanup should follow established procedures. It is essential that you be familiar with the location and the use of the spill kit prior to requiring its use. Spill kits contain all the materials needed to clean up hazardous drug spills and protect health care workers and patients. Spill kits contain protective gear, eye protection, a respirator, utility and latex gloves, a disposable gown or coveralls, and shoe covers. They also contain the equipment needed to clean up the spill: a disposable scoop, a puncture- and leak-resistant plastic container for disposing of glass fragments, absorbent spill pads, gauze and disposable toweling, absorbent powder, and sealable, thick plastic waste disposal bags. Hazardous waste must be stored in leak-resistant containers until it is disposed of in accordance with government and institution policy.

In the event of a spill, put up a warning sign to alert other people in the area of the hazard. Put on all of the protective equipment, including latex gloves covered by utility gloves. Put broken glass in the puncture- and leak-resistant plastic container. Absorb liquids with disposable towels or spill pads. Remove powders with dampened towels or gauze. Rinse the contaminated surface with water, wash it with detergent, and then rinse it again. Start at the outside of the spill and work toward the center. Place all the contaminated materials in sealable plastic disposal bags. In all cases, it is important that the circumstances and the handling of the spill be documented in writing, including completion of an incident report, and kept on file.

If the area is carpeted, refer to institutional policies and procedures for handling spills in carpeted areas. Absorbent powder and "hazardous drug only" vacuum cleaners are often used to clean up spills in these areas.

If a large spill occurs in a BSC, additional steps must be taken. Use the spill kit described above and be sure to seal all contaminated materials in hazardous waste containers while the materials are still inside the BSC. Use utility gloves when handling any broken glass. Thoroughly clean the drain spillage trough and decontaminate the BSC if necessary. Transfer these containers to leak-resistant containers.

Total Parenteral Nutrition Solutions

Total parenteral nutrition (TPN), also known as hyperalimentation, refers to the IV administration of nutrients needed to sustain life. TPN contains carbohydrates, protein, fats, water, electrolytes, vitamins, and trace elements, hence the designation "total."

TPN therapy is indicated for patients who cannot meet their nutritional needs from oral or other gastrointestinal means. TPN may be used for patients who can't eat (e.g., after head and neck surgery, if comatose, or before or after surgery), who will not eat (e.g., patients with chronic diseases or psychologic disorders, or geriatric patients), who should not eat (e.g., patients with esophageal obstruction or inflammatory bowel disease), or who cannot eat or absorb enough to sustain their nutritional needs because their medical condition has increased their nutritional requirements (e.g., patients with cancer, burns, or trauma). Whenever the patient has a functional gastrointestinal system, it should be used preferentially over TPN, unless there is a medical contraindication.

Components of Parenteral Nutrition Solutions

TPN solutions contain base components and additives. Base components are usually mixed first and make up much of the volume of the TPN. They are composed of dextrose (carbohydrates) and amino acids (protein) and may also include fat and water. Additives are usually mixed with the base component and include life-sustaining nutrients, such as electrolytes, vitamins, trace elements (micronutrients) and may also include drugs such as heparin, insulin, and H_2 antagonists.

Carbohydrates are usually administered in the form of dextrose because of its low cost and easy availability. The commercially available concentrations of dextrose vary from 5 to 70%. Usually a 50% or 70% solution is used in TPN preparation, and the final dextrose concentration in the TPN is usually around 25% for solutions administered via a central vein. The dextrose concentration is significantly less for infusions intended for peripheral administration, usually a maximum of 10–12.5%.

Protein is required for tissue synthesis and repair, transport of body nutrients and waste, and maintenance of immune function. Protein is usually given as commercially available synthetic crystalline amino acid formulations. These solutions are available in concentrated forms, such as 8.5%, 10%, or 15% and diluted during the compounding process. A number of special formulations are available for pediatric patients and patients who have kidney disease, liver disease, or are in a high stress situation (e.g., intensive care patients).

Fats (or lipids) are usually administered as fat emulsions. Emulsions are needed since fat is insoluble in water. Administering fat emulsions not only prevents essential fatty acid deficiency, but provides a source of calories. They are commercially available as 10%

or 20% emulsions that may be dispensed in a separate container that can be given through a peripheral IV line. Alternatively, fats can be added to the TPN solution. In this type of TPN, called a 3-in-1 solution or total nutrient admixture (TNA), the fat emulsion is considered a third base component, along with dextrose and amino acids. The 3-in-1 technique offers several nutritional advantages but has certain mixing, stability and compounding disadvantages (see the Preparation section). Thirty percent fat emulsions are available for compounding admixtures only and should not be given as a separate IV infusion.

Water is in all preparations and is usually derived from the components used in the preparation. Sterile water for injection may be added to obtain the desired final concentration or volume. The purpose of adding water is to offset normal bodily losses and to prevent dehydration. In addition to the TPN solution, separate fluids may be given for fluid replacement or for administration of medications.

Electrolytes are needed to meet daily metabolic needs and prevent deficiencies. The electrolytes usually included in TPNs are sodium, potassium, chloride, acetate, phosphate, magnesium, and calcium. Electrolytes are usually administered as a specific salt of the product. For example, sodium may be admixed as sodium chloride, sodium acetate, sodium phosphate, or sodium lactate. Potassium can be given as potassium chloride, potassium acetate, or potassium phosphate. The patient's clinical condition and blood chemistries determine the amount and form of electrolytes required. It is important that the technician pay close attention when electrolytes are added to the TPN. Precipitation may occur if the wrong sequence or concentrations of electrolytes are added to the bag. Alert the pharmacist if a cloudy film or solid clumping develops when the electrolytes are added. This is more apparent in 2-in-1 TPNs where the lipid component has not been added.

Vitamins are usually administered in a standard formulation of fat and water-soluble vitamins and are often abbreviated as "MVI," for multiple-vitamin infusion. Commercial formulations include vitamins A, D, C, E, B_1, B_2, B_6, and B_{12}, folic acid, pantothenic acid, biotin, and niacin. Vitamin K (phytonadione) is sometimes given separately as an intramuscular injection. However, some institutions add vitamin K to the TPN or use vitamin preparations that contain vitamin K.

Trace elements are required for proper enzymatic reactions and for use of energy sources in the body. Typical elements administered are copper, zinc, chromium, manganese, selenium, iron, and iodine. Commercial products are available that include combinations of trace elements and allow administration of a few milliliters to meet the daily requirements. It is extremely important to note that there are many trace element products and concentrations. Care must be taken to prevent incorrect dosing due to selection of the inappropriate product.

Other additives may be added to TPN preparations for consistency and ease of administration. These include, but are not limited to, octreotide, heparin, insulin, H_2 blockers (such as ranitidine), and iron. As with any additive, stability references should be checked before any admixture is prepared.

Orders for TPN Solutions

Procedures for ordering and dispensing TPN solutions vary and are specific to each institution. Many institutions use a standardized TPN ordering form to make the orders straightforward and consistent, yet patient specific (figure 16–28). Often a specific cutoff time for order changes or new orders is used to maximize efficiency and minimize waste. Since setting up to make just one TPN can be costly, this approach saves time and money by allowing multiple bags to be prepared consecutively.

TPN solutions are ordered specifically to meet a patient's metabolic and nutritional needs. These solutions are usually administered by means of a pump to maximize safety.

An order for a central TPN solution might look like this:

Dextrose	250 g
Amino acids	42.5 g
Sodium chloride	60 mEq
Potassium chloride	40 mEq
Potassium phosphate	20 mEq
Calcium gluconate	1 g
Magnesium sulfate	1 g
Trace elements	2 mL
MVI	10 mL
Total volume	1000 mL

Infuse at 100 mL per hour.

Also give: Vitamin K 10 mg intramuscularly (IM) every week, 10% fat emulsion 500 mL intravenously three times per week.

ADULT TPN/PPN PHYSICIAN ORDERS

NOTE: All TPN orders (formula and rate) must be received in the Central Pharmacy by 12 Noon to be activated the same day. Orders received after 12 Noon will be activated the following day. A bag containing 24 hours of TPN will be sent.The adult hang time is 9 p.m.

DO NOT THIN FROM CURRENT CHART

Time Processed

Clerk's Initials

1. SELECT ONE:	☐ REGULAR FORMULA	☐ LOW K FORMULA	☐ NO K FORMULA	☐ LOW ACET HIGH Cl	☐ LOW Na FORMULA	☐ PERIPHERAL FORMULA	☐ SPECIAL FORMULA
AMINO ACIDS	6%	6%	6%	6%	6%	3%	*
DEXTROSE	☐ 15% ☐ 25%	☐ 15% ☐ 25%	☐ 15% ☐ 25%	☐ 15% ☐ 25%	☐ 15% ☐ 25%	10%	+
SODIUM -mEq/L	45	45	45	45	20	45	
POTASSIUM-mEq/L	40.5	20	0	40	40.5	40.5	
CHLORIDE -mEq/L	57.5	59	69	89	44	57.5	XXX
ACETATE -mEq/L	92.8	81.7	52.2	52.2	72.6	66.8	XXX
CALCIUM - mEq/L	5	4.5	5	5	5	5	
MAGNESIUM - mEq/L	8	5	0	8	8	8	
PHOSPHORUS -mM/L	15	7.5	0	15	15	15	

* Other Amino Acid Concentrations Available -- 3% (Renal), 4.25% + Other Dextrose Concentration Available – 35%

2. RATE: 25 ml/hour for 8 hours, then 50 ml/hour for 8 hours, then ____ ml/hour for 8 hours, to a final rate of____ml/hour.
   Note: All solutions containing > 3% amino acids or > 10% dextrose must be given through a central line.
3. **Vitamins** (10 ml) and **trace elements** (5 ml) are added to TPN daily, unless otherwise ordered.
4. **Vitamin** K 10 mg is added to TPN every Monday, unless otherwise ordered.
5. (optional) **Regular Insulin Human** ____________ units/**liter** of TPN.
6. (optional) **Cimetidine**__________mg/**bag** of TPN.
7. **FAT EMULSION:** Infuse over 12 hours.

☐ 20% 250 ml. ☐ Every day
☐ 20% 500 ml. ☐ Every _________

ORDERS

1. STAT portable chest x-ray to verify central line placement, if not previously obtained. Infuse D5W at 20 cc/hr through central line until placement verified.
2. Label TPN catheter. On multi-lumen catheters, white port is designated for TPN. Do not draw blood, take CVP readings, or administer other fluid or drugs through TPN catheter/port.
3. Strict I&O's every 8 hours. Weigh ICU patients three times a week and floor patients weekly.
4. Hang fat emulsion at 0900; hang TPN at 2100. Discard unused portion of TPN.
5. Notify primary service, before hanging first bag of TPN, if blood sugar is >250 mg/dl or if phosphorus is<2.0 mM/dl.
6. Once TPN is hung, do not increase rate if blood sugar is >250 mg/dl.
7. Change TPN and fat emulsion administration sets every 24 hours.
8. Change central line dressing for TPN catheter every 96 hours or as needed per nursing policy (NS-21).
9. LABS: a. Astra-9, Magnesium, Hitachi, Ionized Ca, PT/PTT, CBC with diff with initiation of TPN, then every Monday and Thursday.
   b. Fasting triglyceride before first bottle of fat emulsion hung, then every Monday. (Draw at least 6 hours after fat emulsion infusion completed.)
   c. Obtain 24 hour urine for urea nitrogen (UNU) and creatinine (UCr) on first day of TPN, then every Monday (from 0600 - 0600).
10. Indirect Calorimetry per Nutrition Support Service
11. Finger stick for glucose every 6 hours. Follow designated sliding scale using regular insulin subcutaneously.

A.		OR	B.	
200-249 mg%	5 u		200-249 mg%	______ u
250-299 mg%	10 u		250-299 mg%	______ u
300-349 mg%	15 u		300-349 mg%	______ u
350-399 mg%	20 u		350-399 mg%	______ u
400 mg%	Call MD		400 mg%	Call MD

Supervising Physician Signature:______________________________

Physician Signature :_______________________ Physician Name Printed:_______________________

Beeper #:_________ Date:____________ Time:____________

WHITE-Chart CANARY-Pharmacy PINK-Nursing

Figure 16–28. Example of a TPN order form.

Here is an example of an order for a 3-in-1 central TPN solution:

Dextrose	250 g
Amino acids	85 g
Fat emulsion	50 g
Sodium chloride	80 mEq
Potassium chloride	60 mEq
Potassium phosphate	60 mEq
Calcium gluconate	1 g
Magnesium sulfate	1 g
Trace elements	2 mL
MVI	5 mL
Total volume	2000 mL

Infuse over twenty-four hours. Give vitamin K 10 mg IM every week.

Preparation of TPN Solutions

Preparation of TPN solutions has changed considerably in the past ten to fifteen years. In the past, many of the components required preparation from nonsterile powders. Today, most TPN ingredients are available as sterile solutions, reducing the need for extemporaneous preparation. Most TPNs are made by gravity fill or by means of an automated compounding device.[8]

Gravity Fill

Gravity fill involves equipment that is normally part of an IV program. As the name implies, gravity is used to transfer the base components (dextrose and amino acids plus IV fat emulsion in a 3-in-1 solution) into the final container. The disadvantages of this method are that it limits flexibility in the volumes of base components used, it takes longer than automated methods, and volumes cannot usually be measured accurately. There are two gravity methods of filling bags, the empty bag method and the underfill method.

The empty bag method involves starting with an empty sterile bag that will be used as the final container. Commercially available bags for this purpose have leads that can be connected to bottles or bags of the base components. The desired amounts flow into the empty bag by gravity. This method can be used for either traditional or 3-in-1 preparations.

The underfill method uses commercially available underfilled bags or partial fills, which are partially filled with concentrated dextrose solution. A bottle of amino acids is connected to the underfilled bag by a tubing set and infused into the partially filled bag to make the final mixture.

With either method, other components are added by drawing each up into a syringe and injecting them through an injection port into the final container. This step is usually the final step before labeling and dispensing. Great care must be taken, both in technique and accuracy, since the potential for errors is high and their ramifications are serious. Each additive must be added in the correct amount; if even one is incorrect, the entire solution for that patient must be remade, and the solution made in error is likely to be wasted. Each step must be checked by the pharmacist. To prevent waste, some institutions require that the pharmacist check the calculations and amounts of additives in syringes before they are added to the bag.

Automated Compounding

Automated compounding involves the use of specialized equipment to prepare the TPN solution. There are two primary versions of TPN compounders available. One version provides a separate compounder for the base solutions and the electrolytes while the other version uses one compounder to infuse all the compounded ingredients (bases and electrolytes). In the former, three primary pieces of equipment are used, sometimes together and sometimes individually. An automated compounder prepares the base components dextrose, amino acids, and possibly fat emulsion and water; a second automated compounder adds most or all of the additives or other components; and a computer with software maintains the orders for the ingredients and controls the two compounders (figure 16–29).

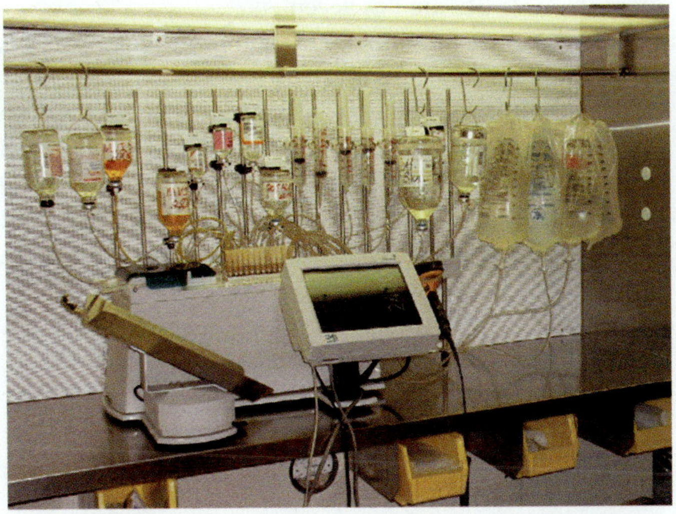

Figure 16–29. Example of the components of an automated TPN preparation device. The devices are (from L to R): The base nutrient compounder control and pump modules, micronutrient compounder, and computer for programming both compounders.

The base compounder uses special tubing that can withstand the pumping action of the machine in allocating large volumes of solutions. It accounts for the specific gravity of the solutions being used and actually weighs the amount pumped into the final container. Some compounders also weigh the original container from which solutions are pumped. It stops pumping when the selected amount has been added. The base compounder can be used with the computer, or it can be used alone. When the base compounder is used alone, the operator enters the desired volume and specific gravity of the base solution components. The device weighs the correct amounts as described above. In the latter, the compounder provides both the base solutions and the additives.

The additives compounder also uses special tubing that delivers exact amounts of the solutions in very small quantities. It weighs the solutions to ensure proper volumes and flushes the line between injections to avoid incompatibility problems. The additives compounder must be used with the computer and cannot be programmed alone.

The computer software controls the system and offers many safeguards. It performs many of the calculations that would otherwise be done by hand and prone to human error, it allows the user to enter maximum safe quantities for different components, and it alerts the user to potential entry errors and inappropriate orders. Alarms are available to detect free-flowing ingredients and air bubbles in the line. The final products are subsequently checked by comparing the anticipated weight of the product against the actual weight of the product. Variances of more than +/– 3% are not accepted.

The accuracy provided by the automated compounders can't totally substitute for all checks and balances in ensuring quality of the product. Checks and balances must be built into each step of the TPN ordering, preparation, and administration process. Calculations should be verified and double-checked, and solutions and their ingredients should be checked and double-checked, regardless of the system used. The many additives that go into a TPN solution make it complicated with respect to compatibility and stability. For example, certain concentrations of electrolytes (e.g., calcium and phosphate) will precipitate when put together and warrant that all solutions be inspected carefully before they are dispensed. For this reason, software programs are designed to analyze key components of the order for potential incompatibilities. Admixture references should also be used before a solution is mixed.

Automated compounders are used inside the LAFW and must be cleaned daily according to the manufacturer's instructions. These systems require routine maintenance and calibration to ensure accurate compounding. To minimize the potential for errors, the compounders should be observed during operation. Quality control procedures may be implemented to verify final contents of the product. These systems are occasionally used for compounding other solutions. Great care should be taken to avoid compounding errors.

Administration

Most TPN solutions are made for administration through a central line (see the Basic Continuous Intravenous Therapy section). This route is used because it results in immediate dilution of the solution being administered, and therefore a very concentrated solution can be administered. Administering a concentrated solution often allows an adult patient to receive their daily nutritional needs with 2000 to 3000 mL of TPN solution.

Occasionally, parenteral nutrition is administered through a peripheral IV line. Peripheral parenteral nutrition (PPN) contains many of the same components as TPN. However, to be administered peripherally, the PPN admixture can't be as concentrated (or have as high of an osmolarity) as TPN. Since these solutions are more dilute, they may not meet all the patient's nutritional needs; that is, they are not "total" nutrition. Consequently, they are often used as either nutritional supplementation or for short-term nutritional intake.

Pediatric Parenteral Drug Administration

Pediatric patients receive many of the same products as adults, including intermittent medications, continuous infusions, chemotherapy, TPN, and analgesics. The unique aspect of this group of patients, of course, is that doses and solutions are much more individualized to meet their specific needs. Standardization of doses is not as common in pediatric patients as it is in adults. Doses are usually calculated based on patients' body weight, resulting in much smaller doses compared to adults. The volume of solution, too, is limited since their blood volume is considerably less than that of an adult.

Intermittent doses are usually given by syringe through a volume control chamber or by using a syringe pump. These systems are used to maximize the accuracy of administration and minimize the amount of fluid given along with the dose of medication. Calculations should be checked and double-checked for these dilutions. A decimal point error could result in a ten-fold overdose or underdose of the drug, which could be significant, especially in a pediatric patient.

Epidural Administration

Epidural administration of drugs involves placing a special catheter into the epidural space of the spine. Some anesthetics, analgesics, and anti-inflammatories are injected into the epidural space to act on the nerve endings and provide the patient with pain relief. The placement of the catheter is a very delicate procedure and is typically performed by an anesthesiologist or a neurosurgeon. Because the drug is injected at the nerve ending, the dose needed for pain relief is greatly reduced as are many of the side effects (e.g. respiratory depression).[9]

Preparing parenterals for epidural administration requires the same aseptic technique as other parenteral products. Good technique is of utmost importance with these products since an infection in the epidural space could be life threatening. Most epidurals must be prepared by the pharmacy and dispensed in syringes or special reservoirs designed to be used with special pumps. All solutions given epidurally must be free of preservatives, meaning that the drug can't be obtained from a multi-dose vial, to prevent toxicity in the spinal column. Dosage calculations should be checked and double-checked. The doses needed are very small, and an error resulting in an inadvertent overdose could have severe consequences.

Epidural patient controlled analgesia. The most common use of epidural analgesia is the administration of a loading dose to initiate pain control, followed by subsequent doses as needed and administered via a PCA pump. This method is very effective in attaining the benefits of both epidural analgesia and PCA. Pump programming is similar to that for IV PCA with doses appropriate for the epidural route.

Continuous infusions. Continuous infusions of epidural analgesics are given with a device that delivers solution at a controlled rate per hour through the epidural catheter.

Bolus injections. Bolus epidural injections of analgesics are often used to initiate therapy or when short-term therapy is required. Bolus dosing may be sufficient to control pain without the use of a pump or continuous infusion device.

Admixture Programs

Many of the practices described in this chapter are elements of an overall pharmacy-coordinated IV admixture program. The need for such well-developed programs is reinforced whenever there is a report of a patient who is harmed by an improperly prepared parenteral product. In almost all of the cases reported, the proper equipment was not used, the ingredients were not correct, personnel preparing the product where not properly trained, or some other preventable reason led to the unfortunate outcome. Although an admixture program does not guarantee that problems will not occur, it does minimize risk to the patient by considering all factors that could potentially cause problems. The true benefit of a formal IV admixture program is that if it is well designed and managed, the whole will be greater than the sum of the parts. That is, each element alone will improve the quality of the products prepared, but with all the components working in concert, the improvement in quality will be even greater. This provides for the best possible outcome for the patient.

All IV admixture programs should comply with USP 797 first and foremost, OSHA regulations of safe practice as well as ASHP Technical Assistance Bulletins and guidelines.[6,7,12]

Components of a Program

The basic components of a formal IV admixture program are listed below. The need or presence of some components will depend on the scope of services provided and the type of patients served. For example, the structure of a program meeting the needs of a 100-bed hospital will differ from that of a home care pharmacy or a large teaching hospital. Each basic component is described below, along with how they are superior to a system that does not utilize a formal program.

Policies and Procedures

Written policies and procedures that are detailed and comprehensive serve as an important part of the foundation for an IV admixture program.[10] The policy portion of the document serves as a basis for decision making, while the procedure portion serves as a description of how the task or function should be carried out.

Space

A coordinated program ideally has a space appropriate for the preparation of sterile products. Standards developed by ASHP and USP describe the desirable room layout, wall, floor, and ceiling surfaces, air quality, cleanliness, maintenance, housekeeping, and processing areas needed as part of a formal program.[11] In many cases, an admixture service is operated from a room that is smaller than ideal; therefore, the space must be well planned for movement of people, LAFW requirements, and flow of patient orders.[4] The heating and cooling requirements of the room need to be properly assessed. The combination of people in the room and the heat generated by the LAFWs can result in an uncomfortably warm environment. If possible, the room should be on its own cooling unit rather than part of a zone in the building. This will allow the room to be cooled without affecting other areas unnecessarily. The area should be well lit and located in a low-traffic area. The floors, walls, and ceiling should have smooth surfaces that cannot easily harbor bacteria and can readily be cleaned and disinfected. Items like cardboard boxes can produce particulates when handled and therefore should not be brought into the IV preparation area. It is ideal to have easily cleaned, moveable supply carts that can be removed from the room for restocking. A room that is clean, organized, and structured within these guidelines will be the safest and most efficient for preparation of sterile products within the hospital.

Training

Pharmacists and technicians who work with sterile products and prepare them on a daily basis should be knowledgeable about the process.[4] Pharmacy technicians who work with these products should be trained to understand basic aseptic technique (including handling supplies, hand washing, garb, etc.), sources of contamination, how to work within a LAFW, how to prepare standard types of parenteral products, and how to prepare non-standard types of preparations as needed. Technicians should demonstrate competency after learning from written training materials, videotapes, and hands-on demonstrations. They should not only demonstrate proper technique, but also have a sample product tested for sterility and accuracy.

Equipment

Selection and maintenance of proper equipment is important in any function, but especially important when it is relied upon to provide a clean work environment for sterile product preparation (such as with an LAFW). LAFWs should be cleaned before use, HEPA filters should be inspected every six months and have their prefilters changed regularly. Compounding equipment (such as syringe pumps used in compounding and automated TPN compounders) should be inspected, calibrated, and maintained according to manufacturers' recommendations. Temperature control equipment, such as refrigerators and freezers, should be monitored for temperature and be equipped with an alarm that sounds when the temperature is outside USP guidelines. All equipment (including tables, chairs, etc.) should be made of materials that are easily cleaned and disinfected (e.g., laminate or stainless steel). All equipment maintenance should be maintained on a schedule and documented.[11] Older recommendations stated that printers be located outside the IV room due to the dust generated from the impact of the printing mechanism. With new thermal and laser printers, this is less absolute. It is recommended that sinks not be located in the IV room due to the microbial growth that they create.

Computers are used for a number of functions related to TPN production, including maintaining patient profiles, generating labels, screening for incompatibilities and duplicate orders, accessing patient information (e.g., labs or diagnosis), charging, and maintaining records.[4]

Standard and Non-Standard Preparations

An IV admixture program makes many different types of products, both standard (routine) and non-standard. Using the expertise of those who work in such an environment can assure that both types receive the same attention and care needed. Non-standard preparations present challenges and, since they are often unusual, may result in errors when made by persons not familiar with them. The use of a coordinated program, references, procedures, and general knowledge will reduce the likelihood of one of these products being prepared incorrectly. Such a program also promotes consistency in preparation and labeling.

Labeling

Countless medication errors can be attributed to poor labeling of medications. An important benefit of a pharmacy IV admixture program is that it allows for consistent, complete labeling of products prepared.[11] The labeling formats must be clear and consistent.

Handling

Order flow and delivery are standardized in a formal IV program. This allows for proper storage (e.g. temperature control, etc.), retrieval of unused preparations (for potential reuse) and delivery of products. This effort improves the product integrity and reduces waste by promoting use of products before they pass their expiration date.[11]

Quality Assurance

Having all sterile products prepared in one department (and often in one area) aids in the development of a coordinated, meaningful quality assurance program. In large institutions requiring compounding of sterile products at satellite sites, a standardized quality assurance program is recommended. Attempting to monitor and evaluate the quality of sterile products that are being prepared in numerous locations throughout a hospital or other setting would be difficult and inefficient without the use of common guidelines.

Quality Assurance Program. All IV admixture programs should have a quality assurance program to ensure that products and services are of desired quality. ASHP's *Technical Assistance Bulletin on Quality Assurance for Pharmacy-Prepared Sterile Products*[12] provides recommendations for preparation, expiration dating, labeling, facilities, equipment, personnel education, training, evaluation, and end-product testing. Some common methods of ensuring quality include air sample testing in the IV room and sampling of end products by the lab using pyrogen testing, flame testing, or tests for microbial contamination.

Revisions to USP introduced in 2008 provide detailed recommendations for the development and implementation of quality assurance programs in intravenous admixture programs. Refer to USP Chapter 797, "Pharmaceutical Compounding—Sterile Preparations" for a full description of recommendations and regulations regarding IV admixture programs.[6]

USP Chapter 797 describes three different levels of risk for products. USP Chapter 797 also defines a fourth class, immediate-use CSPs. Products are classified into one of three risk levels based on how they are prepared, how long they can be stored, whether they are prepared for a single patient or as part of a batch, and whether they are from a sterile or non-sterile source.

Pharmacists are likely to be held responsible for ensuring compliance with the guidelines and other standards of practice, but technicians' work habits and activities will be affected as well. Areas of USP 797 that affect the technician include training, policies and procedures, garb, aseptic technique, process validation, and end-product evaluation. The first four areas are covered in other sections of this chapter, but process validation and end-product evaluation require further explanation.

Process Validation. Process validation means procedures that ensure that the processes used in sterile product preparation consistently result in sterile products of acceptable quality. For most aseptic processes, validation is actually a method for evaluating the aseptic technique of personnel. Validation may be accomplished through process simulation. Process simulation is carried out just like a normal sterile product preparation process except that a microbial growth medium is substituted for the products that would normally be used. Once the sterile product is prepared, the growth medium is incubated and evaluated for microbial growth over a period of time. No microbial growth indicates that the person performing the preparation did not contaminate the product. Individuals should complete a process validation program before being allowed to prepare sterile products, and technique should be re-evaluated regularly.

End-Product Evaluation. End-product evaluation is the final inspection made by the pharmacist before the product is allowed to leave the pharmacy. It includes an inspection for leaks, cloudiness, particulate matter, color, solution volume, and container integrity. In some instances, the growth medium fill procedure, described above, should be supplemented with a program of end-product sterility testing, and a method of recalling products not meeting specifications should be in place. The pharmacist also verifies compounding accuracy with respect to the correct ingredients and quantities. This check of the technician's work is an important step in ensuring that only quality products are sent for patient use.

Summary

Aseptic technique, along with its application to different dispensing and administration systems and dosage types requires special training and practice. This chapter has explained the basics of this technique and described the necessary procedures for compounding sterile preparations and preparing parenteral products. There are potential risks of parenteral therapy, and it is important to remember that using the proper techniques and applying appropriate caution when preparing these products is critical for patient safety. Pharmacy technicians play a key role in this process.

Self-Assessment Questions

1. Intravenous drug therapy is used
   a. when the patient is unable to take needed medications by mouth
   b. when a drug is not needed emergently
   c. when a drug is well absorbed in the stomach
   d. when the patient is afraid of needles
2. Parenteral drug products should
   a. contain pyrogens
   b. be non-sterile
   c. be free of particulate matter
   d. be cloudy
3. In a typical IV setup, an LVP is attached to a primary set that is then attached to the catheter and inserted into the patient. Drugs injected via IV push intermittently are usually given
   a. through another IV line (not through the one used for the LVP)
   b. through a Y-site injection port or flashball on the primary set
   c. by adding them to the LVP solution
   d. continuously through the same IV line as the LVP
4. Large volume parenteral solution containers with potent drugs that need to be infused with a high degree of accuracy and precision are usually administered with the aid of a
   a. roller clamp
   b. electronic infusion device
   c. these solutions are not given IV
   d. LAFW
5. The space between the HEPA filter and the sterile product being prepared is referred to as the
   a. hot spot
   b. backwash zone
   c. zone of turbulence
   d. critical area
6. All manipulations inside a LAFW should be performed at least ______ inches inside the hood to prevent _________ .
   a. twelve inches; smoke
   b. six inches; backwash
   c. ten inches; contamination
   d. two inches; breakage from falling on the floor.
7. Before working in the LAFW
   a. interior surfaces should be wiped with 70% isopropyl alcohol.
   b. the hood should be operated for at least sixty minutes.
   c. hands don't need to be washed since gloves are worn.
   d. interior surfaces should be wiped down with soap and water.
8. Items inside a LAFW should be placed away from other objects and the walls of the hood to prevent
   a. zones of turbulence
   b. dead spaces
   c. windows of contamination
   d. laminar air
9. It is permissible to touch any part of the syringe while making sterile products as long as you are wearing sterile gloves.
   a. True
   b. False
10. A 30 mL syringe with 1 mL calibrations on its barrel can be used to accurately measure 15.5 mL of a solution for injection.
    a. True
    b. False
11. To assure sterility of a new needle
    a. the user should make sure the package was intact and not damaged
    b. wipe the needle with 70% isopropyl alcohol to disinfect it
    c. apply additional silicone so the needle self-sterilizes upon insertion into a vial
    d. only touch the needle while wearing gloves
12. To prevent core formation when entering a vial diaphragm:
    a. only small needles should be used
    b. needles should be inserted quickly before a core is formed
    c. the needle should be inserted with the bevel tip first, then pressing downward and toward the bevel so the bevel tip and heel enter at the same point
    d. the needle should be inserted straight into the vial diaphragm

Self-Assessment Questions

13. Ampules differ from vials in that they
    a. are closed systems
    b. require the use of a filter needle
    c. can be opened without risk of breakage
    d. ampules do not differ from vials
14. Prior to compounding a product for parenteral administration, one should do all of the following *except:*
    a. gather all needed supplies
    b. gather supplies anticipated for the entire shift and place them into the LAFW
    c. inspect all materials for signs they might be defective
    d. disinfect injection sites before entry
15. Labels for IV products
    a. should be handwritten to show personal touch
    b. should not include anything but the drug name and the patient's name, so the patient doesn't become alarmed when reading the label
    c. should be in a format that is consistent and easily understood
    d. are not necessary if the nurse knows what's in the IV
16. Preservatives in parenteral products
    a. kill organisms and therefore eliminate the need for aseptic technique and LAFWs
    b. are harmless and non-toxic in any amount
    c. are present in multi-dose vials
    d. should be used in epidural dosage forms to assure sterility
17. An IV system that uses a threaded drug vial that is screwed into a corresponding receptacle on an IV bag is called
    a. Drug-o-matic
    b. piggyback vial
    c. Add-Vantage®
    d. LVP
18. Buretrol is a common name for a
    a. piggyback system
    b. Add-Vantage®
    c. Volume Control Chamber
    d. small volume parenteral
19. Chronic contact with cytotoxic drugs has the potential to cause
    a. a latex allergy
    b. a positive test for tuberculosis
    c. nightmares
    d. possible chromosome damage, impaired fertility, or cancer
20. Protective apparel for those preparing cytotoxic or hazardous injections in a BSC includes
    a. a low permeability, solid front gown with tight fitting elastic cuffs and latex gloves
    b. a helmet
    c. a self-contained respirator
    d. scrubs
21. After a cytotoxic agent is prepared in the pharmacy, delivery
    a. should be done immediately
    b. can be done by anyone in the pharmacy
    c. can be expedited with systems like pneumatic tubes
    d. includes making the transporter aware of what they are carrying and what the procedure would be in the event of a spill
22. Contents of a "Chemo Spill Kit" include each of the following *except:*
    a. gloves
    b. goggles
    c. a loudspeaker
    d. disposable gown
23. Electrolytes are added to TPN solutions to meet metabolic needs and correct deficiencies. Examples include:
    a. amino acids
    b. potassium chloride
    c. vitamin D
    d. lipid emulsions
24. Lipid or fat emulsions are typically administered by all of the following methods *except:*
    a. as a 10% emulsion given IV through a peripheral line
    b. as a 20% emulsion given IV through a peripheral line
    c. as part of a 3-in-1 TPN solution
    d. IV push

Self-Assessment Questions

25. Dextrose is the base component of TPN solutions most commonly given as a source of carbohydrates. Which of the following statements are true?
    a. It is available as a 5% solution that is commonly used in TPN solutions.
    b. It is available in a concentrated form (50% or more) that is diluted in the final TPN solution to approximately 25%.
    c. It is available as a 70% solution that is commonly given as a separate infusion for calories and energy.
    d. It doesn't matter what the dextrose concentration is when it is given into a peripheral vein.
26. Which of the following is FALSE concerning the gravity fill method of preparing TPN solutions?
    a. The final solution can be either a traditional formulation (amino acids and dextrose as the base) or a 3-in-1 solution (with amino acids, dextrose and fats as the base).
    b. It involves using an empty bag/bottle or using an underfilled container as the final container.
    c. It involves pumping ingredients into the final container; "gravity" really refers to the administration process for these solutions.
    d. It involves numerous checks in the system since so many additives are being measured and injected, leaving a greater potential for error.
27. Automated compounding of TPN solutions
    a. eliminates the need for a pharmacist to double check TPN solutions
    b. may use a device that accurately measures small quantities of electrolytes and injects them into the final container
    c. still requires a technician to manually operate the compounding device
    d. doesn't require the use of aseptic technique in a LAFW since it is automated
28. TPN solutions are typically given through a
    a. central IV line
    b. hand vein
    c. piggyback system
    d. syringe
29. Policies and procedures for a formal IV program typically include all of the following *except:*
    a. personnel training guidelines
    b. quality assurance for the area
    c. environmental monitoring procedures
    d. names of staff working in the area
30. Space and facilities used for sterile product preparation
    a. should be set up to meet recommendations of ASHP and USP
    b. can be anywhere as long as it is within the pharmacy
    c. should be carpeted to minimize noise disturbances
    d. should have a good breeze to keep workers cool

Self-Assessment Answers

1. a. Intravenous drug therapy offers some benefits in drug delivery since it provides rapid blood levels of the medication and since many drugs are not stable or absorbed in the stomach. On the other hand, there are risks associated with parenteral therapy since it is being injected directly into the body. Parenteral therapy is more expensive than oral therapy due to the need for sterility and special equipment. Therefore, the oral route should be attempted first and if not possible then the parenteral route may be used.
2. c. A basic premise required for the safe administration of any parenteral drug is that it be sterile (free of living microorganisms), free of particulate matter (undesirable particles), and free of pyrogens (by-products of organisms that cause fever, chills, and low blood pressure). Many aspects of a good IV admixture program are aimed at producing a product that meets these criteria. Products that do not meet these criteria should not be administered to the patient.
3. b. Intermittent drugs (e.g., antibiotics, anti-ulcer drugs) are often given every six or eight hours through a designated location on the primary set. These locations include Y-sites (shaped like a "Y") or flashball injection sites. The only reason that another site might be required for the administration of these types of drugs would be if they were incompatible with the LVP solution, or if the LVP contained a critical drug that could not be interrupted by the intermittent drug.
4. b. Potent drugs that are adjusted for their effect on the patient must be controlled carefully by the caregiver. Only the use of an electronic infusion device allows this type of control. A roller clamp does control the rate of flow, but only allows the approximate rate of flow and can easily be affected by the movement of the patient.
5. d. A key principle in the use of a LAFW is that nothing passes between the HEPA filter, which is blowing highly purified air and the product being prepared. This area has been termed the "critical area" because of its importance.
6. b. Care must be taken so that manipulations are done well inside the hood (at least six inches) to prevent backwash (i.e., unfiltered room air entering the work surface). Air movement is minimal by the time it reaches the outside of the hood, and any movement or draft could allow room air to move into the hood. By working well inside the hood, this occurrence is minimized. Some users have a tendency to work on the outside edge because it is quieter than working well within the hood, but this obviously eliminates the benefits of using the hood.
7. a. The hood should be operated for about fifteen to thirty minutes so that room air is purged from the work area. The interior surfaces of the hood should be wiped down with 70% isopropyl alcohol to disinfect them. Hands should be washed in bactericidal soap so that bacteria on the hands are minimized.
8. a. Materials placed within the laminar flow workbench disturb the patterned flow of air blowing from the HEPA filter. This zone of turbulence created behind an object could potentially extend outside the hood, pulling or allowing contaminated room air into the aseptic working area (see figure 16–15). When laminar airflow is moving on all sides of an object, the zone of turbulence extends approximately three times the diameter of that object. When laminar airflow is not accessible to an object that is placed adjacent to a vertical wall, a zone of turbulence is created that may extend six times the diameter of the object.
9. b. The barrel of the syringe can be touched and handled, but the syringe tip and plunger should never be touched. Wearing sterile gloves while preparing sterile products does not guarantee sterility since the gloves are no longer sterile once they have touched a non-sterile container or surface.
10. a. Syringes are accurate to one half of the calibrated markings. In this example, that would be one half of one milliliter. Since the needed volume is at that mark, it would be accurate.
11. a. Needles are sterile from the manufacturer as long as the protective overwrap is not damaged. Needles have a silicone lubricant that allows easier penetration into vials. Needles should not be wiped off because it will remove this silicone coating.

12. c. Answer c best describes the special technique that should be used to prevent a core. The other answers describe techniques that would potentially lead to a core.

13. b. Ampules are made of glass and when opened, become an open system (air can pass freely). After they are opened, there could be glass fragments in the solution; therefore, the use of a filter needle is required. Opening ampules can cause injury to the user if not handled carefully. Vials are closed systems, do not have a risk of glass fragments, and therefore do not require the use of a filter needle and do not break on opening.

14. b. Only items needed for the preparation itself should be in the hood. Other items will introduce particulate matter unnecessarily into the work area and will create zones of turbulence, disrupting the effectiveness of the LAFW.

15. c. The label can play a big role in preventing medication errors. As much information as possible should be included on the label, including drug name, strength, hang time, solution, volume, patient name, room number, infusion instructions, frequency of administration, storage requirements, and so forth. This information should be typed or computer generated so that it is readable and should be consistent in format.

16. c. Preservatives are added to retard the growth of microorganisms in multiple dose vials. The presence of these substances should not give a false sense of security that the solution is self-sterilizing, because it is not. Strict aseptic technique is still needed. Also, if doses of drugs are significantly higher than those originally intended, larger volumes of the drug solution are given that result in larger amounts of the preservative being present which might be toxic. Therefore, if preparations involve large amounts of drug solution that contain a preservative or a diluent with a preservative, the pharmacist should be consulted to verify that the total amount of preservative to be administered to the patient will not be toxic. Solutions with preservatives should not be used in preparations for neonates, epidural, or intrathecal dosage forms due to their toxicity.

17. c. An IV system that uses a threaded drug vial that is screwed into a corresponding receptacle on an IV bag is called Add-Vantage®.

18. c. Buretrol is a common name for a Volume Control Chamber.

19. d. Cytotoxic agents require special handling and attention due to their potentially toxic effects. All handlers should be familiar with these special techniques and should be aware of the consequences of improper handling. Potential effects of chronic exposure to one of these agents include possible chromosomal damage, impaired fertility, or cancer.

20. a. Protective apparel is doubly important with cytotoxic agents since you are not only protecting the product from contamination, but also protecting the preparer from exposure. Those handling cytotoxics should wear a non-permeable gown that ties in the back and has some type of tight fitting cuffs. They should also wear latex gloves that are non-powdered. If the gloves have powder on them from the manufacturer, they should be wiped clean with 70% isopropyl alcohol before use. This will prevent the powder from becoming a particulate contaminant. Use of a respirator is not needed when preparing products in a BSC because the hood filters and recycles the air.

21. d. Delivery of cytotoxic agents does not have to occur immediately. Once prepared, the product can receive an expiration date like any other sterile product with consideration for sterility and stability. Special handling and packaging should be used to prevent the container from breaking or leaking while in transit. Mechanical devices such as pneumatic tubes should not be used since they often jar the product, and any leakage or a spill inside a tube system would be very difficult to decontaminate. It is very important that the transporter is aware of what they are carrying and what to do in the event of a spill.

22. c. Chemo spill kits are available commercially or can be compiled with existing pharmacy stock. Spill kits should be assembled containing all the materials needed to clean up hazardous drug spills and protect health care workers and patients. Spill kits should contain the following protective gear: eye protection, a respirator, utility and latex gloves, a disposable gown or coveralls, and shoe covers. They should also contain the equipment needed to clean up the spill: a disposable scoop and a puncture- and leak-resistant plastic container for disposing of glass fragments, absorbent spill pads, gauze and disposable toweling, absorbent powder, and sealable, thick plastic waste disposal bags.

23. b. The electrolytes added to TPN solutions usually include sodium, potassium, chloride, acetate, phosphate, magnesium, and calcium. Electrolytes are usually administered (and calculated) by using a specific salt of the product. For example, sodium is frequently given as sodium chloride. Potassium can be given as potassium chloride, potassium acetate, or potassium phosphate. The patient's clinical condition and laboratory values usually determine the amount and form of electrolytes. The other components listed are commonly in TPN solutions but are not electrolytes.

24. d. Fat emulsions are administered to prevent essential fatty acid deficiency and to provide a source of calories. They are commercially available as 10% or 20% emulsions and are isoosmolar and can be given through a peripheral IV line. Alternatively, fats can be added to the TPN solution. In this case, the fat emulsion is considered a third base component along with dextrose and amino acids, and the TPN is called a 3-in-1 solution or a total nutrient admixture. The 3-in-1 technique offers several nutritional advantages but has certain mixing, stability, and compounding disadvantages.

25. b. Commercially available concentrations vary from 5% to 70%. Usually a 50% or 70% solution is used for TPNs, and the final dextrose concentration in the TPN is usually around 25% for solutions administered via a central vein. The dextrose concentration is significantly less for infusions intended for peripheral administration.

26. c. All of the answers are true except for c. Gravity is used to transfer base solutions into the final container. This process can be slow since the dextrose is very thick in its concentrated form.

27. b. Automated compounding involves the use of specialized equipment to prepare the TPN solution. Three primary pieces of equipment are used, sometimes together and sometimes individually: an automated compounder that prepares the base components, a second automated compounder that adds most or all of the additives or other components, and a computer with software that maintains the orders and controls the two compounders. The base compounder pumps the base components into the final container. The additives compounder also uses special tubing that delivers exact amounts of the solutions in very small quantities. It weighs the solutions to ensure proper volumes and flushes the line between injections to avoid incompatibility problems. The additives compounder must be used with the computer and cannot be programmed alone. The computer and software control the system and offer many safeguards, because they perform many of the calculations that would otherwise be done by hand and be prone to human error. They also allow the user to enter maximum safe quantities for different components and alert the user to potential entry errors and inappropriate orders. The automated compounders are used inside the LAFW and must be cleaned daily according to the manufacturer's instructions.

28. a. Most TPN solutions are made for administration through a central line. This route is used because it results in immediate dilution of the solution being administered, and therefore a very concentrated solution can be administered. This route also allows the medical team to completely meet the adult patient's nutritional needs each day with 2000 to 3000 mL of TPN solution, depending on the weight and needs of the patient. Concerns over the adverse effects of a TPN solution that infuses too quickly require that a pump or other electronic infusion device be used to control its rate of administration.

29. d. Policies and procedures for IV programs typically include sections on personnel training and evaluation, acquisition, storage and handling of supplies, maintenance of the facility and equipment, personnel conduct and dress, product preparation methods, environmental monitoring, process validation, expiration dating practices, labeling guidelines, end product evaluation, housekeeping procedures, quality assurance, and documentation records. Any specific information on individuals would not fall within the purpose of these documents.

30. a. A coordinated program ideally has an appropriate space for the preparation of sterile products. Standards developed by the ASHP and USP describe the desirable room layout, wall/floor/ceiling surfaces, air quality, cleanliness, maintenance, housekeeping, and process areas needed as part of a formal program. While ideal space and facilities are still not available in some institutions, the presence of such a program will serve to show the need for such facilities. In most hospitals, there is no better place to prepare these types of products.

Resources

Achusim LE, et al. Comparison of automated and manual methods of syringe filling. *Am J Hosp Pharm.* 1990;47:2492–2495.

Power L, Jorgensen J. *Safe Handling of Hazardous Drugs DVD and Workbook.* Bethesda, MD: American Society of Health-System Pharmacists, 2006.

American Society of Parenteral and Enteral Nutrition. Safe practices for parenteral nutrition formulations. *JPEN.* 1998;22:49–66.

Brier KL. Evaluating aseptic technique of pharmacy personnel. *Am J Hosp Pharm.* 1983;40:400–403.

Cohen MR. Proper technique for handling parenteral products. *Hosp Pharm.* 1986;21:1106.

Hasegawa GR, editor. Caring about stability and compatibility. *Am J Hosp Pharm.* 1994;51:1533153–4.

Leff RD, Roberts RJ. *Practical Aspects of Intravenous Drug Administration.* 2nd ed. Bethesda, MD: American Society of Hospital Pharmacists; 1992.

McDiarmid MA. Medical surveillance for antineoplastic drug handlers. *Am J Hosp Pharm.* 1990;47:1061106–6.

USP <797> "Pharmaceutical Compounding–Sterile Preparations. *United States Pharmacopeia (USP31).* Rockville, MD: United States Pharmacopeia; 2008.

References

1. Plumer AL. *Principles and Practice of Intravenous Therapy.* Boston, MA: Little, Brown and Co.; 1982.
2. Lindley CM, Deloatch KH. *Infusion Technology Manual: A Self-instructional Approach and Videotape.* Bethesda, MD: American Society of Hospital Pharmacists; 1993.
3. Turco S, King RE. *Sterile Dosage Forms, Their Preparation and Clinical Application.* 4th ed. Philadelphia, PA: Lea & Febiger; 1994.
4. Hunt ML. *Training Manual for Intravenous Admixture Personnel.* 5th ed. Chicago, IL: Pluribus Press; 1995.
5. Compounding Sterile Preparations: ASHP's Video Guide to Chapter <797>. Bethesda, MD: American Society of Health-System Pharmacists; 2009.
6. USP <797>. "Pharmaceutical Compounding–Sterile Preparations. United States Pharmacopeia (USP31). Rockville, MD: United States Pharmacopeia; 2008.
7. American Society of Hospital Pharmacists. Technical assistance bulletin on handling cytotoxic and hazardous drugs. *Am J Hosp Pharm.* 1990;47:1033–1049.
8. Abramowitz PW, Hunt ML, Jr. *Principles and Advantages of Automated Compounding: A Pharmacy Education Guide.* Deerfield, IL: Clintec Nutrition; 1992.
9. Littrell RA: Epidural infusions. *Am J Hosp Pharm.* 1991;48:2460–2474.
10. Hethcox JM. The policy and procedure manual. In: Brown TR, editor. *Handbook of Institutional Pharmacy Practice.* 3rd ed. Bethesda, MD: American Society of Hospital Pharmacists; 1992: 53–62.
11. Buchanan EC., Schneider PJ. *Compounding Sterile Preparations*, 3rd ed. Bethesda, MD: American Society of Health-System Pharmacists; 2009: 174–176, 342–344.
12. American Society of Health-System Pharmacists. ASHP guidelines on quality assurance for pharmacy-prepared sterile products. *Am J Health-Syst Pharm.* 2000;57:1150–1169.

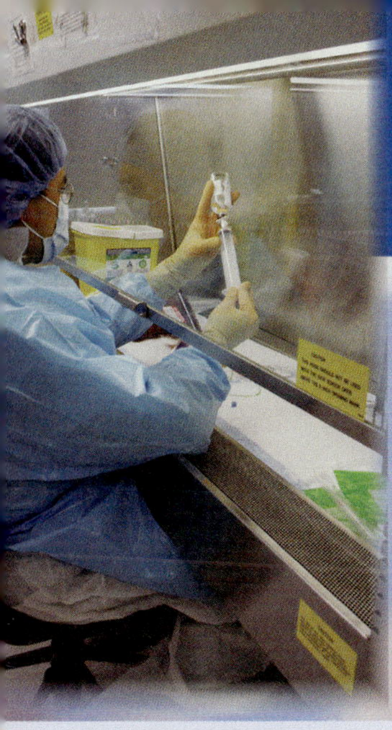

Chapter 17

Medication Errors

Jacqueline Z. Kessler

Learning Outcomes

After completing this chapter you will be able to

- List eleven different types of medication errors.
- Identify causes or factors that contribute to medication errors.
- List five "high alert" medications.
- Describe methods of preventing medication errors from occurring.
- List examples of common medication errors.
- Describe the possible consequences of actual medication errors.
- Explain the steps to be taken when an error has been identified.
- Explain the role of quality assurance monitoring of medication errors.

Key Terms

compliance error An error occurring when patients do not follow their dosing regimen.

deteriorated drug error Use of an expired medication or one whose properties have been compromised.

failure mode and effects analysis (FMEA) A process that evaluates where errors might occur and estimates their potential impact.

high alert medications Medications that have a high risk of causing patient harm when used in error.

improper dose error A dose that is greater than or less than that ordered by the prescriber.

medication error Any error occurring in the medication use process.

medication misadventure A general term to describe drug-related incidents.

monitoring error Failure to review a medication order or associated clinical laboratory values.

omission error A scheduled dose that is omitted entirely.

prescribing error Error occurring during the prescribing process.

root cause analysis (RCA) A process for retrospectively analyzing an error.

unauthorized drug error An error occurring when a drug given to or taken by a patient was not ordered by an authorized prescriber.

wrong administration technique error An error occurring when a medication is given or taken by the wrong route or the use of an improper procedure.

wrong dosage form error Use of the incorrect medication dosage form.

wrong time error Administration of a medication dose outside of an established scheduled time.

Pharmacists are responsible for the safe and appropriate use of medications in all pharmacy practice settings. As part of the multidisciplinary health care team, the pharmacist's role is to establish patient-specific drug therapy regimens designed to achieve predefined therapeutic outcomes without subjecting the patient to undue harm.

As pharmacists become more involved in patient-specific care, technicians are permitted to perform tasks that were previously restricted to pharmacists. As their responsibilities expand, the role of technicians in ensuring medication safety also increases. As a result, they need to be aware of potential causes of medication errors and the significance of their role in preventing those errors.

Numerous terms are used to describe drug-related incidents. The term **medication misadventure** is used to describe adverse drug reactions (unintended responses to drugs used at normal doses), adverse drug events (an injury from a medicine or lack of an intended medicine) and medication errors (errors related to the medication use process that may or may not result in adverse drug outcomes).[1] This chapter focuses on errors that occur during the medication use process, which includes the prescribing, dispensing, and administration phases of medication use; monitoring the patient for expected and unexpected outcomes; and patient compliance.

Types of Medication Errors

Medication errors can occur at any point during the medication use process. They do not occur only in the pharmacy. For example, medication errors can occur when a prescriber writes an order (during the prescribing process), when a nurse transcribes a medication order, when office personnel phone in a prescription to the pharmacy, or when patients do not take their medication as directed (i.e. patient compliance in adhering to the drug regimen).

Pharmacy technicians need to be aware of and concerned with all types of errors, not just those specifically occurring in the pharmacy. It is possible for a pharmacist to miss an error but a technician to notice it. According to the *ASHP Guidelines on Preventing Medication Errors in Hospitals*, medication errors can be categorized into eleven types, including:[2]

- Prescribing Errors
- Omission Errors
- Wrong Time Errors
- Unauthorized Drug Errors
- Improper Dose Errors
- Wrong Dosage Form Errors
- Wrong Drug Preparation Errors
- Wrong Administration Technique Errors
- Deteriorated Drug Errors
- Monitoring Errors
- Compliance Errors

Note that the specific category to which an error belongs is not always obvious because of the complex nature of the medication use process. Errors can occur because of multiple factors, and therefore may fit into several categories.

Prescribing Errors

A **prescribing error** occurs at the time a prescriber orders a drug for a specific patient. Errors can include the selection of an incorrect drug, dose, dosage form, route of administration, length of therapy, or number of doses. Other prescribing errors include inappropriate rate of administration, wrong drug concentration, and inadequate or incorrect instructions for use. When evaluating whether a medication was prescribed in error, it is important to consider patient characteristics, such as allergies, weight, age, medical indication (condition being treated), and concurrent drug therapy, among other factors. For example, a prescription for amoxicillin 250 mg PO TID may be appropriate to treat a middle ear infection in a five-year-old child, but the dose would be too high for a twelve-month-old infant and thus would be considered a prescribing error. Prescriptions that are filled incorrectly because of illegible handwriting are also considered prescribing errors.

Omission Errors

Failure to administer an ordered dose to a patient in a hospital, long-term care facility, or other facility before the next scheduled dose is considered an **omission error**. An omission error occurs when a dose is completely omitted as opposed to administered late. An example would be when a patient forgets to take their morning dose of acarbose (Precose). If a dose is ordered to be held for medical reasons, it is not considered an error. Examples of times when an omitted dose is not an error are when the patient cannot take anything by mouth (NPO) prior to a procedure or when health care providers are waiting for drug level results to be reported. In addition, not administering medications because a patient refuses to take them is not considered an error.

Wrong Time Errors

Timing of administration is critical to the effectiveness of some medications. Maintaining an adequate blood level of some drugs, such as antibiotics, frequently depends on evenly spaced, around-the-clock dosing. Administering doses too early or too late can affect the drug blood level and consequently the efficacy of the drug.

Long-term care facilities and hospitals frequently establish standardized administration times to maintain consistency because it could be harmful to a patient if a daily dose is administered inconsistently. It would, however, not be realistic to expect all morning doses to be administered at, for example, exactly 0800; therefore, an acceptable interval surrounding the scheduled time is usually established. An institution may determine that administering medications within thirty minutes of the scheduled time (thirty minutes before or after) is acceptable. Medications administered outside this window would be considered **wrong time errors**. For example, if an order were written for cefazolin 1g IV to be given within thirty minutes of the beginning of surgery, but the dose is given sixty minutes prior to surgery, a wrong time error would occur. Wrong time errors are occasionally unavoidable because the patient is away from the patient care area for a test or the medication is not available at the time it is due.

Unauthorized Drug Errors

Administration of a medication to a patient without proper authorization by the prescriber is categorized as an **unauthorized drug error**. An unauthorized drug error might occur if a medication for one patient was given mistakenly to another patient or if a nurse gave a medication without a prescriber order. Another cause is when patients "share" prescriptions at home. In some states, refilling a prescription that has no refills remaining without authorization from the prescriber is another example of an unauthorized drug error.

Some health care facilities establish guidelines or protocols that allow flexibility in administering medications on the basis of specific patient parameters. For example, a post-surgical protocol may allow a nurse to administer an infusion of potassium chloride when a patient's blood potassium level falls below a specified level. The dose of potassium chloride may vary depending on how low the blood level is. Administration of a medication outside established guidelines is another example of an unauthorized drug error.

Improper Dose Errors

Improper dose errors occur when a patient is given a dose that is greater or less than the prescribed dose. This type of error can occur when there is a delay in documenting a dose, or absence of documentation, that results in an additional dose being administered. Inaccurate measurement of an oral liquid is also an improper dose error. Excluded from this category are doses that cannot be accurately measured or are not specified, as in topical applications. Variances that occur from apothecary to metric conversions are excluded as well.

Wrong Dosage Form Errors

Doses administered or dispensed in a different form than ordered by the prescriber are classified as **wrong dosage form errors**. Depending on state laws and health care facility guidelines, dosage form changes may be acceptable to accommodate particular patient needs. For example, dispensing a liquid formulation without a specific prescription to a patient who has difficulty swallowing tablets might be an acceptable dosage form change.

Wrong Drug Preparation Errors

Drugs that require reconstitution (adding liquid to dissolve a powdered drug), dilution, or special preparation prior to dispensing or administration are subject to wrong drug preparation errors. Examples include reconstituting an azithromycin oral suspension with an incorrect volume of water, using bacteriostatic saline instead of sterile water to reconstitute a lyophilized powder for injection, and not activating an ADD-Vantage® IV admixture bag. Using the wrong base product when compounding an ointment is another example of a wrong drug preparation error.

Wrong Administration Technique Errors

Doses that are administered using an inappropriate procedure or incorrect technique are categorized as **wrong administration technique errors**. For example, a subcutaneous injection that is given too deep and an intravenous (IV) drug that is allowed to infuse via gravity instead of using an IV pump are classified in this category. Instilling eye drops in the wrong eye is another example of an error in this category.

Deteriorated Drug Errors

Although sometimes cumbersome, monitoring expiration dates of products is very important. Drugs used past their expiration date may have lost potency and may be less effective or ineffective. Refrigerated drugs stored at room temperature may decompose to the point at which their efficacy is less than optimal. Medications that are dispensed or administered beyond their expiration date and medications that have deteriorated because of improper storage are considered to be **deteriorated drug errors**.

Monitoring Errors

Monitoring errors result from inadequate drug therapy review. For example, ordering serum drug levels for a patient taking phenytoin to prevent seizures, but not reviewing them or not responding to a level outside of the therapeutic range is a monitoring error. Not ordering drug levels when required or prescribing an antihypertensive agent, which lowers blood pressure, and failing to check blood pressure are monitoring errors as well.

Compliance Errors

Medication errors are committed by patients when they fail to follow or adhere to a prescribed drug regimen. This is referred to as a **compliance error.** Compliance errors can be detected when a patient requests refills for prescriptions at unreasonable intervals (too long after or too soon before a refill is due) without a reasonable explanation. An example of a compliance error is when a patient taking antibiotics to treat an infection discontinues therapy before all the doses are taken.

Other Errors

Errors that cannot be placed into one of the preceding eleven categories are grouped together in a miscellaneous category. A medication that is dispensed without adequate patient education might be considered an error in this category. For example, a prescription for alendronate (Fosamax) that is dispensed without informing the patient (either verbally, by the use of an auxiliary label, or by the distribution of a medication teaching guide) that they must not lie down for a minimum of thirty minutes after taking their dose would be considered a miscellaneous error.

✔ Some of the errors as defined in the ASHP guidelines seem to apply primarily to patients in health care facilities. These same definitions, however, can be applied to home health care, clinic, and physician office settings, as well as the outpatient pharmacy practice settings.

Incidence

Although medication errors are common, determining their actual numbers is difficult. Few studies provide a complete and thorough evaluation of errors within the entire medication use process. It is difficult to project data from studies on medication errors because of the different methods used to detect errors and the various definitions of errors. In addition, the focus of some studies is on just physician, nursing, or pharmacy errors or just one component of the medication use process.

Medication errors can occur at any point in the medication use process. Millions of doses are administered daily in health care facilities and patient homes, and the volume of prescriptions filled annually in community-based pharmacies, including mail order, is approximately 3.54 billion.[3] On the basis of these estimates alone, it is apparent that even with a high rate of accuracy, a small percentage of errors can result in a large number of medication errors. In addition, the number of new drugs and dosage forms available continues to grow, making it difficult to keep up with new developments in pharmacy. Staying abreast of technological advances and complex medication regimens requires professional commitment.

✔ Medication error awareness and prevention must be a high priority in all health care facilities and pharmacies.

Medication Error Rates

This section describes medication error rates reported in some studies. It provides an overview of the complexity of studying medication errors owing to the different monitoring, measuring, and reporting techniques used. It also reviews differences in the studies that contribute to varying medication error rates reported in the literature.

The Harvard medical practice study that analyzed the incidence of adverse events in hospitalized patients found that 19% of the adverse events that occurred in hospitalized patients were related to drug complications.[4] This study demonstrates that complications from drugs, including those caused by errors, are a significant cause of medical management injuries in hospitalized patients.

Physician prescribing error rates in hospital and community settings have been reported to be 0.3 to 1.9%.[5–7] One study determined that almost one-third (28.3%) of the prescribing errors were potentially harmful if not followed up by a pharmacist.[6] An evaluation of causes of prescribing errors in hospitals found that the majority of potentially serious prescribing errors were made because of performance lapses (knowing the right thing to do, but accidentally doing something else) by the physician or because of failure to adhere to established procedures.[8] Further, it has been observed that errors occurring earlier in the medication use process (in the prescribing phase) are more likely to be detected and corrected than those occurring later in the process (in administration).[9]

Physician prescribing is only the first step in the medication use process. Other studies have evaluated medication errors occurring at other stages. Error rates of pharmacists dispensing in the outpatient setting have been reported to be approximately 12%.[10,11] There are conflicting data evaluating the relationship between the number of serious errors and the number of prescriptions filled.[10,11] The medication error rate in hospitals has been estimated to be one error per patient per day.[12] One study evaluated the number of errors occurring in the drug administration phase in thirty-six hospitals and skilled nursing facilities and found that 19% of all doses were not administered correctly. The majority (43%) of errors were due to wrong time of administration.[13] The Institute of Medicine estimates that approximately 1.5 million people are harmed by medications each year. As many as 400,000 of these adverse events are considered to be preventable.[14]

Medication error studies report different error rates. Pharmacy technicians should recognize that the differences in error rates may be due to differences in how studies were performed, the various techniques and definitions used, and the scope of the study. Many errors are identified and corrected before medications reach the patient and these errors might not be accounted for. Studies also show that a small percentage of errors lead to adverse events in patients.[15]

Medication Error Reporting

The rate of medication errors is often based on incident reports. Ideally, health care providers complete incident reports when a medication error is discovered. That does not always happen, however, because many health care personnel lack the knowledge to identify errors, lack the time to document them, or are afraid of negative consequences.

Many times errors are discovered when a pharmacist checks a prescription or medication order prior to dispensing, and the error is corrected promptly before the medication reaches the patient. Often, the error is not documented because it is not recognized as an error or the reporting process is cumbersome. For these reasons, the number of medication errors is probably higher than reported.

Reporting medication errors can sometimes be a frightening experience. Health care personnel may be afraid of disciplinary or punitive actions or of the backlash of reporting an error made by a coworker. They may also be concerned about liability issues should a negative outcome occur because of an error.

It is apparent that medication errors occur every day in all practice settings. Fortunately, most of these errors are detected and corrected before the medication ever reaches the patient. Some medication errors do, however, reach the patient, and some errors result in negative outcomes.

Impact of Medication Errors

The outcomes of medication errors range from no effect to minor discomfort to devastating long-term disability or death.[16,17] Often, predicting the outcome and significance of a medication error is difficult because so many factors are involved. Such factors include the type of medication error, the health status of the patient, the pharmacologic classification of the drug involved, the route of drug administration, the timing of drug administration, the cost to the health care system, and the damage to the patient's trust in care providers.

Impact on the Patient

In a report of five pediatric patients who received overdoses of vincristine (a chemotherapy drug), three patients died and two recovered.[18] Of the three patients who died, two received a tenfold overdose, and the third was very ill with advanced stage leukemia. The two children who recovered were in remission (i.e., their leukemia was under control) at the time and received smaller overdoses. In this situation, the health status of the patients and magnitude of the overdose helped determine the significance of the error.

Sometimes, not receiving a drug or receiving it late can harm patients as well. Administration of a dose of phenytoin to prevent seizures was delayed twenty-eight hours in an elderly patient, resulting in the patient experiencing a seizure.[19] The patient subsequently underwent extensive surgery to repair a jaw fracture that resulted from a fall during the seizure. These events can be attributed to one medication error—late administration of the phenytoin. Many case reports describe adverse drug events caused by medication errors.

Financial Implications

Not only can medication errors lead to negative patient outcomes, they can prolong hospital stays and increase health care expenses.[20] Treating adverse events is estimated to cost billions of dollars annually.[14,16,21,22] It was estimated that $1.5 million was spent in a single year to treat adverse drug events at one hospital.[21] Another study evaluated the cost of drug-related patient injury and death in the ambulatory setting. That study estimated that the United States spends $76.6 billion annually to manage those drug-related occurrences, some of which were due to medication errors.[22] Not only must the cost of additional medical management be considered, but also the legal fees and out-of-court settlements resulting from malpractice claims.

Medication errors or the use of contaminated drugs that result in patient disability or death are categorized as "never events" by the National Quality Forum, a nonprofit organization represented by numerous health care, consumer advocate, and philanthropic groups. Some states have revised Medicaid reimbursement to include provisions that will not reimburse hospital expenses associated with treating conditions that result from never events.[23]

Loss of Trust

Patients can lose faith in the medical community as a result of experiencing or reading about an adverse drug event. They may choose to switch pharmacies or physicians or even hesitate to seek medical help for fear of not receiving quality care. Patients may also seek nonconventional treatments from outside the medical community. Personnel responsible for medication errors that result in significant patient injury also can lose confidence in themselves as practitioners.

Fortunately, most medication errors are detected and corrected before the medication is dispensed to the patient or the patient care area. Medication errors do occur, however, and can result in reversible or permanent negative patient outcomes. They can also be associated with a financial impact to an individual, an institution, and the overall health care system.

Causes of Medication Errors

Medication errors can be attributed to a number of different causes. It would be unfair to place blame solely on an individual without considering factors that can contribute to an error. Administrators of health systems constantly strive to decrease the presence of factors in the medication use system that contribute to medication errors. In turn, each health care worker must also strive to minimize the occurrence of medication errors. One of the best ways to do this is to become familiar with the most common causes of medication errors. Medication errors are most often attributed to one or more of the following: calculation errors, improper use of zeros and decimal points, inappropriate use of abbreviations, careless prescribing, illegible handwriting, missing information, drug product characteristics, compounding/drug preparation errors, prescription labeling, work environment and personnel issues, and deficiencies in medication use systems.

Calculation Errors

Reports show that numerous medication errors are caused by errors in mathematical calculations. Miscalculation of doses can lead to serious patient harm or even death.[17,24] Calculation errors are made by prescribers, pharmacists checking doses for appropriateness or calculating doses, technicians compounding products, and nurses preparing or administering doses. Even with the use of calculators and computers, health care personnel frequently make calculation errors.[25]

The pediatric population is particularly at risk for calculation errors. It is not uncommon for pediatric doses to be determined by the patient's weight, requiring an interim step to calculate the final dose. Many drugs are not available in pediatric formulations, so adult formulations must be diluted or manipulated multiple times to get the appropriate dose.

Personnel with multiple years of experience are just as likely to make mathematical errors as inexperienced personnel.[26,27] Calculation errors are often made by using the wrong concentration of stock solutions, misplacing a decimal point, or using wrong conversions. Personnel also neglect to double-check their work, or rely on their memory instead of looking up a conversion. In some cases, they fail to ask themselves, "Does the answer seem reasonable?"

Safety First

Always double-check calculations and look up conversions instead of relying on memory. Think about whether the answer makes sense.

Another way to decrease the risk of a calculation error is to ask a pharmacist or another technician to double-check the calculation prior to preparing the product. The calculation should be performed independently and should be compared with the original answer. This system is an effective way to prevent calculation errors. (See Chapter 14, Pharmacy Calculations.)

Decimal Points and Zeros

Misplacing a decimal point by one place results in errors tenfold greater than or less than intended. For drugs with a narrow therapeutic range (e.g., digoxin, phenytoin, warfarin, gentamicin), the consequences can be significant.

Decimal point errors can occur as a result of a miscalculation, as described above, and also when writing orders or instructions. Failure to write a leading zero in front of a number less than one (e.g., .1 mg instead of 0.1 mg) can result in the number being read as a whole number (1 mg). Writing unnecessary trailing zeros can also be confusing (e.g., 10.0 mg instead of 10 mg, which could be misinterpreted as 100 mg). Medication order sheets with lines can sometimes cause a decimal point to be overlooked on the copy that is sent to the pharmacy. Medication orders that are received via fax should be reviewed carefully since artifact (insignificant markings on the page) might cause the order to be misinterpreted.

When writing numbers, a leading zero should always be used with a decimal point for numbers less than one (0.1 mg, not .1 mg) and a decimal point and trailing zero should never be used for whole numbers (10 mg, not 10.0 mg). Technicians must be aware of the potential for decimal point errors due to misplaced or missing decimal points when interpreting orders, and questionable orders should be brought to the attention of the pharmacist.

Rx for Success

A good general rule to follow is to question any dose that requires less than one-half or more than two of the dosage unit (tablet, capsule, teaspoonful). This rule often helps catch calculation errors.

Abbreviations

The abbreviation of medical terms and drug names can lead to medication errors. For example, the use of the abbreviation "AZT" for zidovudine (Retrovir), an antiretroviral agent used to treat HIV infection, could also be interpreted as azathioprine (Imuran), an immunosuppressant agent, which would cause harm to the patient if an error was made.

Another example of an abbreviation error is the use of "U" as an abbreviation for units. This abbreviation could result in a tenfold error if the "U" were read as a "zero" (e.g., 10 U insulin could be read as 100 insulin). A daily order written as "QD" instead of "daily" may be troublesome because it could be read as "QID" (four times a day) or "OD" (every other day).

The Joint Commission has developed a list of dangerous abbreviations and dose designations that should not be used (table 17-1).[28] This "do not use" list applies to physician orders and medication documentation that is handwritten or printed on preprinted order forms. The Institute for Safe Medication Practices (ISMP) has a

Table 17-1. The Joint Commission Official "Do Not Use" List

Do Not Use	Potential Problem	Use Instead
U (unit)	Mistaken for "0" (zero), the number "4" (four) or "cc"	Write "unit"
IU (International Unit)	Mistaken for IV (intravenous) or the number 10 (ten)	Write "International Unit"
Q.D., QD, q.d., qd (daily)	Mistaken for each other	Write "daily"
Q.O.D., QOD, q.o.d, qod (every other day)	Period after the Q mistaken for "I" and the "O" mistaken for "I"	Write "every other day"
Trailing zero (X.0 mg)* Lack of leading zero (.X mg)	Decimal point is missed	Write X mg Write 0.X mg
MS	Can mean morphine sulfate or magnesium sulfate	Write "morphine sulfate" Write "magnesium sulfate"
MSO_4 and $MgSO_4$	Confused for one another	

[1] Applies to all orders and all medication-related documentation that is handwritten (including free-text computer entry) or on preprinted forms.

***Exception:** A "trailing zero" may be used only where required to demonstrate the level of precision of the value being reported, such as for laboratory results, imaging studies that report size of lesions, or catheter/tube sizes. It may not be used in medication orders or other medication-related documentation.

Additional Abbreviations, Acronyms and Symbols (For possible future inclusion in the Official "Do Not Use" List)		
Do Not Use	**Potential Problem**	**Use Instead**
> (greater than) < (less than)	Misinterpreted as the number "7" (seven) or the letter "L" Confused for one another	Write "greater than" Write "less than"
Abbreviations for drug names	Misinterpreted due to similar abbreviations for multiple drugs	Write drug names in full
Apothecary units	Unfamiliar to many practitioners Confused with metric units	Use metric units
@	Mistaken for the number "2" (two)	Write "at"
cc	Mistaken for U (units) when poorly written	Write "mL" or "ml" or "milliliters" (mL is preferred)
µg	Mistaken for mg (milligrams) resulting in one thousand-fold overdose	Write "mcg" or "micrograms"

more extensive list of abbreviations and terms that have been misinterpreted and led to medication errors. This list is available on their website.[29]

There are many accepted abbreviations in health care, and use of abbreviations can be efficient if everyone understands and agrees on the definitions. The Joint Commission's 2009 National Patient Safety Goals include a recommendation that organizations create a list of abbreviations, acronyms, and symbols that should *not* be used.[30] This list should include the terms on the official "do not use" list and any additional terms that the organization feels might contribute to medication errors. Being unaware of the accepted interpretation of abbreviations can lead to errors, and creating new abbreviations that others may not understand should be avoided.[31] ASHP recommends that an approved list of abbreviations be developed by the organization's Pharmacy and Therapeutics Committee or its equivalent.[2] Abbreviations not on the approved list should be reviewed carefully before processing an order.

Rx for Success

Write out directions for medications rather than using nonstandard or ambiguous abbreviations. The complete drug name, preferably the generic, should be used.

Technicians should become familiar with the list of abbreviations approved at their facility. Community pharmacies generally do not have a formal, approved list of abbreviations. Posting a list of commonly accepted medical abbreviations in the pharmacy, however, is beneficial. Technicians should also be familiar with the abbreviations and dose designations that are considered dangerous and pay particular attention to them when filling orders. See Appendix A at the end of this book for a list of medical abbreviations.

High Alert Medications

Several medications or drug classes have been categorized as **high alert medications** because of their high risk of causing serious harm to patients when given in error. Errors with drugs designated as high alert do not necessarily occur more frequently than others. According to the ISMP, the following medications are examples of high alert medications:[32]

1. heparin
2. narcotics and opiates (e.g., morphine, hydromorphone, oxycodone)
3. potassium chloride injection
4. insulin
5. chemotherapeutic agents (e.g., methotrexate, vincristine, doxorubicin)
6. neuromuscular blocking agents (e.g., vecuronium, cisatracurium, succinylcholine)

A complete list of high alert medications and drug classes can be found on the ISMP website.[32]

Pharmacies should evaluate how high alert medications are handled and institute specific error reduction strategies as appropriate. Such strategies might include limiting the number of strengths or vial sizes of medications stocked, use of special auxiliary labeling, strategic storage locations, double-checks, and the use of standardized or preprinted orders.

Rx for Success

Become familiar with medications designated as "high alert" in your organization (e.g., heparin, fentanyl, paralyzing agents) and make sure to follow any extra precautions that have been established specifically for these products.

Prescribing Issues

Medication errors can result from the way a drug is prescribed. Issues associated with the prescribing component of the medication use processes that may contribute to an error include verbal orders, confusion regarding the concentration of a product, illegible handwriting, missing information, use of the apothecary system, and writing doses based on the course of therapy as opposed to a daily dose. This section describes how these prescribing issues can lead to errors, in addition to ways to minimize such errors.

Verbal and Telephone Orders Oral orders (orders given orally by a prescriber) can lead to medication errors when they are heard incorrectly or when they are transcribed to writing or entered into a computer incorrectly.[33] This can occur when an order is orally communicated in a face-to-face situation (verbal order) or when an order is given over the telephone (telephone order). The use of cellular phones and poor quality connections can make telephone orders even more difficult to understand. With the number of similar sounding products available, it is easy to misunderstand an oral order. In one case report, a telephone order from a physician for Prograf (tacrolimus), an immunosuppressant, 10 mg daily was misunderstood by the pharmacist as Prozac (fluoxetine), an antidepressant. As the pharmacist was counseling the patient on the use of fluoxetine, it became apparent that there had been a mix-up.[34]

Verbal or telephone orders should only be used in situations when it is impossible or impractical for the prescriber to write the order or submit it electronically. A written copy of the order should be placed in the pharmacy's prescription file or the patient's medical record. Institutional pharmacies routinely require the prescriber to confirm verbal or telephone orders by signature. The use of oral orders should particularly be avoided in chemotherapy prescribing because of the complexity of these orders and the potentially lethal impact of mistakes with these drugs.

✔The recipient of a verbal or telephone order should immediately write down the order and read it back to the prescriber to ensure clarity of the order.

Although cell phones, unfamiliar terminology, accents, and poor connections can make taking an oral order difficult, it is the responsibility of the technician to ask the other party to clarify parts of the order that are not clear. Simply asking the other party to spell the names of the medications and other words that are unclear and repeating the order back to the other party can help ensure that the right order is received. When reading back numbers that may be easily misunderstood, it is helpful to say each numeral. For example, 50 should be stated as "fifty as in five zero."

✔Many states limit the acceptance of verbal medication orders to registered pharmacists. State law and pharmacy policy should be consulted to determine what role, if any, technicians may play in accepting verbal orders.

Drug Concentration. Failure to include the concentration of a liquid formulation in a prescription can result in a wrong dose being dispensed. For example, an order for amoxicillin suspension 1/2 tsp (2.5 mL) TID does not specify the concentration of the suspension, causing confusion as to the actual dose ordered. It could be interpreted as 62.5 mg (1/2 tsp of 125 mg/5 mL) or 125 mg (1/2 tsp of 250 mg/5 mL).

Writing "1 amp," "1 vial," or "1 cap" can lead to errors when products come in multiple strengths, doses, or vial sizes. An order for one "vial" of magnesium sulfate might be filled with a 2 mL vial (8 mEq), a 20 mL vial (16 mEq), or a 10 mL vial of 50% concentration (40 mEq). The pharmacist should clarify ambiguous doses before the technician processes the order.

Illegible Handwriting. The poor handwriting of physicians frequently is the subject of jokes; however, illegible handwriting of any health care provider is no laughing matter when it contributes to medication errors. With the many sound-alike and look-alike drug names on the market, it is easy to understand how illegible handwriting can lead to errors. One report describes a poorly written order for Aredia (pamidronate), a blood calcium lowering agent, 60 mg IV that was filled and administered as Adria, a commonly spoken term for Adriamycin (doxorubicin), a chemotherapy agent. The patient received approximately 20% of the dose before the error was noticed and experienced bone marrow toxicity (decrease in blood cell counts) as a consequence.[35] Both agents are reasonable medications for a cancer patient and are prescribed in doses of 60 mg, but the poorly written medication name led to the mix-up. Facsimile transmission of handwritten orders can further complicate interpretation of illegible handwriting.

The entire order should be carefully evaluated when trying to decipher illegible handwriting. Sometimes the dose or route of administration is helpful in determining what medication was ordered. Assistance should be obtained from a pharmacist when orders are difficult to interpret because of illegible handwriting. The pharmacist should contact the prescriber to clarify orders that are difficult to interpret. In some practice settings, technicians may play a role in obtaining order clarifications.

Using standardized, preprinted order forms for complex drug regimens is one way to minimize illegible handwriting.[2] Computer generated and typewritten labels reduce medication errors by making the medication labels easier to read for both health care personnel and patients. The use of upper- and lowercase lettering (as opposed to all uppercase) also improves readability.

Missing Information. Lack of complete medical information about the patient, such as age, weight, height, allergies, and diagnosis, can contribute to medication errors. Medical information is important because dose often depends on the indication and severity of the condition. Unfortunately, physicians do not routinely write the indication on prescriptions, and patients do not always fully understand their conditions. In some hospital pharmacies, medical information is available only in the chart because the pharmacy computer system does not interface with the main hospital computer.

Thorough and complete medication profiles should be maintained for all patients. These profiles should include at a minimum, current prescription and nonprescription medications, allergies, age, height, and weight of the patient. Previous medication use is also helpful. Profiles should be kept current and referred to routinely. It may be necessary to question the patient or contact the prescriber to obtain this information, because pharmacists often need it to check for appropriateness. See Chapter 13,

Processing Medication Orders and Prescriptions, for additional information on this topic.

Apothecary System. The apothecary system is an outdated system of measurement that some prescribers continue to use. This system can lead to errors because it is unfamiliar to many health care personnel and must be converted to the metric system. The fact that "1 gr" (grain) may be interpreted as 60 mg or 65 mg is confusing enough, but if it is written sloppily, it could be misread as "1 gm" (1 gram = 1000 mg). Prescribers should be discouraged from using the apothecary system.

Apothecary conversion charts should be readily available in the pharmacy, and technicians should become familiar with commonly used apothecary symbols and their metric equivalents, which are available in Chapter 14, Pharmacy Calculations.

Course Dose vs. Daily Dose. Chemotherapy medication regimens are commonly prescribed on a per course or cycle of treatment basis as opposed to a per dose basis. This practice increases the risk of medication errors because the orders are often difficult to interpret.[36] Many chemotherapy treatments require a patient to receive medication over several days and then rest (receive no medication treatment) for several days or weeks. This allows time for the patient to recover from the side effects and for the medications to work in the optimal phase of the tumor cell cycle. One course of treatment may consist of several medications given on one or more days during a specified time period.

An example of a chemotherapy course dose is fluorouracil 4 g/m^2 IV days one, two, three, and four. This order could be misinterpreted as 4 g/m^2 of fluorouracil daily for four days—a total of 16 g/m^2—or as 4 g/m^2 to be divided into four daily doses (1 g/m^2 daily on days one, two, three, and four). Errors such as this can result in massive overdoses, leading to prolonged illness or death.

Drug Product Characteristics

Characteristics of drug products that can contribute to medication errors include look-alike and sound-alike drug names, the use of numbers or letters as part of the drug name, product labeling, color coding, and advertising.[37] Drug product problems identified by the USP are forwarded to pharmaceutical manufacturers so they can address the problems by making appropriate modifications to the drug products.

Look-Alike and Sound-Alike Drug Names. Many case reports deal with medication errors caused by confusion surrounding drug names.[38–43] Hundreds of drug names either sound or look like other trade or generic drug names. The USP provides an easy to use search tool called USP's Drug Error Finder on their Web site.[44] This search tool contains over 1,400 sound-alike and look-alike medication names that have been identified in error reports. For medication errors that were reported through the USP Reporting Program, the severity of the error is also provided. ISMP also maintains a list of "confused" medication names on their website (see Appendix B).[45]

Sometimes errors occur because medication names look and sound similar and may even be used to treat a common condition. For example, nelfinavir (Viracept) and nevirapine (Viramune) are two antiretroviral agents used in the treatment of HIV infection. Both the brand and the generic names are similar, increasing the risk for confusion.[46] Sloppy handwriting and misspelling also can contribute to drug name confusion. An order carelessly written for interferon, an immunologic agent, 1 mL was interpreted and prepared as Imferon (iron dextran) 1 mL.[38] In this case, the patient's mother questioned the dark brown coloring of the drug before it was administered and the mix-up was corrected before the patient received the wrong drug.

The likelihood of confusing two drugs with similar names is increased when the dosages of both drugs are the same. Lanoxin (digoxin) and Levoxine (levothyroxine) have similar looking and sounding names and both may be prescribed at a dose of 0.125 mg daily.[40] Because of these similarities, the pharmaceutical manufacturer of Levoxine changed the trade name to Levoxyl in an effort to avoid confusion with Lanoxin.

A frequently reported mix-up occurs between quinine, an antimalarial, and quinidine, an antiarrhythmic. The names are similar, routine doses are the same, and they are frequently stocked next to each other. It is easy to see how one medication could be picked instead of the other.

Confusion with sound-alike and look-alike medication names is a growing issue with the increasing number of medication products available. In a review of medication errors associated with look-alike and sound-alike medications reported over a four-year period, the USP found that each of the top ten selling medications in the U.S. have been identified in a look-alike or sound-alike pairing.[47] Pharmaceutical manufacturers are responsible for carefully selecting medication product names, keeping patient safety in mind. Approximately 30% of all new medication names reviewed by the FDA are rejected because they may lead to confusion.[48] Table 17-2 lists examples of medication names that were changed to reduce the risk of prescribing errors. Health care providers can help identify potentially confusing drug names by notifying the USP or FDA with their concerns.

Numbers and Letters as Part of Medication Names. Manufacturers sometimes include numbers and letters as prefixes and suffixes to brand names (e.g., Tylenol #3, Percocet-5, Effexor-XR). Although the intent may be to indicate strength or that a product is an extended release formulation, it can lead to errors. One case of such an error reported in the literature describes an ice pack applied to the chest of a patient hospitalized with pneumonia instead of administration of the antibiotic azithromycin. The physician wrote for a "Z-Pak," commonly prescribed this way on outpatient prescriptions. The specific dosage regimen was not written out because the product is available as a blister pack containing the entire course of therapy and is labeled with dosing instructions. The patient's pneumonia worsened until the error was discovered two days later and appropriate treatment was initiated.[49]

Numbers in the medication name can be misinterpreted as the dose. For example, the prescription in figure 17-1 could be misinterpreted to take five tablets of Percocet every four hours as needed instead of one tablet of Percocet-5 every four hours as needed. A patient could become extremely drowsy or confused after taking five tablets of Percocet-5.

Letters or numbers that are omitted from brand names when writing an order can contribute to errors. For example, the immediate release form of venlafaxine (Effexor) could be dispensed instead of the extended release formulation because the "XR" part of the name was omitted in the prescription shown in figure 17-2. The extended release formulation is designed to release the drug slowly over the entire day, whereas the immediate release form releases the entire dose at once.

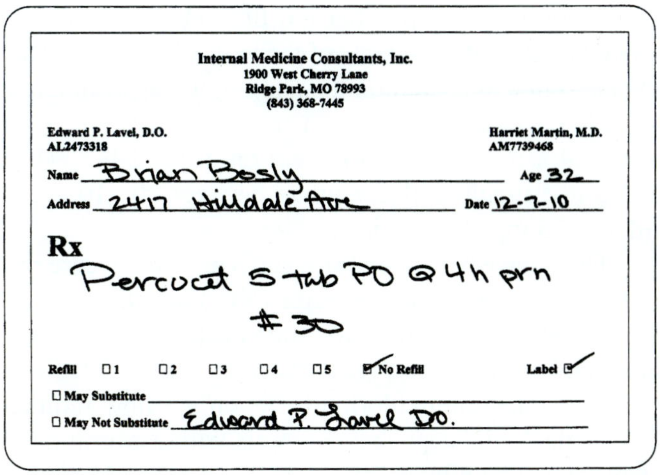
Internal Medicine Consultants, Inc.
1900 West Cherry Lane
Ridge Park, MO 78993
(843) 368-7445
Edward P. Lavel, D.O.
AL2473318
Harriet Martin, M.D.
AM7739468
Name Brian Bosly Age 32
Address 2417 Hilldale Ave Date 12-7-10
Rx
Percocet 5 tab PO q 4h prn
#30
Refill ☐1 ☐2 ☐3 ☐4 ☐5 ☑ No Refill Label ☑
☐ May Substitute
☐ May Not Substitute Edward P. Lavel DO.

Figure 17-1. Example of a medication name that includes a number.

Product Labeling. As a marketing strategy, product labels often emphasize a manufacturer's name or logo, potentially making it difficult to readily identify the drug name and dose. Manufacturers often use the same labeling scheme, including letter size, print, and background color, to associate the product with the manufacturer. Sometimes this strategy, which makes all labels look alike, can be detrimental.

The dosage strength and total contents of liquid formulations are not always labeled clearly. Different vial sizes of injections may be similarly labeled with the

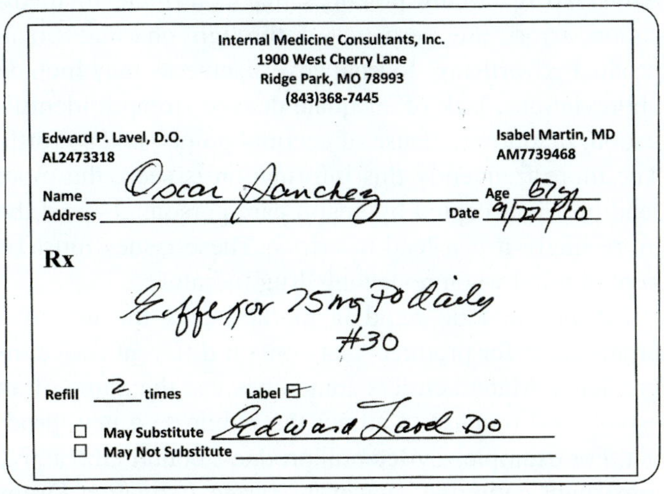
Internal Medicine Consultants, Inc.
1900 West Cherry Lane
Ridge Park, MO 78993
(843)368-7445
Edward P. Lavel, D.O.
AL2473318
Isabel Martin, MD
AM7739468
Name Oscar Sanchez Age 67 y
Address Date 9/22/10
Rx
Effexor 75 mg PO daily
#30
Refill 2 times Label ☑
☐ May Substitute Edward Lavel DO
☐ May Not Substitute

Figure 17-2. Example of a prescription for "Effexor XR" where the "XR" was omitted.

Table 17-2. Examples of Drug Product Names Changed to Reduce the Risk of Prescribing Errors

Former Trade Name	Confused With	New Trade Name
Clonopin	Clonidine	Klonopin
Omacor	Amicar	Lovaza
Losec	Lasix	Prilosec
Microx	Micro-K	MyKrox
Reminyl	Amaryl	Razadyne

concentration (mg/mL), but too little emphasis may be placed on the total contents of the vial. When midazolam (Versed) first appeared on the market, it was available in a 5 mg/mL concentration in 1 mL and 2 mL size vials. The vial size was not prominent on either label, which made it difficult to differentiate between the 10 mg (2 mL) and 5 mg (1 mL) vials.

There have been numerous cases of a health care provider using a potassium chloride (KCl) injection to flush an IV line instead of normal saline because the vial sizes and labeling of the two products were similar. Manufacturers of potassium chloride injection are now required to use black vial caps and overseals with a warning that states "must be diluted."[50]

Color Coding. Relying on the color of product packaging is not a safe practice. Manufacturers may change their packaging color scheme at any time, and color-coding schemes for similar products may differ among manufacturers. Sometimes there is too little difference between colors in a color scheme, which leads to mix-ups. Medication products with similar colors can be misplaced in the stock areas and could easily be dispensed in error. For example, both daunorubicin 20 mg and doxorubicin 10 mg are packaged in vials that are shaped similarly and have dark blue vial caps. They are both lyophilized powders that turn into red solutions upon reconstitution. Relying on the color of the vial cap or of the diluted solution could lead to very serious errors. The ISMP recommends that color coding medications be used cautiously because it has not been scientifically shown to prevent medication errors and several problems have been identified by its use.[51]

Advertising. Many practices that contribute to medication errors are perpetuated through pharmaceutical product advertising. Journal advertisements may include abbreviations, lack of adequate dosage strength identification, inappropriate use of decimal points, and so forth. The more frequently this information is seen, the more readily it is accepted by health care personnel—and the more likely it can lead to errors. These issues must be kept in mind when reviewing drug literature.

A problematic trend in marketing is the use of a brand name for products that contain different active ingredients. Manufacturers sometimes use the name of an established product to attract the public to a new product. For example, Zyrtec oral products contain the active ingredient cetirizine; however, Zyrtec Itchy Eye Drops contain the active ingredient ketotifen. Similarly, Claritin oral products contain loratadine as the active ingredient and Claritin Eye contains ketotifen. Another example of a manufacturer's attempt to draw upon the use of a familiar brand name is Pepcid versus Pepcid Complete. Pepcid contains the active ingredient famotidine, but Pepcid Complete is a combination product containing famotidine, calcium carbonate, and magnesium hydroxide. These examples demonstrate the importance of carefully reading product labels.

Compounding/Drug Preparation Errors

Errors can occur during the compounding and drug preparation phase. These errors can be difficult for others to catch, so it is essential that technicians take steps to decrease the risk of error when compounding and preparing drug products. Such an approach includes reading the product labels carefully, not processing more than one prescription at a time, labeling prescriptions properly, storing drugs properly, maintaining a safe work environment, and keeping up with changes in the medical profession.

Reading the Label. Reading drug product labels carefully when filling an order is a step that should not be neglected. This step is extremely important because of the number of product names that sound and look alike, have similar product packaging, small print, and color coding.

> **Rx for Success**
>
> Read the label at least three times to help prevent medication errors: when you remove it from the shelf, as it is being prepared, and as the finished product is set aside for the pharmacist to check.

Processing Multiple Products. Processing more than one prescription or order at the same time can result in errors. For example, it is easy to add a medication to the wrong IV bag if several orders are being compounded simultaneously in the laminar flow hood. Filling a prescription for the wrong patient or confusing the quantities to be dispensed is also possible.

Technicians should process only one prescription or common batch (e.g., all 0800 cefazolin 1 g IVPB orders) at a time. Supplies for multiple prescriptions should not be mixed together. Each prescription should be completed before starting the next one.

✔ Completed prescriptions waiting for a pharmacist check should be clearly separated from each other, from those that have not yet been completed, and from those that have already been checked by the pharmacist.

Labeling Technicians should be familiar with the labeling requirements for prescriptions in their pharmacy as dictated by state law and pharmacy policies and procedures. If a label is handwritten, it should be neat and legible. Ink and toner cartridges and printer ribbons should be changed before the print is too faded to read, the label should be free of smudges, and the print should be aligned on the label appropriately. Labels that are difficult to read can result in miscommunication and medication errors.

Auxiliary labels give the patient and nursing personnel useful information. For example, in figure 17-3, some pharmacies affix a warning label to neuromuscular blockers, "warning – paralytic agent." Another example is the use of a "shake well" label for oral suspensions as shown in figure 17-4. This information can be important in helping to prevent medication errors. Many pharmacy computer systems are designed to identify the appropriate auxiliary labels for prescriptions, and other pharmacies use reference charts as aids. Auxiliary labels should be placed carefully on the drug container so they do not cover up other pertinent information.

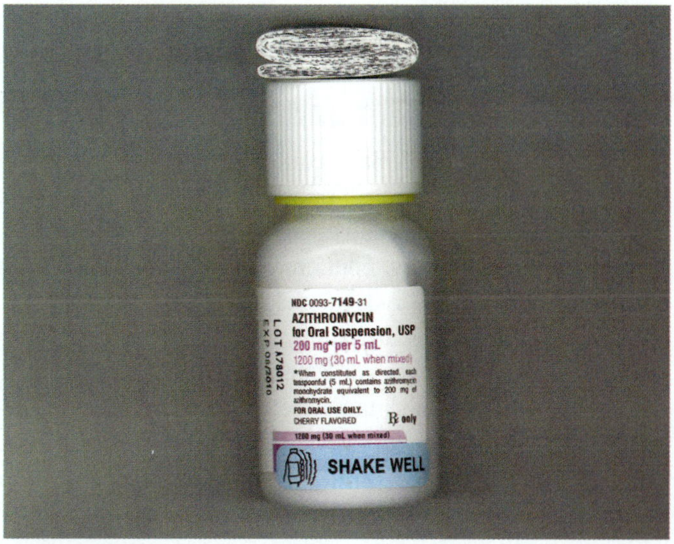

Figure 17-4. Example of an auxiliary label identifying a medication that must be shaken prior to use.

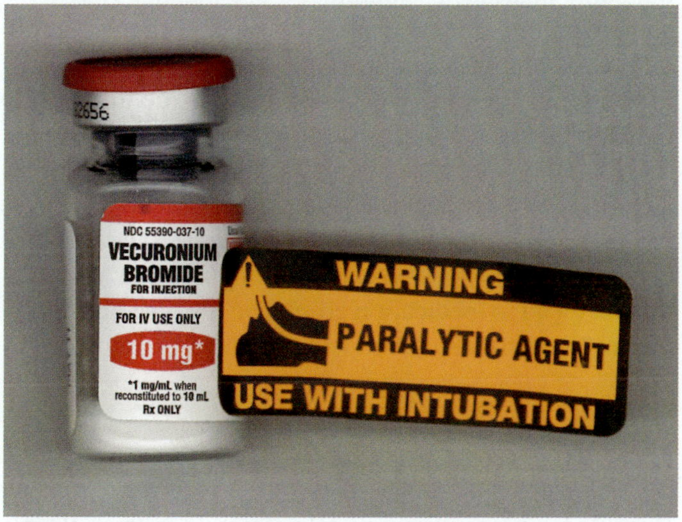

Figure 17-3. Example of an auxiliary label identifying a neuromuscular blocking agent which is considered a high alert medication.

Deteriorated Medications. Because expired medications and improperly stored medications may have lost their potency and thus, their effectiveness, technicians should take steps to keep these medications out of the dispensing stock. In many cases, it is the technician's responsibility to rotate stock. Technicians should be familiar with the pharmacy's regular system for checking for expired medications. Although checking expiration dates is sometimes viewed as a tedious job, it is important because it reduces the risk of making deteriorated drug errors.

When replenishing stock, always remove expired medications and place the stock with the earliest expiration date near the front to be used first. Some drugs have a short expiration date once the container has been opened. Pharmacies usually have procedures that require the date of opening or the expiration date to be written on the label to help prevent use of an expired drug. Examples of drugs that usually require dating include reconstituted oral suspensions and injectable drugs.

Rx for Success

Technicians should be familiar with the drugs that have short expiration dates and the procedures for indicating date of first use or expiration. Marking opened containers with an "X" to readily identify the container that should be used first is also recommended.

Medications that require special storage conditions, such as refrigeration or freezing, should be stored in those conditions as long as possible prior to use. Drugs stored under refrigeration may be stable for only a short time out of the refrigerator. When filling an order for a pharmacist to check, the technician must comply with the institution's policy. Some pharmacies/pharmacists require that refrigerated medications be left in the refrigerator and not on the counter, whereas others allow them to stay on the counter briefly.

Work Environment and Personnel Issues

Factors within the workplace can contribute to medication errors. Inadequate lighting,[52] poorly designed work spaces, and inefficient workflow can make it difficult to perform assigned duties accurately. Cluttered work spaces and stock areas can increase the risk of picking up the wrong drug. The many distractions and interruptions, including phone calls, in a busy pharmacy can cause loss of concentration.[53]

Many modern pharmacies rely on specialized equipment and computers to assist in filling prescriptions. Improper maintenance of this equipment can result in unacceptable performance or may necessitate the use of older, unfamiliar, or cumbersome manual systems when the equipment breaks down. For example, failure to properly maintain a balance can result in an inaccurate measure of medication components for a compounded prescription and ultimately a wrong dose error. Routine maintenance schedules should be followed to prevent equipment malfunction. Technicians should be trained on the use and maintenance of such equipment. Operating manuals should be available in the pharmacy for troubleshooting when a problem occurs.

Scheduling of staff members and the frequency of rotating shifts have been shown to correlate with error rates.[54] Other factors, such as staffing levels and amount of supervision, are also work environment issues to consider.

The frequency with which drug products are changed because of changes in purchasing contracts may lead to unfamiliarity with products among the staff. Significant changes should be communicated to the staff, and product labels should be read carefully.

Untrained, inadequately trained, or inexperienced personnel may be unfamiliar with drug names, doses, or uses of agents, which limits their ability to recognize inappropriate orders and circumstances. New technological advances make keeping up with drug use difficult even for experienced health care practitioners. The important thing is for technicians to recognize their limits and work within them, just as nurses, pharmacists, and physicians are trained to do. Relying on memory instead of checking references (e.g., dilution charts, maximum dosage ranges) or performing complicated calculations without a double-check stage can result in errors. It is a technician's responsibility to help prevent medication errors by questioning unusual or unfamiliar orders. When abnormal or unfamiliar situations arise, it is always best to consult references and others before making a decision or taking action. Being aware of a potential error and not knowing what to do about it, thinking that someone else will catch it, or feeling intimidated by a pharmacist or supervisor increases the chances that an actual error will take place.

The lack of knowledge of medication errors and how to avoid them also contributes to medication errors. Not being familiar with common errors or medications most frequently involved in errors might cause one to think that medication errors are infrequent. The medication errors most frequently reported to the USP in 2002 involved albuterol, insulin, morphine, potassium chloride, heparin and warfarin. Of these six medications, all but albuterol were most frequently involved in errors that were associated with patient harm or death.[55]

Deficiencies in Medication Use Systems

Medication errors cannot be attributed to human error alone. Errors are frequently due in part to defective or inadequate systems.[56] For example, stocking dangerous drugs in patient care areas (i.e., open floor stock) increases the risk of an error because the drugs are available to nurses without a pharmacy check. Floor stock mix-ups, such as between heparin injection and normal saline injection for flushing IV tubing, potassium chloride and furosemide injections, and premixed lidocaine in D5W 500 mL and plain D5W 500 mL bags, can lead to serious consequences.

Advances in technology such as automated dispensing cabinets, bar coding, robots, and computerized order entry have been shown to reduce medication errors.[57–60] The use of such technology in pharmacies is increasing, but some pharmacies continue to use manual systems to some extent.[61] The unavailability of or difficulty in obtaining patient data, such as current body weight, allergy information, or laboratory results, also contributes to medication errors.

Inefficient processes with too many or too few checks along the way or checks at inappropriate times can cause errors. Lack of standardized procedures or outdated procedures can also lead to errors. Being familiar with factors that lead to medication errors and ways of preventing them is the first step in reducing medication errors.

Prevention of Medication Errors

It is impossible to eliminate all potential for error. People are not perfect, and even the most conscientious and knowledgeable staff members can make mistakes. There are several systems and methods that help to prevent medication errors, including failure mode and effects analysis, systems designed to prevent medication errors, legal requirements, policies and procedures, multiple check systems, standardized order forms, education and training, and computerization and automation.

Failure Mode and Effects Analysis

Sometimes the systems that people work within present numerous opportunities for errors. **Failure mode and effects analysis (FMEA)**, also called failure mode effect and criticality analysis (FMECA), is a systematic evaluation of a process or system used to predict the opportunity for and severity of errors at various steps in the process.[62,63] FMEA focuses on finding flaws within a system that create opportunities for individuals to make errors. It evaluates the "how" and "why" of an error instead of the "who."

The first step in evaluating a system or process using FMEA is to describe in detail the individual steps involved in the overall process from start to finish. Use of a flow diagram is helpful to create a visual representation of the process. The next step is to list the potential opportunities for failure at each stage. Then, the effects of these failures on the process and their root causes are described. The severity, likelihood of occurrence, and probability of actually identifying the failure are then estimated. The criticality index is determined by multiplying these three estimates. Steps that have the highest criticality index should be addressed first because improvements in these areas have the greatest potential for reducing the risk for error. After making changes to the process, FMEA should be performed again to determine the effectiveness of these changes.

An acute care hospital in California used the FMEA system to reduce IV pump-related medication errors. One year after implementation of several error reduction strategies identified during the FMEA, it was noted that pump-related medication errors had decreased significantly.[64]

Systems Designed to Prevent Medication Errors

There are many ways to reduce the risk of a medication error. Institutions help minimize medication errors by fostering a well-trained and knowledgeable staff, maintaining a favorable work environment, and instituting effective policies and procedures, among other things.

✔ Technicians must be familiar with the systems designed to provide additional checks in the medication use process. It is also essential that technicians ask questions when they are not familiar with the proper procedures.[5]

Well-designed systems help prevent medication errors. Such systems adhere to legal requirements and include licensed personnel, policies and procedures, multiple check systems, standardized order forms and checklists, and quality assurance activities and monitoring systems, which are addressed later in this chapter.

Another system designed to help prevent medication errors in the outpatient setting is patient counseling. When a patient or designee drops off a prescription to be filled at the pharmacy, the pharmacist or pharmacy technician asks if the patient is allergic to any medications and asks for the proper spelling of the patient's name and address, among other things. When the prescription is picked up, the pharmacist and the patient discuss how to take the medication, any possible side effects, and why it is important for the patient to take the medication exactly as the physician has prescribed it. The patient has the opportunity to ask questions or discuss any concerns about the medication with the pharmacist. Patient counseling plays a very important role in reducing medication errors because it increases the likelihood that patients will take their medication as prescribed.

Legal Requirements

Pharmacy laws are designed to protect the public by ensuring that a knowledgeable individual double-checks the results of the prescribing process and oversees the use of medications. The laws, which are covered in detail in Chapter 2, Pharmacy Law, help prevent medication errors.

Policies and Procedures

Policies and procedures formally establish a system to prevent medication errors. Therefore, technicians should be familiar with the workplace's policies and procedures. A study of dispensing errors in an outpatient pharmacy concluded that approximately 33% of the errors discovered were due to noncompliance with company or department policies and procedures.[11]

Multiple Check Systems

Another system designed to prevent medication errors is a multiple check system. This can include the pharmacist reviewing a physician order, a pharmacy technician preparing a medication for the pharmacist to check, a nurse inspecting the dose from the pharmacy, and a patient asking questions and examining the medication before taking it. A multiple check system is especially important with potentially lethal drugs, such as cancer chemotherapeutic agents.[36]

Advocate Lutheran General Hospital

Cancer Chemotherapy Order Form/ADULT

Part 1 - Chemotherapy

Orders must be received in pharmacy by 2100 for administration between 2300 and 0900

☐ Protocol # ______ 1 2 3 4 5 6 7 8 Course (Circle One)	Diagnosis	BSA m² ☐ Dose reduction____ %	Height	Weight

CHEMOTHERAPY

Provide dose, select a route and designate the frequency and duration for each chemotherapy ordered. Designate day number, sequence and time in column A. Cont. Inf. = Continuous Infusion over 24 hours

A	DRUG	DOSE	ROUTE		FREQUENCY/DURATION	Total Dose per Course
	Asparaginase	units/m² = U	☐ IVPB over 30 min	☐ SC ☐ IM	q X doses	unit
	Bleomycin	units/m² = U	☐ IVP over 10 min ☐ IVPB over h	☐ Cont Inf	q X doses	unit
	Carboplatin	AUC of ____ = mg/m² = mg	☐ IVPB over 30 min Creat= mg/dl		q X doses	mg/m²
	Carmustine	mg/m² = mg	☐ IVPB over 60 min in GLASS container	☐ Cont Inf	q X doses	mg/m²
	Cisplatin	mg/m² = mg	☐ IVPB over 60 min ☐ IVPB over ____ h with g mannitol	☐ Cont Inf	q X doses	mg/m²
	Cyclophosphamide	mg/m² = mg	☐ IVP over 5 - 10 min ☐ IVPB over 30 - 60 min	☐ Cont Inf	q X doses	mg/m²
	Cytarabine	mg/m² = mg	☐ Intrathecal ☐ IVPB over h	☐ Cont Inf	q X doses	mg/m²
	Dacarbazine	mg/m² = mg	☐ IVP over 2-3 min ☐ IVPB over 15 - 30 min	☐ Cont Inf	q X doses	mg/m²
	Daunorubicin	mg/m² = mg	☐ IVP over 2 - 3 min ☐ IVPB over 15 min		q X doses	mg/m²
	Docetaxel	mg/m² = mg	☐ IVPB over 60 min in glass container		q X doses	mg/m²
	Doxorubicin	mg/m² = mg	☐ IVP over 10 - 15 min ☐ IVPB over 30 min	☐ Cont Inf	q X doses	mg/m²
	Etoposide	mg/m² = mg	☐ IVPB over 1 -2 h	☐ Cont Inf	q X doses	mg/m²
	Fluorouracil	mg/m² = mg	☐ IVP over 2 - 3 min ☐ IVPB over 30 - 60 min		q X doses	mg/m²
	Gemcitabine	mg/m² = mg	☐ IVPB over h ☐ IVPB over 30 min	☐ Cont Inf	q X doses	mg/m²
	Idarubicin	mg/m² = mg	☐ IVPB over 15 min		q X doses	mg/m²
	Ifosfamide	mg/m² = mg	☐ IVPB over 30 - 60 min	☐ Cont Inf	q X doses	mg/m²
	Mesna	mg/m² = mg	☐ IVPB over 15 -20 min, 30 min prior to, 4h & 8h after start of ifosfamide	☐ Mix with ifosfamide	q X doses	mg/m²
	Mesna	mg/m² = mg	☐ IVPB over 15 - 20 min, 4h and 8h after last ifosfamide			
	Methotrexate	mg/m² = mg	☐ Intrathecal ☐ IVPB over h	☐ Cont Inf	q X doses	mg/m²
	Leucovorin	mg/m² = mg	☐ IVP over 3 min ☐ 24 h after methotrexate ☐ Prior to fluorouracil	☐ PO	q X doses	mg/m²
	Vinblastine	mg/m² = mg	☐ IVP over 2 - 3 min	☐ Cont Inf	q X doses	mg/m²
	Mitoxantrone	mg/m² = mg	☐ IVPB over 15 min		q X doses	mg/m²
	Paclitaxel	mg/m² = mg	☐ IVPB over h in GLASS container	☐ Cont Inf	q X doses	mg/m²
	Vincristine	mg/m² = mg	☐ IVP over 2 - 3 min	☐ Cont Inf	q X doses	mg/m²
	Topotecan	mg/m² = mg	☐ IVPB over 30 min	☐ Cont Inf	q X doses	mg/m²
	Vinorelbine	mg/m² = mg	☐ IVP over 6 - 10 min		q X doses	mg/m²

Other:

Date:	Time:	Prescriber's signature	Pager #:

91-4123-1 06/09
Page 1 of 3

Figure 17–5. Example of a preprinted order form for chemotherapy.

Standardized Order Forms

Standardized, preprinted order forms are used to prevent medication errors by making medication orders easier for the prescriber to read and easier for the pharmacist and nurse to interpret. Figure 17-5 is an example of a standardized, preprinted order form. Note that the chemotherapy agents are listed in alphabetical order with the exception of those beginning with the letter "v." Vinblastine, vinorelbine, and vincristine are separated on the form because of the similarity in their names. Also note that the nonchemotherapy agents, mesna and leucovorin, are listed next to their companion chemotherapy drugs to prompt the physician to remember to order them when appropriate.

Chemotherapeutic agents have been designated as high alert medications by ISMP, making them ideal drugs to be included on a standardized order form.[32] The use of preprinted order forms for other complicated drug therapies and high-risk drugs can also be beneficial. Preprinted forms are neatly typed and therefore legible. They make it easier for other health care personnel to double-check the prescriber's order and calculations. The forms help reduce errors primarily associated with illegible handwriting and also informally educate the prescriber about which medications are on the hospital formulary.

Checklists can be included on a standard preprinted order form. This system ensures that personnel use a systematic, thorough procedure to check medications before they are prescribed, dispensed, or administered to a patient.[36]

Education and Training

Education and training are important in reducing medication errors. Training can include pharmacy calculations, compounding techniques, pharmacy abbreviations, preparation of IV medications, and computer operation skills. Health care personnel should be familiar with the classes of medications, their generic and trade names, and their forms and doses.

The Joint Commission requires organizations to prove that their personnel are competent. Ideally, on-the-job training includes instruction and demonstrations. After technicians have been instructed and have witnessed a demonstration of a task, they are usually asked to perform the task while the educator observes. This procedure allows for documentation of the technicians' competency.

To complement formal and on-the-job training, technicians should read pharmacy literature, participate in local pharmacy organizations, and attend continuing education lectures to improve their knowledge base. At a minimum, these programs and activities help technicians keep up with changes in formulations and recognize the differences among various medication products.[2]

Computerization and Automation

The proper use of computerization and automation are effective ways to prevent medication errors.[57–60] Many health care facilities use bar coding, automated dispensing cabinets (ADCs), and robots to reduce medication errors. The technology reduces the number of health care personnel who handle the medications, which can in turn reduce the risk for human error.[65] Pharmacy-generated medication administration records and labels are recommended to assist nurses in interpreting and documenting medication activities.[2]

Computerized physician (or prescriber) order entry (CPOE) has been shown to reduce the rate of serious errors in an inpatient setting by 55%.[66] CPOE is also being investigated at some institutions to decrease the number of personnel involved in the ordering process and medication errors in the transcription process (when medication orders are re-written to another document

Technology Topics

Packaging is getting more sophisticated and many products are available in bar-coded unit-dose packaging for use with automated dispensing cabinets, robots, and bar-coded medication administration. Bar coding patient ID bands helps prevent health care personnel from mistaking one patient for another. Computerized pharmacy systems utilize decision support tools that enable automated checking of doses, duplicate therapies, allergies, drug interactions, and other alerts.

such as a medication administration record by a nurse or unit clerk). Computer systems with clinical decision support (automatic alerts that warn prescribers about possible allergies, drug interactions, or overdoses) have been shown to prevent potential adverse events before the order reaches the pharmacist.[67,68] Although computerized order entry has many advantages, it is important to recognize that new opportunities for errors may arise.[69–71]

The Quality Assurance Process

Despite efforts to prevent medication errors, they do occur, in which case it is important to document and evaluate the circumstances involved in the error so that healthcare personnel can be educated on how to prevent such errors from occurring in the future.

What to Do When an Error Occurs

When a potential medication error occurs—for example, a pharmacy technician incorrectly fills a medication order—and the pharmacist catches the error in the pharmacy, usually the pharmacist will talk to the technician about the error and ask for it to be corrected. It is important for the technician to realize that the pharmacist's intent is to make the mistake a learning experience for the technician as well as to give the technician an opportunity to ask questions. Although making a mistake is frustrating, learning what factors may have contributed to the error and focusing on ways to avoid such an error in the future are important.

Whatever the circumstances surrounding an actual medication error, the pharmacy technician has a responsibility to inform the pharmacist about any known details. Pharmacists usually investigate the error, the severity of the consequences, and gather the details before contacting the physician.

If the error is caught before the patient receives the medication, it can be corrected within the pharmacy. If the patient has received the medication, the course of action depends on the details of the error. The pharmacist may refill the medication for free and have it delivered to the patient or send a formal letter of apology to the patient. Additional monitoring of the patient may be needed until any residual effects have been resolved. When informing the patient about an error, an explanation of how the error occurred and the possible short-term and long-term effects should be provided.

Pharmacies should have written procedures in place that describe when and how to inform patients of errors. The procedures should also include who is responsible for informing the patients, what follow-up procedures should be taken, and what documentation is required.

Documentation. When a medication error occurs, the organization's medication error reporting form should be completed according to the organization's established reporting procedures. Figure 17-6A, B is an example of a medication error reporting form.

The medication error reporting form should be completed and reviewed by those involved in the error to ensure that the content is accurate and correct. Once the form is complete, it is usually sent to the pharmacy supervisor or manager and, if necessary, to the risk management department for review. These forms are reviewed periodically by the organization's designated committee (quality assurance, for example), which may consist of pharmacy, medicine, nursing, risk management, quality, staff educators, and legal counsel staff members.[2]

Root Cause Analysis. Once an error has occurred, it is important to thoroughly examine the error to learn why it occurred and how such an error can be avoided in the future. A **root cause analysis (RCA)** is a process that examines the contributing factors regarding why and how an error (or near miss) occurred. There are usually several factors that led to the error.[56]

A root cause analysis consists of five steps:

1. Establish a team of appropriate personnel to conduct the root cause analysis. This team may include pharmacists, technicians, nurses, prescribers, risk management representatives, or other allied health personnel. The team should seek management support and establish meeting times and locations.

MEDI-CATION ERRORS REPORTING PROGRAM

USP MEDICATION ERRORS REPORTING PROGRAM

Presented in cooperation with the Institute for Safe Medication Practices

USP is an FDA MEDWATCH partner

Reporters should not provide any individually identifiable health information, including names of practitioners, names of patients, names of healthcare facilities, or dates of birth (age is acceptable).

Date and time of event:

Please describe the error. Include description/sequence of events, type of staff involved, and work environment (e.g., code situation, change of shift, short staffing, no 24-hr. pharmacy, floor stock). If more space is needed, please attach a separate page.

Did the error reach the patient? ☐ Yes ☐ No

Was the incorrect medication, dose, or dosage form administered to or taken by the patient? ☐ Yes ☐ No

Circle the appropriate Error Outcome Category (select one—see back for details): A B C D E F G H I

Describe the direct result of the error on the patient (e.g., death, type of harm, additional patient monitoring).

Indicate the possible error cause(s) and contributing factor(s) (e.g., abbreviation, similar names, distractions, etc.).

Indicate the location of the error (e.g., hospital, outpatient or community pharmacy, clinic, nursing home, patient's home, etc.).

What type of staff or healthcare practitioner made the initial error?

Indicate if other practitioner(s) were also involved in the error (type of staff perpetuating error).

What type of staff or healthcare practitioner discovered the error or recognized the potential for error?

How was the error (or potential for error) discovered/intercepted?

If available, provide patient age, gender, diagnosis. Do not provide any patient identifiers.

Please complete the following for the product(s) involved. (If more space is needed for additional products, please attach a separate page.)

	Product #1	Product #2
Brand/Product Name (If Applicable)		
Generic Name		
Manufacturer		
Labeler		
Dosage Form		
Strength/Concentration		
Type and Size of Container		

Reports are most useful when relevant materials such as product label, copy of prescription/order, etc., can be reviewed.

Can these materials be provided? ☐ Yes ☐ No Please specify:

Suggest any recommendations to prevent recurrence of this error, or describe policies or procedures you instituted or plan to institute to prevent future similar errors.

Name and Title/Profession | Telephone Number ( ) | Fax Number ( )

Facility/Address and Zip | E-mail

Address/Zip (where correspondence should be sent)

Your name, contact information, and a copy of this report are routinely shared with the Institute for Safe Medication Practices (ISMP). Copies of reports will be sent to third parties such as the manufacturer/labeler, and to the Food and Drug Administration (FDA). You have the option of including your name on these copies.

In addition to releasing my name and contact information to ISMP, USP may release my identity to these third parties as follows (check boxes that apply):

☐ The manufacturer and/or labeler as listed above ☐ FDA ☐ Other persons requesting a copy of this report ☐ Anonymous to all third parties

Signature | Date

Return to:
USP CAPS
12601 Twinbrook Parkway
Rockville, MD 20852-1790

Submit via the Web at www.usp.org/mer
Call Toll Free: 800-23-ERROR (800-233-7767)
or FAX: 301-816-8532

Date Received by USP | File Access Number

PSF116G

WEPDF

Figure 17–6A. Example of a medication error reporting form.

NCC MERP Index for Categorizing Medication Errors

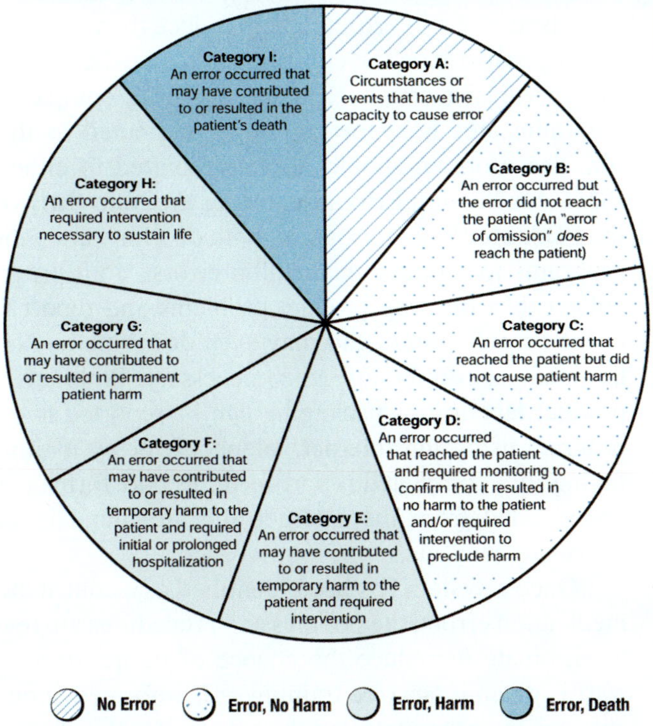

NCC MERP Index for Categorizing Medication Errors Algorithm

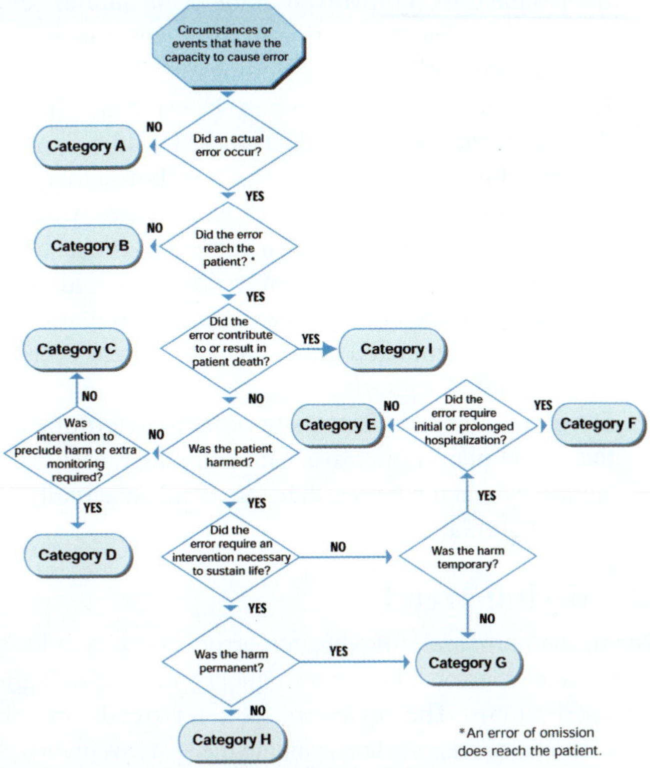

Full-size copies are available: **INDEX**—www.nccmerp.org/010612_color_index.pdf; **ALGORITHM**—www.nccmerp.org/010612_color_algo.pdf

National Coordinating Council for Medication Error Reporting and Prevention Definitions

Harm
Impairment of the physical, emotional, or psychological function or structure of the body and/or pain resulting therefrom.

Monitoring
To observe or record relevant physiological or psychological signs.

Intervention
May include change in therapy or active medical/surgical treatment.

Intervention Necessary to Sustain Life
Includes cardiovascular and respiratory support (e.g., CPR, defibrillation, intubation, etc.).

U.S. Pharmacopeia
12601 Twinbrook Parkway
Rockville, MD 20852-1790

NO POSTAGE NECESSARY IF MAILED IN THE UNITED STATES

BUSINESS REPLY MAIL
FIRST-CLASS MAIL PERMIT NO 39 ROCKVILLE MD

POSTAGE WILL BE PAID BY ADDRESSEE:

THE USP CENTER FOR THE ADVANCEMENT OF PATIENT SAFETY
12601 TWINBROOK PARKWAY
ROCKVILLE MD 20897-5211

Figure 17–6B. Back page of the USP Medication Error Reporting Form with information to assist in completing the form.

Part 3

2. Describe the event in detail. As much information as possible about the event should be obtained, and the people directly involved in the event should be interviewed. The description of the event is then revised to include any new findings.
3. Diagram the steps that led up to the error to help determine the root cause. The steps should be described in chronological order and thoroughly examined for inconsistencies or weaknesses. Based on this information, propose a summary of causes.
4. Develop a specific action plan to address the identified causes of the error. Some of the action plans might be implemented immediately, whereas others may be more long term.
5. Develop outcome measures in order to determine if the action plan is effective. The outcome measures should evaluate whether the actions taken actually prevent similar errors.

Identifying Trends

One of the purposes of medication error review is to look for medication errors that occur frequently or involve high-risk medications. The reviewers look for trends among medication error reports and evaluate the systems involved in the errors. Many quality assurance committees focus on the pharmacy's processes (e.g., staff orientation and education) instead of on individual staff members, because most medication errors are due to poor drug distribution systems, miscommunication, faulty pharmaceutical packaging, labeling, nomenclature, and lack of information rather than any one person. Education is important to prevent other associates from making similar mistakes. When there is a chance of serious errors, action is taken to improve the system and minimize the possibility of errors.[72]

Making Necessary Changes

Once a trend has been identified, action must be taken to reduce the possibility of future errors. Changes may involve educating staff, purchasing a more appropriately labeled medication from another company, revising department policies and procedures, or purchasing a piece of equipment.

Three ways the pharmacy department can educate its staff on a continual basis about actual medication errors are by publishing summaries of errors that have occurred in staff newsletters, conducting educational programs, and discussing medication errors as a regular agenda item at staff meetings. It is important for technicians to pay close attention to newsletters, educational programs, and discussions of errors to help reduce them.

If product labeling contributed to a medication error, the pharmacist usually contacts the drug company and communicates how the labeling contributed to the error. The problem should also be reported to either the ISMP Medication Errors Reporting Program (MERP) or the FDA MedWatch Program, both of which are national programs to monitor medication errors. Both programs collect data on drug product problems and report them to the manufacturers and may even distribute an alert to the medical community when necessary. Problems with product labeling or packaging can be reported to either program using the Internet, telephone, or by mailing or faxing in a completed report form. Report forms can be downloaded from the Internet and are found in many pharmacy journals.

Once a system has been identified as a contributor to medication errors, the policies and procedures are revised to eliminate or reduce the chance of future errors. The staff is given in-service training or is informed about the changes in procedures and the reasons for the changes.

Monitoring the Impact of Change

After a system has been modified, it is important to continue to monitor for medication errors to determine the impact of the changes.[72]

Liability Issues

Technicians and pharmacists need to be informed about how to prevent medication errors. In addition to the liability to the institution or company, technicians and pharmacists may be held personally accountable for a medication error involving injury to a patient.[73]

Summary

The ultimate goal of pharmacy services must be the safe use of medications by the public.[74] Medication errors can occur in many ways and also can be prevented in many ways. Pharmacy technicians play an important role in ensuring the safe use of medications.

Self-Assessment Questions

1. A medication error is defined as "an error made by a pharmacist or pharmacy technician at any time during the dispensing process."
   a. True
   b. False
2. Which of the following actions might increase the likelihood of a medication error?
   a. Reading the drug label carefully when selecting the drug from the shelf
   b. Reviewing recent medication errors at a pharmacy staff meeting
   c. Asking another pharmacy technician to double-check a calculation
   d. Having a nurse phone in a prescription order that was communicated verbally by the doctor
3. Manufacturers are required to print the warning, "MUST BE DILUTED," on the container cap and label for which of the following products?
   a. Potassium chloride injection vial
   b. Vincristine injection
   c. Digoxin oral liquid
   d. Amoxicillin suspension
4. Kedeisha Banks received the following prescription for an antibiotic to treat a respiratory tract infection on January 1:

   Amoxicillin 500 mg PO TID for 10 days

   After taking the drug for three days, Ms. Banks felt much better and stopped taking her medication.

   On January 12, Ms. Banks presents to the pharmacy with the following prescription for another antibiotic:

   Azithromycin 500 mg PO daily for 3 days

   The medication error described above would be categorized as which of the following medication error type?
   a. Patient noncompliance
   b. Prescribing error
   c. Wrong drug dispensed
   d. Deteriorated drug error
5. The pharmacist asks you to prepare the following medications:

   Gentamicin 1 g IVPB every 8 hours

   Cefazolin 60 mg IVPB every 12 hours

   After obtaining the necessary supplies from the shelf, you are puzzled by the number of vials needed for the gentamicin dose (13 vials). You should:
   a. Prepare the doses as requested, but ask another technician to check your calculations
   b. Question the pharmacist about the order because you have never had to use so many vials to prepare a gentamicin dose before
   c. Prepare the doses as requested because the order has already been reviewed by a pharmacist
   d. Contact the doctor to clarify the order
6. Katie Loden presents to your pharmacy with the prescription in figure 17-7 and Lanoxin (digoxin), a heart medication, is dispensed. She calls the pharmacy several hours later and asks why her thyroid medication is a yellow instead of a light brown round tablet.

   How would this medication error most likely be categorized?

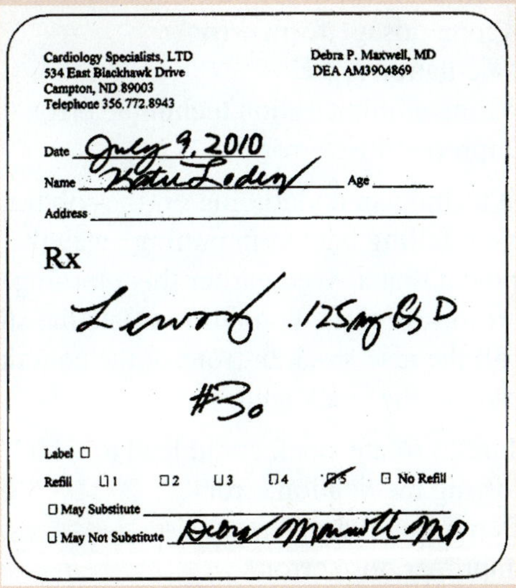
Cardiology Specialists, LTD
534 East Blackhawk Drive
Campton, ND 89003
Telephone 356.772.8943

Debra P. Maxwell, MD
DEA AM3904869

Date July 9, 2010
Name Katie Loden Age ______
Address ______

Rx

[illegible] .125mg QD

#30

Label ☐
Refill ☐ 1 ☐ 2 ☐ 3 ☐ 4 ☐ 5 ☐ No Refill
☐ May Substitute ______
☐ May Not Substitute Debra Maxwell MD

Figure 17-7. Prescription to use when answering question 6.

Self-Assessment Questions

a. Patient compliance error
b. Prescribing error
c. Wrong drug preparation error
d. Physician error

7. Amina Shah was in the radiology department when the nurse came to her room to administer the 0900 dose of captopril 25 mg PO three times daily (scheduled for 0900, 1600 and 2200). Because of the complexity of the procedure and a number of delays in radiology, Ms. Shah did not return to her room until 1500, at which time her captopril was administered.

   Which of the following is a TRUE statement regarding Ms. Shah's captopril?
   a. A nursing error has been committed.
   b. An omission error occurred.
   c. The medication delay resulted in a wrong time error for the 0900 dose.
   d. No medication error has occurred.

8. When compounding the following order, the technician inadvertently used 1 mL of the 40 mg/mL concentration solution instead of the pediatric concentration (10 mg/mL).

   Gentamicin 10 mg IVPB every 8 hours

   Identify the category in which this error could be classified.
   a. Wrong dosage form error
   b. Calculation error
   c. Wrong administration technique error
   d. Improper dose error

9. As a technician undergoing on-the-job training, you are falling behind in putting away the drug shipment that arrived earlier this morning. In an effort to save time, you fail to rotate the stock and put all the new stock in front of the containers already in the stock area.

   Failure to rotate stock could lead to which of the following medication errors?
   a. Deteriorated drug error
   b. Improper dose error
   c. Compliance error
   d. Monitoring error

10. Experienced pharmacy technicians are less likely than technicians-in-training to make calculation errors.
    a. True
    b. False

11. Which of the following can lead to a calculation error?
    a. Not verifying that the final answer is reasonable
    b. Using an inaccurate conversion
    c. Misplacing the decimal point
    d. All of the above

12. Which of the following is LEAST likely to lead to a wrong dose error?
    a. 4 mg
    b. .4g
    c. 4U
    d. 4.0 units

13. Using abbreviations that have been published in reputable medical journals is acceptable because only widely accepted abbreviations are used in publications.
    a. True
    b. False

14. Identify four things from the order in figure 17-8 that could contribute to a medication error.

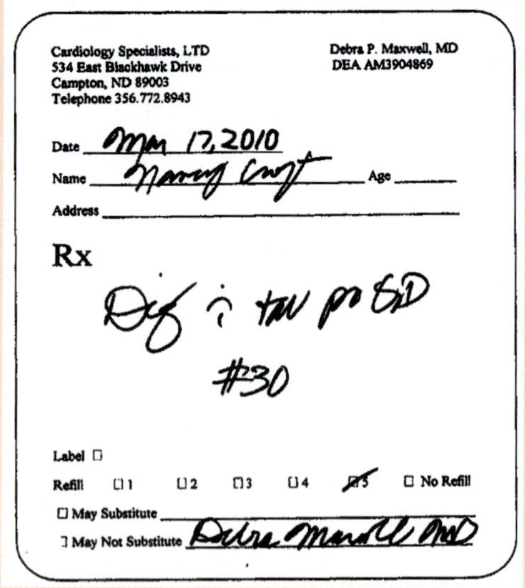
Cardiology Specialists, LTD
534 East Blackhawk Drive
Campton, ND 89003
Telephone 356.772.8943

Debra P. Maxwell, MD
DEA AM3904869

Date ______
Name ______ Age ______
Address ______

Rx

#30

Label ☐
Refill ☐1 ☐2 ☐3 ☐4 ☐5 ☐ No Refill
☐ May Substitute ______
☐ May Not Substitute ______

Figure 17-8. Prescription to use when answering question 14.

Self-Assessment Questions

15. One morning you are busy preparing IVPB antibiotic orders for the 1000 delivery. The orders are:

    Pat Carlson Cefazolin 1 g IVPB every 8 hr

    Paul Cariton Ceftazidime 1 g IVPB every 8 hr

    You decide to prepare both orders simultaneously to save time and avoid missing the delivery.

    List four reasons why the risk of making an error this morning is increased.

16. Name at least five things the pharmaceutical manufacturer could do to improve labeling of the new drug product shown in figure 17-9.

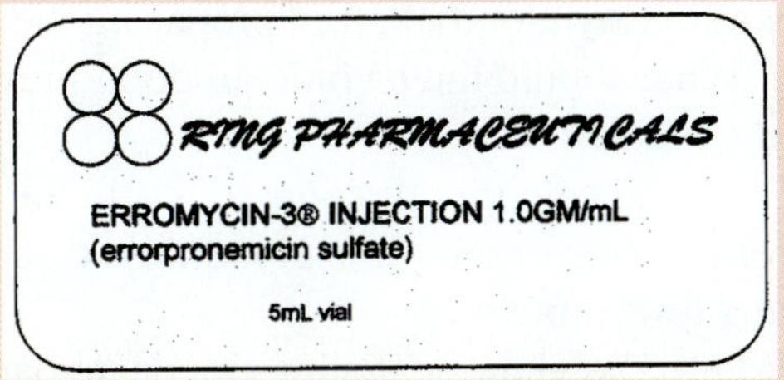

Figure 17-9. Drug product label for question 16.

17. Which of the following statements are TRUE regarding the practice of color coding drug product packaging and its relationship to medication errors?
    a. Color coding the vial caps red for all injectable solutions that turn red upon reconstitution would decrease the likelihood of medication errors.
    b. Developing a color coding scheme unique to a specific manufacturer would decrease the likelihood of a mediation error.
    c. Color coding saves time because you do not have to read the product label.
    d. In general, color coding is an unsafe practice.

18. Which could be considered a contributing factor(s) to medication errors?
    a. Performing routine maintenance procedures on the tablet counting machine
    b. Failing to read current pharmacy literature about new drug products
    c. Scheduling additional staff to work during periods of heavy workload
    d. Always using leading zeros

19. Why are published medication error rates probably underestimated?
    a. Only errors that result in patient injury are reported
    b. Some errors go undetected
    c. Few errors are identified and corrected during the prescribing phase
    d. Efficient anonymous reporting systems are common

20. Which of the following statements is TRUE regarding the impact of medication errors on health care expenses?
    a. Medication errors are usually insignificant, easily corrected, and inexpensive.
    b. Medical costs for treating negative outcomes due to medication errors are usually paid for by the health care worker responsible for the error.
    c. Health care expenses associated with medication errors cost billions of dollars each year.
    d. Malpractice claims for medication errors are usually dismissed in court.

21. Omission errors are less likely to result in negative outcomes than improper dose errors because the patient is not receiving a harmful dose.

    True or False

22. Lisa Kim, a technician working in the unit dose cartfill area, notices the 25 mg and 50 mg strengths of diphenhydramine (Benadryl) are mixed together in the same storage bin. What can Lisa do to correct this problem?
    a. Make no changes, because technicians are responsible for reading labels carefully and will notice the different strengths
    b. Modify the stock shelf so each strength has its own section or bin

Self-Assessment Questions

c. Change the label to indicate that both strengths are in the bin
d. Store the 25 mg capsule under "Benadryl" and the 50 mg capsule under "Diphenhydramine"

23. A technician compounds a continuous infusion of heparin 25,000 units in 500 mL of 5% Dextrose in Water (D5W) and places the bag on the counter for the pharmacist to check. The technician then begins to fill other medication orders. One of the orders the technician fills is for two heparin 5,000 unit syringes for subcutaneous injection. The technician notices the same patient name on the continuous infusion label and the subcutaneous injection labels. What should the technician do?
    a. Fill the medication orders and assume the pharmacist will notice the duplication
    b. Inform the pharmacist that both heparin prescriptions have the same patient name and ask if both orders are correct
    c. Ask another technician what the standard dose of heparin is and fill both orders
    d. Check the patient's medication profile and fill both orders for heparin

24. A technician fills a medication order for a 20 mg prednisone tablet with a propranolol 20 mg tablet. The pharmacy technician supervisor notices the error before the pharmacist checks all the filled medication orders. What should the technician supervisor do to prevent the wrong medication from leaving the pharmacy?
    a. Tactfully call the error to the attention of the technician who made the error and ask him to correct it
    b. Quickly correct the mistake before the pharmacist also notices the error
    c. Don't tell the technician to avoid embarrassment
    d. Leave it up to the pharmacist to find and correct the error

25. A newly employed technician begins training in the pharmacy. A senior technician is assigned to discuss technician responsibilities with the new employee. Which of the following ideas can the senior technician discuss or demonstrate that can prevent medication errors?
    a. Discuss experiences the senior technician has had with making and preventing medication errors
    b. Demonstrate the use of the credit card verification machine
    c. Demonstrate how to fill medication orders and talk on the telephone at the same time
    d. Medication error prevention should not be discussed because the employee is new

26. A technician compounding an IV preparation of calcium gluconate and 5% Dextrose in Water (D5W) notices the calcium gluconate injection looks slightly cloudy before preparing the IV bag. What should the technician do to prevent a medication error?
    a. Place the calcium gluconate vials in the refrigerator to see if the cloudiness disappears in a few minutes
    b. Return the vial of calcium gluconate back to the shelf and use another vial that looks clear
    c. Place the calcium gluconate vial in a tub of warm water for fifteen minutes
    d. Inform the pharmacist that the calcium gluconate vials look cloudy and inspect all the calcium gluconate vials in stock

27. Nancy Andrews, a pharmacy technician, notices that the carvedilol tablets in the automated counting machine are almost gone. She also notices that there are no more carvedilol tablets in the pharmacy to restock the machine. What is the next action she can take to reduce the chance of a medication error?
    a. Inform the technician on the next shift that the carvedilol tablets are almost gone
    b. Remind herself to order carvedilol tablets the next time she is scheduled to work
    c. Inform the pharmacist that the pharmacy is almost out of carvedilol tablets
    d. Determine the immediate needs of the patients and inform the purchasing personnel of the situation

Self-Assessment Questions

28. Match the medications in the first column that are commonly mistaken with the ones in the second column:

Hydroxyzine 25 mg tablet	Percodan tablet
Potassium Chloride 20 mEq injection	Quinidine 200 mg tablet
Desipramine 25 mg tablet	Lidocaine 1 g prefilled syringe
Quinine 200 mg capsule	Dimenhydrinate 50 mg capsule
Epinephrine 1:1000 injection	Hydralazine 25 mg tablet
Percocet tablet	Furosemide 20 mg injection
Diphenhydramine 50 mg capsule	Imipramine 25 mg tablet
Lidocaine 100 mg prefilled syringe	Epinephrine 1:10,000 injection

29. The pharmacy receives a prescription for hydrocortisone 2.5% cream. The technician notices the pharmacy is out of stock of the cream. The pharmacy can substitute hydrocortisone 2.5% ointment without calling the doctor.
    a. True
    b. False
30. A nurse discovers that the continuous infusion of IV fluids being administered to Mr. Williams contains potassium chloride 40 mEq. Because of Mr. Williams' kidney problems, the IV fluids prescribed for him were supposed to be without potassium chloride. After the nurse discontinues the incorrect bag and hangs the correct fluids (without potassium), the nurse is required to call the physician.
    a. True
    b. False
31. A pharmacy technician notices that two different looking tablets are mixed together in the ciprofloxacin 500 mg tablet bin in the automated counting machine. The filling log indicates that the machine was refilled the day before and the lot number is significantly different than the previous refill log entries. What should the technician do?
    a. Remove the tablets that look different and discard them
    b. Nothing—assume the manufacturer has changed the look of the tablets
    c. Inform the pharmacist of the situation immediately
    d. Nothing—the person who refilled the machine rarely makes mistakes
32. A pharmacy technician supervisor notices several technicians making the same calculation error. At the next staff meeting, the supervisor discusses the errors with the group without mentioning who made the mistakes. The supervisor also demonstrates how to perform the calculations correctly. This practice can help prevent medication errors.
    a. True
    b. False
33. The purpose of a national medication error reporting program is to share experiences among health care personnel so patient safety can be improved. It also can contribute to educational efforts to prevent future medication errors.
    a. True
    b. False
34. Name at least five departments or members of a quality assurance committee that are responsible for reviewing reports of medication errors.
35. Name three ways a pharmacy can educate the staff about actual medication errors on a continuous basis.
36. Technicians and pharmacists can be held legally responsible for a medication error that causes harm to a patient.
    a. True
    b. False

Self-Assessment Answers

1. False. A medication error can occur any time during the medication use process—prescribing, transcription, dispensing, or administration—and can be made by anyone involved in the medication use process, including physicians, nurses, pharmacy staff, patients, or their caregivers.
2. d. Verbally transmitted orders can easily be misunderstood, especially with the number of sound-alike drug names on the market. In this case, the order was verbally communicated twice—from the physician to the nurse and then again to the pharmacist.
3. a. Undiluted potassium chloride injection should never be injected directly into a patient's vein because of the potential for an irregular heartbeat and possibly death. The USP implemented this labeling requirement in response to the many potassium chloride injection errors reported.
4. a. Patients have a responsibility in the medication use process to take their medication as instructed. Not taking the entire prescription could have led to inadequate treatment, with symptoms reappearing a short time later. The newer, more costly agent may have been prescribed because the physician was not aware that Ms. Banks had stopped taking her amoxicillin after three days. This may have led the physician to believe that amoxicillin was ineffective and an alternate agent was required. It is assumed that the pharmacist counseled Ms. Banks adequately when the amoxicillin was dispensed.
5. b. Technicians should not feel intimidated about questioning a pharmacist if something does not seem right. Pharmacists make errors just like everyone else.
6. b. The error was made because Levoxyl (levothyroxine) was poorly written by the prescriber and misread as Lanoxin (digoxin).
7. c. An omission error occurred because the 0900 dose was not administered until the next scheduled dose was due. The patient would likely receive only two doses that day instead of three.
8. d. Improper dose error is the best classification for this error. The patient would have received 40 mg instead of the 10 mg prescribed. The 40 mg/mL gentamicin could have been used to prepare the IVPB accurately; however, by using 0.25 mL instead of 1 mL this could be classified as a calculation error.
9. a. Failure to rotate stock can result in drugs with longer expiration dates being used first. Older drugs on the back of the shelf may expire before being used.
10. False. Number of years of pharmacy experience does not correlate with frequency of calculation errors.
11. d. All examples can lead to calculation errors.
12. a. The amount ".4 g" could be interpreted as 4 g and would best be written as 0.4 g or 400 mg. Both c and d would be best written as "4 units." Abbreviations should be avoided whenever possible because the "U" in "4U" could be read as "40." Trailing zeros after the decimal point should be avoided for the same reason.
13. False. Many times authors make up abbreviations for disease states or drug names/combinations to avoid having to write out lengthy terms numerous times. This practice is acceptable when writing an article for publication, provided the full term is spelled out the first time the abbreviation is used. It is not an acceptable practice for writing medication orders or prescription labels.
14. 1. The use of "dig" as an abbreviation for digoxin
    2. "QD" could be interpreted as QID, OD, or QOD and should therefore be written out as "daily"
    3. "1 tab" is not appropriate because digoxin is available in two strengths
    4. Poor handwriting
15. 1. The drug names are similar
    2. More than one order is being prepared at the same time
    3. The patients' names are similar
    4. It is a rushed work environment
16. 1. Make the manufacturer name/logo less prominent (smaller)
    2. Omit the trailing zero in the concentration strength
    3. Enlarge the total contents of the vial

4. Enlarge the drug name
5. Change the trade name to something that does not sound like erythromycin or E-Mycin
6. Use "g" as the abbreviation for gram

17. d. Matching vial cap colors with solution colors would not aid drug identification. Color coding unique to a manufacturer would be confusing, as manufacturers may change with each new drug purchasing contract. Drug product labels should always be read carefully.
18. b. Technicians have a responsibility to continuously learn about new drugs and therapies.
19. b. There is no way to account for errors that are not detected. Reasons might be that errors that are corrected before the drug is administered to the patient are frequently not reported, and health care personnel may be uncomfortable reporting errors.
20. c. Costs of treating adverse events caused by medication errors, out-of-court settlements, and legal fees add up to billions of dollars annually.
21. False. Omission errors can be just as dangerous as wrong dose errors, because the medical treatment for which the drug is prescribed has been withheld.
22. b. Medications with the same generic name but different strengths should be stored in separate bins next to each other on the shelf. There is an increased chance of error when different strengths are stored together in the same bin.
23. b. The technician should question the pharmacist about the duplicate orders. One order may have been for another patient, or an order to discontinue the continuous infusion may have been overlooked.
24. a. The second technician should tactfully point out the error to the first technician and allow the first technician to correct it. This gives the first technician a chance to learn from the mistake and may prevent similar mistakes in the future. Checking the stock bin to see if additional propranolol tablets were incorrectly placed in the prednisone bin can also prevent future mistakes.
25. a. Generally, discussing previous medication errors and error correction from a senior technician's experience can help teach the new technician about medication errors. Answer c is wrong because it is important to concentrate on correctly filling medication orders without doing two things at once. Performing one task at a time can reduce the chance of medication errors.
26. d. The technician has a responsibility to be observant and inform the pharmacist about any potential medication errors. The technician should compound this IV admixture only if the calcium gluconate looks clear. The technician also has the responsibility to alert appropriate personnel so that all calcium gluconate vials in the pharmacy can be inspected for the cloudy appearance.
27. d. The technician has the responsibility to make sure the pharmacy has enough carvedilol capsules to prevent patients from missing their scheduled doses. If the pharmacy runs out of a medication, an error of omission may occur.
28. Hydroxyzine—Hydralazine

    Potassium Chloride—Furosemide

    Desipramine—Imipramine

    Quinine—Quinidine

    Epinephrine—Epinephrine

    Percocet—Percodan

    Diphenhydramine—Dimenhydrinate

    Lidocaine—Lidocaine
29. False. The physician must be contacted, and the prescription would need to be changed with physician approval before the ointment can be dispensed. Dispensing a cream instead of an ointment, or vice versa, is a common mistake. In many cases, the packaging only differs by one word (ointment or cream). Many pharmacies store ointments separately from creams in an effort to prevent mistakes.
30. True. The nurse should immediately contact the physician and inform the physician about the medication error. The physician will determine if further action is needed.
31. c. Inform the pharmacist of the situation immediately. The pharmacist can help investigate and provide direction according to established policies and procedures.

32. True. This practice can educate the staff about the correct way to make the calculation and prevent future medication errors.

33. True. The FDA MedWatch Program is an example of a national program.

34. The committee should have representatives from pharmacy, medicine, nursing, risk management, quality assurance, those involved in staff education, and legal counsel.

35. The pharmacy can educate staff about actual medication errors with periodic newsletters, educational programs, and by reviewing medication error reports at staff meetings.

36. True. Technicians and pharmacists both contribute to the safe use of medications by the public. If their actions result in patient harm, they may be held legally liable for their actions, along with the institution and others involved.

Resources

American Society of Hospital Pharmacists. ASHP guidelines on preventing medication errors in hospitals. *Am J Hosp Pharm.* 1993;50:305–14.

Manasse, Jr HR, Thompson KK, eds. *Medication Safety: A Guide for Health Care Facilities.* Bethesda, MD: American Society of Health-System Pharmacists, Inc; 2005.

Bates DW. Preventing medication errors: A summary. *Am J Health-Syst Pharm.* 2007;64(S9):S3–9.

Brennan TA, Leape LL, Laird NM et al. Incidence of adverse events and negligence in hospitalized patients–results of the Harvard medical practice study I. *N Engl J Med.* 1991;324: 370–6.

Cohen JR, Anderson RW, Attilio RM et al. Preventing medication errors in cancer chemotherapy. *Am J Health-Syst Pharm.* 1996;53:737–46.

Cohen MR, Senders J, Davis NM. Failure mode and effects analysis: a novel approach to avoiding dangerous medication errors and accidents. *Hosp Pharm.* 1994;29:319–24, 326–28, 330.

Cohen MR, ed. *Medication Errors.* 2nd ed. Washington, DC: American Pharmaceutical Association; 2007.

Johnson JA, Bootman JL. Drug-related morbidity and mortality and the economic impact of pharmaceutical care. *Am J Health-Syst Pharm.* 1997;54:554–8.

Kistner UA, Keith MR, Sergeant KA et al. Accuracy of dispensing in a high-volume, hospital-based outpatient pharmacy. *Am J Hosp Pharm.* 1994;51:2793–7.

Allan EL, Barker KN. Fundamentals of medication error research. *Am J Hosp Pharm.* 1990;47:555–71.

Kenagy JW, Stein GC. Naming, labeling, and packaging of pharmaceuticals. *Am J Health-Syst Pharm.* 2001;58:2033–41.

Recommended Web Sites

American Society of Health-System Pharmacists (ASHP): www.ashp.org

MedWatch: The FDA Safety Information and Adverse Event Reporting Program: www.fda.gov/Safety/MedWatch/default.htm

Name Differentiation Project: www.fda.gov/Drugs/DrugSafety/MedicationErrors/ucm164587.htm

FDA MedWatch Safety Information and Adverse Event Online Reporting Form: www.fda.gov/downloads/Safety/MedWatch/DownloadForms/UCM082725.pdf

Institute for Safe Medication Practice (ISMP): www.ismp.org

ISMP Medication Errors Reporting Program (MERP): https://www.ismp.org/orderforms/reporterrortoISMP.asp (to report an error online)

The Joint Commission: www.jointcommission.org

The Joint Commission National Patient Safety Goals: www.jointcommission.org/patientsafety/nationalpatientsafetygoals/

United States Pharmacopeia: www.usp.org

References

1. ASHP Report. Suggested definitions and relationships among medication misadventure, medication errors,

adverse drug events, and adverse drug reactions. *Am J Health-Syst Pharm.* 1998;55:165–6.
2. American Society of Hospital Pharmacists. ASHP guideline on preventing medication errors in hospitals. *Am J Hosp Pharm.* 1993;50:305–14.
3. National Association of Chain Drug Stores. 2008 community pharmacy results. Available from: http://www.nacds.org/user-assets/pdfs/pharmacy/2008CommunityPharmacyResults.pdf Accessed June 26,2010.
4. Brennan TA, Leape LL, Laird NM et al. Incidence of adverse events and negligence in hospitalized patients—results of the Harvard medical practice study I. *N Engl J Med.* 1991;324:370–6.
5. Lesar TS, Briceland LL, Delcoure K et al. Medication prescribing errors in a teaching hospital. *JAMA.* 1990;263:2329–34.
6. Rupp MT, DeYoung M, Schondelmeyer SW. Prescribing problems and pharmacist interventions in community practice. *Medical Care.* 1992;30:926–40.
7. Blum KV, Abel SR, Urbanski CJ et al. Medication error prevention by pharmacists. *Am J Hosp Pharm.* 1988;45:902–3.
8. Dean B, Schachter M, Vincet C et al. Causes of prescribing errors in hospital inpatients: a prospective study. *Lancet.* 2002;359:1373–8.
9. Bates DW, Cullen DJ, Laird N et al. Incidence of adverse drug events and potential adverse drug events. *JAMA.* 1995;274:29–34.
10. Guernsey BG, Ingrim NB, Kokanson JA et al. Pharmacists' dispensing accuracy in a high-volume outpatient pharmacy service: focus on risk management. *Drug Intell Clin Pharm.* 1993;17:42–6.
11. Kistner UA, Keith MR, Sergeant KA et al. Accuracy of dispensing in a high-volume, hospital-based outpatient pharmacy. *Am J Hosp Pharm.* 1994;51:2793–7.
12. Allan EL, Barker KN. Fundamentals of medication error research. *Am J Hosp Pharm.* 1990;47:55–71.
13. Barker KN, Flynn EA, Pepper GA et al. Medication errors observed in 36 health care facilities. *Arch Intern Med.* 2002;162:1897–1903.
14. Institute of Medicine. *Preventing medication errors: quality chasm series.* Washington, DC: National Academy Press; 2006.
15. Bates DW, Boyle DL, Vander Vliet MB et al. Relationship between medication errors and adverse drug events. *J Gen Intern Med.* 1995;10:199–205.
16. Leape LL. Error in medicine. *JAMA.* 1994;272:1851–7.
17. Phillips J, Beam S, Brinker A et al. Retrospective analysis of mortalities associated with medication errors. *Am J Health-Syst Pharm.* 2001;58:1835–41.
18. Kaufman A, Kung FH, Koenig HM et al. Overdosage with vincristine. *J Pediatr.* 1976;89:671–4.
19. Davis NM. Preventing omission errors. *Am J Nursing.* 1995;95:17.
20. Classen DC, Pestotnik SL, Evans RS et al. Adverse drug events in hospitalized patients. *JAMA.* 1997;277:301–6.
21. Schneider PJ, Gift MG, Lee Y et al. Cost of medication-related problems at a university hospital. *Am J Health-Syst Pharm.* 1995;52:2415–8.
22. Johnson JA, Bootman JL. Drug-related morbidity and mortality. A cost of illness model. *Arch Intern Med.* 1995;55:1949–56.
23. Department of Health & Human Services. Patient Safety: CMS initiatives addressing never events. Available at: http://www.cms.hhs.gov/SMDL/downloads/SMD073108.pdf. Accessed May 10, 2010.
24. Lesar TS, Briceland L, Stein DS. Factors related to errors in medication prescribing. *JAMA.* 1997;277:312–17.
25. Koren G, Barzilay Z, Modan M. Errors in computing drug doses. *Can Med Assoc J.* 1983;129:721–3.
26. Bindler R, Bayne T. Medication calculation ability of registered nurses. *IMAGE: J Nursing Scholarship.* 1991;23:221–4.
27. Glover ML, Sussmane JB. Assessing pediatrics residents' mathematical skills for prescribing medication: a need for improved training. *Academic Medicine.* 2002;77:1007–10.
28. The Joint Commission. The official "*Do Not Use List*" of abbreviations. Available at: http://www.jointcommission.org/PatientSafety/DoNotUseList. Accessed May 10, 2010.
29. Institute for Safe Medication Practices. List of error-prone abbreviations/symbols and dose designations. Available at: http://www.ismp.org/Tools/errorproneabbreviations.pdf. Accessed May 10, 2010.
30. Joint Commission. 2009 National Patient Safety Goals. Available at: http://jointcommission.org/NR/rdonlyres/31666E86-E7F4-423E-9BE8-F05BD1CB0AA8/0/HAP_npsg.pdf. Accessed May 10, 2010.
31. Robertson WO. Alphabet soup: more or less? *JAMA.* 1980;244:1902. Letter.
32. Institute for Safe Medication Practices. High alert medications. Available at: www.ismp.org/Tools/highalertmedications.pdf. Accessed May 10, 2010.
33. Allinson RR, Szeinbach SL, Schneider PJ. Perceived accuracy of drug orders transmitted orally by telephone. *Am J Health-Syst Pharm.* 2005;62:78–83.
34. Institute for Safe Medication Practices. *Sound-alike names. ISMP Medication Safety Alert.* 2007;12(24):1.
35. Davis NM. Confusion over illegible orders. *Am J Nursing.* 1994;94(1):9.
36. Cohen JR, Anderson RW, Attilio RM et al. Preventing medication errors in cancer chemotherapy. *Am J Health-Syst Pharm.* 1996;53:737–46.
37. Kenagy JW, Stein GC. Naming, labeling, and packaging of pharmaceuticals. *Am J Health-Syst Pharm.* 2001;58:2033–41.

38. Davis NM. A well-informed patient is a valuable asset. *Am J Nursing.* 1994;94:16.
39. Rodriquez G, Poretsky L. Toradol instead of tapazole. *Am J Health-Syst Pharm.* 1995;52:1098. Letter.
40. Pourmotabbed G. The naming of drugs is a difficult matter. *N Engl J Med.* 1994;331:1163.
41. Chu G, Mantin R, Shen Y et al. Massive cisplatin overdose by accidental substitution for carboplatin. *Cancer.* 1993;72:3707–14.
42. Malcolm KE, Hogan TT, Wyatt TL. Is the prescription really for selegiline? *Am J Hosp Pharm.* 1994;51:930. Letter.
43. Cohen MR, Davis NM. Trademark similarities can cause problems. *Am Pharm.* 1993;NS33:16–7.
44. United States Pharmacopeia. USP's drug error finder. Available at: http://www.usp.org/hqi/similarProducts/drugErrorFinderTool.html. Accessed May 10, 2010.
45. Institute for Safe Medication Practices. ISMP's list of confused drug names. Available at: http://www.ismp.org/Tools/confuseddrugnames.pdf. Accessed May 10, 2010.
46. Raffalli J, Nowakowski J, Wormser GP. "Vira something": a taste of the wrong medicine. *Lancet.* 1997;350:887. Letter.
47. Cousins DD, Heath WM eds. Stop, look and listen: highlights of USP's 8th annual MEDMARX data report related to look-alike, sound-alike drug errors. Available at http://www.usp.org/pdf/EN/patientSafety/capsLink2008-04-01.pdf. Accessed May 10, 2010.
48. Food and Drug Administration. Consumer updates: drugs. Available at: http://www.fda.gov/ForConsumers/ConsumerUpdates/ucm048644.htm. Accessed June 26, 2010.
49. Lawyer C, Despot J. 'Z-Pak' vs ice pack: need for clarity and continuous quality assurance. *JAMA.* 1997;278:1405. Letter.
50. Rheinstein PH, McGinnis TJ. Medication errors. *Am Fam Physician.* 1992;45:2720–22.
51. A spectrum of problems with using color. http://ismp.org/Newsletters/acutecare/articles/20031113.asp Accessed May 10, 2010.
52. Buchanan TL, Barker KN, Gibson JT et al. Illumination and errors in dispensing. *Am J Hosp Pharm.* 1991;48:2137–45.
53. Flynn EA, Barker KN, Gibson JT et al. Impact of interruptions and distractions on dispensing errors in an ambulatory care pharmacy. *Am J Health-Syst Pharm.* 1999;56:1319–1325.
54. Gold DR, Rogacz S, Bock N et al. Rotating shift work, sleep and accidents related to sleepiness in hospital nurses. *Am J Public Health.* 1992;82:1011–4.
55. Hicks RW, Cousins DD, Williams RL. Selected medication-error data from USP's MEDMARX program for 2002. *Am J Health-Syst Phar.* 2004;61:993–1000.
56. Leape LL, Bates DW, Cullen DJ et al. Systems analysis of adverse drug events. *JAMA.* 1995;274:35–43.
57. Maviglia SV, Yoo JY, Franz C et al. Cost-benefit analysis of a hospital pharmacy bar code solution. *Arch Intern Med.* 2007;167:788–94.
58. Helmons PJ, Wargel LN, Daniels CE. Effect of bar-code-assisted medication administration on medication administration errors and accuracy in multiple patient care areas. *Am J Health-Syst Pharm.* 2009;66:1202–10.
59. DeYoung JL, VanderKooi ME, Barletta JF. Effect of bar-code-assisted medication administration on medication error rates in an adult medical intensive care unit. *Am J Health-Syst Pharm.* 2009;66:1110–15.
60. Poon EG, Cina JL, Churchill W et al. Medication dispensing errors and potential adverse drug events before and after implementing bar code technology in the pharmacy. *Ann Intern Med.* 2006;145:426–34.
61. Pedersen CA, Schneider PJ, Scheckelhoff DJ. ASHP national survey of pharmacy practice in hospital settings: dispensing and administration-2008. *Am J Health-Syst Pharm.* 2009;66:926–46.
62. Cohen MR, Senders J, Davis NM. Failure mode and effects analysis: a novel approach to avoiding dangerous medication errors and accidents. *Hosp Pharm.* 1994;29:319–24, 326–28, 330.
63. Williams E, Talley R. The use of failure mode effect and criticality analysis in a medication error subcommittee. *Hosp Pharm.* 1994;29:331–2, 334–7.
64. Adachi W, Lodolce AE. Use of failure mode and effects analysis in improving the safety of i.v. drug administration. *Am J Health-Syst Pharm.* 2005;62:917–20.
65. Borel JM, Rascati KL. Effect of an automated, nursing unit-based drug dispensing device on medication errors. *Am J Health-Syst Pharm.* 1995;52:1875–9.
66. Bates DW, Leape LL, Cullen DJ et al. Effect of computerized physician order entry and a team intervention on prevention of serious medication errors. *JAMA.* 1998;280:1311–16.
67. Raschke RA, Gollihare B, Wunderlich RA et al. A computer alert system to prevent injury from adverse drug events: development and evaluation in a community teaching hospital. *JAMA.* 1998;280:1317–20.
68. Kaushal R, Shojania KG, Bates DW. Effects of computerized physician order entry and clinical decision support systems on medication safety: A systematic review. *Arch Intern Med.* 2003;163:1409–1416.
69. Koppel R, Metlay JP, Cohen A et al. Role of computerized physician order entry systems in facilitating medication errors. *JAMA.* 2005;293:1197–1203.
70. Santell JP, Kowiatik JG, Weber RJ et al. Medication errors resulting from computer entry by nonprecribers. *Am J Health-Syst Pharm.* 2009;66:843–53.

71. Zhan C, Hicks RW, Blanchette CM et al. Potential benefits and problems with computerized prescriber and order entry: analysis of a voluntary medication error-reporting database. *Am J Health-Syst Pharm.* 2006;63:353–58.
72. Cohen MR. Risk management of medication errors must include a careful look at the specific systems involved. *Hosp Pharm.* 1996;31:454, 458, 461–2.
73. Brushwood DB. Patient injury and attempted link with pharmacist's negligence. *Am J Hosp Pharm.* 1993;50:2382–5.
74. Brodie DC. *The Challenge to Pharmacy in Times of Change—A Report of the Commission on Pharmaceutical Services to Ambulant Patients by Hospitals and Related Facilities*. Washington, DC: American Pharmaceutical Association and American Society of Hospital Pharmacists; 1966.

Part Four

Business Applications

This section includes the chapters related to the business end of the practice of pharmacy, including purchasing, inventory, billing and reimbursement of products and services. There is also a chapter on Durable and Nondurable Medical Equipment in this section since many pharmacies offer these products for their patients.

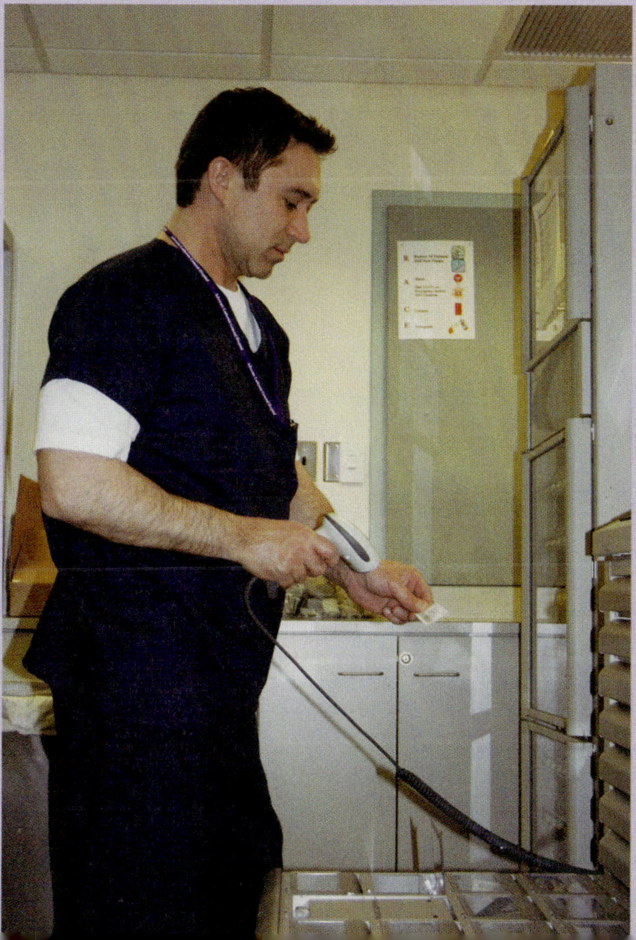

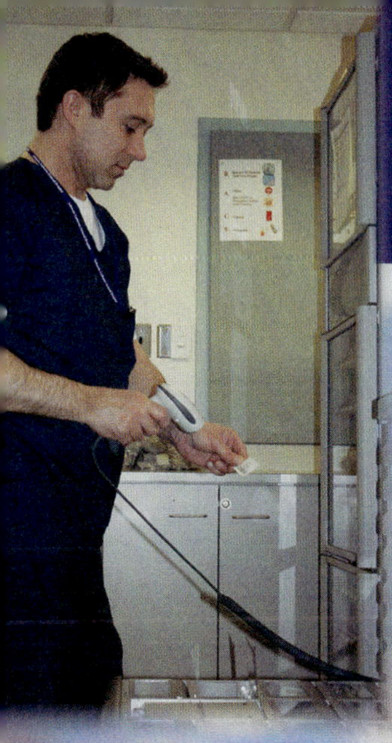

Chapter 18

Durable and Nondurable Medical Equipment, Devices, and Supplies

Daphne E. Smith-Marsh

Learning Outcomes

After this chapter you will be able to:

- Describe the characteristics of durable and nondurable medical equipment.
- Identify the various types of blood glucose meters and continuous glucose monitoring systems.
- Describe the steps in measuring blood glucose.
- Describe the nondurable medical supplies used in insulin delivery, blood glucose, and lab monitoring.
- Explain the methods of insulin delivery using syringes, continuous infusion pumps, and insulin pens.
- Identify the various types of blood pressure monitors and explain the methods of measuring blood pressure.
- Identify commonly used pedometers and heart rate monitors.
- List the advantages and disadvantages of home diagnostic products and identify commonly used products.
- Identify orthopedic support products.
- Describe the purpose of ostomy products.

Key Terms

aneroid blood pressure monitor Type of monitor that indicates varying blood pressure using a pointer in a gauge.

CLIA-waived The Clinical Laboratory Improvement Amendment of 1988 established that some clinical tests be exempted from certain laboratory requirements.

colostomy Surgical formation of an artificial anus by connecting the colon to an opening in the abdominal wall.

continuous subcutaneous insulin infusion Delivery of insulin through a pump device that provides the medication 24 hours a day.

control solution A type of solution that mimics blood and that is used to test the accuracy of a blood glucose meter and test strips.

durable medical equipment Reusable equipment used for the treatment of illness or injury (e.g. wheelchairs, walkers, blood glucose meters).

hemoglobin A1c Blood test that measures the amount of glucose attached to hemoglobin in red blood cells. Provides an estimate of blood glucose control over the previous 2–3 months.

insulin pen Portable device that contains a prefilled cartridge of insulin.

lancet A sharp-pointed instrument used to make small incisions, commonly used to obtain blood samples for blood glucose monitoring.

nondurable medical equipment Single-use equipment for a medical purpose (e.g. gloves, dressings, syringes and needles).

orthotic Device designed for the support of weak or ineffective joints or muscles.

orthopedic devices Equipment used for a deformity, disorder, or injury of skeleton and associated structures.

orthotic devices Equipment that can prevent or correct a physical deformity or malfunction, or that can support a weak or deformed portion of the body.

ostomy An operation (as a colostomy, ileostomy, or urostomy) to create an artificial passage for bodily elimination.

pedometer An instrument that records the distance a person covers on foot by responding to the body motion at each step.

stoma An artificial permanent opening, especially in the abdominal wall, made in surgical procedures.

test strip Specifically designed strip with reagent used to measure blood glucose.

urostomy An ostomy for the elimination of urine from the body.

Durable medical equipment, devices, and supplies are reusable products, used for the treatment of an illness or injury, that are typically ordered by a physician or other health care provider for use in a patient's place of residence.[1,2] Nondurable medical equipment, devices, and supplies are manufactured for one-time use only and are disposable. This chapter introduces common durable and nondurable medical equipment, used for monitoring blood glucose and blood pressure, and the administration of insulin through insulin pumps and insulin pens. Select heart rate monitors, pedometers, home diagnostic products, orthopedic devices, and ostomy products are also described. Certain types of durable and nondurable medical equipment and supplies are available in pharmacies. A 2008 survey of independent community pharmacists reports that 40% of those pharmacists provided durable medical equipment to patients.[3] Pharmacy technicians in various practice settings should be able to identify durable and nondurable medical equipment and supplies.

Durable and Nondurable Medical Equipment

Medicare defines **durable medical equipment (DME)** as medical supplies that are

- able to withstand repeated use
- primarily and customarily used to serve a medical purpose
- generally not useful to a person in the absence of an illness or injury
- appropriate for use in the home

This equipment is also known as durable medical equipment, prosthetics, orthotics, and supplies.[4-6] The elderly and persons with physical disabilities may need to use durable medical equipment to improve mobility. Wheelchairs, walkers, canes, and crutches are types of durable medical equipment that are used as mobility aids. Durable medical equipment can be used to monitor vital signs, such as blood glucose, blood pressure, and heart rate, or can be used to administer medications, such as a nebulizer or an infusion pump.

Nondurable medical equipment consists of medical supplies that must be discarded after use and often can be used at home or in a medical facility. Examples of commonly used durable and nondurable medical equipment are listed in Table 18-1.

Table 18-1. Common Durable and Nondurable Medical Equipment

Durable Medical Equipment		Nondurable Medical Equipment
Wheelchairs	Home oxygen equipment	Exam gloves
Walkers	Hospital beds	Diapers
Canes	Infusion pumps	Absorbent bed pads
Crutches	Braces	Insulin syringes and pen needles
Scooters	Blood glucose meters	Blood glucose test strips and lancets
Suction pumps	Blood pressure monitors	Dressing materials (bandages, gauze dressings, tape)
Commode and shower chairs	Nebulizers	Ostomy supplies

The Role of the Pharmacy Technician

Pharmacies that supply durable medical equipment, prosthetics, orthotics, and supplies can provide an important service for patients. The use of durable and nondurable medical equipment can improve a patient's quality of life. Persons with impaired mobility often use durable medical equipment. Patients who have diabetes or hypertension can self-monitor their blood glucose and blood pressure at home with medical equipment. The pharmacist can provide education for the use of medical equipment.

✔ The pharmacy technician can assist the pharmacist in maintaining adequate supplies and equipment and be involved in the process of billing insurance for these items.

Billing and Reimbursement

The Centers for Medicare and Medicaid Services require that all suppliers of durable medical equipment, prosthetics, orthotics, and supplies be accredited to bill Medicare Part B. As of January 1, 2010, pharmacies that supply this type of equipment must be Medicare accredited.[7] Medicare Part B covers 80% of this type of equipment and supplies. The patient must pay 20%, the remaining cost. Persons with Medicaid can have their 20% coinsurance covered. For more information, refer to Chapter 20, Billing and Reimbursement.

Clinical Laboratory Improvement Amendments Act (CLIA)

Several devices that are introduced in this chapter are classified as **CLIA-waived** products. The Clinical Laboratory Improvement Amendments Act of 1988 (CLIA) established that some clinical tests could be waived from certain laboratory requirements. On February 28, 1992, regulations were published stating that waived tests were defined as simple laboratory examinations and procedures that are approved by the Food and Drug Administration (FDA) for home use.[8] Therefore, certain home diagnostic tests using blood or urine samples can be used without maintaining requirements as strict as those for laboratory tests.

Durable and nondurable medical equipment and supplies are commonly used in the management of certain diseases, such as diabetes mellitus. Diabetes mellitus is a disease in which there are elevated levels of glucose (sugar) in the blood, which is caused by insulin deficiency and/or insulin resistance (the body not using insulin properly). Diabetes is a prevalent disease; there are currently 23.6 million persons in the United States with diabetes, which is approximately 7.8% of the U.S. population.[9] In 2007, the estimation of health care costs for the treatment of diabetes was $174 billion.[9] There are 57 million Americans who have pre-diabetes, which places them at risk for developing diabetes in the future.[9] Blood glucose monitoring and insulin therapy are commonly used to manage diabetes and incorporate the use of specific durable and nondurable medical equipment and supplies.

Blood Glucose Monitoring

Blood glucose meters are used to monitor blood glucose, which is also called blood sugar. Self-monitoring of blood glucose provides valuable information to evaluate the impact of lifestyle changes and/or medication therapy in a person with diabetes. Maintaining blood glucose levels that are near normal minimizes complications of diabetes, such as an increase risk of heart disease, stroke, blindness, kidney failure, nerve damage, and amputations. According to the American Diabetes Association, plasma blood glucose levels before meals should be 70–130 mg/dL and <180 mg/dL 1–2 hours after meals.[9] Blood glucose readings that are consistently higher than goal levels increase the risk of complications.

✔ Monitoring blood glucose is very important to determine if diabetes is under control. Hyperglycemia (high blood glucose) and hypoglycemia (low blood glucose) can be identified with the use of blood glucose meters.

Meters and Supplies

Blood glucose meters are considered to be durable medical equipment; however, in order to obtain the measurement of glucose, the use of nondurable supplies is required. Those supplies include test strips, lancets, and control solution.

Blood glucose meters have similar features, such as an area for a test strip to receive a blood sample and a display of the glucose measurement. Blood glucose meters in the United States display the glucose measurement in milligrams per deciliter (mg/dL). Most meters measure whole blood glucose versus plasma levels of glucose, which is typically 10–15% higher than whole blood. There are meters that calculate a plasma equivalent measure from whole blood. Blood glucose meters vary in features, such as the size of blood sample needed for testing, calibration, testing time, and memory of test results.[10,11] A meter is chosen based on its features and the needs of the patient. There are advantages to using meters that require small blood samples, have automatic calibration, and provide test results in 5 seconds. Meters that are smaller are more convenient to carry. There are audible blood glucose meters that can be used by persons who have visual impairments.

A **test strip** used in blood glucose monitoring contains a reagent that interacts with a blood sample to generate a blood glucose measurement. Biosensor technology allows the blood sample to be drawn onto the test strip, instead of the blood sample being placed on top of the test strip.[10] Test strips are designed to be used with a specific meter and cannot be interchanged.

Some test strips are stored in a vial, with one strip removed at a time and placed into the meter for each test. Two meters, the Bayer Breeze 2 and Accu-chek Compact Plus, store multiple test strips in a drum or disc, which is placed into the meter.[12] The Breeze 2 uses a disc that contains 10 strips, and the Compact Plus uses a drum that contains 17 strips. For these meters, one test strip is obtained from the meter at the time of testing and discarded after the reading has been generated. The entire drum or disc is removed from the meter when all of the strips are used, and a new drum or disc is then placed in the meter. The meter also keeps track of how many test strips remain in the drum or disc. Test strips should be stored away from heat and humidity and not used after their expiration date. The expiration of test strips can range from 3 to 18 months, depending upon the type of meter.

A **lancet** (small needle) is used for one-time use to puncture the skin to obtain a blood sample. Lancets can be used with a lancet device, and the depth of puncture can be adjusted. Adjustment in depth of puncture can allow different sizes of blood samples to be obtained. A smaller depth of puncture produces a smaller blood sample. A larger depth of puncture produces a large blood sample and is usually more painful. Some lancets are designed to be used with specific lancet devices, whereas others can be used with most lancet devices. The gauge size (which determines the thickness of the needle) of lancets can vary from 21–33 gauge.[11] Lancets with higher numbers are thinner, with the 33-gauge lancet being the thinnest available. Thinner lancets are less painful for patients and can allow for a smaller blood sample to be obtained.

One product, Accu-chek Multiclix, provides six preloaded lancets in a drum.[13] The drum is placed in the Multiclix lancet device that is designed to prevent the reuse of lancets. The lancet device also provides 11 depth settings. The lancet drum is discarded after the six lancets have been used.

Blood obtained from the fingertip has traditionally been used for testing blood glucose. However, alternate site testing is now available for newer blood glucose meters. The alternate sites include the palm of the hand, the forearm, the thigh, and the calf. A special cover is placed over a lancet device to obtain a blood sample at an alternate site. Blood glucose readings obtained from alternate sites can vary compared with fingertip readings when glucose levels rapidly change, such as after a meal, after injecting insulin, during exercise, and when a person is ill or under stress.[12] Blood samples should be obtained from the fingertip if a person has symptoms of low blood glucose or if the results obtained from the alternate site are out of their usual range of blood glucose.

Control solution is a type of solution that mimics blood and that is used to test the accuracy of a blood glucose meter and test strips.[12] The solution is applied to a test strip; it generates a reading that should be within a certain range. The control solution is specific for a particular meter and may come as low, normal, or high control. The solutions can be categorized as "Level 1" or "Level 2," representing low or high control. The ranges for each type of control are provided in meter instructions or on the bottle of solution. Control solutions are used to check blood glucose meters at their first use and can be used weekly to determine the accuracy of test strips. The solutions can also be used if a person is unsure whether the meter is providing a correct blood glucose reading. The expiration date of the control solution varies by manufacturer and can range from 3 to 6 months.

Blood Glucose Monitoring Process

The steps for monitoring blood glucose are as follows:[12]

1. Gather materials used for test: meter, test strips, lancets, and alcohol preps.
2. Wash hands or clean finger/area of skin to be used for test with alcohol prep.
3. Place test strip in meter or obtain test strip from meter.
4. Lance (stick) the area of skin to obtain blood sample.
5. Apply blood sample to test strip.
6. Record blood glucose reading in log book.
7. Discard lancet in hard, plastic, puncture-resistant container.

> **Rx for Success**
>
> Being aware of the various types of blood glucose meters and supplies available allows pharmacy technicians to assist patients with product selection. Check to make sure patients receive the appropriate supplies for their specific blood glucose meter.

Insulin Delivery

Insulin is a hormone that is produced in the pancreas, which promotes the utilization of glucose, synthesis of protein, and the formation and storage of lipids (fat).[2,15] Different types of insulin vary in their onsets, peaks, and durations of action. Insulin is classified according to its action (rapid-acting, short-acting, intermediate acting, or long-acting). More than one type of insulin may be

Table 18-2. Insulin products

Name of insulin	Type of Action
Insulin lispro (Humalog)	Rapid-Acting
Insulin aspart (Novolog)	Rapid-Acting
Insulin glulisine (Apidra)	Rapid-Acting
Regular Human (Humulin R, Novolin R)	Short-Acting
NPH (Humulin N, Novolin N)	Intermediate-Acting
Insulin glargine (Lantus)	Long-Acting
Insulin detemir (Levemir)	Long-Acting

needed to control blood glucose levels. Depending on the type of insulin, it is injected with or before meals or administered once daily. The insulin concentration that is most commonly used contains 100 units/mL and is available in 3-mL or 10-mL sizes. Various types of insulin are available; the most common are listed in Table 18-2.

Insulin is injected subcutaneously (under the skin). Traditionally, insulin has been administered using an insulin syringe; however, it can also be administered with insulin pens or as a continuous infusion using a pump. Sites of injection include the abdomen (which is the fastest site of absorption), the back of the arm, the outer thigh, and the hip/buttocks area.[16] The sites of injection should be rotated (inject within a larger area for 1–2 weeks and then move to another area).

Safety First It is important to rotate injection sites because frequent injections into a specific area of skin can cause a fatty buildup of tissue under the skin that can affect the absorption of insulin.[15]

Injection with Syringes

Insulin stored in a vial is injected into the skin using syringes. Insulin syringes are available in 30-unit (3/10 mL), 50-unit (0.5 mL), and 100-unit (1 mL) sizes (Figure 18-1).[17] A syringe should be chosen that is close to the number of insulin units injected. Using a smaller volume syringe (3/10 mL) for a small amount of insulin (less than 30 units) allows for more accurate dosing. The 30-unit and 50-unit syringes have 1-unit markings. The 30-unit (3/10 mL) syringes are also available with half-unit markings. The markings on the 100-unit (1 mL) syringes are 2 units each.

The length of the insulin syringe needle can vary from 5/16 inch to 1/2 inch, and the gauge can range from 28 to 31. Longer needle lengths can be used for persons injecting larger amounts of insulin (>50 units per injection). Higher gauge needles are thinner and can therefore be less painful.

For subcutaneous injection of insulin, the individual is advised to "pinch" a large fold of skin and inject the needle into that area of skin at a 45- or 90-degree angle. This method minimizes the likelihood of insulin being injected into a muscle. Most persons inject insulin into the skin at a 90-degree angle. However, persons who are thin or who are very muscular may inject insulin at a 45-degree angle.

The steps of insulin injection using a syringe are as follows:[16]

1. Wash hands; gather materials (insulin vial, syringe, alcohol prep).
2. Clean site of injection with alcohol prep.
3. Remove needle cover; draw air into syringe that is equivalent to number of insulin units.
4. Inject air into insulin vial.
5. Invert insulin vial, withdraw insulin units, and check for air bubbles while syringe needle remains in vial.
6. If air bubbles are present, push insulin back into vial and withdraw insulin units again. Repeat until there are no large air bubbles present in syringe.

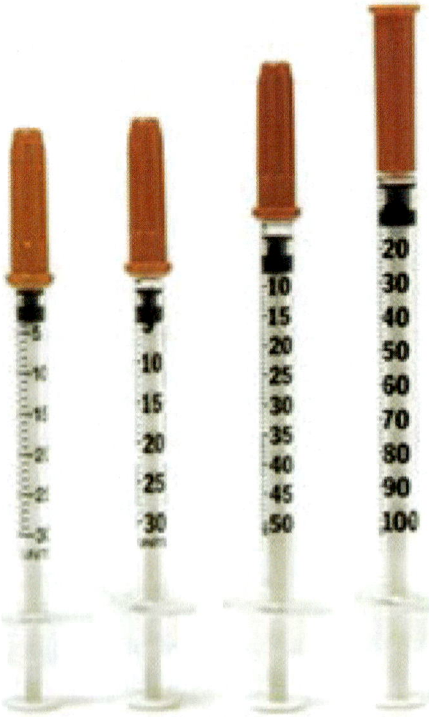

Left to right:

- 3/10 cc syringe with half-unit markings
- 3/10 cc syringe with whole unit markings
- 1/2 cc syringe
- 1 cc syringe

Figure 18-1. BD syringes. (Courtesy of BD, Becton, Dickinson, and Company, 2010.)

7. Remove syringe from vial.
8. Pinch fold of skin, inject at 45- or 90-degree angle.
9. Keep needle in skin for a few seconds; then release skin fold and remove needle from skin.

> **Safety First** Insulin syringes should be discarded after single use. Risk of infection or scarring are increased when an insulin syringe is reused. Syringes should be discarded in hard, puncture-resistant containers.

Insulin Pens

Insulin pens are a portable, discreet and convenient delivery device for insulin administration. The components of insulin pens include an insulin cartridge, a dose indicator, and a dose knob, which allows insulin to be administered. Durable insulin pens are reusable and require that an insulin cartridge be placed into the device. The insulin cartridges are available in 1.5-mL (150 units) or 3-mL (300 units) sizes.[18]

Disposable insulin pens are prefilled and allow the user to discard the entire device when it is empty or when the insulin contained in the pen has reached its expiration date. Most disposable insulin pens contain 3 mL, or 300 units of insulin.[18]

Therefore, these devices contain less insulin than insulin vials, which are available in 10-mL sizes. Figure 18-2 displays various insulin pens.[18-20] This figure is not inclusive of all insulin pens and these products continue to be updated with newer models.

Instead of using a syringe, pen needles are attached to the pen before the injection and removed immediately after the injection. Pen needles are available in various lengths and gauge sizes. Becton Dickinson pen needles are compatible with all insulin pens sold in the United States. Other brands of pen needles include NovoFine, SureComfort, Ulticare, and Unifine Pentips.

The lengths of pen needles are 4 mm (5/32"), 5 mm (3/16"), 6 mm (1/4"), 8 mm (5/16"), and 12.7 mm (1/2"). The shorter needle (5-mm size) are recommended for very thin or muscular persons and for children. The mini-needle is used as a "no pinch required" approach; the mini-needles are so small that they do not reach muscle tissue when injecting without pinching a fold of skin.[21]

Becton Dickinson pen needles are displayed in Figure 18-3.

Insulin pens or cartridges are stored in the refrigerator until first use. Once in use, the insulin pen should remain at room temperature until the expiration date of insulin. The expiration date of insulin contained in a cartridge or pen can range from 10–42 days.[18] The Food and Drug Administration issued a warning in May 2009 regarding the sharing of insulin pens.[23] Using an insulin pen in more than one person increases the potential risk of transmitting bloodborne pathogens, substances that can cause disease. Therefore, insulin pens should not be shared between persons.

Advantages of using insulin pens include the following:[16,18,22]

- Portable, discreet, and convenient for injections away from home.
- Insulin prefilled in self-contained cartridges.

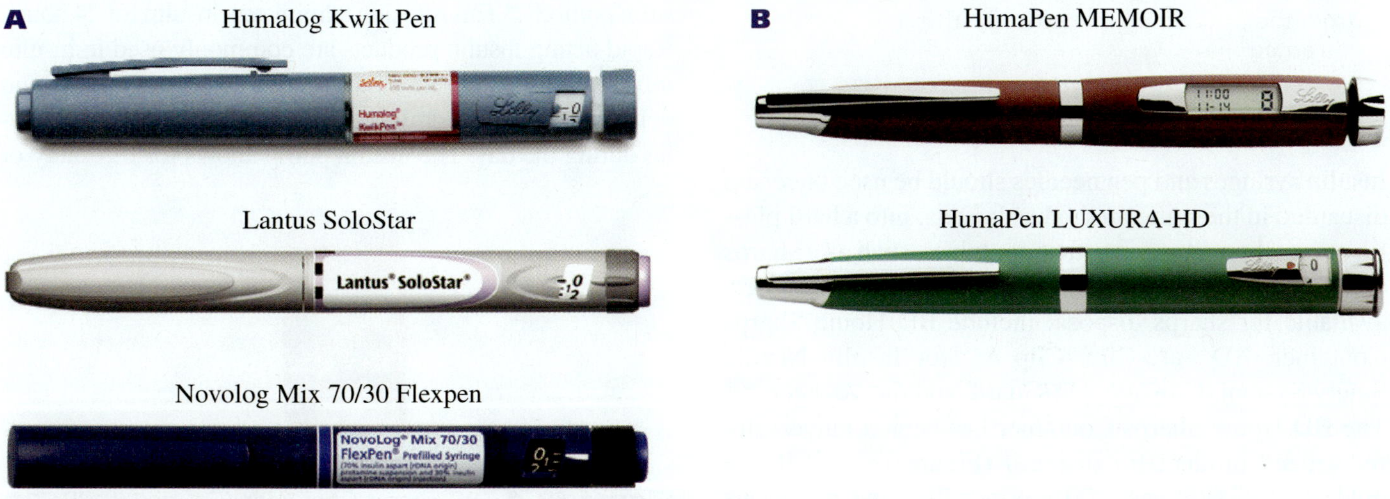

Figure 18-2. A. Disposable Insulin Pens. **B.** Durable Insulin Pens.

5 mm, 31 gauge
BD Mini pen needle

8 mm, 31 gauge
BD Short pen needle

12.7 mm, 29 gauge
BD Original pen needle

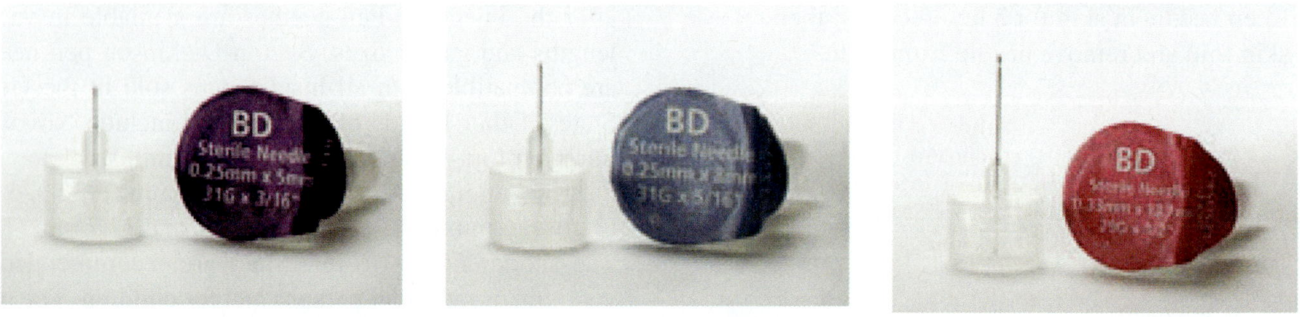

Figure 18–3. BD pen needles. (Courtesy of BD, Becton, Dickinson, and Company, 2010.)

- Dosage dial allows more accurate dosing, particularly for persons with vision impairment and dexterity limitations.

Disadvantages of using insulin pens include the following:[16,18,22]

- Typically more expensive than using an insulin vial and syringe.
- Limited to commercially available products (no manual mixing of insulin).
- Each injection is limited to a maximum number of units (varies per device).
- Must not be used for multiple patients.

Safety First Insulin pens should never be shared or used for multiple patients, and, to prevent transmission of infectious diseases, pen needles should not be reused. Pen needles should be removed from the insulin pen immediately after injection and discarded.

Sharps Disposal

Insulin syringes and pen needles should be used once and discarded in the same method as lancets, into a hard plastic or metal puncture-resistant container, such as a sharps container or empty liquid detergent bottle. Products available for sharps disposal include BD Home Sharps Container, BD Safe-Clip, Clip & Stor Insulin Needle Safety System, UltiCare, UltiGuard, and the Voyager.[24-26] The BD Home Sharps Container has been a universally recognized product for disposal (Figure 18-4).[24] It can hold 70–100 syringes, 300 pen needles, and numerous lancets. The container can also be disposed of through the BD Sharps Disposal by Mail program, which provides a postage-paid cardboard box that allows a person to send full home containers back to the company for proper disposal.

The BD Safe-clip, Clip & Stor system, and the Voyager allow needles to be clipped and contained in the device. The Voyager completely clips the needle and part of the syringe; however, it cannot be used to dispose of pen needles.[26] The UltiMed product line has devices for pen needles (UltiCare) and syringes (UltiGuard). Each product has 100 syringes or pen needles, with a dispenser and disposal unit.[25] Regulations for home sharps disposal vary by state.[24]

Continuous Infusion

Continuous subcutaneous insulin infusion is another method of administering insulin. This type of infusion is provided through a catheter attached to an insulin reservoir within an insulin pump.[27-29] This infusion administers insulin for 24 hours. Rapid-acting insulin products are commonly used in insulin infusion pumps. Patients may choose this method of insulin delivery if they are administering multiple injections of insulin during the day. The insulin pump allows for flexibility of

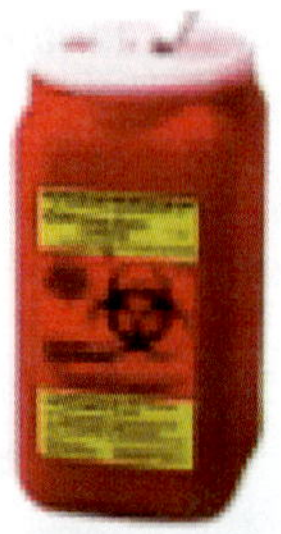

Figure 18–4. BD Sharps Container. (Courtesy of BD, Becton, Dickinson, and Company, 2010.)

meals and physical activity. Frequent blood glucose monitoring is required with the use of insulin pumps.

Advantages of insulin pump therapy include the following:[27-29]

- Elimination of individual insulin injections
- More accurate insulin delivery than injections
- Improvement of hemoglobin A1c level
- Fewer variations in blood glucose levels and reduction in episodes of low blood sugar
- Ability to administer additional insulin based upon carbohydrate intake and blood glucose levels
- Flexibility in mealtimes and physical activity

Disadvantages of insulin pump therapy include the following: [27-29]

- Weight gain
- Diabetic ketoacidosis (DKA), a severe, life-threatening reaction that can occur in the absence of insulin, if the catheter is removed or occluded
- Expense
- Device attached to body at all times
- Extensive education required
- Infection resulting from improper care

Insulin pumps vary by several features, such as basal rates, battery life, and degree of water resistance. Insulin administered by pump provides both basal and bolus delivery. Basal insulin delivery mimics the continuous, steady insulin release of the pancreas, which occurs 24 hours a day. Bolus insulin delivery occurs around meals to control the increase of blood glucose after ingesting food. The amount of insulin used in the insulin pump is determined by averaging the total units of insulin used per day. This total dose is divided into 40–50% for basal and 50–60% for bolus insulin.[28,29] The basal portion is divided by 24 to determine an initial hourly basal rate. The basal rate is adjusted based upon physical activity and blood glucose patterns. Insulin to carbohydrate ratios are also determined, and correction boluses are used to provide additional insulin when blood glucose is too high.

Those who choose insulin pump therapy must be educated regarding nutrition, the importance of frequent blood glucose monitoring, and the action of insulin in their body and during specific situations. Education is also needed for health care professionals to provide assistance with adjustment of insulin doses.

Infusion sets are used to deliver insulin through the insulin pump, usually containing cannula and tubing. The cannula is injected into the skin with straight or slanted insertion of a needle.[27] The length of tubing varies for children and adults. Most infusion sets have a luer lock connection that can be used on most pumps. However, some pumps require infusion sets that are compatible with their product. The infusion sets can also vary by needle gauge and length and by how the set is disconnected from the pump. Figure 18-5 illustrates an insulin pump and infusion sets.[27]

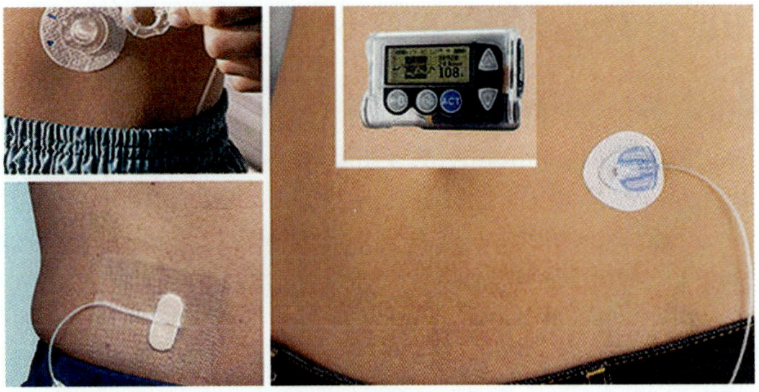

Figure 18–5. Infusion sets and insulin pump.

Blood Pressure Monitoring

Hypertension (high blood pressure) is a major risk factor for heart disease, stroke, congestive heart failure, and kidney disease. One aspect of hypertension management is regular monitoring of blood pressure. A health care professional may suggest that patients obtain a blood pressure monitor so that their blood pressure can be measured at home. Home blood pressure monitoring can help determine whether an adjustment in lifestyle and/or medication therapy is necessary to maintain normal blood pressure. A blood pressure reading, measured in millimeters of mercury (mmHg), comprises the systolic and diastolic blood pressure. The first, or upper, number (systolic blood pressure) is the pressure in the arteries when the ventricles of the heart contract and eject blood from the heart. The second, or lower, number (diastolic blood pressure) is the pressure in the arteries when the ventricles of the heart relax and fill with blood.[30-32] Normal blood pressure is considered to be <120/80 mmHg. High blood pressure for adults is defined as a systolic blood pressure of 140 mmHg or higher, or a diastolic blood pressure of 90 mmHg or higher.[30] Goals for blood pressure vary based upon whether a person has other health conditions.

Blood Pressure Monitors

Both aneroid and digital blood pressure monitors are available. **Aneroid blood pressure monitors** have a built-in stethoscope, a gauge with a dial where numbers are read, and a cuff that is manually inflated. The cuff consists of an inner and outer layer. The inner layer is made of rubber that fills with air and squeezes the arm. An outer layer is usually made of nylon and has a fastener to hold the cuff in place. Aneroid blood pressure monitors are less expensive than digital monitors and require adequate hearing, sight, and dexterity to obtain an accurate reading.

Digital blood pressure monitors are easy to read and can be manually or automatically inflated. However, these devices can be expensive, particularly when extra features are included, such as a printout of blood pressure readings. The accuracy of digital blood pressure monitors can be changed by body movements or irregular heart rates.

Accuracy of blood pressure is affected by the size of the cuff used with the monitor. Arm cuffs are available in large sizes.

There are several manufacturers of blood pressure monitors, including Omron, Panasonic, Homedics, Samsung, Microlife, and ReliOn. Selected blood pressure monitors are shown in Figure 18-6.[33]

Automatic arm inflation/digital monitor

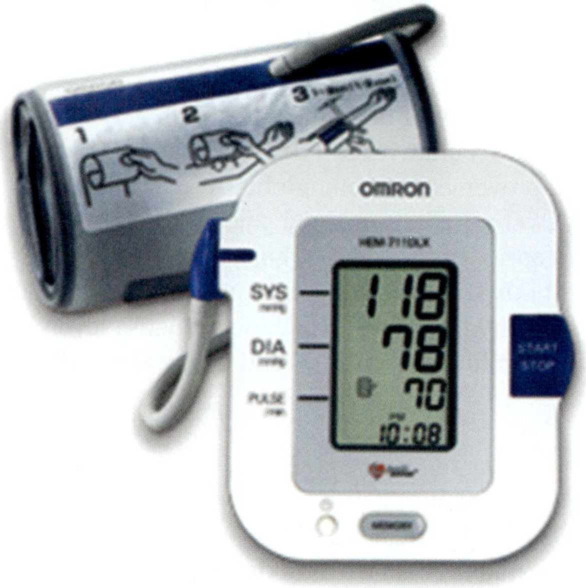

Manual inflation monitor

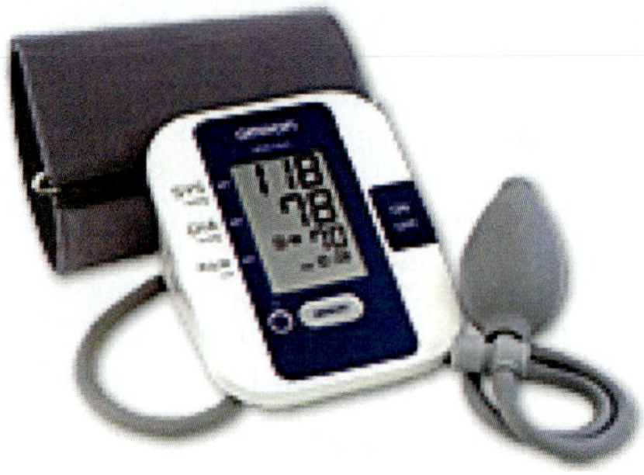

Wrist monitor

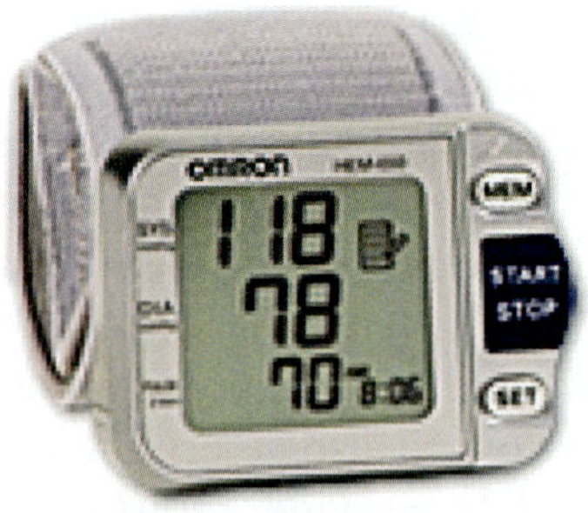

Figure 18–6. Select Omron blood pressure monitors. (Courtesy of Omron Healthcare, Inc., 2010.)

Monitoring Process

The steps for monitoring blood pressure include the following:[31,32]

1. Avoid food, caffeine, tobacco, and alcohol for 30 minutes before taking a measurement. Eating, drinking caffeine or alcohol, or using tobacco can increase blood pressure readings. Empty your bladder before measuring blood pressure; a full bladder can increase blood pressure slightly.
2. Sit quietly for 3–5 minutes in a comfortable position, with your legs and ankles uncrossed and your back supported against a chair, before measuring blood pressure.
3. Rest your arm, raised to the level of your heart, on a table, desk, or chair arm. You may need to place a pillow or cushion under your arm to elevate it enough. Place the cuff on bare skin, not over clothing. Rolling up a sleeve until it tightens around your arm can result in an inaccurate reading, so you may need to slip your arm out of the sleeve.
4. Place the arm cuff over the brachial artery. There is usually a guide on the cuff for appropriate placement. Make sure to use a cuff that is the correct size for your arm. If a cuff is too small, the blood pressure reading can be falsely elevated. If the cuff is too large, the blood pressure can be lower than the actual measurement.
5. Measure blood pressure by following the directions for the specific monitor.

6. Remain quiet (i.e., don't talk) while taking your blood pressure.
7. If your monitor doesn't automatically log blood pressure readings or heart rates, write the measurements down in your own log.
8. Take a repeat reading 2–3 minutes after the first one to check accuracy. You can wait as little as one minute between readings.

Wrist and finger monitors are smaller devices that are also used to monitor blood pressure. However, these monitors are considered to be less accurate than ones in which a cuff is placed over the arm.[32] The arm should be at heart level when wrist monitors are used.

Rx for Success

The appropriate arm cuff size should be given to persons obtaining blood pressure monitors. Blood pressure monitors should be selected based upon ease of use and cost.

Heart Rate Monitoring

A heart rate monitor is a device that allows users to measure their heart rate in real time.[34,35] Persons may want to self-monitor their heart rate when being physically active. Knowing the heart rate before, during, and after exercise can help determine whether an exercise program is appropriate and goals are being met. Normal heart rate ranges for adults, 18 years of age or older, are 60–100 beats per minute.[34] Heart rate monitors usually consist of two elements: a strap transmitter and a wrist receiver (which usually doubles as a watch). Traditionally, the monitors used a chest strap. However, strapless heart rate monitors are available. Advanced models can average heart rate over the exercise period, record the time a person is in a specific heart rate zone, track calories burned, and perform a detailed logging that can be downloaded to a computer.[35] Heart rate monitors are also available for specific sports or training.[35]

Electrodes within the monitor are in contact with the skin to monitor the electrical voltages in the heart. When a heart beat is detected, a radio signal is transmitted, which the receiver uses to determine the current heart rate. This signal can be a simple radio pulse or a unique coded signal from the chest strap; the latter prevents one user's receiver from picking up signals from other nearby transmitters.

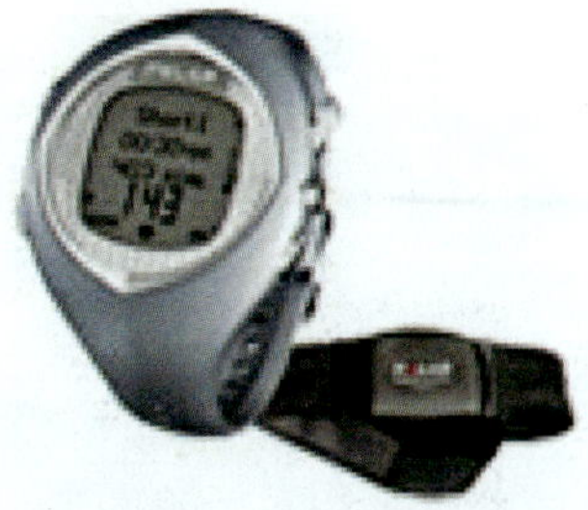

Figure 18-7. Polar heart rate monitor with chest transmitter.

Manufacturers of heart rate monitors include Polar (Figure 18-7), New Balance, Omron, Acumen, Timex, Oregon Scientific, and Garmen.

Regular physical activity can improve blood glucose control, reduce cardiovascular risk factors, contribute to weight loss, and improve well-being.[36,37] Incorporating exercise into daily schedules can be challenging. Therefore, monitoring the distance that a person walks or the amount of steps taken can help determine the amount of exercise done during the day.

Monitoring Distance with Pedometers

A **pedometer** is a device that records each step a person takes by detecting the motion of the hips.[36,37] The distance of each person's step varies, so calibration is needed to record a standardized distance, such as the number of miles walked. The recommended number of steps per day for weight loss is 10,000.[36] The use of a pedometer is associated with significant increases in physical activity and significant decreases in body mass index and blood pressure.[36]

Pedometer technology includes a mechanical sensor and software to count steps. Early forms of the device used a mechanical switch to detect steps, together with a simple counter. More advanced pedometers rely on microelectromechanical system (MEMS) inertial sensors and sophisticated software to detect steps. The use of MEMS inertial sensors permits more accurate detection of steps and fewer false-positives.[28] A false-positive occurs when the pedometer incorrectly records a step when the device is bumped or moved.

The pedometer should be worn on a belt to provide an accurate measurement of steps. The simplest pedometers only count steps and display the number of steps and/or distance. However, there are pedometers that also provide calorie estimates, clocks, timers, stopwatches, speed estimators, and 7-day memory, as well as monitor heart

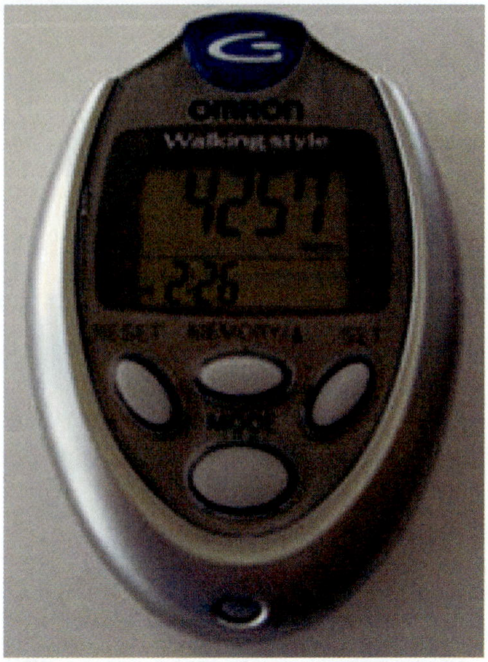

Figure 18-8. Omron digital pedometer. (Courtesy of Omron Healthcare, Inc., 2010.)

rate. An example of an advanced pedometer is shown in Figure 18-8.[38]

Home Diagnostic Products

Several nondurable products are available for people to measure lab values and diagnose certain conditions at home, such as kits to measure cholesterol and hemoglobin A1c, determine whether a person has been exposed to HIV, and detect pregnancy or ovulation.

✔ Home diagnostics are convenient for patients; however, it is important for patients to follow up and discuss any results with their health care provider.

Measuring Cholesterol

High cholesterol is a major modifiable risk factor for heart disease, the leading cause of death in the United States.[39] An estimated 102.3 million American adults (more than 60% of all adults aged 20 years and older) have total blood cholesterol levels of 200 milligrams per deciliter (mg/dL) and higher, which is above desirable levels.[39] Of these, 41.3 million (more than 1 of every 5 adults) have levels of 240 mg/dL or higher, which is considered high risk for coronary heart disease. A 10% decrease in total blood cholesterol levels can reduce the incidence of heart disease by as much as 30%.[39,40]

Many people are unsure of their cholesterol levels. Home testing of cholesterol can be used to determine health risk status for heart disease.[41] Available nondurable medical products that measure cholesterol include the Home Access Instant Total Cholesterol Test kit, Accutech CholesTrak, Biosafe, and CheckUp America Cholesterol Panel test.[41,42] These cholesterol kits use a blood sample that is obtained through fingerstick by using a lancet. The Home Access and CholesTrak measure total cholesterol levels and provide results within 10–15 minutes using a grid that looks similar to that of a thermometer (Figure 18-9). The BioSafe Full Lipid Panel Cholesterol test provides levels for total cholesterol, high density lipoprotein (HDL), low density lipoprotein (LDL), and triglycerides. The sample used for the BioSafe kit is mailed to a laboratory and processed within three days, with the results sent back to the patient and/or the health care provider. The CheckUp America kit uses a serum-based test, which is considered a "good standard" for professional results.[41] This kit provides a comprehensive laboratory report to the user that compares results against the National Cholesterol Education Program, which is used to evaluate cholesterol levels and determine appropriate treatment. Patients who use home cholesterol tests should discuss the results with their physician.

Measuring Hemoglobin A1c

A **hemoglobin A1c** test gives individuals information about their average blood glucose control for the past 2–3 months in order to determine how well their diabetes treatment plan is working.[43-46] The measurement gives an assessment of blood glucose control over a longer period than the readings obtained through blood glucose meters. Patients may want to monitor their hemoglobin A1c levels between physician visits to monitor their

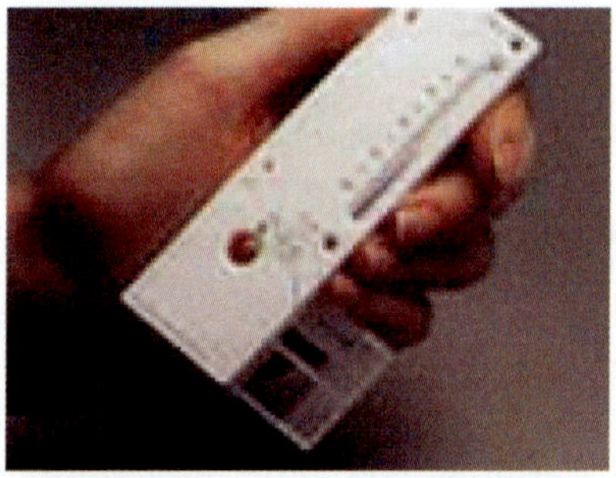

Figure 18-9. CholesTrak Home Cholesterol Kit. (Courtesy of AccTech, LLC., 2010.)

blood glucose control. Currently available nondurable medical products include AccuBase A1c Glycohemoglobin test kit, A1c at Home kit, the Biosafe Hemoglobin A1c test kit, and A1CNOW Self Check.[43-46]

A blood sample is obtained from a fingertip using a lancet. The samples used in each of these kits must be mailed to a reference laboratory, and the results are sent back to the patient by mail, by fax, or electronically (Biosafe test kit is mail only). For the AccuBase A1c kit, the lab procedure screens for abnormal hemoglobins, such as S, C, F, abnormal peaks, and/or red blood cell disturbances (anemia), and reports an interference-free A1c answer.[44] The A1c readings should be reviewed with a person's physician to discuss need for adjustment of diabetes therapy.

HIV Testing

The rates of human immunodeficiency virus (HIV) in the United States are rapidly increasing. At the end of 2007, an estimated 1,051,875 persons in the United States were living with HIV/AIDS, with 21% undiagnosed and unaware of their HIV status.[47] The earliest symptoms of HIV infection occur while the body begins to form antibodies to the virus (known as seroconversion), between 6 weeks and 3 months after infection with the HIV virus. Individuals who show early HIV symptoms may develop flu-like symptoms that can include fever, rash, muscles aches, and swollen lymph nodes and glands. However, for most people, there are no symptoms.

Individuals may choose to use a home HIV test to test in the privacy of their home because there could be concern for maintaining confidentiality. The FDA has approved home HIV testing products, including the Home Access HIV-1 Test System.[48,49] The Home Access standard kit provides results seven days after the blood sample arrives at a designated laboratory. The results are recorded anonymously; the patient is assigned a code number with each kit. Results are retrieved by calling a toll-free number. The kit is considered to be 99.9% accurate. Follow-up with a physician is important when results are obtained. Partner(s) should also be tested, particularly if a positive result is obtained.

Pregnancy Testing

The first home pregnancy tests were marketed in the mid-1970s and have been one of the most popular products for home diagnostic testing.[50,51] The most common home pregnancy tests involve placing a drop of urine on a prepared chemical strip or placing the strip in an urine stream for 5–10 seconds. The strip is designed to detect a pregnancy hormone called human chorionic gonadotropin (hCG). If a woman is pregnant, which is considered a positive result, there is a color change or symbol appears. Other tests use a collection cup in which urine contacts a test disk that changes colors for a positive result. The results for these home tests are considered to be up to 99% accurate. However, false-negatives and false-positives have been reported.

False-negative results can occur if home pregnancy tests are done very early in the pregnancy.[50] False-positive results can be caused by having soap in the urine collection cup, testing equipment in a very warm environment, protein or blood in the urine, or the hCG hormone in the urine from another cause.[50]

Common brands for home pregnancy tests include Clear Blue Easy, First Response Early Result, and E.P.T.[51]

Ovulation Testing

Ovulation testing is used in family planning to determine when a woman is most fertile and able to become pregnant. Ovulation is the discharge of a mature egg from the ovary. When an egg is released, a woman's ability to become pregnant is increased. Ovulation predictor tests work by allowing a woman to detect her monthly luteinizing hormone (LH) surge, which is present in urine just before ovulation. LH is the hormone that facilitates ovulation (the release of the egg). The best time for fertilization of the egg to occur is within 6 to 24 hours after ovulation.[52]

Orthopedic Devices

Orthopedic devices are types of durable medical equipment that are used by patients of all ages. These devices are also used by athletes to provide support or aid in recovery from injuries.

Orthopedic devices, such as braces, supports, and splints, can be used for rehabilitation and pain management that result from a vast range of conditions. **Orthotic devices** are types of medical equipment that can prevent or correct a physical deformity or malfunction, or that can support a weak or deformed portion of the body. Thousands of people depend on such devices to help them manage various physical challenges, whether through use of temporary devices for a short time or permanent devices that are used across the span of a person's life. Some braces and supports can be purchased "off-the-shelf," whereas others require a custom-fitting process. In every

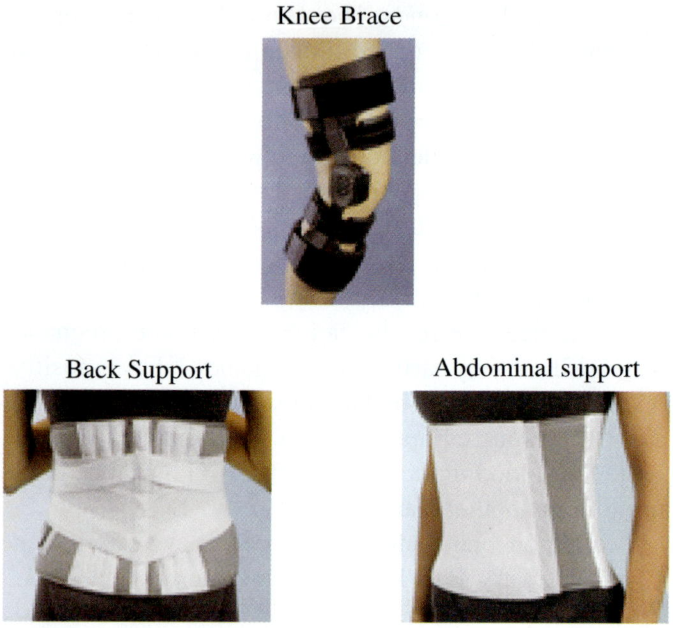

Figure 18–10. Orthopedic Devices.

case, the decision to use a brace or support and to monitor its use carefully should be made with the assistance of a certified orthotist.[59]

Braces and supports fall into five general categories:

1. Spinal (neck and back)
2. Lower extremity (feet, knees, legs, hips)
3. Pediatric (children between birth and age 18)
4. Upper extremity (hand, wrist, arm, elbow, shoulder)
5. Mastectomy (breast replacement or support)

Figure 18-10 displays selected orthopedic products.

Ostomy Products

An **ostomy** is a surgically created opening in the body. There are several times of ostomies, depending upon the type of surgery performed. A sigmoid or descending colostomy is the most common type of ostomy surgery, in which the end of that portion of the colon is brought to the surface of the abdomen.[60] A **colostomy** is performed in order to bypass or remove the lower colon and rectum. This surgery is performed in persons with certain types of cancer of the bowel or anus. The procedure generally involves creating a passage, called a **stoma**, through the abdominal wall, that is connected to the colon. The feces pass through this passage and are eliminated. Patients must learn how to care for the stoma and keep the area clean.

An ileostomy involves the small intestine. An Ileoanal reservoir (also known as a J-Pouch) is the most common alternative to the conventional ileostomy. There is no stoma with this procedure. The colon and most of the rectum are removed, and an internal pouch is formed out of the terminal portion of the ileum.[54] An opening at the bottom of the pouch is attached to the anus so that the existing anal sphincter muscles can be used for continence.

An **urostomy** is a procedure that diverts urine from the bladder. A continent urostomy allows for a reservoir or pouch to be created inside the abdomen using a portion of the small or large bowel.

There are several commercially available pouches that are placed over the stoma. The pouch systems include a skin barrier and a collection pouch. One-piece systems consist of a skin barrier and pouch contained in a single unit. With two-piece systems, the skin barrier remains on the skin, and a collection pouch is changed. Both of these types of pouches can be drainable or closed. Closed ended pouches are usually discarded after one use and arc most commonly used by those who can irrigate clean stool directly out of the colon through the stoma.[55]

There are various types of skin barriers, cleaners, deodorants, and accessories that can be used for ostomies. Ostomy belts, pouch covers, tape, and adhesive remover are some of the types of products available.

Summary

Durable and nondurable medical equipment, devices, and supplies are beneficial for home monitoring and screening of certain conditions and for rehabilitation. Blood glucose meters and products used for insulin delivery can improve the management of diabetes. Durable and nondurable medical equipment, devices, and supplies can assist in the administration of medication, provide support for persons with limited mobility, and improve the management of daily ostomy care. This type of medical equipment and supplies can improve the quality of life of patients. Patient-specific characteristics, such as age, degree of mobility, and disease states, should be considered when these products are recommended to patients. Pharmacy technicians can assist patients with selection of durable and nondurable equipment and supplies and and provide information regarding insurance coverage of these items. Therefore, knowledge of the types of durable and nondurable medical supplies is beneficial in pharmacy practice.

Self-Assessment Questions

1. Which of the following products are types of durable medical equipment?
   a. Bandages
   b. Diapers
   c. Exam gloves
   d. Blood glucose meters
2. Medicare covers 100% of the cost of durable medical equipment.
   a. True
   b. False
3. Which of the following supplies are used to obtain a blood sample for blood glucose monitoring?
   a. Pen needles
   b. Syringes
   c. Lancets
   d. Control solution
4. Control solutions are used to monitor the accuracy of a blood glucose meter.
   a. True
   b. False
5. Which of the following statements are true?
   a. The forearm is an alternate site for testing blood sugar.
   b. Lancets with smaller gauge sizes are thinner.
   c. Lancets can be used for insulin injections.
   d. A smaller depth of lancet puncture produces a larger blood sample.
6. The steps of insulin injection with syringe include all of the following *except* the following:
   a. Wash hands, gather materials.
   b. Clean site of insulin injection.
   c. Draw air into syringe equivalent to insulin units.
   d. Inject air into skin.
7. Advantages of using insulin pens include the following:
   a. Insulin is prefilled in cartridges.
   b. Less expensive than insulin vials.
   c. Can be used in multiple patients.
   d. Contains large quantity of insulin compared to insulin vials.
8. Insulin pens are stored at room temperature when in use.
   a. True
   b. False
9. Wrist blood pressure monitors are more accurate than those used on the arm.
   a. True
   b. False
10. Which of the following should *not* be done before monitoring blood pressure?
    a. Sit quietly for three to five minutes
    b. Urinate
    c. Avoid eating
    d. Drink caffeine
11. A pedometer is a device that records the numbers of steps that a person walks.
    a. True
    b. False
12. A heart rate monitor usually consists of a transmitter and receiver.
    a. True
    b. False
13. Home cholesterol tests can help determine health risk status for heart disease.
    a. True
    b. False
14. The Home Access HIV-1 product is an FDA-approved kit for home HIV-1 testing.
    a. True
    b. False
15. Which of the following can cause a false positive result in home pregnancy testing?
    a. Having testing equipment at room temperature.
    b. Having blood in urine.
    c. Taking test very early in pregnancy.
    d. Absence of protein in urine.
16. An ovulation test is used to determine if a women is pregnant.
    a. True
    b. False

Self-Assessment Questions

17. Advantages of insulin pump therapy include the following:
    a. Weight gain
    b. Expense
    c. Flexibility
    d. Device attached to body at all times
18. Regulations for home sharps disposal vary by each state.
    a. True
    b. False
19. There are five general categories for braces and supports.
    a. True
    b. False
20. Closed-ended pouches are usually discarded after one use.
    a. True
    b. False

Self-Assessment Answers

1. d. Blood Glucose Meters are considered durable medical equipment. Bandages, diapers, and exam gloves are nondurable medical equipment because they are single-use, disposable supplies.
2. b. False. Medicare Part B covers 80% of durable medical equipment and supplies. The patient must pay the remaining 20% of the cost.
3. c. Lancets are used to get a sample of blood for blood glucose testing. Pen needles and syringes are used to administer insulin.
4. a. True. Control solutions are used to test the accuracy of blood glucose meters.
5. a. The forearm is an alternate site for testing blood sugar. Lancets are used to get blood samples for testing, not for administering insulin. Lancets with the largest gauge sizes are the thinnest. A smaller depth of lancet puncture produces a smaller blood sample.
6. d. Air should never be injected into the skin; the air is injected into the vial before the dose is withdrawn.
7. a. A main advantage of insulin pens is that the insulin is available as prefilled cartridges. Pens are more expensive than vials and should never be used in multiple patients. Insulin pens contain a smaller volume of insulin compared to insulin vials.
8. a. True. Insulin pens should be stored at room temperature.
9. b. False. Wrist blood pressure monitors are *less* accurate than those worn on the arm.
10. d. Eating and drinking caffeinated beverages should be avoided before blood pressure is monitored. In addition, it is best to empty the bladder beforehand and sit quietly for 3–5 minutes prior to the reading.
11. a. True. A pedometer is a device that records the numbers of steps.
12. a. True. A heart rate monitor usually consists of a transmitter and receiver.
13. a. True. Home cholesterol tests can help determine health risk status for heart disease, in conjunction with a health care provider.
14. a. True. The Home Access HIV-1 product is an FDA-approved kit for home HIV-1 testing.
15. b. Having blood or protein in the urine can cause a false positive test, as well as testing equipment that is in too warm of an environment. Taking the test very early in the pregnancy can cause a false-negative result.
16. b. False. Ovulation tests are used to determine if a women is ovulating or in the most fertile stage of her cycle. They are not used to detect pregnancy.
17. c. Flexibility of meals and physical activity is an advantage of insulin pumps. Disadvantages of

insulin pumps include the following: the device is attached to the body at all times, there is more weight gain, and the expense is greater.

18. a. True. Regulations for home sharps disposal vary by state.
19. a. True. There are five general categories for braces and supports: spinal (neck and back); lower extremity (feet, knees, legs, hips); pediatrics (<18 years of age); upper extremity (hand, wrist, arm, elbow, shoulder); and mastectomy (breast replacement or support).
20. a. True. Closed-ended pouches are usually discarded after one use.

References

1. American Society of Health-System Pharmacists (ASHP). Glossary: durable medical equipment. Available at: http://www.ashp.org/Import/PRACTICEANDPOLICY/PracticeResourceCenters/PharmaceuticalReimbursement/Glossary.aspx Accessed May 11, 2010.
2. *Stedman's Medical Dictionary* (26th ed). Baltimore, MD: Williams and Wilkins; 1995.
3. Radford A, Richardson I, Mason M, Rutledge S. The key role of sole community pharmacists in their local healthcare delivery systems. Findings Brief. The North Carolina Rural Health Research & Policy Analysis Center and the RUPRI Center for Rural Health Policy Analysis. Available at: http://www.shepscenter.unc.edu/rural/pubs/finding_brief/FB88.pdf. Accessed May 11, 2010.
4. Medicare Interactive US. What is durable medical equipment (DE)? Available at: http://www.medicareinteractive.org/page2.php?topic=counselor&page=script&slide _id=188. Accessed May 11, 2010.
5. Centers for Medicare & Medicaid Services. Medicare coverage of durable medical equipment and other devices. CMS Publication No. 11045. Revised December 2008. Available at: http://www.medicare.gov/publications/pubs/pdf/11045.pdf. Accessed May 11, 2010.
6. Pray WS. Durable medical equipment: a challenging practice. *U.S. Pharmacist.* 2008;33(6):10–15.
7. Khani J, Coster J. NCPA, NACDS fight to preserve patient access to needed DMEPOS. *Pharmacy Times.* Available at: http://www.pharmacytimes.com/issue/pharmacy/2009/December2009/CCPA-1209. Accessed May 11, 2010.
8. United States Food and Drug Administration: Medical Devices. Clinical Laboratory Improvement Amendments (CLIA). Available at: http://www.fda.gov/cdrh/clia/cliawaived.html. Accessed May 11, 2010.
9. American Diabetes Association: Diabetes Statistics. Available at: http://www.diabetes.org/diabetes-basics/diabetes-statistics/. Accessed May 11, 2010.
10. Brown, LC. Self monitoring of blood glucose: the role of the pharmacist. Available at: http://www.pharmacytimes.com/issues/articles/2002-10_271.asp. Accessed May 11, 2010.
11. Diabetes Network. Blood glucose meters. Available at: http://www.diabetesnet.com/diabetes_technology/blood_glucose_meters.php. Accessed May 11, 2010.
12. Bunker K. Blood glucose meters. *Diabetes Forecast.* Available at: http://forecast.diabetes.org/magazine/features/blood-glucose-meters. Accessed May 11, 2010.
13. Roche Diagnostics. Accu-Chek Multiclix lancet device. Available at: http://www.accu-chek.com/us/rewrite/content/en_US/2.1.6.1:10/article/ACCM_general_article_2836.htm. Accessed May 11, 2010.
14. LifeScan, Inc. Control solution. Available at: http://lifescan.com/products/teststrips/solution. Accessed May 11, 2010.
15. Leahy J, Cefalu WT. *Insulin Therapy*. New York: Marcel Dekker, Inc.; 2002.
16. Becton, Dickinson and Company. How to inject insulin. BD Diabetes Education Center. Available at: http://www.bd.com/us/diabetes/page.aspx?cat=7001&id=7257. Accessed May 11, 2010.
17. Becton, Dickinson and Company. Insulin syringe size. Available at: http://www.bd.com/us/diabetes/page.aspx?cat = 7001&id=7251. Accessed May 11, 2010.
18. Gebel E. Insulin pens. *Diabetes Forecast.* Available at: http://forecast.diabetes.org/magazine/features/insulin-pens. Accessed May 11, 2010.
19. Eli Lilly and Company. Insulin pens. Available at: http://www.lillydiabetes.com/content/lilly-product-info.jsp. Accessed May 11, 2010.
20. Sanofi-Aventis. The Lantus Solostar Insulin Pen. Available at: http://www.lantus.com/solostar/solostar_insulin_pen.aspx. Accessed May 11, 2010.
21. Becton, Dickinson and Company. BD pen needles. Available at: http://www.bd.com/us/diabetes/page.aspx?cat=7002&id=7409. Accessed June 28, 2010.
22. American Association of Clinical Endocrinologists. Insulin pens and safety. AACE Patient Safety Exchange. Available at: http://www.aacepatientsafetyexchange.com/editorial/index.php?id=6. Accessed May 11, 2010.
23. Food and Drug Administration. Insulin pens: risk of transmission of blood-borne pathogens from shared use. Available at: http://www.fda.gov/Safety/MedWatch/SafetyInformation/SafetyAlertsforHumanMedicalProducts/ucm127783.htm. Accessed May 11, 2010.
24. Becton, Dickinson and Company. Disposal products. Available at: http://www.bd.com/us/diabetes/page.aspx?cat=7002&id=7413. Accessed May 11, 2010.
25. UltiMed disposal products. Available at: http://www.ulti-care.com/. Accessed May 11, 2010.

26. Home Medical Supplies, Inc. Voyager: diabetic needle disposal. Available at: http://www.homemedicalsupplies inc .com/Home_Medical_Supplies_products_needle_dispos .htm. Accessed May 11, 2010.
27. Neithercott T. Insulin pumps and infusion sets. *Diabetes Forecast.* Available at: http://www.forecast.diabetes.org/ insulin-pumps. Accessed May 11, 2010.
28. American Diabetes Association. Insulin pumps. Available at: http://www.diabetes.org/living-with-diabetes/treatment-and-care/medication/insulin/insulin-pumps.html. Accessed May 11, 2010.
29. American Diabetes Association. Position statement: continuous subcutaneous insulin infusion. *Diabetes Care.* 2004;27(suppl 1):S110.
30. Centers for Disease Control and Prevention. High blood pressure facts. Available at: http://www.cdc.gov/blood pressure/facts.htm. Accessed May 11, 2010.
31. Family doctor.org. Blood pressure monitoring at home. Available at: http://familydoctor.org/online/famdocen/home/ common/heartdisease/treatment/128.html. Accessed May 11, 2010.
32. Mayo Clinic.com. Get the most out of home blood pressure monitoring. Available at: http://www.mayoclinic. com/health/high-blood-pressure/HI00016. Accessed May 11, 2010.
33. Omron Health Care. Blood pressure monitors. Available at: http://www.omronhealthcare.com/products/ 186-home-products-blood-pressure-monitors. Accessed May 11, 2010.
34. The Cleveland Clinic Miller Family Heart & Vascular Institute. Pulse and target heart rate. Available at: http:// my.clevelandclinic.org/heart/prevention/exercise/pulsethr .aspx. Accessed May 11, 2010.
35. Heart Rate Monitors USA. Available at: http://www .heartratemonitorsusa.com/heartratemonitor-viewall.html. Accessed May 11, 2010.
36. Bravata DM. et al. Using pedometers to increase physical activity and improve health: a systematic review. *JAMA.* 2007;298(19):2296–2304.
37. Mayo Clinic.com. Walking for fitness? Make it count with a pedometer. Available at: http://www.mayoclinic.com/ health/walking/SM00056_D. Accessed May 11, 2010.
38. Omron Health Care. Measure walking distance with Omron Digital Pedometers. Available at: http://www.gosmartpe dometers.com. Accessed May 11, 2010.
39. U.S. Department of Health and Human Services. *A Public Health Action Plan to Prevent Heart Disease and Stroke.* Atlanta, GA: U.S. Department of Health and Human Services, Centers for Disease Control and Prevention; 2003.
40. Cohen JD. A population-based approach to cholesterol control. *Am J Med.* 1997;102:23.
41. Test Country. Cholesterol Tests. Available at: http://www .testcountry.com/categories.html?cat=12&left. Accessed May 11, 2010.
42. Health Check Systems. CholesTrak Home Cholesterol Test. Available at: http://www.healthchecksystems.com/ cholestrak.htm. Accessed May 11, 2010.
43. Bayer Diabetes Care. A1CNOW. Available at: http:// www.a1cnow.com/. Accessed May 11, 2010.
44. Diabetes Technologics, Inc. AccuBase A1c Test Kit. Available at: http://www.diabetestechnologies.com. Accessed May 11, 2010.
45. Flexsite Diagnostics. Diabetes Test A1c at home. Available at: http://www.flexsite.com. Accessed May 11, 2010.
46. A1CNOW Self Check System. Available at: http://www .simplewins.com/site/Adults/Monitor/Pages/Bayer-Products/A1C-Meter. Accessed May 11, 2010.
47. Centers for Disease Control and Prevention. HIV/AIDS statistics and surveillance. Available at: http://www .cdc.gov/hiv/topics/surveillance/index.htm. Accessed May 11, 2010.
48. United States Food and Drug Administration. HIV home test kits. Available at: http://www.fda.gov/BiologicsBlood Vaccines/SafetyAvailability/HIVHomeTestKits/default .htm. Accessed May 11, 2010.
49. Home Access Health Corporation. The Home Access HIV-1 test. Available at: http://www.homeaccess.com/ HIV_Test.asp. Accessed May 11, 2010.
50. Food and Drug Administration. Home pregnancy tests: how to use a popular test wisely. Available at: http:// www.fda.gov/MedicalDevices/Safety/AlertsandNotices/ TipsandArticlesonDeviceSafety/ucm109396.htm. Accessed May 11, 2010.
51. Consumer Search. Compare pregnancy tests. Available at: http://www.consumersearch.com/www/family/pregnancy-tests/compare. Accessed May 11, 2010.
52. Early Pregnancy Tests.com. Ovulation tests. Available at: http://www.early-pregnancy-tests.com/ovulationtests .html. Accessed May 11, 2010.
53. Prosthetics & Orthotics Hanger, Inc. Orthotics, braces and supports. Available at: http://www.hanger.com/Pages/ default.aspx. Accessed May 11, 2010.
54. United Ostomy Associations of America, Inc. What is an ostomy? Available at: http://www.uoaa.org/ostomy_info/ whatis.shtml. Accessed May 11, 2010.
55. *New York Times.* Colon cancer. Available at: http://health .nytimes.com/health/guides/disease/colon-cancer/surgery .html. Accessed May 11, 2010.

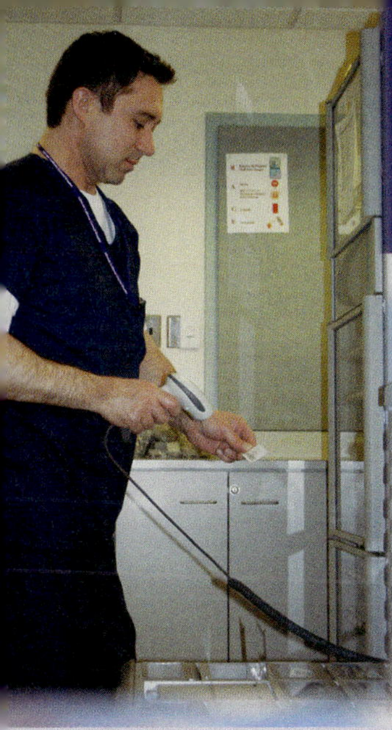

Chapter 19

Purchasing and Inventory Control

Jerrod Milton

Learning Outcomes

After completing this chapter you will be able to:

- Demonstrate an understanding of the formulary system and its application in a purchasing and inventory system.
- Execute lending and borrowing pharmaceutical transactions between pharmacies.
- Apply the proper principles and processes when receiving and storing pharmaceuticals.
- Identify key techniques for reviewing packaging, labeling, and storage considerations when handling pharmaceutical products.
- Demonstrate an understanding of pharmaceutical products that require special handling within the purchasing and inventory system.
- Demonstrate both an understanding and the application of appropriate processes for maintaining and managing a pharmaceutical inventory.
- Complete the appropriate processes in the handling of pharmaceutical recalls and the disposal of pharmaceutical products.

Key Terms

bar code medication administration (BCMA) A process in which the nurse scans a bar code on a patient's ID band and the bar code specific to the medication prior to medication administration. Documentation of the administration is automatically entered into the patient's electronic health record.

direct purchasing Buying directly from a manufacturer. It typically involves the execution of a purchase order from the pharmacy to the manufacturer of the drug.

group purchasing organization (GPO) An organized group that contracts with manufacturers to purchase pharmaceuticals at discounted prices, in return for a guaranteed minimum purchase volume. Hospitals, independent community pharmacies, and other retail chain pharmacies become members of a GPO to leverage buying power and take advantage of the lower prices that manufacturers offer to the GPOs.

just-in-time inventory management An inventory method in which products are ordered and delivered at just the right time—when they are needed for patient care. The goal is minimizing wasted steps, labor, and cost.

manufacturer A company that manufacturers or makes products such as drugs.

maximizing inventory turns An inventory turn occurs when stock is completely depleted and reordered. Ideally, products should not sit on the shelf unused for long periods; they should be purchased and used many times throughout the course of a year. Inventory turns can be calculated by dividing the total purchases in a period by the value of physical inventory taken at a reasonable single point in time.

par-level system An inventory management system in which predetermined stock minimum and maximum quantities to be maintained are established. Once the stocked quantity goes below the par level, more product is ordered.

perpetual inventory process An inventory method in which medications, specifically controlled substances, and investigational drugs are inventoried and tracked continuously. Each dose or packaged unit, such as a tablet, vial, or milliliter of fluid volume, is accounted for at all times.

prime vendor A wholesaler from which a pharmacy purchases 90 to 95% of its pharmaceuticals according to an established arrangement or contract.

purchase order A document executed by a purchaser and forwarded to a supplier that is considered a legal offer to buy products or services.

recall When a product is removed from the market by the manufacturer on its own accord or at the direction of the FDA, for safety or quality reasons, such as mislabeling, contamination, lack of potency, lack of adherence to acceptable Good Manufacturing Practices, or other situations that may present a significant risk to public health.

stock rotation Placing the products that will expire the soonest in the front of the shelf or bin and those with later expiration dates behind them.

tall man lettering An error prevention technique used to differentiate look-alike medication names. A portion of the letters are capitalized (e.g., niCARdipine and NIFEdipine).

wholesaler A large-scale warehouse with drugs and supplies located in various geographic regions that exist to help bring pharmaceutical products closer to the market.

Pharmaceutical products flow into the pharmacy through a sophisticated and highly regulated distribution channel. Once they arrive in the pharmacy, these (often expensive) items become assets, and the inventory management process begins. Proper storage and availability of these products are essential to the delivery of patient care and the efficient operation of the pharmacy.

An effective pharmaceutical purchasing and inventory control system requires the understanding and active participation of all pharmacy staff. Certain staff members are often designated to be responsible for managing the pharmacy inventory and purchasing activities. Pharmacy technicians are often the principal buyers of medications and supplies for the pharmacy. Many hospitals strive to maintain accreditation of The Joint Commission. Its standards on medication management are intended to guide operational procedures and promote consistently safe practices related to the procurement, storage, dispensing, and administration of pharmaceuticals. Because pharmacy technicians are such an important part of preparation and dispensing of medications, their knowledge and performance are critical to the success of purchasing and inventory control procedures.

This chapter describes the basic principles of pharmaceutical purchasing and inventory control. It applies to all types of pharmacy settings, including institutional, home infusion, and ambulatory care pharmacy operations. For technicians who are interested in pursuing a specialized position within purchasing and inventory control, and for readers desiring more in-depth study, a reading list is included in the Resources section of this chapter.

Ordering Pharmaceuticals

Some pharmacies employ a dedicated purchasing agent to manage the procurement and inventory of pharmaceuticals. Others employ a more general approach, whereby several staff members are involved in ordering pharmaceuticals. The state-of-the-art practice involves the use of automated technology to manage the processes of purchasing and receiving pharmaceuticals from drug wholesalers. This technology includes using bar codes and handheld scanning devices for online procurement, purchase order generation, and electronic receiving processes (figure 19-1). Some pharmacies use sophisticated inventory management carousel systems to manage portions of their inventory (figure 19-2). Using computer and mechanical technology for these purposes has many benefits, including up-to-the-minute product availability information, comprehensive reporting capabilities, accuracy, reduced training time, and improved operational efficiency. It also encourages compliance with various pharmaceutical purchasing contracts.

The National Drug Code

All commercial pharmaceutical manufacturers are required to register pharmaceuticals with the Food and Drug Administration (FDA). This FDA Drug Registration and Listing System (DRLS) is a database that utilizes a unique identification number, called the National Drug Code (or NDC number), to identify drug products that are intended for human consumption or use.

The NDC number appears on the manufacturer's label and follows a 10-digit format, either 4-4-2 (four digits-four digits-two digits), 5-3-2, or 5-4-1, as shown in figure 19-3. The first set of digits identifies the specific drug manufacturer or labeler of the product and is assigned by the FDA. The next segment of digits is the

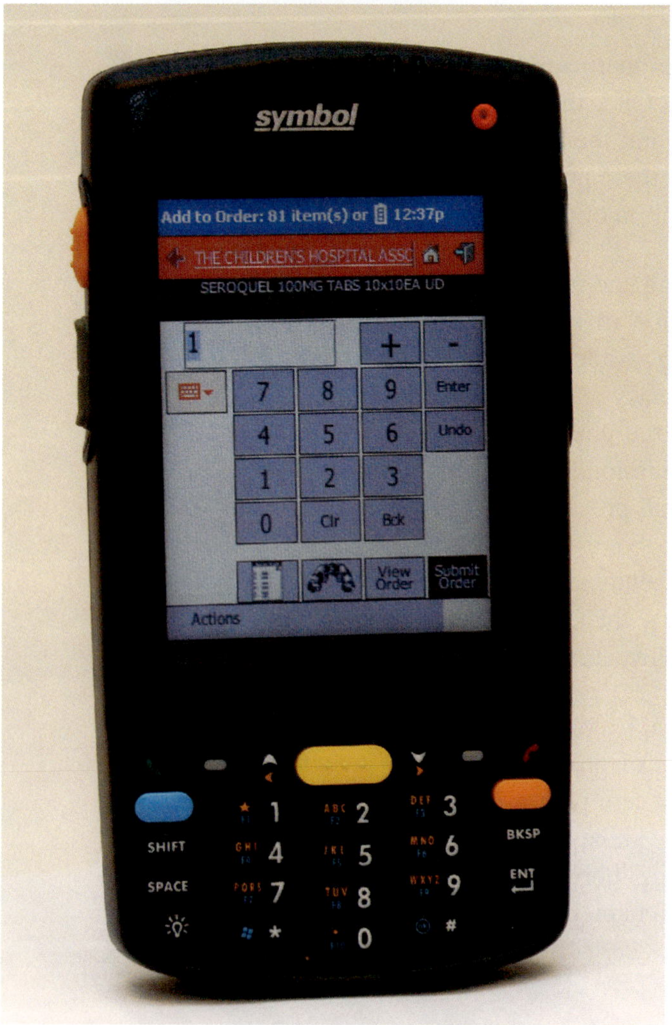

Figure 19–1. Handheld bar code scanning device.

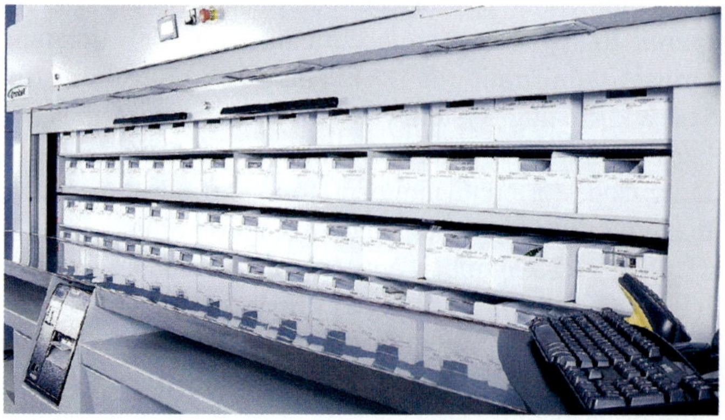

Figure 19–2. Medication dispensing carousel.[1]

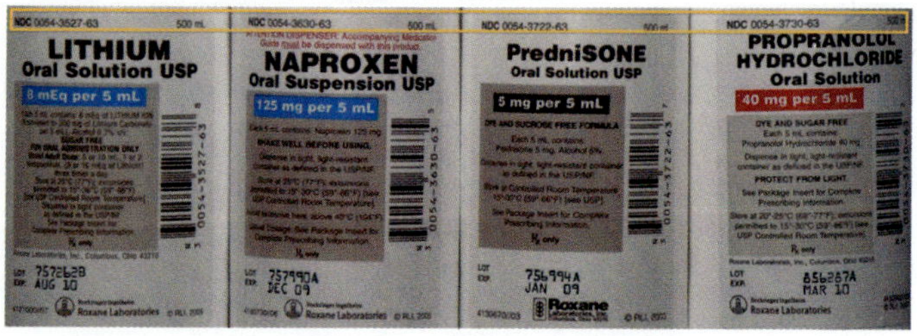

Figure 19–3. NDC numbers.

product code, denoting the formulation, dosage form, and strength. The final segment identifies package type and size. The NDC number is particularly useful in precisely identifying drug products in the processes of dispensing, placing orders, and addressing drug recalls.

The Formulary System

Most hospitals and health care systems develop a list of medications that may be prescribed for patients in the institution or health care system. This list, usually called a formulary, serves as the cornerstone of the purchasing and inventory control system. The formulary is developed and maintained by a committee of medical and allied health staff called the Pharmacy and Therapeutics (P&T) Committee. This group generally comprises physicians, pharmacists, nurses, and administrators, although individuals from other disciplines may be present, such as dieticians, risk managers, and case managers. They collaborate to ensure that the safest, most effective, and least costly medications are included on the formulary. The products on the hospital formulary dictate what the hospital pharmacy should keep in inventory.

Third-party prescription pharmacy benefits managers (PBMs) also establish plan-specific formularies for their ambulatory patients. In serving their patients, community (retail) pharmacy staff frequently encounter drug formularies that are specific to particular insurance plans; they adjust their inventory accordingly. Most retail pharmacies do not restrict items in their inventory as a hospital pharmacy does because, in this setting, inventories are largely dependent on the dynamic needs of their patient population and, to some degree, their patients' respective insurance plans. Therefore, the concept of formulary management differs greatly depending on the pharmacy setting (e.g., hospital versus retail pharmacy).

Formats and Updates. The hospital formulary is usually available electronically and/or in print form. The formulary is produced exclusively for health practitioners involved in prescribing, dispensing, administering, and monitoring medications. It is generally formatted to inform users of product availability, the appropriate therapeutic uses, and recommended dosing and administration of medications. Some formularies are organized alphabetically by the generic drug's name, which is typically cross-referenced with the trade name products; others may be organized by therapeutic drug class. In most cases, the drug storage areas in the pharmacy are arranged alphabetically, by either the generic or trade name of the drug. Therefore, the formulary can help the pharmacy technician determine whether a product is stocked in the pharmacy and where it would be located.

It is important for pharmacy technicians to understand how the formulary is updated and, how and when changes to the formulary are communicated to the staff. Drugs are added and deleted from the formulary on a regular basis, but the frequency of these changes varies among organizations. Printed formularies are typically updated every 12 to 18 months. Loose-leaf formularies and those maintained online can be updated continuously in a more timely manner, whereas bound formulary handbooks rely on supplementary updates or publication of serial editions. A sample formulary listing is shown in figure 19-4.

Other important information that may be available in the formulary, specified under each listing, is the dosage form, strength, and concentration; package size(s); common side effects; and administration instructions. Some institutions also indicate the actual or relative cost of a given item. When selecting a drug product from inventory, the technician must consider all product characteristics, such as name, dosage form, strength or concentration, and package size. Detailed review and consideration of each listing helps minimize errors in product selection.

Non-Formulary Protocol. In keeping with the standards and controls created by an organized formulary system, most hospitals employ a formal procedure to manage appropriate drug use. The use of products that are not on the official hospital formulary is considered *non-formulary* drug use. Typically, when a prescriber orders a non-formulary product, the pharmacist requests verbal or written justification for its use and challenges the request, as appropriate, if a comparable or therapeutically equivalent product is available on the hospital formulary. In certain cases, the utilization of a non-formulary product is warranted when its benefit is believed to be superior to that of the other alternative formulary items that may exist (usually for a patient-specific or disease-specific reason).

Isotretinoin

Brand Names Accutane®

Therapeutic Class 84:36 Skin and Mucous Membrane Agents, Miscellaneous

Use Treatment of severe recalcitrant cystic and/or conglobate acne unresponsive to conventional therapy; used investigationally for the treatment of children with metastatic neuroblastoma or leukemia that does not respond to conventional therapy

Pregnancy Risk Factor X

Contraindications Sensitivity to parabens, vitamin A or other retinoids

Warnings Not to be used in women of childbearing potential unless woman is capable of complying with effective contraceptive measures; therapy is normally begun on the second or third day of next normal menstrual period; effective contraception must be used for at least 1 month before beginning therapy, during therapy, and for 1 month after discontinuation of therapy

Precautions Use with caution in patients with diabetes mellitus

Adverse Reactions

Central nervous system: Fatigue, headache, dizziness

Dermatologic: Pruritus, hair loss, cheilitis, photosensitivity

Endocrine & metabolic: Hypertriglyceridemia, hyperuricemia

Gastrointestinal: Xerostomia, anorexia, nausea, vomiting, inflammatory bowel syndrome

Hematologic: Increase in erythrocyte sedimentation rate, decrease in hemoglobin and hematocrit

Hepatic: Hepatitis

Neuromuscular & skeletal: Bone or joint pain, muscle aches

Ocular: Conjunctivitis, corneal opacities

Miscellaneous: Epistaxis

Drug Interactions Avoid other vitamin A products; may interfere with medications used to treat hypertriglyceridemia

Food Interactions Increased isotretinoin bioavailability when given with food or milk

Mechanism of Action Reduces sebaceous gland size and reduces sebum production; regulates cell proliferation and differentiation

Pharmacokinetics

Absorption: Oral: Demonstrates biphasic absorption

Distribution: Crosses the placenta; appears in breast milk

Protein binding: 99% to 100%

Metabolism: In the liver; major metabolite: 4-oxo-isotretinoin (active)

Half-life, terminal: 10-20 hours for isotretinoin, and 11-50 hours for its metabolite

Peak serum levels: Within 3 hours

Elimination: Excreted equally in urine and feces

Usual Dosage Oral: 0.5-2 mg/kg/24 hours in 2 divided doses for 15-20 weeks

Monitoring Parameters CBC with differential and platelet count, baseline sed rate

Patient Information Avoid pregnancy during therapy; use birth control; discontinue therapy if visual difficulties, abdominal pain, rectal bleeding, diarrhea; exacerbation of acne may occur during first weeks of therapy; avoid use of other vitamin A products; decreased tolerance to contact lenses may occur; do not donate blood for at least 1 month following stopping of the drug; effective contraceptive measures must be used since this drug may harm the fetus; there is information from manufacturers about this product that you should receive; there is a copy of patient information which can be given to patient or for your information; do not double next dose if dose is skipped

Dosage Forms Capsule: 10 mg, 20 mg

Figure 19–4. Sample formulary listing.

The pharmacy's non-formulary procedure may or may not restrict the use of various dosage forms of a given chemical entity, so pharmacy technicians need to understand the policy in place at their specific institutions. The P&T committee regularly reviews non-formulary drug utilization to identify trends and review concerns, and this process may prompt the addition of new products to the formulary over time.

Pharmaceutical Purchasing Groups

Most health system pharmacies are members of a **group purchasing organization (GPO).** The GPO contracts with manufacturers to purchase pharmaceuticals at discounted prices, in return for a guaranteed minimum purchase volume. Hospitals, independent community pharmacies, and other retail chain pharmacies typically become members of a GPO to leverage buying power and take advantage of the lower prices that manufacturers offer to the GPOs.

Purchasing contracts can involve sole-source or multisource products. Sole-source *branded* products are available from only one **manufacturer**, whereas multisource *generic* products are available from numerous manufacturers. Although sole-source products may be produced by only one manufacturer, they may be included in what is known as a competitive market basket. For example, the echinocandin antifungal agent class contains all of the sole-source branded competing products in the market basket, including caspofungin (Cancidas), micafungin (Mycamine), and anidulofungin (Eraxis).

GPOs negotiate purchasing contracts that are mutually favorable to members of the group and to manufacturers. In addition to lower prices, pharmacies also benefit because this reduces the time staff spent establishing and managing purchasing contracts with product vendors. A GPO guarantees the price of pharmaceuticals over the established contract period, which may be one year or more. With the purchase price predetermined, the pharmacy can order the product directly from the manufacturer or from a wholesale supplier.

Occasionally, manufacturers are unable to supply a given product that the pharmacy is buying on contract, which may require the pharmacy to buy or substitute a competing product that is not on contract at a higher cost. Most purchasing contracts include provisions that protect the pharmacy from incurring additional expenses in the event this occurs. Generally, the manufacturer is responsible for rebating the difference in cost back to the pharmacy when this occurs. Therefore, it is important that the pharmacy technician documents any resulting off-contract purchases and communicates the information to the pharmacist-in-charge for reconciliation with the contracted product vendor.

Direct Purchasing

Direct purchasing from a manufacturer involves the execution of a purchase order (PO) from the pharmacy to the manufacturer of the drug. A **purchase order** is a document, executed by a purchaser and forwarded to a supplier, that is considered a legal offer to buy products or services. It usually indicates descriptive information, such as the item description, package size, desired quantity, and listed price. The advantages of direct purchasing include not having to pay handling fees to a third-party wholesaler, the ability to order on an infrequent basis (e.g., once a month), and a less demanding system for monitoring inventory. Some disadvantages include the following: a large storage capacity is needed; a large amount of cash is invested in inventory; the pharmacy's return/credit process becomes more complicated; and staff resources required in the pharmacy and accounts payable department to prepare, process, and pay purchase orders to more companies are increased. Other disadvantages include the likelihood that the manufacturer's warehouse is not local in relation to the pharmacy, which creates a dependency on the shipping firms used by the manufacturers to ship products reliably. In addition, the delivery schedule is often unpredictable or not available on weekends, and there may be delays in delivery.

For most pharmacies, the disadvantages of direct ordering outweigh the advantages. As a result, most pharmacies primarily purchase through a drug wholesaler. The **wholesaler** (also known as distributor) usually operates a large-scale warehouse in various geographic regions and exists to help bring pharmaceutical products closer to the market. This helps local pharmacies buy in smaller quantities and receive drugs in a timely manner (i.e., often same day), as opposed to ordering products directly from the manufacturer, in which case shipping and product delivery may take many days. It helps pharmacies manage their expenses and more effectively turn over their shelf inventories. Some drugs, however, can only be purchased directly from the manufacturers. These products generally require unique control or storage conditions and may be very costly, relative to others. An example is Botulinum Immune Globulin Intravenous (also known as BabyBIG®. This product is used to treat suspected infant botulism and must be ordered under a strict protocol from the Infant Botulism Treatment and Prevention Program (IBTPP), operated by the State of California. Once the BabyBIG® treatment indication is established and approved (on a patient-by-patient basis), the ordering pharmacy must complete an invoice and purchase agreement in order to initiate shipment of this life-saving product. In 2010, the current price per vial of BabyBIG® was approximately $45,300. Once purchased, funds must be wired to the IBTPP within five business days to satisfy the terms of the order. Consequently, most pharmacies use a combination of direct purchases from manufacturers and drug wholesalers.

Drug Wholesaler and Prime Vendor Purchasing

Purchasing from a drug wholesaler permits the acquisition of drug products from different manufacturers through a single vendor. When a health system pharmacy agrees to purchase most (e.g., 90 to 95%) of its pharmaceuticals from a single wholesale company, a **prime vendor** arrangement is established, and, customarily, a contract between the pharmacy and the drug wholesaler is developed. Usually, wholesalers agree to deliver 95 to 98% of the items on schedule and offer a 24-hour/7-day-per-week emergency service. They also provide the pharmacy with electronic order entry/receiving devices, a computer system for ordering, bar coded shelf stickers, and a printer for order confirmation printouts. They may also offer a highly competitive discount (minus 1 to 2%) below product cost/contract pricing and competitive alternate contract pricing.

Some wholesalers offer even larger discounts to pharmacies that may prefer a prepayment arrangement. In these situations, the wholesaler monitors the aggregate purchases of the pharmacy (e.g., a rolling three-month average) and bills the pharmacy this amount in advance (prepayment). This may be attractive to both the wholesaler and the pharmacy because it creates larger cash flow and investment capital for the wholesaler while saving the organization money on its pharmaceutical purchases through discounted pricing.

These wholesaler services make the establishment of a prime vendor contract appealing and result in the following advantages: more timely ordering and delivery, less time spent creating purchase orders, fewer inventory carrying costs, less documentation, computer-generated lists of pharmaceuticals purchased, and overall simplification of the credit and return process. Purchasing through a prime vendor customarily allows for drugs to be received shortly before use, supporting a just-in-time ordering philosophy (which is described later in the chapter). Purchasing from a wholesaler is a highly efficient and cost-effective approach toward pharmaceutical purchasing and inventory management.

Borrowing Pharmaceuticals

No matter how effective a purchasing system is, there are times when the pharmacy must borrow drugs from other pharmacies. Most pharmacies have policies and procedures addressing this situation. Borrowing or lending drugs between pharmacies is usually restricted to emergency situations and limited to authorized staff. Borrowing is also limited to products that are commercially available, thus eliminating items such as compounded products or investigational medications. Most pharmacies have developed forms to document and track merchandise that is borrowed or loaned (figure 19-5). These forms also help staff document the details that are needed to prevent errors in the transactions.

Community Pharmacy
555-3779

Borrowed From: ______________________ Lent To: ______________________
Drug: ______________________
Amount: ______________________
(# of vials, tablets, etc. and bulk or unit dose packaging)
Date: ______________________ By: ______________________
****
Date ordered: ____________ From: ____________ By: ____________
Date returned: ______________________ By: ______________________
Date in Loan Book: ______________________ By: ______________________
Value: $________

Figure 19-5. Sample borrow/lend form.

The pharmacy department's borrow and lend policies and procedures should provide detailed directions on how to borrow and lend products, which products may be borrowed or loaned, sources for the products, and reconciliation of borrow and lend transactions (the payback process). Securing the borrowed item may require the use of a transport or courier service or may include the use of security staff or other designated personnel. Some states have established strict limits on the quantities of products that can be borrowed or loaned under *casual sale* protocol, such as interpharmacy borrowing, lending, or even donating to a charity cause such as a legitimate medical mission. This information is vital for pharmacy technicians to understand so that they can fulfill their responsibility when borrowing or lending products.

Rx for Success

Purchasing and inventory staff should keep up with returning borrowed items in order to remain in good standing with those pharmacies that participate in this practice. Reconciliation of these items should be done at least quarterly.

Receiving and Storing Pharmaceuticals

One of the most useful experiences for a new pharmacy technician is to observe the way that the pharmacy department receives pharmaceuticals. This experience is useful for a number of reasons:

- It helps the pharmacy technician become familiar with the various processes involved with the ordering and receiving of pharmaceuticals.
- It helps the technician become familiar with formulary items.
- It demonstrates the system used to ensure that only formulary items are put into inventory.
- It familiarizes the technician with the various locations in which drugs are stored.

Receiving is one of the most important parts of the pharmacy operation. A poorly organized and executed receiving system can put patients at risk and elevate health care costs. For example, if the wrong concentration of a product were received in error, it could lead to a dosing error or a delay in therapy. Misplaced products or out-of-stock products also jeopardize patient care, as well as the efficiency of the department—both are undesirable and costly outcomes. To avoid these unfavorable outcomes, pharmacy technicians need to become familiar with the process of receiving and storing pharmaceuticals.

The Receiving Process

Some pharmacies create processes whereby the person receiving pharmaceuticals is different from the person ordering them. This process is especially important for controlled substances, because it effectively establishes a check in the system to minimize potential drug diversion opportunities. Drug diversion is the theft of a pharmaceutical by an individual for illicit personal use or gain.

In a reliable and efficient receiving system, the receiving personnel verify that the shipment is complete and intact (i.e., they check for missing or damaged items) before putting items into circulation or inventory. The receiving process begins with the verification of the boxes containing pharmaceuticals delivered by the shipper. The person receiving the shipment begins the process by verifying that the name and address on the boxes are correct and that the number of boxes matches the shipping manifest. Many drug wholesalers use rigid plastic totes because they protect the contents of each shipment better than foam or cardboard boxes. These totes are also environmentally friendly; they are returned to the wholesaler for cleaning and reuse. Each tote should be inspected for gross damage.

Products with a cold storage requirement (i.e., refrigeration or freezing) should be processed first. The shipper is responsible for taking measures to ensure that the cold storage environment is maintained during the shipment process and generally packages these items in a shippable foam cooler that includes frozen cold packs to keep products at the correct storage temperature during shipment.

Receiving personnel play a critical role in protecting the pharmacy from financial responsibility for products damaged in shipment, products not ordered, and products not received. Any obvious damage or other discrepancies with the shipment, such as a breach in the cold storage environment or an incorrect product, should be noted on the shipping manifest, and, if warranted, that part of the shipment should be refused. Ideally, identifying gross shipment damage or incorrect tote counts should be performed in the presence of the delivery person and should be well documented when signing for the order. Other

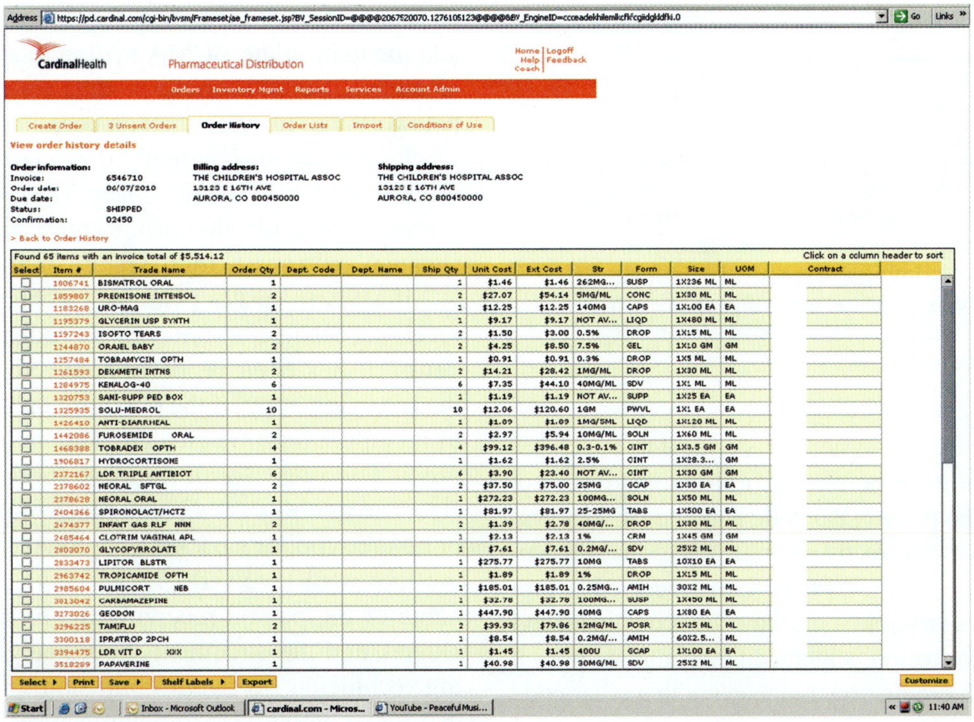

Address https://pd.cardinal.com/cgi-bin/bvsm/Frameset/ae_frameset.jsp?BV_SessionID=@@@@2067520070.1276105123@@@@&BV_EngineID=ccceadekhilemkcfkfcgidgkldfki.0

CardinalHealth Pharmaceutical Distribution

Home | Logoff
Help | Feedback
Coach

Orders Inventory Mgmt Reports Services Account Admin

Create Order | 3 Unsent Orders | Order History | Order Lists | Import | Conditions of Use

View order history details

Order information:
Invoice: 6546710
Order date: 06/07/2010
Due date:
Status: SHIPPED
Confirmation: 02450

Billing address:
THE CHILDREN'S HOSPITAL ASSOC
13123 E 16TH AVE
AURORA, CO 800450000

Shipping address:
THE CHILDREN'S HOSPITAL ASSOC
13123 E 16TH AVE
AURORA, CO 800450000

> Back to Order History

Found 65 items with an invoice total of $5,514.12

Click on a column header to sort

Select	Item #	Trade Name	Order Qty	Dept. Code	Dept. Name	Ship Qty	Unit Cost	Ext Cost	Str	Form	Size	UOM	Contract
	1006741	BISMATROL ORAL	1			1	$1.46	$1.46	262MG...	SUSP	1X236 ML	ML	
	1059807	PREDNISONE INTENSOL	2			2	$27.07	$54.14	5MG/ML	CONC	1X30 ML	ML	
	1183268	URO-MAG	1			1	$12.25	$12.25	140MG	CAPS	1X100 EA	EA	
	1195379	GLYCERIN USP SYNTH	1			1	$9.17	$9.17	NOT AV...	LIQD	1X480 ML	ML	
	1197243	ISOPTO TEARS	2			2	$1.50	$3.00	0.5%	DROP	1X15 ML	ML	
	1244870	ORAJEL BABY	2			2	$4.25	$8.50	7.5%	GEL	1X10 GM	GM	
	1257484	TOBRAMYCIN OPTH	1			1	$0.91	$0.91	0.3%	DROP	1X5 ML	ML	
	1261593	DEXAMETH INTNS	2			2	$14.21	$28.42	1MG/ML	DROP	1X30 ML	ML	
	1284975	KENALOG-40	6			6	$7.35	$44.10	40MG/ML	SDV	1X1 ML	ML	
	1320753	SANI-SUPP PED BOX	1			1	$1.19	$1.19	NOT AV...	SUPP	1X25 EA	EA	
	1325935	SOLU-MEDROL	10			10	$12.06	$120.60	1GM	PWVL	1X1 EA	EA	
	1426410	ANTI-DIARRHEAL	1			1	$1.09	$1.09	1MG/5ML	LIQD	1X120 ML	ML	
	1442086	FUROSEMIDE ORAL	2			2	$2.97	$5.94	10MG/ML	SOLN	1X60 ML	ML	
	1468388	TOBRADEX OPTH	4			4	$99.12	$396.48	0.3-0.1%	OINT	1X3.5 GM	GM	
	1906817	HYDROCORTISONE	1			1	$1.62	$1.62	2.5%	OINT	1X28.3...	GM	
	2372167	LDR TRIPLE ANTIBIOT	6			6	$3.90	$23.40	NOT AV...	OINT	1X30 GM	GM	
	2378602	NEORAL SFTGL	2			2	$37.50	$75.00	25MG	GCAP	1X30 EA	EA	
	2378628	NEORAL ORAL	1			1	$272.23	$272.23	100MG...	SOLN	1X50 ML	ML	
	2404366	SPIRONOLACT/HCTZ	1			1	$81.97	$81.97	25-25MG	TABS	1X500 EA	EA	
	2474377	INFANT GAS RLF NNN	2			2	$1.39	$2.78	40MG/...	DROP	1X30 ML	ML	
	2485464	CLOTRIM VAGINAL APL	1			1	$2.13	$2.13	1%	CRM	1X45 GM	GM	
	2803070	GLYCOPYRROLATE	1			1	$7.61	$7.61	0.2MG/...	SDV	25X2 ML	ML	
	2833473	LIPITOR BLSTR	1			1	$275.77	$275.77	10MG	TABS	10X10 EA	EA	
	2963742	TROPICAMIDE OPTH	1			1	$1.89	$1.89	1%	DROP	1X15 ML	ML	
	2985604	PULMICORT NEB	1			1	$185.01	$185.01	0.25MG...	AMIH	30X2 ML	ML	
	3013042	CARBAMAZEPINE	1			1	$32.78	$32.78	100MG...	SUSP	1X450 ML	ML	
	3273026	GEODON	1			1	$447.90	$447.90	40MG	CAPS	1X80 EA	EA	
	3296225	TAMIFLU	2			2	$39.93	$79.86	12MG/ML	POSR	1X25 ML	ML	
	3300118	IPRATROP 2PCH	1			1	$8.54	$8.54	0.2MG/...	AMIH	60X2.5...	ML	
	3394475	LDR VIT D XXX	1			1	$1.45	$1.45	400U	GCAP	1X100 EA	EA	
	3518289	PAPAVERINE	1			1	$40.98	$40.98	30MG/ML	SDV	25X2 ML	ML	

Select ▸ | Print | Save ▸ | Shelf Labels ▸ | Export | Customize

Figure 19–6. Electronic purchase order.

problems identified after delivery personnel have left, such as mispicks (i.e., products sent in error by the vendor), product dating, or internally damaged goods, must be resolved according to the vendor's policies. Most vendors have specific procedures to follow in reporting and resolving such discrepancies. The technician can also identify packages that are received containing broken tablets, defective seals, etc., so that the wholesaler/shipper can be alerted to weaknesses in the delivery system. Quality issues can often be identified first by the technicians working the receiving area.

The next step of the receiving process entails checking the newly delivered products against the receiving copy of the purchase order. This generally occurs after the delivery person has left. A purchase order, created when the order is placed, is a complete list of the items that were ordered. Some pharmacies may still use a traditional paper purchase order. However, the state-of-the-art practice employs electronic, Web-based technology to place orders with respective wholesale distributors (figure 19-6). In this case, the order is transmitted and received in an instant, and the wholesaler's inventory of particular products is available in near real-time. This technology allows for more efficient operations and effective communication between the pharmacy and wholesaler and simplifies order reconciliation and billing processes.

TECHNOLOGY TOPICS

The contemporary practice of receiving employs bar code technology, which simplifies the process of receiving—to the extent that invoice reconciliation against the contents of shipment totes can be accomplished with a bar code scanner.

The person responsible for checking products into inventory uses the receiving copy of the purchase order that is included in each wholesaler tote to ensure that the products ordered have been received. The name, brand, dosage form, size of the package, concentration or strength, and quantity of product must match the purchase order.

Once the accuracy of the shipment is confirmed, the packing list is generally signed and dated by the person receiving the shipment. At this point, the product's expiration date should be checked to ensure that it meets the department's minimum expiration date requirement. Frequently, departments require that products received have a minimum shelf life of 6 months remaining before they expire.

Technology Topics

Bar Code Medication Administration (BCMA) is a novel technology that has slowly emerged in health care institutions. It is meant to improve the safety of medication administration at the bedside and improve medication administration documentation in the patient's electronic health record.

If a hospital uses a BCMA system, it is critical that each bar code be scanned at the time that each product is received. This ensures that the product bar code is in the BCMA system so that it can scan correctly when it gets to the bedside. This applies even if the product has been received before from the same manufacturer. Some bar codes contain lot and expiration date information, which could change with each manufacturer batch production. In the event that a bar code does not scan, it is customary for the receiving technician to add the item to the BCMA system manually or to overlay an internal bar code on the product prior to shelving it. It is noteworthy to mention that, on occasion, the manufacturer/wholesaler may inadvertently ship an excess quantity of an ordered product to the pharmacy. The ethical response is to immediately notify the manufacturer or wholesaler of this situation and arrange for the return of any excess quantity.

If a pharmacist or pharmacy technician other than the receiving technician removes a product from a shipment before it has been properly received and cannot locate the receiving copy of the purchase order, a written record of receipt should be created. This is done by listing the product, dosage form, concentration/strength, package size, and quantity on a blank piece of paper (figure 19-7) or on the supplier's packing slip/invoice and checking off the line item received (figure 19-8). In both cases, the name of the person receiving the product should be included, and the document should be given to the receiving technician, to avoid confusion and an unnecessary call to the wholesaler or manufacturer.

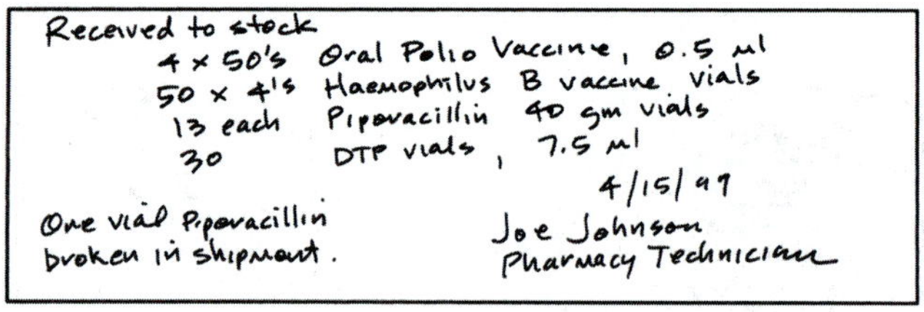
Received to stock
4 x 50's Oral Polio Vaccine, 0.5 ml
50 x 4's Haemophilus B vaccine vials
13 each Piperacillin 40 gm vials
30 DTP vials, 7.5 ml
4/15/97
One vial Piperacillin broken in shipment.
Joe Johnson
Pharmacy Technician

Receipt on blank piece of paper must include precise detail of the amount, product description, person receiving product, and the date of receipt.

Figure 19-7. Receipt of pharmaceutical on blank paper.

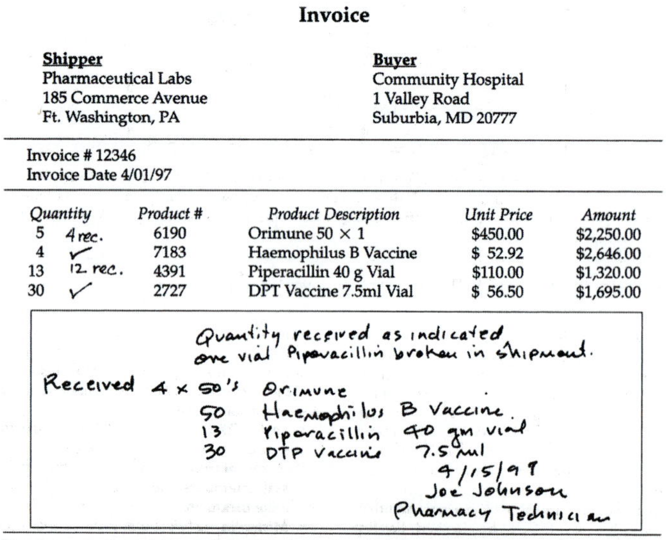
Invoice

Shipper
Pharmaceutical Labs
185 Commerce Avenue
Ft. Washington, PA

Buyer
Community Hospital
1 Valley Road
Suburbia, MD 20777

Invoice # 12346
Invoice Date 4/01/97

Quantity		*Product #*	*Product Description*	*Unit Price*	*Amount*
5	4 rec.	6190	Orimune 50 × 1	$450.00	$2,250.00
4	✓	7183	Haemophilus B Vaccine	$ 52.92	$2,646.00
13	12 rec.	4391	Piperacillin 40 g Vial	$110.00	$1,320.00
30	✓	2727	DPT Vaccine 7.5ml Vial	$ 56.50	$1,695.00

Quantity received as indicated, one vial Piperacillin broken in shipment.
Received 4 x 50's Orimune
50 Haemophilus B Vaccine
13 Piperacillin 40 gm vial
30 DTP vaccine 7.5 ml
4/15/97
Joe Johnson
Pharmacy Technician

Receipt on an invoice or packing slip can be done the same way as receipt on a blank piece of paper or the quantities can be checked or modified as received.

Figure 19-8. Receipt of pharmaceutical on packing slip/invoice.

The Storing Process

Once the product has been received properly, it must be stored properly. Depending on the size and type of the pharmacy operation, the product may be placed in a bulk central storage area or into the active dispensing area of the pharmacy. In any case, the expiration date of the product should be compared with that of the products currently in stock. Products already in stock that have expired should be removed. Products that will expire in the near future should be highlighted and placed in the front of the shelf or bin. This is a common practice known as **stock rotation.** The newly acquired products generally have longer shelf lives and should be placed behind packages that will expire before them.

✔ Stock rotation is an important inventory management principle that encourages the use of products before they expire and helps prevent the use of expired products and waste.

Table 19-1 identifies the optimal storage temperatures and humidity.

The use of automated dispensing devices in in-patient hospital nursing units, clinics, operating rooms, and emergency rooms has facilitated the use of computers for inventory management. Similar devices are evolving in retail pharmacy and hold promise for not only making the dispensing process safer and more efficient, but also serving to assist in inventory management. These devices are essentially repositories, or *pharmaceutical vending machines*, for medications that are dispensed directly from a patient care area.

A variety of manufacturers of automated dispensing devices are in the current market. The Pyxis Medstation and Omnicell are common examples of devices available to institutions. These machines generally are networked via a dedicated computer file server within the facility, and they allow both unit-dose and bulk pharmaceuticals to be stocked securely on a given patient care unit location. Each unit's inventory is configurable and allows for variation and flexibility from device to device, depending on the unit's location.

Product Handling Considerations

Pharmacy technicians usually spend more time handling and preparing medications than the pharmacists. This presents pharmacy technicians with the critical responsibility of assessing and evaluating each product from both a content and labeling standpoint. It also provides the technician with an opportunity to confirm that the receiving process was performed properly.

Just as checking the product label carefully when a prescription or medication order is filled is important, taking the same care when receiving pharmaceuticals and accurately placing them in their storage location are essential. The pharmacy technician should read product packaging carefully rather than relying on the general appearance of the product (e.g., packaging type, size or shape, color, logo), because a product's appearance can change frequently and may be similar to that of other products. Technicians play a vital role in minimizing dispensing errors that can occur because of human fallibility. They are generally the first in a series of checks involved in an accurate dispensing process.

When performing purchasing or inventory management roles, the technician must pay close attention to the product's expiration date. For liquids or injectable products, the color and clarity of the items should also be checked for consistency with the product standard. Products with visible particles, an unusual appearance, or a broken seal should be reported to the pharmacist.

Table 19–1. Defined Storage Temperatures and Humidity†

Freezer	–25° to –10° C	–13° to 14° F
Cold (Refrigerated)	2° to 8° C	36° to 46° F
Cool	8° to 15° C	46° to 59° F
Room Temperature	The temperature prevailing in a working area.	
Controlled Room Temperature	20° to 25° C	68° to 77° F
Warm	30° to 40° C	86° to 104° F
Excessive Heat	Any temperature above 40°C (104° F)	
Dry Place	A place that does not exceed 40% average relative humidity at controlled room temperature or the equivalent water vapor pressure at other temperatures. Storage in a container validated to protect the article from moisture vapor, including storage in bulk, is considered a dry place.	

† United States Pharmacopeia 26/The National Formulary 21, pp. 9–10;2003. United States Pharmacopeial Convention, Inc., Rockville, MD.

Look-Alike/Sound-Alike Products

Because pharmacy technicians handle so many products each day, they are in an ideal position to identify packaging and storage issues that could lead to errors. Technicians should pay close attention to these three main issues of product similarity:

1. Similar *drug names*. Various drugs with similar names (e.g., niCARdipine, NIFEdipine, cycloSPORINE, cycloSERINE) can cause problems when stored in an immediately adjacent shelf position. Although the use of **tall man lettering** can help draw attention to the dissimilarities in the product name, extra precaution in shelf positioning may be warranted (figure 19-9).
2. *Similar package sizes.* Stocking products of similar name, color, shape, and size can result in error if someone fails to read the label carefully. Sometimes the company name or logo is emphasized on the label instead of the drug name, concentration, or strength (figure 19-10). Pharmacy repackaged items often look the same as a result of the nature of the packaging process implemented.
3. *Similar label format.* Storing products that are similar in appearance adjacent to one another can result in error if someone fails to read the label (figure 19-11).

Safety First The convention of labeling pharmaceuticals with tall man lettering is also known as mixed case labeling, and it is an important tactic employed in the interest of calling attention to similarities in drug names. Research on this approach has demonstrated effectiveness in distinguishing similarities and preventing look-alike, sound-alike drug mix-ups.[2]

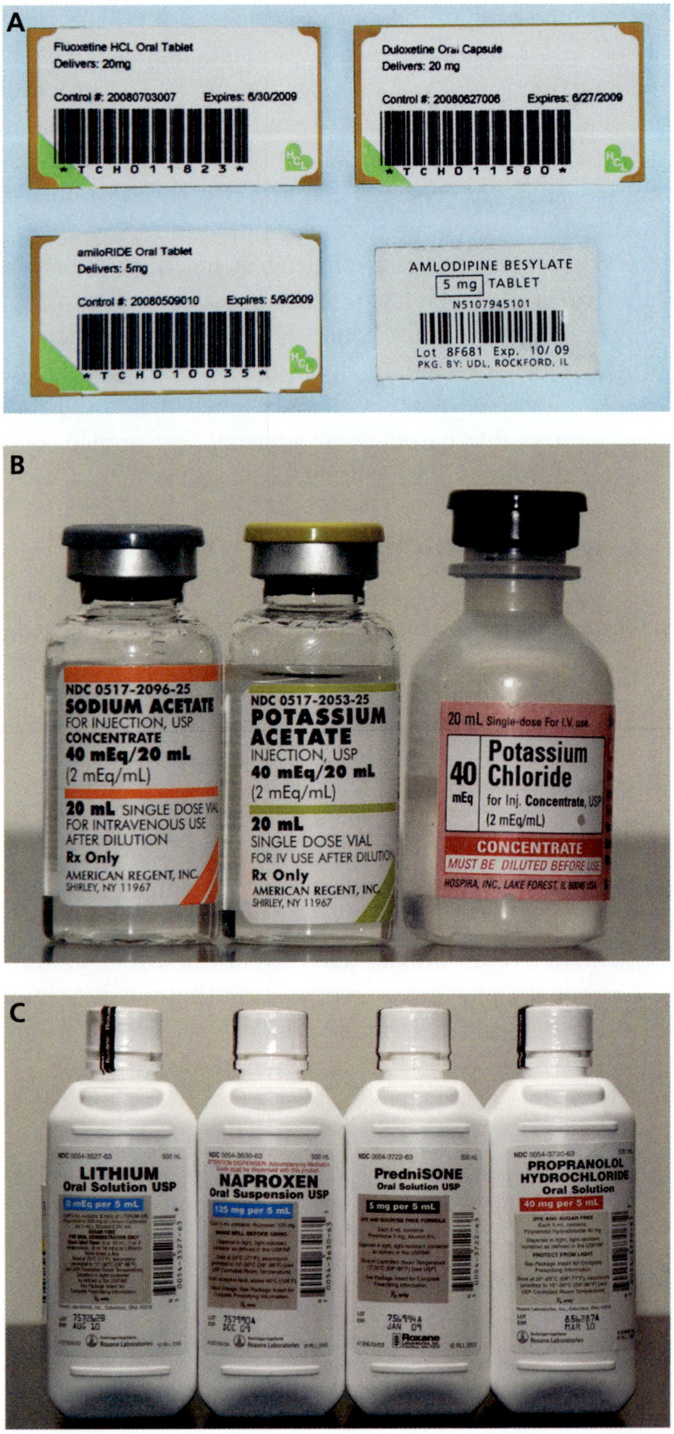

Figure 19–9. Look-alike/sound-alike product names.

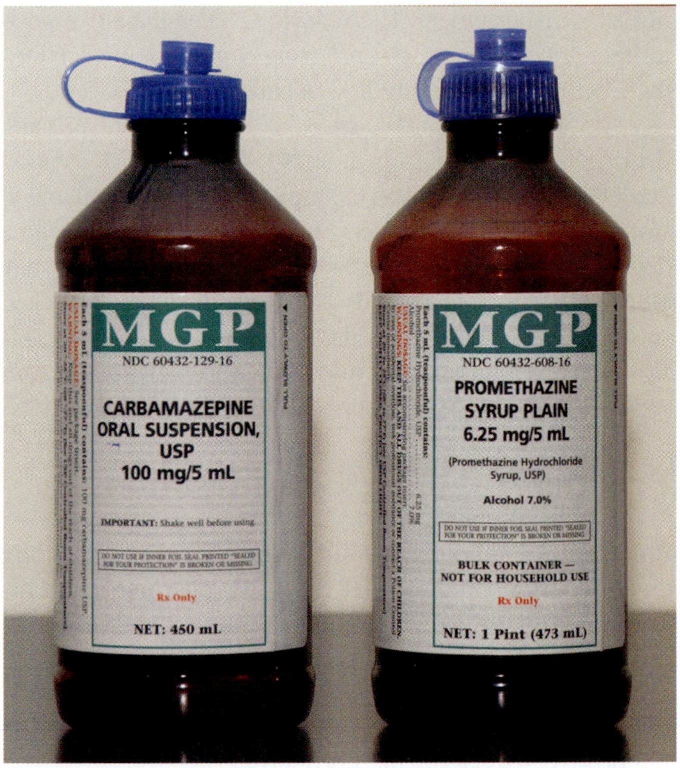

Figure 19–10. Product labeling, showing emphasis on manufacturer name.

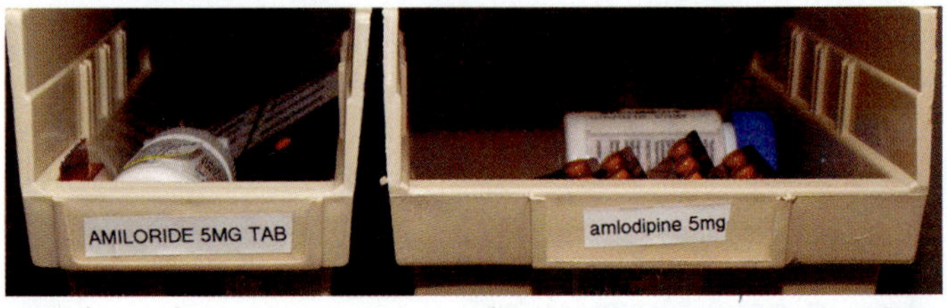

Figure 19–11. Product inventory: label format and shelf position.

Alerting other staff members to products that fall into one of these categories is essential. Some pharmacies routinely discuss product handling considerations at staff meetings or in departmental newsletters. Dispensing errors can be averted by simply relocating a look-alike/sound-alike product or by placing warning notes (i.e., auxiliary labeling or highlights) on the shelf or directly on the product itself. Pharmacy technicians should also discuss their concerns with coworkers and advocate changes to products with poor labeling.

Products Requiring Special Handling

The principles discussed in the prior section of this chapter generally apply to all pharmaceutical products. The procurement, receipt, and storage of certain classes of pharmaceuticals, such as controlled substances, investigational drugs, chemotherapy, radiopharmaceuticals, compounded drugs, and some other products, require the knowledge of additional requirements.

Controlled Substances. Controlled substances have specific ordering, receiving, storage, dispensing, inventory, record-keeping, return, waste, and disposal requirements established under the law. The *Pharmacist's Manual: An Informational Outline of the Controlled Substances Act of 1970* and the *ASHP Technical Assistance Bulletin on Institutional Use of Controlled Substances* provide detailed information on the specific handling requirements for controlled substances.[3,4]

It is critical for pharmacy technicians to know two principles regarding controlled substances:

1. Ordering and receiving Schedule II controlled substances require special order forms and additional time (1 to 3 days).
2. Controlled substances are inventoried and tracked continuously. This type of inventory method is referred to as a **perpetual inventory process**, whereby each dose or packaged unit, such as a tablet, vial, or milliliter of fluid volume, is accounted for at all times.

In some pharmacies, pharmacy technicians work with pharmacists to manage inventory and order, dispense, and store controlled substances. See Chapter 2, Pharmacy Law, for more information on controlled substances.

Controlled substances require additional processing when ordering, receiving, dispensing, storing, and inventorying occurs. These procedures are required by Drug Enforcement Administration (DEA) regulations and, in many cases, the State Board of Pharmacy. These regulations create the chain of accountability in the interest of minimizing drug diversion, illicit drug use, and public safety. State and federal regulations vary regarding length of storage requirements for purchase orders, invoices, and dispensing records. It is best to check both sets of regulations and comply with the stricter requirements.

Regulations specific to Schedule II controlled substances require DEA form 222 to be completed to initiate procurement of these products. Form 222 is a triplicate, handwritten form, and each copy has a specific intent, as specified by the DEA. On receipt of DEA Schedule II products, the pharmacy must separately file the appropriate copy of form 222, along with the supplier's copy of the invoice and packing slip accompanying each shipment. Alternatively, the pharmacy can be registered with the DEA to place Schedule II orders online through the wholesaler's electronic process.

✔A perpetual inventory of Schedule II products is maintained by the pharmacy, so an exact accounting should be performed whenever a product is added or removed from the inventory.

Schedule III, IV, and V controlled substances are generally obtained in a manner identical to that for other noncontrolled substances. However the receipt and storage requirements of these products may depend on state regulation or on the specific employer's policy. For example, state regulation may require a pharmacy to file separately the receipts of all controlled substances ordered during a particular year and to maintain them in a readily retrievable manner for inspection. Some pharmacies may require all controlled substances inventories to be shelved separately from other legend drugs, whereas others may store them together.

Chemotherapy. Because of the hazards inherent with human exposure to antineoplastic or chemotherapy products, care and precaution must be exercised in the receipt, handling, and storage of these products. The distributor generally ships antineoplastic drugs separately and apart from other products (e.g., in their own container). Special care should be exercised when opening and unpacking totes containing these products. Although the distributor takes appropriate measures to pack and pad the items properly inside totes, it is still possible for damage to occur. As an additional safety precaution, many pharmacy operations keep the inventory locations of these products completely separate from those of other medications (usually in a dedicated satellite pharmacy, or the area where the antineoplastic drugs are prepared for patient administration). Pharmacy technicians should be familiar with the organization's chemotherapy and hazardous materials spill management protocol. Most hospitals have a "chemotherapy spill kit" on hand to be used in the management and cleanup of an accidental spill.

Investigational Drugs. Investigational drugs also require special ordering, inventorying, and handling procedures. Generally, the use of investigational drugs is categorized into two distinct areas: 1) use under a formal protocol approved by the site's institutional review board (IRB), and 2) the compassionate use of investigational drugs for a single patient as may be authorized by the manufacturer and the FDA. Compassionate drug use is legal, although the drug is technically still being scientifically tested by the manufacturer (usually in a late stage of drug development) and will eventually be considered by the FDA for licensure as it shows promising health benefits. In both cases, the physician or primary investigator may be responsible for ordering the product, whereas the pharmacy staff generally handles the inventory management and distribution of the investigational drug once it is received. Most research protocols require very rigorous investigational drug inventory and dispensing records, including maintaining a perpetual inventory of the product. Maintaining a perpetual inventory is similar to that required for DEA Schedule II drugs; it means that the pharmacy follows procedures to ensure a complete and accurate accounting of the precise quantity on hand for the drug (down to the single unit of measure). Other record-keeping in this context involves evidence of proper cold chain storage—a complete daily log of product refrigeration temperatures and actions that is taken if the storage temperature range deviated from those required by the product. Research Site Monitors (regulatory administrators) invariably ask to see these records during their periodic site visits. Investigational drug products are typically required under protocol to be stored in a secured area of the pharmacy, physically separate and apart from those noninvestigational products, simply as a matter of preventing an inadvertent dispensing error.

Some pharmacies associated with academic institutions that conduct clinical research have organized investigational drug services that are formally managed by a pharmacist who is principally dedicated to pharmaceutical research activities. In these cases, the investigational drug service pharmacist may have been delegated authority to order, dispense, and manage the inventory of investigational drugs in full compliance with the research protocol.

Pharmacy technicians often prepare or handle investigational drugs and participate in the perpetual inventory record-keeping system.

Rx for Success

Pharmacy technicians must learn department procedures for investigational drugs and be competent in the proper handling, storage, dispensing, and inventory systems involved.

Restricted Drug Distribution System (RDDS). The intent of the restricted drug distribution system is to ensure that specific drugs identified as high risk are safely procured, prescribed, dispensed, and administered. The FDA, the manufacturer, and the distributor collaborate to establish tighter controls over designated products.

If improperly administered, certain drugs can cause serious adverse effects, such as blood disorders, birth defects, or changes in cardiovascular status. For example, the drug thalidomide can cause severe birth defects. If the clinical benefit of using a restricted drug is perceived to outweigh the risks, the pharmacy can obtain it under prescription if proper screening, education, and monitoring requirements are satisfied.

Satisfying the requirements necessary to obtain these drugs may be limited to the presence of a specific disease state being treated by a physician who is registered under the RDDS. As a matter of satisfying restricted distribution requirements, the physician may have to attest to patient-specific criteria. This might include a failed treatment response to other medications, contraindications to other therapy, or evidence from laboratory data. In other cases, physicians may need to commit to administering the medication under controlled conditions, such as in their office. In most cases, the RDDS requires registration of the prescribing physician, dispensing pharmacy, patient name and other demographic information, a patient agreement form for liability purposes, the specific indication for the medication, its dose and quantity to be dispensed. In some programs, lab results, adherence to a robust patient counseling or outreach protocol, and reimbursement information guaranteeing payment are required (table 19-2). The primary goal of RDDS is safe, effective product use and reduced risk to the patient.

Compounded Products. Unlike drugs ordered from an outside source, compounded products are extemporaneously prepared in the pharmacy as indicated by scientific compounding formulas. These products may include oral liquids, topical preparations, solid dosage forms, and sterile products.

The use of compounded products requires that prescribing patterns and expiration dates be monitored closely. These products typically have short expiration dates, ranging from days to months. Because pharmacy technicians likely identify usage patterns and determine stock and product needs, procedures for monitoring patient use, product expiration dates, and additional stock needs must be well-known and adhered to by technicians in order to prevent stock shortages. Specific pharmacy technicians may initiate compounding activities, but this may vary according to departmental procedures.

Table 19-2. Examples of Restricted Distribution Products

Drug	Physician Enrollment and Training	Patient Enrollment	Specific Requirements: Requires Registration of Retail Pharmacy to Dispense	Specialty Distributor or Centralized Pharmacy	Adminis-tration in Medical Setting	Requires Lab Test Prior to Distribution
Abarelix (Plenaxis)	X		X*		X+	
Alosetron (Lotronex)	X					
Ambrisentan (Letairis)	X	X	X			X^^
Bosentan (Tracleer)	X	X		X		
Clozapine (Clozaril)	X	X	X			X^
Deferasirox (Exjade)	X			X		
Dofetilide (Tikosyn)	X	X	X		X++	
Getfitinib (Iressa)	X	X		X		
Isotretinoin (Accutane)	X	X	X			X^^
Lenalidomide (Revlimid)	X	X		X		X^^
Mifepristone (Mifeprex)	X				X+	
Natalizumab (Tysabri)	X			X**		
Sodium Oxybate (Xy-rem)	X	X		X		
Thalidomide (Thalomid)	X	X	X			X^^

* dispensed by registered hospital pharmacy
** dispensed only to authorized infusion sites
\+ administered in doctor's office
++ 3-day in-patient hospital stay required upon initiation
^ white blood cell count
^^ negative pregnancy test

As described in Chapter 15, Nonsterile Compounding and Repackaging, many pharmacies extemporaneously prepare (or compound) pharmaceutical products from raw materials. The skill of compounding pharmaceutical products is both an art and a science. Materials used in the process often include commercially available pharmaceuticals, chemicals, suspending agents, sweeteners, and levigating agents. Some of these raw materials are not routinely available through the pharmaceutical wholesaler and must be procured through a specialty supply house. Pharmaceutical-grade raw materials require a pharmacy or medical license prior to shipment.

All chemicals are shipped according to the Department of Transportation (DOT) and company safe practice standards and include a materials safety data sheet (MSDS) for each chemical. Strong acids and alkaline chemicals and other toxic raw materials are frequently used in the process of compounding pharmaceuticals. The receiving pharmacy technician should be familiar with the utility and safe product handling and storage requirements of these chemicals.

✔ The MSDS information must be made available to all staff who may be exposed to the chemical. MSDS sheets are often maintained in a central location, accessible to all pharmacy staff for immediate reference.

Chemical inventories should be completely separate from commercially available pharmaceuticals, preferably in another room in a designated shelving section or storage cabinet, in the interest of patient and staff safety.

Repackaged Pharmaceuticals. Although manufacturers supply many drugs in prepackaged unit-dose forms, the pharmacy staff is responsible for packaging some products. These items are generally unit-dose tablets and capsules, unit-dose oral liquids, and some bulk packages of oral solids and liquids (also see Chapter 15, Nonsterile Compounding and Repackaging).

Each pharmacy establishes stocking mechanisms for these products and relies on pharmacy technicians to identify and respond to production and stock needs. Generally, designated technicians coordinate repackaging activities, but some pharmacies may integrate repackaging with other responsibilities of the pharmacy technician. Knowledge of the department's procedures for repackaging is required to prevent disruptions in dispensing activities.

Non-Formulary Items. Non-formulary items also require special handling. No matter how much planning is devoted to formulary management, some patients still need medications that are not routinely stocked in the pharmacy. The pharmacist usually determines when a non-formulary medication should be ordered. However, the pharmacy technician is often in the best position to monitor the supply and determine when and if additional quantities should be ordered.

Non-formulary medications generally are not mixed into the shelving system of formulary products in the pharmacy; they fall outside normal inventorying mechanisms. Often, manual tracking mechanisms and computer system queries of active non-formulary orders are the two most common techniques used to monitor and order these products.

Medication Samples. Traditional inventory management and handling practices do not work well with medication samples for two reasons:

1. Medication samples are not ordered by the pharmacy—they are usually provided to physicians on request by the drug manufacturer and are free of charge. This often occurs without the pharmacy's knowledge.
2. Samples are not usually dispensed by the pharmacy.

Both of these factors make it difficult to know whom to contact if a medication sample is recalled and difficult to ensure that medication samples are not sold. Because of difficulties in controlling samples, organizations may allow samples to be stored and dispensed in ambulatory clinics only after being registered with the pharmacy for tracking purposes. These difficult logistical and control factors have led many organizations to adopt policies that simply disallow medication samples.

If an organization allows samples, the samples are likely stored outside the pharmacy and requires that pharmacy personnel to register and inspect the stock of medication samples. Pharmacy technicians are sometimes involved in inspecting medication sample storage units. These technicians are often responsible for determining whether a sample is registered with the pharmacy, stored in acceptable quantities, labeled with an expiration date that has not been exceeded, and, generally, stored under acceptable conditions. The technician should review the department's policies and procedures regarding medication samples to learn the role of the pharmacy technician in this regard.

Radiopharmaceuticals. Radiopharmaceutical agents are typically used in diagnostic imaging as contrast media and can include oral and injectable products. Other radiopharmaceutical products are used therapeutically to treat diseases of the thyroid gland and forms of cancer. Technically speaking, these drugs are radioactive and potentially hazardous to humans and the environment because they emit low to moderate levels of radiation. Therefore, special procedures aimed at minimizing exposure are warranted. Pharmacy technicians should become intimately familiar with and closely follow policies and procedures associated with the procurement, handling, and storage of radiopharmaceutical products. See Chapter 6, Specialty Pharmacy Practice, for additional information.

Maintaining and Managing Inventory

An inventory management system is an organized approach designed to maintain just the right amount of pharmaceutical products in the pharmacy at all times. A variety of inventory management systems are used, ranging from simple to complex. They include employing an order book in which pharmacy staff write down what is necessary to order (aka the "eyeball" method); the minimum/maximum (par) level; the Pareto (ABC) Analysis; and the fully automated, computerized system.

Business Philosophies and Models

The Pareto ABC Analysis, also known as the 80/20 rule, essentially groups inventory products, by aggregate value and volume of use, into three groupings: A, B, and C (figure 19-12). This analysis is useful in determining where inventory control efforts are best directed. For example, group A may include 20% of all items that make up 65% of the inventory cost. Tighter inventory control over these items would be sensible. Group B may include

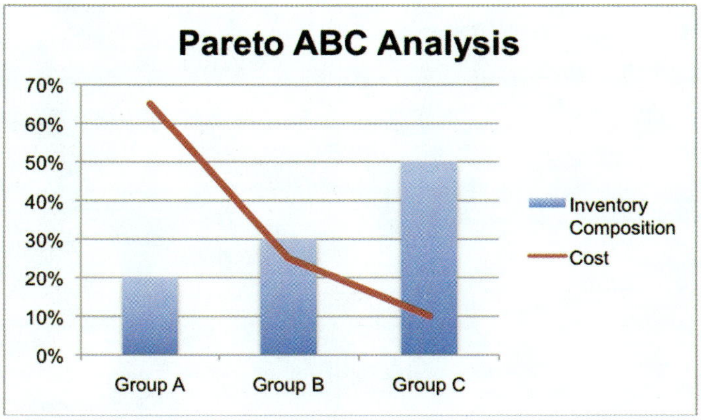

Figure 19–12. Pareto ABC analysis.

30% of items and 25% of the inventory cost. An automatic order cycle might be useful for B items, based on well-established par levels. Group C may include 50% of items and 10% of the inventory cost. Less aggressive monitoring of C items may be reasonable.

Manual Systems

Manual inventory models require the active oversight of pharmacy technicians and are usually based on a minimum/maximum, or par-level, system. The **par-level system** uses predetermined stock minimum and maximum quantities to be maintained. Once item par-levels are established, they are usually identified on or near the shelf label of individual pharmaceutical items kept in inventory. For example, based on average production demand, the average daily consumption of 1-gram vials of cefazolin injection might be 57, but it may range from as low as 50 to as many as 150 per day, depending on seasonal patient volume. If the pharmacy can obtain cefazolin from its wholesaler routinely within 24 hours, in this case, it may be reasonable to maintain daily inventory levels at a minimum quantity of 75 vials and a maximum of 100 vials. If the minimum and maximum par-level quantities appear on the shelf where the product is stored, staff can more readily assess and order products to avoid shortages and interruption in patient care, and par-level quantities can be changed on a day-by-day basis, depending on seasonal demand.

Staff members can create a pharmaceutical order using a handheld bar code scanning device, or they can enter product stock numbers directly into a personal computer. They strive to maintain physical pharmaceutical inventories within the minimum to maximum range to avoid running short on a product or overstocking. Running short on a product can affect patient care, and overstocking adds unnecessary operational expense.

Manual systems require pharmacy staff to scan inventory levels routinely and place orders accordingly. With both electronic and manual systems, pharmacy staff should be aware that the diversity of their patients' specific needs or dynamic seasonal volume may require modification in a particular product's par-level. In contrast to a manual system, with an automated perpetual inventory system, each dispensing transaction is subtracted from the perpetual inventory that is maintained electronically in a computerized database; conversely, quantities of products received are automatically added to the inventory on hand in the computerized system. When the quantity of a pharmaceutical product in stock reaches a predetermined point (often called *par*), a purchase order is automatically generated to order more of the product. The system does not depend on any one employee to monitor the inventory or reorder pharmaceuticals.

The technology for having a computerized inventory in most pharmacies is available, but interfacing a computerized inventory system with existing pharmacy computer systems designed for dispensing and patient management systems is often difficult. In addition, other variables, such as product availability, contract changes, and changing use patterns (either up or down), make relying on the fully computerized model challenging. Consequently, even the most sophisticated electronic and automated systems still require human oversight.

Automated dispensing devices are capable of tracking perpetual inventory at the product level. They also limit access to only authorized personnel and record the identities of individuals who access inventory, as well as how much of a specific drug was removed for a given patient. A useful feature in many of these systems allows pharmacy personnel to generate automatically a fill-list of what needs to be replenished on the basis of a par-level system. In essence, the nursing and medical personnel who use these automated dispensing devices have a computerized inventory and billing system that the pharmacy staff manages. Medications used to restock these devices may be taken from the pharmacy's main inventory, or a separate purchase order may be executed for each device on a periodic basis.

The par-level inventory system relies on a predetermined order quantity and an order point. These systems typically include shelf labels that correspond to each product and that are placed on the storage bin or shelf to

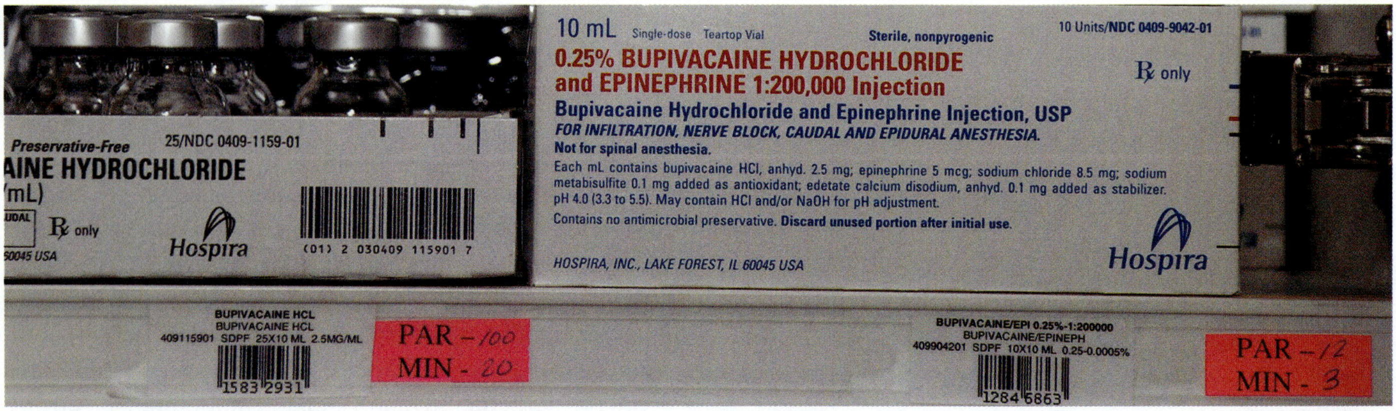

Figure 19–13. Shelf labels correspond to each product and are placed on the storage bin or shelf. The minimum and maximum inventory level is written on this label, and the information is used as a relative guide for pharmacy staff involved in purchasing pharmaceuticals.

alert staff to the minimum stock quantity (figure 19-13). The minimum and maximum inventory level is written on this label, and the information is used as a relative guide for pharmacy staff involved in purchasing. When removing a product, the pharmacy technician should always determine whether the minimum stock quantity has been reached and inform the appropriate purchasing personnel or list the item in a designated order book as described in the following. An assigned staff member performs a periodic inventory of the stock to identify products that have a stock level at or below the reorder point. When the inventory is reduced to or is below the order point, designated pharmacy personnel initiate or electronically transmit a purchase order to a drug wholesaler.

Just-in-time inventory management is a philosophy that simply means products are ordered and delivered at just the right time—when they are needed for patient care—with a goal of minimizing wasted steps, labor, and cost. Pharmaceuticals are neither overstocked nor understocked. In pharmacy, this business philosophy couples responsible financial management of pharmaceutical purchasing with the clinical aspects of patient care.

A related business philosophy is known as **maximizing inventory turns**. This is important because a product is technically a business asset that should not sit on the shelf unused for long periods.

✔ Specific drug inventory is ideally purchased and used many times throughout the course of a year; therefore, the inventory is turned over every time the stock is depleted and reordered.

A simple means of calculating total inventory turns in a given period is to divide the total purchases in that period by the value of physical inventory taken at a reasonable single point in time.

For example, if total pharmaceutical purchases in a 12-month calendar period or other fiscal year (FY) business accounting cycle were $10,24,590 and the physical inventory value on 12/31/2009 was $521,550, the calculated inventory turns for FY2010 would be 19.6 times ($10,243,590/$521,550 = 19.6). This method assumes a relatively constant volume of pharmaceutical purchases and constant residual inventory over time. The economic principle is simple: avoid buying pharmaceuticals that won't be used in a timely manner. Minimizing inventory carrying costs (or holding costs) is an important aspect of sound business administration. Carrying cost can be defined as all costs associated with inventory investment and storage costs, which might include interest, insurance, taxes, and storage expenses.

Regardless of the inventory system used, pharmacy technicians are vital contributors to its success. The pharmacy technician may frequently identify changes in use or prescription patterns of pharmaceuticals. Examples of reasonable stocking up might include high use of asthmatic medications by the emergency department, high doses of a particular IV benzodiazepine sedative by a critically ill patient who is likely to be hospitalized for an extended period, a long-acting pain reliever used by one or more oncology patients, or the seasonal utilization of a drug such as palivizumab to prevent serious viral infections in high-risk infants during the winter months. The converse is true as well; specific product inventory par-levels should be managed downward when a high-use patient is discharged. Alerting purchasing staff to orders for unusual amounts of medications helps avoid out-of-stock situations and facilitates optimal inventory management.

> **Rx for Success**
>
> Pharmacy technicians are in an ideal position to identify trends in pharmaceuticals. Be aware of the need to order more of a specific medication in response to high use by specific patients, as well as the need to reduce stock of pharmaceuticals that are rarely used or tend to expire before use.

Automated Systems

Many pharmacies use a simple order book system, also called a *want list* or *want book*. When pharmacists or pharmacy technicians determine that a product should be reordered—the "eyeball" approach—they write the item in the order book. Although this approach is simple, it provides the least amount of structured control over inventory because par-levels are generally not established. Its success is highly dependent on the participation of the staff. Therefore, the order book system is usually not the sole method of inventory management and is often used in conjunction with one of the other systems mentioned previously.

A most effective system for inventory management is the automated or computerized system that supports a just-in-time product inventory. Automated systems automatically maintain a perpetual computerized inventory of drug products stocked within them. An example of this type of application is the *pharmacy workflow system* marketed by Omnicell.[5] This system allows for complete integration of the remote supply distribution cabinets, central dispensing carousel systems, and bar code packaging systems. It automates the ordering, receiving, stocking, and picking process and relies heavily on bar code product technology. In addition to facilitating the inventory management process, this program can also help the pharmacist capture product expiration dates and lot numbers upon dispensing. This system is very effective as long as the wholesale product delivery systems are efficient and the electrical power supply to the units themselves is maintained. Imagine the difficulty in reverting to a manual process if the power went out! Backup systems are highly recommended as business continuity measures in the event of technological or other utility failure.

Although automated inventory management modalities are available, they have not become the mainstay of current practice. Generally, a combination of manual and automated inventory systems is employed.

Proper Disposal and Return of Pharmaceuticals

Despite the most efficient systems, well-developed policies and procedures, and the best intentions of staff to manage the pharmaceutical inventory properly, it is nearly impossible to avoid encountering inventory items that expire and require proper disposal for one reason or another.

Expired Pharmaceuticals

The most common reason that drugs are returned to the manufacturer is because they have expired. The process for returning drugs in the original manufacturer packaging is relatively simple and not particularly time-consuming when done routinely. Returning expired products to the manufacturer or wholesaler prevents the inadvertent use of these products and enables the department to receive either full or partial credit for them. Some wholesalers limit credit given on returns of short-dated products. Generally, wholesalers do not give full credit on returns of products that expire within six months.

To return products, pharmacy personnel must complete the documentation required by the product's manufacturer or wholesaler and package the product so that it can be shipped. Many wholesalers have implemented electronic documentation systems to further simplify the return process. Technicians often perform these duties under the supervision of a pharmacist. Some pharmacies contract with an outside vendor, a reverse distributor, who completes the documentation and coordinates the return of these products for an agreed-upon fee. In that case, the pharmacy technician need only assist the vendor with the location and packaging of expired pharmaceuticals.

Expired pharmaceuticals compounded or repackaged by the pharmacy department cannot be returned and, for safety reasons, must be disposed of after they have expired. Proper disposal prevents the use of subpotent products or products without guaranteed sterility. The precise procedure for disposal depends on the type and content of the product. Many states are now enforcing regulations issued in the 1970s by the Environmental Protection Agency under the Resource Conservation and Recovery Act (RCRA) that govern the proper disposal mechanisms of hazardous chemicals, including drugs.[6] Thus, each pharmacy should have detailed procedures governing the proper, legal disposal of pharmaceutical waste. The pharmacy technician should be familiar with these procedures. Disposal of expired, compounded, or repackaged pharmaceuticals by the pharmacy technician should be completed under the supervision of the pharmacist (see the following section on Pharmaceutical Waste Management).

Other expired products that require disposal rather than return are chemicals used in the pharmacy laboratory. Most pharmacies stock a supply of chemical-grade products used in extemporaneous pharmaceutical compounding, such as sodium benzoate or sodium citrate (preservatives); lactose or talc (excipients); buffers; and active pharmaceutical ingredients, such as phenol, hydrocortisone, neomycin, or lidocaine. When such products expire, they should be disposed of in accordance with the pharmacy's hazardous waste procedures and state laws.

Expired controlled substances are disposed of uniquely. These products can't be returned to the manufacturer or wholesaler for credit. They must be destroyed, and the destruction must be documented to the satisfaction of the DEA. The DEA provides a specific form, titled "Registrant's Inventory of Drugs Surrendered" (Form 41), for recording the disposal of expired controlled substances. Ideally, the actual disposal of expired controlled substances should be completed by a company sanctioned by the DEA or by a representative of the state board of pharmacy. In other cases, the DEA may allow the destruction of controlled substances by a pharmacy, provided that the appropriate witness process is followed and documented. The DEA disposal of controlled substances form should be completed properly and submitted to the DEA immediately after the disposal. A copy of the record of disposal form is signed by a DEA representative and returned to the pharmacy, where it is kept on file.

The use and disposition of investigational drugs must also be documented carefully. Expired investigational drugs should be returned to the manufacturer or sponsor of an investigational drug study according to the instructions provided. The pharmacy technician may be responsible, under the supervision of the pharmacist, for the completion of documentation, packaging, and shipment of the expired investigational agents. Investigational drug products that expire because of product instability or sterility issues should never be discarded. These doses should be retained with the investigational drug stock and be clearly marked as expired drug products; the investigational study sponsor needs to review and account for all expired investigational drug products.

Return of Other Pharmaceuticals

Non-expired pharmaceuticals that need to be returned because of an ordering error generally require authorization from the original supplier and completion of the appropriate documentation. The Prescription Drug Marketing Act mandates that pharmacies authorize and retain records of returned pharmaceuticals to prevent potential diversion of pharmaceuticals. The pharmacy technician must be familiar with pharmacy department procedures for returning medications to a supplier; this includes sample medications that may have been provided by a manufacturer. Typically, a pharmacy has a process for returning mistakenly ordered medications to the prime drug wholesaler on a routine basis, which prevents the need for storage in the pharmacy of overstocked or mistaken products. The pharmacy technician may be responsible for relevant documentation, filing paperwork, and packaging returned products under the supervision of the pharmacist.

Pharmaceutical Waste Management

The environmental impact of pharmaceutical waste is becoming a prominent public health issue worldwide. A report following a multiple-month study indicates that trace amounts of pharmaceuticals are present in the drinking water of 24 major U.S. metropolitan cities nationwide.[7] This problem is a concern because many pharmaceuticals maintain potency or pose toxic health threats to humans and other animals, despite water purification through rural and metropolitan treatment facilities. Although some of the contamination comes naturally through human excretion, a larger concern is the routine waste disposal of medication by consumers and pharmacies through the sewer system and landfills. In fact, pharmaceuticals are widely considered chemical pollutants (like pesticides and industrial sewage). Drugs that affect the endocrine system (hormones), antimicrobials, and active byproducts are but a few of the pharmaceuticals found in increasing amounts in waterways and drinking water.

As a result of this increasing concern, the Environmental Protection Agency (EPA) and state health departments are expected to enforce proper pharmaceutical disposal practices more rigorously. Adherence with regulations and pharmaceutical waste-stream management protocols is expensive and operationally challenging, to say the least. However, it is a socially responsible imperative to curb this environmental threat.

✔ It is the obligation of not only the pharmacist, but all others involved in the handling and disposal of medications, to understand the environmental implications of drug waste and to comply with procedures employed to protect the environment, public safety, and future generations.

Drug Recalls

A **drug recall** effectively removes a manufactured product from the market. Manufacturers, on their own accord or at the direction of the Food and Drug Administration (FDA), occasionally **recall** pharmaceuticals for such reasons as mislabeling, contamination, lack of potency, lack of adherence to the acceptable Good Manufacturing Practices, or other situations that may present a significant risk to public health. A pharmacy must have a system for rapid removal of any recalled products.

Role of the Food and Drug Administration

The FDA plays an active role in initiating the drug recall process. Unlike biologics and devices, the FDA has no statutory (legal) authority to recall drugs. Manufacturers voluntarily issue recalls in their duty to protect public health, and the FDA helps manufacturers coordinate drug recall information and develop specific voluntary recall plans. It performs health hazard evaluations to assess public risk associated with products being recalled (**Table 19-3**). When recalls are issued, the FDA classifies recall actions in accordance with the level of risk and works with manufacturers to formulate recall strategies on the basis of the health hazard presented by the product. It decides on the need for public warnings and assists the recalling agency with public notification about the recall as needed.

Table 19–3. FDA Drug Recall Classes[8]

FDA Drug Recall Classes	
Class I	The most serious of recalls; ongoing product use may result in serious health threat or death.
Class II	Moderate severity concern; ongoing product use may pose serious adverse events or irreversible consequences.
Class III	Lowest severity concern; ongoing product use unlikely to cause adverse health threat; however, a marginal chance of injury may exist, so the product is being recalled.

The following were the top reasons for drug recalls in 2007.[9]

1. Correctly labeled product in incorrect package.
2. Temperature abuse.
3. Subpotent (single-ingredient drugs).
4. Chemical contamination.
5. Impurities/degradation products.
6. Failed USP dissolution test requirements.
7. Labeling illegible.
8. Marketed without an approved New Drug Application (NDA)/abbreviated New Drug Application (ANDA).
9. Lack of assurance of sterility.
10. Label mix-up.
11. Stability data that do not support expiration date.
12. Microbial contamination of nonsterile products.

Role of Manufacturers, Distributors, and Pharmacies

Because of their responsibility to protect the public consumer, manufacturers and distributors typically implement *voluntary recalls* when a marketed drug product needs to be removed from the market. This method of recall is more efficient and effective in ensuring timely consumer protection than an FDA-initiated court action or seizure of the product. Recall notices are sent in writing to pharmacies by the manufacturer of the product or by drug wholesalers. These notices indicate the class of recall, the reason for recall, the name of the recalled product, the manufacturer, all affected lot numbers of the product, response required, instructions on the extent of action required in contacting affected patients, and how to return the product to the manufacturer.

On receipt of the recall notice, a pharmacy staff member, usually a pharmacy technician, checks all pharmaceutical inventory stores to determine whether any recalled products are in stock. If none of the recalled products are in stock, a note indicating "none in stock" is written on the recall notice and filed in a recall log to document that the recall was properly addressed. If a recalled product is in stock, all products should be gathered, packaged, and returned to the manufacturer if requested. In some cases, the drug is destroyed. The instructions and product package should be reviewed by the pharmacist-in-charge before returning the drug to the manufacturer or distributor. Any recall action taken should be in accordance with the instructions provided in the recall notice, and these actions should be well-documented for future reference.

If patients have received a recalled product, the pharmacist-in-charge has a duty to follow the action required by the recall notice. Examples of actions taken may be to collect and segregate any remaining inventory of the recalled product and arrange for return through the wholesale distributor; to provide prudent notification of medical providers or other allied health professionals associated with the use of the recalled product; and to contact any patients who may have received the recalled product lot number(s) and to offer proper counseling on what to do.

Upon completion of all activity regarding the product recall, a summary of actions taken should be documented on the recall letter and filed in the pharmaceutical recall log. The FDA has been known to request documentation of all recall activities to ensure compliance and, ultimately, patient safety. The technician should keep in mind that it may be necessary to order replacement stock to compensate for recalled items that were removed from stock. In some instances, the recall may encompass all products, and it is impossible to order replacement stock. The pharmacist-in-charge should be notified in this case in order to decide which, if any, alternative products may be required to place into inventory as therapeutic alternatives to the out-of-stock items.

Drug Shortages

Often, manufacturers are unable to supply a pharmaceutical because of various supply and demand situations, such as the inability to obtain raw materials, manufacturing difficulties related to equipment failure, or the inability to produce sufficient quantities to stay ahead of the market demand for the pharmaceutical. Although unfortunate, drug shortages are a reality that must be managed to avoid compromising patient care. As with drug recalls, the pharmacist-in-charge should be notified in order to communicate drug shortages and recommend alternative therapies effectively to prescribers. Both ASHP and the FDA publish a valuable resource listing on their Web sites that highlights the status of current manufacturers' shortages (see the Resources section at end of the chapter).

Counterfeit Pharmaceuticals

Unfortunately, there is a global concern related to the fraudulent mislabeling and distribution of counterfeit drugs. These products are dangerous because they may not meet standards of quality or potency and are therefore ineffective in treating the disease for which they are intended and can cause harm. These products can range from those containing incorrect ingredients, subpotency, and even toxic ingredients, even though the package or dosage form appears to be legitimate. Obviously, these products are illegal and pose serious threats to the patient and caregiver.

Any pharmaceutical product is at risk for being counterfeited, and developing countries appear to be the most threatened by this malicious activity. Unfortunately, the level of sophistication of individuals engaged in the act of counterfeiting is growing, even in countries with more highly controlled markets, including the United States. In 2009, the U.S. Department of Health and Human Services warned the public of fraudulent H1N1 influenza products.[10] Illegal Internet-based pharmacies were suspected of selling drugs without prescriptions and for selling fraudulent or counterfeit products.

What's being done about this problem? In 2006, the World Health Organization formed an initiative aimed at combating counterfeit medication distribution. It is a global partnership called International Medicinal Products Anti-Counterfeiting Taskforce (IMPACT). The organization has brought together international enforcement and regulatory agencies, customs and police authorities, pharmaceutical manufacturing representatives, wholesale companies, health care providers, and patient delegates to coordinate efforts and raise awareness of this problem. As a result, laws, standards, monitoring and reporting programs, and penal sanctions are being developed and coordinated to minimize the threat of fraudulent medication distribution. In many states, pedigree laws have either been passed or are in the pipeline. Simply stated, these laws require the drug wholesaler to provide a statement of origin or otherwise prove the genealogy of drugs distributed. Every step in the distribution chain has to be documented and verified, from the point of manufacturer origin to the wholesale distribution point. An electronic pedigree (e-Pedigree) ensures, through documentation, that a drug was safely and securely manufactured and distributed.

Through e-Pedigree, complete accountability for the drug chain of custody can occur, and reasonable assurances necessary to protect public interests are provided. Pedigree regulations likely limit the ability of pharmacies to return drugs to distributors. Unfortunately, fraudulent drugs have entered the supply chain as returns to reputable wholesalers.

Pharmacy technicians need to be aware of the existence of counterfeit pharmaceuticals and the methods that are being employed to address the issue. When managing drug shortages and working outside of the routine wholesale distribution channels, it is essential to ensure that pharmaceuticals are being obtained from a reliable source. It is acceptable to obtain and verify the licensing information from alternative drug suppliers or from those purporting to have product when other reputable suppliers do not. The technician should also remain aware of those pharmaceutical products that are known or suspected to be at risk and communicate any concerns when procuring, receiving, and handling these products.

Summary

The movement of pharmaceuticals into and out of the pharmacy requires an organized, systematic, and cooperative approach. The pharmacy technician plays a vital role in maintaining the functionality of these systems because the medication is ultimately used to provide pharmaceutical care. Familiarity with product conditions and uses positions the pharmacy technician to identify quality and care issues that can strengthen the purchasing and inventory control system.

Self-Assessment Questions

1. The formulary contains important information to assist the pharmacy technician in all of the following areas except:
   a. Identification of trade names of products
   b. Identification of product concentration
   c. Identification of package size
   d. Identification of expiration dates
2. Receiving and storing pharmaceuticals should be reserved solely for personnel with subject matter expertise in group purchasing and contracting processing.
   a. True
   b. False
3. When receiving a shipment of pharmaceuticals, use DEA form 106 to check in the order.
   a. True
   b. False
4. Most drug inventories are organized by National Drug Code (NDC).
   a. True
   b. False
5. When documenting the receipt of pharmaceuticals for which the purchase order or manufacturer's invoice cannot be located, which of the following should be recorded?
   a. Product name and amount
   b. Product name, strength, and amount
   c. Date of receipt, product name, and amount
   d. Date of receipt, name of receiver, product name, strength, dosage form, and amount
6. A receiving copy of a purchase order is not required to check in an order if a manufacturer's invoice is available.
   a. True
   b. False
7. Which of the following is not an important consideration in processing a manufacturer's recall notice?
   a. Checking the refrigerator temperature logs
   b. Timely response in checking the inventory and removing affected products
   c. Documenting the inspection and any action required
   d. Receiving proper credit from the manufacturer
8. Restricted distribution products are the same as controlled substances.
   a. True
   b. False
9. Virtually any pharmaceutical product can be counterfeited, and developing countries appear to be the most threatened by this malicious activity.
   a. True
   b. False
10. Which types of pharmaceuticals are found in increasing amounts in waterways and drinking water?
   a. Injectables
   b. Contrast media
   c. Antimicrobials
   d. Over-the-counter products

Self-Assessment Answers

1. d. The formulary serves as a valuable reference in determining all aspects of product information, including the generic and brand names, drug concentration, and package size. It does not contain expiration dates, which vary by product.
2. b. False. Receiving and storing of pharmaceuticals is an important process that should be performed routinely by experienced pharmacy staff. However, it is important for trainees and inexperienced staff to learn the receiving and storing process.
3. b. False. The receiving copy of the purchase order (not DEA form 106) should be used to check in a pharmaceutical order because it documents precisely what was ordered.
4. b. False. In most cases, the drug storage areas in the pharmacy are arranged alphabetically, by either the generic or trade name of the drug.

5. d. It is important to document essential information about the product, the receiver, and the date of receipt.
6. b. False. If a drug was shipped in error, the receiving copy of the purchase order may be different from the manufacturer's invoice. Therefore, a copy of the purchase order should be used to check in a shipment of pharmaceuticals.
7. a. The most critical processes in responding to a manufacturer's recall are reviewing and removing affected products from the hospital's inventory, documenting the inspection and any action required, and receiving proper credit from the manufacturer.
8. b. False. Although the restricted distribution of certain pharmaceuticals is very tightly regulated and may be restricted by the FDA, the manufacturer, or distributor, those pharmaceuticals are distinctly different from controlled substances, which are regulated by the DEA.
9. a. True. Any pharmaceutical product is at risk for being counterfeited, but developing countries appear to be the most threatened by this malicious activity.
10. c. Antimicrobials, drugs that affect the endocrine system (hormones), and active (but metabolized) byproducts are but a few of the pharmaceuticals found in increasing amounts in waterways and drinking water.

Resources

American Society of Hospital Pharmacists. ASHP statement on the formulary system. *Am J Hosp Pharm.* 1983;40: 1384–1385.

American Society of Health-System Pharmacists. Drug shortages. Available at: http://www.ashp.org/shortages.

American Society of Health-System Pharmacists. (2007) Pharmaceutical waste management: issues and options for health systems. Retrieved from ASHP Advantage. Available at: http://symposia.ashp.org/pharmawaste/.

American Society of Health-System Pharmacists. (2007) Pharmaceutical waste management: a discussion guide for health-system pharmacists. Retrieved from ASHP Advantage. Available at: http://symposia.ashp.org/pharmawaste/Discussion_Guide.pdf.

Bicket WJ, Gagnon JP. Purchasing and inventory control for hospital pharmacies. *Top Hosp Pharm Manage.* 1987;7(2): 59–74.

Celia F. (2005, June 6). States move to comply with move to require pedigree laws. Retrieved from Drug Topics. Available at: http://drugtopics.modernmedicine.com/drugtopics/article/articleDetail.jsp?id=163714.

Department of Defense. (2008, August 28). *Drugs subject to restricted distribution or controlled access programs.* Retrieved from Department of Defense Pharmacoeconomic Center. Available at: http://pec.ha.osd.mil/Controlled_Distribution_Drugs.php?submenuheader=0.

Eban, K. (2005). *Dangerous Doses: How Counterfeiters Are Contaminating America's Drug Supply.* Orlando, FL: Harcourt, Inc.

FDA. (2010, April 7). Drug shortages. Retrieved from U.S. Food and Drug Administration. Available at: http://www.fda.gov/Drugs/DrugSafety/DrugShortages/default.htm.

FFF Enterprises. (2010) Drug pedigree laws. Retrieved from FFF. Available at: http://www.fffenterprises.com/Resources/PedigreeMap.aspx.

Hughes TW. Automating the purchasing and inventory control functions. *Am J Hosp Pharm.* 1985;42:1101–1107.

Kroll DJ. The pharmacy technician as a purchasing agent. *J Pharm Tech.* 1985;1(1):29–31.

Roffe BD, Powell MF. Quality assurance aspects of purchasing and inventory control. *Top Hosp Pharm Manage.* 1983;3(3): 62–74.

Soares DP. Quality assurance standards for purchasing and inventory control. *Am J Hosp Pharm.* 1985;42:610–620.

U.S. Food and Drug Administration Center for Drug Evaluation and Research. (2010, April 25). *The National Drug Code Directory.* Retrieved from FDA. Available at: http://www.fda.gov/drugs/informationondrugs/ucm142438.htm.

Wetrich JG. Group purchasing: an overview. *Am J Hosp Pharm.* 1987;44:158–192.

World Health Organization. (2010) Counterfeit medicines. Retrieved from WHO. Available at: http://www.who.int/mediacentre/factsheets/fs275/en/.

Yost RD, Flowers DM. New roles for wholesalers in hospital drug distribution. *Top Hosp Pharm Manage.* 1987;7(2): 84–90.

References

1. Omnicell. *Inventory Management Carousel.* Available at: http://www.omnicell.com/Resources/Datasheets/WorkflowRx.pdf. Accessed May 14, 2010.
2. Institute for Safe Medication Practice. Use of tall man letters is gaining wide acceptance. ISMP Medication Safety Alert; 2008, July 31. Available at: http://www.ismp.org/newsletters/acutecare/articles/20080731.asp. Accessed May 14, 2010.
3. U.S. Department of Justice Drug Enforcement Administration. Pharmacist's manual: an informational outline of the Controlled Substances Act of 1970. April 2004.

8th ed. Washington, DC: DEA. Available at: http://www.deadiversion.usdoj.gov/pubs/manuals/pharm2/2pharm_manual.pdf. Accessed May 14, 2010.

4. American Society of Hospital Pharmacists. ASHP technical assistance bulletin on institutional use of controlled substances. *Am J Hosp Pharm.* 1987;44:580–589.
5. Omnicell. *Pharmacy Workflow System.* Available at: http://www.omnicell.com/Solutions/Central-Pharmacy-Automation/Pharmacy-Workflow/Pages/default.aspx. Accessed May 14, 2010.
6. United States Environmental Protection Agency. Wastes: information resources. *RCRA Online.* Available at: http://www.epa.gov/waste/inforesources/online/index.htm. Accessed May 14, 2010.
7. CBS News Health. *Probe: pharmaceuticals in drinking water.* March 10, 2008. Available at: http://www.cbsnews.com/stories/2008/03/10/health/main3920454.shtml. Accessed May 14, 2010.
8. US Recall News. Product Recall Classes I, II, III. March 7, 2008. Available at: http://www.usrecallnews.com/2008/03/product-recall-classes-i-ii-iii.html. Accessed May 14, 2010.
9. Center for Drug Evaluation and Research. *Improving Public Health Through Human Drugs.* Food and Drug Administration, U.S. Department of Health and Human Services; 2007.
10. U.S. Food and Drug Administration. *FDA, FTC warn public of fraudulent 2009 H1N1 influenza products offending web sites and illegal activity targeted for action.* FDA News Release: May 1, 2009. Available at: http://www.fda.gov/NewsEvents/Newsroom/PressAnnouncements/ucm149576.htm. Accessed May 14, 2010.

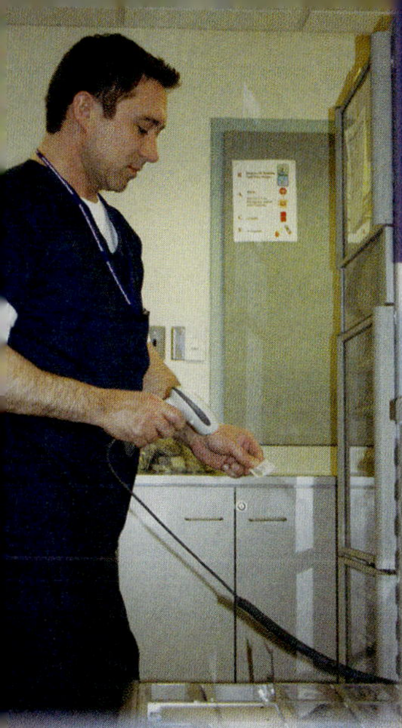

Chapter 20

Billing and Reimbursement

Sandra F. Durley, Margaret Byun, and JoAnn Stubbings

Learning Outcomes

After completing this chapter you will be able to:

- Explain the basic principles of pharmacy billing and reimbursement.
- Define common pricing benchmarks.
- List various payers of pharm Describe the differences in reimbursement processes dependent on aceuticals and pharmacy services.
- payers and patient care settings.
- Describe the categories of information that are needed to submit a third-party claim for a prescription or medication order.
- Use knowledge of third-party insurance billing procedures to identify a reason for a rejected claim.

Key Terms

adjudication Prescription claims adjudication refers to the determination of the insurer's payment after the member's insurance benefits are applied to a medical claim.

average manufacturer price (AMP) The average price paid to manufacturers by wholesalers for drugs distributed through retail pharmacies. This includes discounts and other price concessions that are provided by manufacturers.

average sales price (ASP) Price based on manufacturer-reported selling price data and includes volume discounts and price concessions that are offered to all classes of trade.

average wholesale price (AWP) A commonly used benchmark for billing drugs that are reimbursed in the community pharmacy setting. The AWP for a drug is set by the manufacturer of the drug.

coinsurance A percentage charge for a service, such as a prescription or doctor visit.

copayment An amount that insured individuals must pay for a service, such as a prescription or doctor visit, each time they use the insurance benefit.

cost sharing The amount of insurance costs shared by the employee or beneficiary.

coverage gap Also referred to as the "donut hole." This is a period of no coverage that typically occurs once the individual's total prescription drug spending for the year reaches the initial coverage limit. During the coverage gap, the beneficiary must pay all costs for prescriptions until the total prescription spending for the year reaches the catastrophic coverage threshold.

deductible A fixed amount that must be paid each year by the individual before the insurance starts to pay.

diagnosis-related group (DRG) A set rate paid for an inpatient procedure based on cost and intensity. Drugs provided during an inpatient stay are not separately reimbursed; they are included in the DRG payment.

dispensing fee The amount paid for dispensing the prescription.

federal upper limit (FUL) The maximum of federal matching funds that the federal government will pay to state Medicaid programs for eligible generic and multisource drugs.

fee for service A method of payment in which providers bill separately for each patient encounter or service they provide.

formulary A specific list of drugs that are included with a given prescription drug plan.

health care common procedure coding system (HCPCS) A set of medical codes that identifies procedures, equipment, and supplies for claim submission purposes.

indemnity A system of health insurance in which the insurer pays for the cost of covered services after care has been given on a fee-for-service basis. It usually defines the maximum amounts covered.

institutional patient assistance programs (IPAPs) Programs offering assistance to patients in an institution. Bulk medication replacement is provided to the institution (e.g., pharmacy or clinic) instead of to an individual patient. The institution has the obligation of verifying that each patient who receives medications meets the established criteria.

maximum allowable cost (MAC) Used for generic or multisource drug reimbursement; usually based on the cost of the lowest available generic equivalent.

network A group of pharmacies, physicians, hospitals, or other providers who participate in a certain managed care plan.

patient assistance programs (PAPs) Programs offering certain free drugs to low-income patients who lack prescription drug coverage and meet certain criteria.

pharmacy benefit manager (PBM) An organization that manages pharmacy benefits for managed care organizations, self-insured employers, insurance companies, labor unions, Medicaid and Medicare prescription drug plans, the Federal Employees Health Benefits Program, and other federal, state, and local government entities.

premium The amount the individual pays to belong to a health plan. Premiums are often paid monthly.

prior authorization Requires the prescriber to receive pre-approval from the PBM in order for the drug to be covered by the benefit.

prospective payment The amount to be paid for drugs is predetermined based on the condition that is being treated. It typically includes all costs associated with treating a particular condition, including medications.

quantity limits Set upper limits of an amount of a drug that is covered by the benefit, or the total days of therapy.

retrospective payment Drugs are dispensed and reimbursed later, according to a predetermined formula that is specified in a contract between the pharmacy and the third-party payer, such as the insurance company or pharmacy benefit manager.

revenue Represents the inflow of funds.

step therapy Requiring the use of a recognized first-line drug before a more complex or expensive second-line drug is used. Beneficiaries must try and fail with the first-line drug before a second-line drug can be covered by the benefit.

third-party payer An organization (either private or public) that reimburses a pharmacy or patient for products and/or services.

wholesale acquisition cost (WAC) Represents the "list price" at which the manufacturer sells the drug to the wholesaler.

In addition to providing goods and services, all businesses share a common goal—to make a profit. Even nonprofit organizations need to generate enough revenue to cover their expenses in order to remain viable. Pharmacies are no exception. In many practice settings, pharmacy technicians serve as the patient's first point of contact with the pharmacy billing system, so it is important for them to understand the basic concepts related to billing and reimbursement. This chapter provides a broad overview of the principles of pharmacy billing and reimbursement.

Pharmacy Accounting Basics

Most pharmacies are "hybrid businesses"; that is, they provide both goods and services. Although pharmacists provide many services that help ensure that patients use medications appropriately, the primary source of revenue generation for a pharmacy is the sale of products (i.e., drugs). In simple accounting terms, **revenue** represents the inflow of funds. Money is exchanged for goods and services that are provided. In a typical pharmacy setting, prescription and nonprescription drug sales account for the highest portion of revenue.

The outflow of cash is considered expenses. Before the revenue can be generated, the products (i.e., drugs) must be purchased by the pharmacy. The amount the pharmacy pays to a vendor to buy the drugs for stock is called the acquisition cost. In pharmacy terms, the margin is typically the difference between the selling price of a drug to the patient and the acquisition cost of the drug.

Margin = Amount paid by the patient – acquisition cost of drugs

Example: For a drug with an acquisition cost of $20 and for which the patient paid $50

Margin = $50 – $20 = $30

In addition to drug purchases, there are overhead costs associated with providing pharmaceutical products to patients. Overhead costs often include various expenses such as rent and utilities, personnel costs (i.e., salaries for pharmacists and technicians), equipment (computers, fax, printer), and supplies (labels, vials, etc.). These expenses represent cash outflow. The net profit is the amount of money that is left over after all of the expenses have been paid.

Net Profit = Total revenue – total expenses (i.e., cost of drugs and other expenses)

Example: for a business with total revenue of $10 million and total expenses of $9 million

Net Profit = $10 million – $9 million = $1 million

In order for a pharmacy or any business to make a profit, the total revenue must exceed total expenses. Within the past five years, there have been significant changes in reimbursement for drugs, which affects pharmacy profits. Pharmacy technicians who have knowledge of basic drug reimbursement principles can play a significant role in increasing pharmacy profit margins.

Pharmacy Reimbursement Basics

Reimbursement for pharmaceuticals is complex and widely variable. Fortunately, most pharmacy computer systems have reimbursement rates and formulas programmed into the software application. However, it is important for pharmacy technicians to understand how pharmacies are reimbursed for drugs. The exact methodology that is used to bill and reimburse for drugs varies based on several factors, including the following:

- The practice setting in which the drug is dispensed.
- The type of drug that is being dispensed (e.g., single-source brand products vs. multisource generic products).
- The party who is paying for the drugs.

For example, in institutional settings such as hospitals and hospital-based outpatient clinics, payment for drugs may be prospective, which means that the amount to be paid for drugs is predetermined based on the condition that is being treated. **Prospective payment** typically includes all costs associated with treating a particular condition, including medications. With prospective payment systems, pharmacies are challenged to deliver drugs at or below the predetermined rate in order to ensure that drug costs are covered. More information on prospective payment methods is presented later in this chapter.

In community pharmacy practice, the most common type of payment method is retrospective, or **fee for service**. In the **retrospective payment** model, drugs are dispensed, and later reimbursed, according to a predetermined formula that is specified in a contract between the pharmacy and the **third-party payer,** such as the insurance company or pharmacy benefit manager. The reimbursement rate for third-party prescriptions is based on a formula consisting of various parts: ingredient cost, dispensing fee, and patient copayments. The ingredient cost is the amount paid to the pharmacy for the cost of the drug product, the **dispensing fee** is the amount paid for dispensing the prescription, and the **copayment** (also known as "copay") is the cost-sharing amount paid by the patient or customer. In order for the pharmacy to make a profit, the total reimbursement rate should be greater than the costs to dispense the prescription.

Third-party reimbursement = (ingredient cost + dispensing fee) – copayment

The ingredient cost is based on a payment benchmark, or a standard against which pricing is based. Benchmark prices are often referenced by common acronyms, as described in the following text.[1]

Historically, the **average wholesale price (AWP)** has been the most commonly used benchmark for billing drugs that are reimbursed in the community pharmacy setting. AWP was created in the 1960s and was the first generally accepted standard pricing benchmark. The AWP for a drug is set by the manufacturer of the drug, and the AWP is readily available from several sources, including MediSpan and First Databank. AWP is known as the "sticker price" of a drug that the pharmacy sells to a customer or third-party payer. AWP is usually set at 20–25% above the wholesale acquisition cost (WAC), another common benchmark for billing for drugs.[2]

Wholesale acquisition cost (WAC) is set by each manufacturer. It represents the "list price" at which the manufacturer sells the drug to the wholesaler. However, WAC does not include any discounts or price concessions (e.g., reduced prices for on-time payment) that may be offered to the drug wholesaler. If AWP is the basis for reimbursement, the formula is usually the AWP less some percentage (e.g., AWP – 15%). If WAC is the basis, the formula is usually WAC plus a small percentage (e.g., WAC + 3%).[2]

There is growing recognition that neither AWP nor WAC represents what is actually paid for drugs, and, in recent years, these benchmarks have become widely controversial.[1-2] New benchmarks that are used for drug pricing within the past decade include **average sales price (ASP)** and **average manufacturer price (AMP).** ASP is based on manufacturer-reported selling price data and includes volume discounts and price concessions that are offered to all classes of trade. ASP is explained in further detail in the Medicare section of this chapter. Other third-party payers will likely begin to use ASP as the benchmark for drug pricing in the future.[1]

AMP is the average price paid to manufacturers by wholesalers for drugs distributed through retail pharmacies. AMP includes discounts and other price concessions that are provided by manufacturers. AMP was created by Congress in 1990 to facilitate calculating Medicaid rebates. The Budget Deficit Reduction Act of 2005 (DRA) requires that AMP be used to calculate the **federal upper limit (FUL)** for drugs that are paid through Medicaid. The FUL represents the maximum of federal matching funds that the federal government pays to state Medicaid programs for eligible generic and multisource drugs. With the enactment of the Patient Protection and Affordable Care Act of 2010 (health care reform) on March 23, 2010, the AMP was established as 175% of the ASP.

Typically, the reimbursement formula for a generic product is different than that for a brand product. Sole-source or brand-name drugs are usually reimbursed based on AWP or WAC, whereas generic or multisource drugs are reimbursed based on a **maximum allowable cost (MAC)** schedule, which is usually based on the cost of the lowest available generic equivalent. Commercial insurance companies and Medicaid often use MAC lists for generic reimbursement; however, these lists can present a challenge to pharmacies because they may not be published and are widely variable from one insurance company to another.

Sample formulas include the following:

- Sole-source drug reimbursement = AWP – 15% + $3.50 dispensing fee
- Multisource drug reimbursement = MAC + $3.50 dispensing fee

Here are some examples:

Sole source drug with an AWP of $100
Sole source reimbursement = $100 – $15 + $3.50
= $88.50
Multisource drug with a MAC of $50
Multisource reimbursement = $50 + $3.50 = $53.50

The dispensing fees are widely variable and typically range from $1.50 to $6.00 per prescription. This fee is somewhat unrelated to the actual cost of dispensing a prescription because the fee does not reflect the actual time spent by the pharmacist. The dispensing fee may differ for brand and generic prescriptions.

✔ Some third-party payers may pay a higher dispensing fee for generic drugs or formulary products as an incentive to encourage utilization of preferred products.

Payment for Drugs and Dispensing Services

In 2008, $234 billion were spent on outpatient prescription drugs in the United States. Private insurance paid for 42% of this total, followed by public payers such as Medicare and Medicaid, which paid for 37%. Consumers paid the remaining 21% in the form of out-of-pocket payment for prescriptions or copayments (figure 20-1).[3]

Consumers (Self-Pay)

Although many patients have some form of prescription drug coverage, a significant number of Americans are uninsured or underinsured. Since the implementation of Medicare and Medicaid in the 1960s and the implementation of the Medicare Modernization Act in 2006, the percentage of patients who pay directly for prescription drugs has decreased. However, some patients who lack prescription drug coverage as a medical benefit may still pay directly. In these cases, reimbursement formulas are set by the pharmacy and are similar to those that have been described previously; however, the patient is fully responsible for the amount paid. The amount that is paid by a cash-paying customer is often referred to as the "usual and customary price" or the "cash price." Many third-party contracts indicate that the amount to be paid for a prescription is based on a reimbursement formula (as previously explained) or the usual and customary price. The lower of the two prices is the amount usually paid.

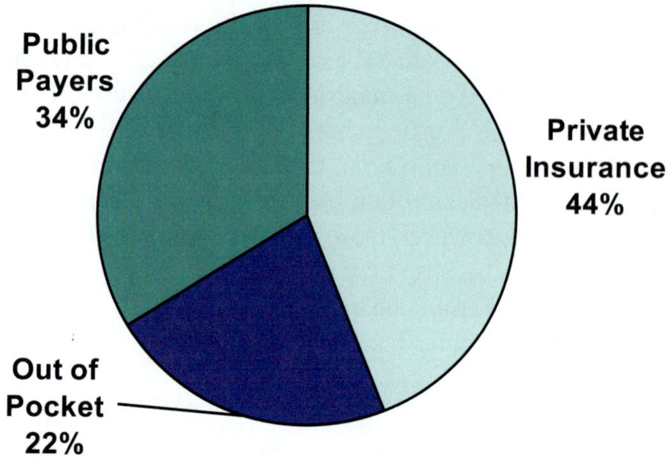

Figure 20-1. Sources of payment for retail prescription drugs in 2008. Data from Kaiser Family Foundation.

Many drug companies offer certain free drugs through **patient assistance programs (PAPs)** to low-income patients who lack prescription drug coverage and meet certain criteria. The criteria for PAPs are widely variable and are determined by individual drug companies. In most cases, the products that are available free to the patient are proprietary drugs, and the patient is required to complete an application that determines eligibility. On approval, the drug company delivers a specified quantity of the drug (usually a 30- to 90-day supply) to a licensed pharmacist or physician on the patient's behalf.

Some companies also offer bulk replacement or **institutional patient assistance programs (IPAPs).** In the IPAP model, medications are provided to an institution (e.g., pharmacy or clinic) rather than to the individual patient. The institution has the obligation of verifying that each patient who receives medications meets the established criteria. In the IPAP model, pharmacies typically receive "replacement" product for medications that have already been dispensed.

Rx for Success

Pharmacy technicians can play an important role in helping pharmacists identify and enroll eligible patients in Patient Assistance Programs.

Copay foundations or independent charity patient assistance programs are other resources that can be used to help patients who can't afford to pay for prescriptions or copays. A list of resources for PAPs and various copay foundations is available at the end of this chapter.

The 340B drug pricing program is another option that can be utilized to assist patients who lack adequate prescription drug coverage. There are several types of facilities that qualify as "covered entities" for 340B pricing, including federal qualified health centers (FQHCs), disproportionate share hospitals (DSH), and state-owned AIDS drug assistance programs. Covered entities that are eligible to participate in the drug pricing program can offer drastically reduced drug prices to eligible patients.

The Office of Pharmacy Affairs, which is located within Health Resources and Services Administration, administers the 340B drug discount program.

Private Insurance

In 2008, 42% of prescription drugs were paid by private insurance.[3] The most common purchasers of private insurance are employers, labor unions, trust funds, and professional associations. Additionally, individuals can purchase private insurance directly from an insurance company. Private insurance can be either managed care (based on a network of providers) or indemnity (non-network-based coverage). Managed care is a type of private health insurance or health care organization that is based on networks of providers, such as pharmacies, doctors, and hospitals. The cost to the employee for managed care plans is typically lower than indemnity insurance, as long as the employee accesses providers within the contracted network. **Indemnity** insurance offers more choices of physicians and hospitals, but the employee's out-of-pocket costs are higher than with managed care. With indemnity insurance, either the patient pays up front or the provider accepts payment after the services are rendered.

Pharmacy Benefit Managers. **Pharmacy benefit managers (PBMs)** are organizations that administer pharmacy benefits for private or public third-party payers, also known as plan sponsors. These organizations may include managed care organizations, self-insured employers, insurance companies, labor unions, Medicaid and Medicare prescription drug plans, the Federal Employees Health Benefits Program, and other federal, state, and local government entities. Some of the major PBMs are CVS Caremark, Medco, Express Scripts, Walgreens Health Initiatives, and Wellpoint Pharmacy Management. About 95% of people who have prescription drug coverage receive their benefit from a PBM.[5]

Once a plan sponsor chooses a PBM to manage the pharmacy benefit, the sponsor pays the PBM a fee that is usually based on the number of beneficiaries (plan members and dependents) who are covered by the pharmacy benefit. The fee should cover the total cost of the pharmacy benefit (including all prescriptions) for the covered beneficiaries. In return for the fee paid by the plan sponsor, the PBM administers the pharmacy benefit under the direction of the sponsor. The PBM designs and manages the pharmacy benefit so that the cost of prescriptions dispensed does not exceed the amount of money paid to the PBM by the sponsor. For example, PBMs and their sponsors develop formularies, negotiate discounts or rebates with pharmaceutical companies, set copays, communicate with providers and beneficiaries, keep track of all prescriptions dispensed, and pay network pharmacies for prescriptions dispensed that are covered by the pharmacy benefit.

The **formulary** is the cornerstone of any PBM activities. It is a specific list of drugs that is included with a given pharmacy benefit. The formulary usually includes both brand and generic drugs in most therapeutic categories. Brand-name drugs can be either preferred (designated by the PBM as the first-choice drugs) or nonpreferred. The PBM may charge different copays for different types of formulary drugs. For example, a typical copay for a generic drug is $10, for a preferred brand-name drug is $26, and for a nonpreferred brand-name drugs is $46. These levels of copays are known as copay tiers.

The PBM can utilize administrative tools within the context of the formulary in order to optimize the clinical and economic performance of the pharmacy benefit. Some of the more common administrative tools are prior authorization, step therapy, and quantity limits.[6] **Prior authorization** requires the prescriber to receive preapproval from the PBM in order for the drug to be covered by the benefit. The prescription is not paid for by the PBM until prior authorization has been given. Prior authorization is often used for newer drugs, such as those that have only been on the market for six months or less, so that the PBM can ensure that the drugs are being prescribed according to guidelines of the FDA and evaluate the impact of these new drugs on the formulary.

Step therapy requires use of a recognized first-line drug before a more complex or expensive second-line drug is used. Beneficiaries must try and fail with the first-line drug before a second-line drug can be covered by the benefit. For example, the PBM might require use of a generic antibiotic before newer, more complex, broad spectrum antibiotics are prescribed.

Quantity limits set upper limits of the amount of a drug that is covered by the benefit, or the total days of therapy. For example, the benefit may limit the duration of therapy with proton-pump inhibitors for the treatment of peptic ulcer disease to eight weeks. In the best interest of the patient, the physician or pharmacist may request an override of any of the restrictions the PBM places on therapy. If the physician or pharmacist requests an override and it is approved, the desired therapy is covered by the pharmacy benefit for that patient. Or the physician can simply prescribe another equivalent medication for the patient that does not have utilization restrictions.

For PBMs, administering the pharmacy benefit is a constant balancing act of managing costs and providing quality service and value to their sponsors and beneficiaries. Many PBMs try to achieve this balance by offering mail service for prescriptions, whereby beneficiaries can get up to a 90-day supply of medication through the mail for a reduced copayment. Some pharmacy benefit plans require beneficiaries to use the PBM mail service for certain prescription refills. Another way that PBMs try to better serve their customers and manage costs is to offer specialty services for beneficiaries who require high-cost drugs, such as the newer biotechnology drugs that patients inject themselves (e.g., some medications for multiple sclerosis and rheumatoid arthritis). These specialty services may include special delivery of the medication to the beneficiary's home at no charge, free nursing visits to help train the patient to inject the medication, a 24-hour hotline for the beneficiary to ask a pharmacist questions about the medication, and prior authorization assistance. Overall, PBMs provide a complex and valuable service for the health care system and assist plan sponsors in administering the pharmacy benefit to millions of beneficiaries.

Processing Private Third-Party Prescriptions. Patients with a prescription drug benefit should have a prescription identification (ID) card. The information on the prescription ID card is necessary in order to submit a claim to the PBM. Figure 20-2 is an example of a typical prescription ID card.

The card identifies the PBM (Any PBM) or drug benefit provider. It shows a telephone number for the PBM customer service department. The employer may be identified (Your Company, Inc.), followed by the Member Name (Jane Doe) and Member ID Number (12345678). If the beneficiary is different from the plan member, such as a dependent child, the Participant's Name may be listed. Finally, the BIN # (000012) is the bank identification number, which is also needed to submit the claim. It references the claims processor or PBM.

Any PBM **1-800- 555-1212**

Your Company, Inc.
GROUP #: XXXXXX
Member Name: Jane Doe
Member ID Number: 123456789
Participant's Name: Sally Doe
BIN# 000012

Figure 20-2. Example of a typical prescription ID card.

Once the technician enters information in the pharmacy computer from the prescription ID card and the prescription, the PBM either accepts or rejects the claim. If the claim is rejected, the PBM responds with a message, commonly known as a rejection code. Such codes are standard across all prescription benefit plans and may include "Missing or Invalid Patient ID," "Prior authorization required," "Pharmacy not contracted with plan on date of service," "Refill too soon," or "Missing or invalid quantity prescribed."[7] The technician must assess the meaning of the rejection code and respond accordingly. The resolution may be simple, such as checking the patient ID and making sure it was entered correctly. Or the pharmacist or physician may need to take further action (such as obtaining prior authorization) in order for the claim to be processed. If the issue can't be resolved or if the rejection code is unclear, the technician may need to call the PBM customer service, which is usually listed on the prescription ID card.

Public Payers

In 2008, 37% of prescription drugs were paid for by public payers. Medicare is the largest public payer, accounting for 60% of prescription charges in 2008, followed by Medicaid at 22%, and other public payers, such as the Department of Veterans Affairs, the Department of Defense, and the Indian Health Service at 12%.[8]

Medicare. Medicare is the federal health program for the elderly, disabled, and people with end-stage renal disease or amyotrophic lateral sclerosis (ALS), otherwise known as Lou Gehrig disease.[9] Most people automatically qualify for Medicare once they turn 65 years of age and are eligible for Social Security payments, and if they or their spouse have made payroll tax contributions to

Medicare for a total of 10 years or 40 quarters. There are four parts to Medicare:

- Part A (hospital insurance)
- Part B (medical insurance)
- Part C (Medicare Advantage plans)
- Part D (prescription drug coverage)

Medicare Part A. Medicare Part A helps cover inpatient care (hospitals, skilled nursing facilities, hospice care, and some home health care). For most people, Part A coverage is pre-paid through payroll taxes. Individuals not entitled to premium-free Part A may purchase coverage by paying a monthly **premium**. Medicare Part A coverage involves a **deductible** and a benefit period of 60 days. A deductible is an out-of-pocket amount that must be paid before insurance coverage begins. Full Medicare coverage applies for the first 60 days; thereafter, the beneficiary is responsible for **coinsurance**, which is a fixed percentage charge for a service.[10–12]

Part A claims are processed by a fiscal intermediary, and the **diagnosis-related group (DRG)** is the basis for reimbursement. A fiscal intermediary acts as an agent for the federal government that processes and pays Medicare claims. A diagnosis-related group is a set rate paid for an inpatient procedure based on cost and intensity. It is important to understand that drugs provided during an inpatient stay are not separately reimbursed; they are included in the DRG payment.

Medicare Part B. Medicare Part B is optional medical insurance for outpatient physician and hospital services, clinical laboratory services, and durable medical equipment, prosthetics, orthotics, and supplies (DMEPOS). Part B coverage involves paying a monthly premium, an annual deductible, and coinsurance. Because Part B coverage is optional, beneficiaries are required to enroll actively in order to receive benefits, and they may incur higher premiums if enrollment is delayed. Part B may cover medical services that Part A does not cover, such as some home health care and physical and/or occupational therapy services.

Medicare Part B pays for medically necessary services and supplies and covers some preventative services, such as pneumococcal vaccines and cancer screenings (cervical, breast, colorectal, and prostate). Medicare Part B benefit categories include specific drug products, such as immunosuppressive drugs (e.g., mycophenolate, cyclosporine) used for transplant patients, erythropoietin stimulating agents (e.g., epoetin, darbepoetin) for home dialysis patients, oral anticancer drugs, and oral antiemetic drugs (in place of intravenous antiemetics).

Medicare does not always pay 100% for Part B covered items. Each Medicare covered item is assigned to a payment category, which determines the amount Medicare pays. Most often, Medicare pays a percentage (e.g., 80%) of the approved amount after the patient's deductible has been met, and the patient is responsible for paying the remaining portion (e.g., 20%), known as coinsurance. Individuals with Part B coverage are responsible for the premium, deductible, copayment, and coinsurance amounts.[12]

If the patient has a secondary insurance, the copayments or coinsurance may be submitted to the secondary insurer. Part B claims are processed by a local Medicare carrier, and DMEPOS items are processed by DME Medicare administrative contractors (DME MACs). If an assigned claim is not filed within one year, Medicare reduces the allowed amount by 10% for payable claims.[12]

Medicare Part C. Medicare Part C is the Medicare Advantage Plan, which combines Part A and B coverage. Under this plan, benefits are provided by Medicare-approved private insurance companies. These private fee-for-service and managed care plans often include prescription drug benefits, called Medicare Advantage Prescription Drug plans or MAPDs; as such, Part C beneficiaries should not enroll in a Part D prescription drug plan. There are five types of Part C plans: health maintenance organizations (HMOs), preferred provider organizations (PPOs), medical savings account plans, private fee-for-service plans, and Medicare special needs plans.

Medicare Part C beneficiaries are required to pay premiums, deductibles, copayments, and coinsurance for services. Medicare Advantage Plans charge one combined premium for Part A and B benefits and prescription drug coverage (if included in the plan).

Medicare Part D. Medicare Part D is a federal prescription drug program that is paid for by the Centers for Medicare and Medicaid Services (CMS) and by individual premiums. It was enacted as part of the Medicare Prescription Drug, Improvement, and Modernization Act of 2003. Medicare Part D offers a voluntary insurance benefit for outpatient prescription drugs.

✔ Everyone who is eligible for Medicare Part A or Part B is also eligible for Medicare Part D. Individuals must enroll in Medicare Part D by joining a Medicare prescription drug plan or a Medicare Advantage plan that includes coverage for prescription drugs.

Medicare prescription drug plans are administered by private PBMs or other companies approved by Medicare. Each plan varies in terms of cost and drugs covered.

There are four times during the year at which a Medicare beneficiary can join, switch, or drop a Medicare prescription drug plan.[13] These are the following:

- When the beneficiary turns 65 years of age and becomes eligible for Medicare.
- When the beneficiary receives Medicare as a result of a disability.
- During the period from November 15 through December 31 of any year. This is known as the open enrollment period.
- When the beneficiary qualifies for Extra Help.

A Medicare beneficiary can join a Medicare prescription drug plan online at www.medicare.gov or by calling 1-800-MEDICARE. If Medicare beneficiaries do not join a Medicare prescription drug plan during any of these available times, they may incur a late enrollment penalty. This may happen if they become eligible for Medicare when they turn 65 years of age but decide *not* to join a Medicare prescription drug plan because their prescription usage is low or because they want to avoid paying a premium. The penalty amounts to a monthly charge of 1% of the national base beneficiary premium (calculated by CMS) for every month that the beneficiary does not join a Part D plan. Some Medicare beneficiaries do not join a Medicare prescription drug plan because they have creditable coverage, which is, coverage that is at least as good as the Standard Medicare Drug Benefit. Creditable coverage can be from a current or former employer, union, Veterans Administration, Department of Defense, or Federal Employees Health Benefits Program, for example. Individuals with creditable coverage avoid a late enrollment penalty as long as their creditable coverage is in effect. If their creditable coverage is discontinued for any reason, such as an employer discontinuing coverage, the beneficiary should join a Medicare prescription drug plan in order to avoid the late enrollment penalty. Technicians may advise customers to contact their employee benefits manager or CMS (1-800-MEDICARE or www.medicare.gov) if they have questions about joining Medicare Part D.

Individuals with Medicare Part D typically pay a monthly premium, an annual deductible, and either coinsurance or copayments for each prescription. Table 20-1 shows the Standard Medicare Part D prescription drug benefit that serves as the reference point for all Medicare prescription drug plans. Each insurance company or PBM that offers a Medicare prescription drug plan must offer at least the standard level of coverage offered in the Standard Medicare Part D benefit.

Most Medicare prescription drug plans have a **coverage gap,** sometimes referred to as a "donut hole." This is a period of no coverage that typically occurs once the individual's total prescription drug spending for the year reaches the initial coverage limit. During the coverage gap, the beneficiary must pay all costs for prescriptions until the total prescription spending for the year reaches the catastrophic coverage threshold. The coverage gap can be considered the "deductible in the middle" of the Medicare prescription drug plan. Some individuals never reach the coverage gap, whereas others reach it within the first few months of the year—it all depends on the total prescription spending for the individual. Individuals

Table 20-1. Medicare Part D Standard Benefit, 2010

Benefit Parameters	Total Spending	Beneficiary Pays
Annual deductible	$310	100%
Initial coverage limit	$275.01 – $2,830	25%
Coverage gap	$2,830 – $6,440	100%
Catastrophic coverage	$6,440 and over	5%

*Amounts may increase each year

Source: Centers for Medicare and Medicaid Services, Announcement of calendar year (CY) 2010 Medicare Advantage capitation rates and Medicare Advantage and Part D payment policies. Page 37. Available at: http://www.cms.hhs.gov/MedicareAdvtgSpecRateStats/Downloads/Announcement2010.pdf. Accessed on April 23, 2010.

must continue to pay their premium every month, even when they are in the coverage gap. Also, the Medicare prescription drug plan starts over every year in January, with a new deductible, premium, copay or coinsurance, and coverage gap. Beneficiaries receive a notice in October from their prescription drug plan that outlines how their plan will change for the following year. They can then decide to remain with their plan for the following year or switch to another plan during the open enrollment period from November 15 through December 31.

Special populations can receive Extra Help to pay for the Medicare prescription drug plan. Individuals are automatically enrolled in Extra Help, also known as the Low-income Subsidy, if they already receive full Medicaid benefits (referred to as "dual eligibles"), Medical Savings Programs (MSP), or Supplemental Security Income (SSI).[14] Some people may qualify for Extra Help if they meet certain income and asset standards, but they must apply for Extra Help through the Social Security Administration. People who qualify for Extra Help do not pay premiums or deductibles, they have reduced or no copayments, and they are not affected by the coverage gap (table 20-2). Dual eligibles do not pay premiums or deductibles, have low fixed copays, and are not affected by the coverage gap. Although Extra Help is available, there are over 2 million people in the United States who are eligible but have not applied.[14] Technicians can help customers who may be eligible by suggesting that they apply for Extra Help. They can apply at any time during the year, whether or not they are currently enrolled in a Medicare prescription drug plan.

Table 20-2. Extra Help: Copayments for Prescriptions, 2010

	Generic	Brand-Name
Institutionalized beneficiaries	$0	$0
Dual eligibles	$1.10	$3.30
Other Extra Help	$2.50	$6.30

*Amounts may increase each year

Source: Centers for Medicare and Medicaid Services, Announcement of calendar year (CY)

2010 Medicare Advantage capitation rates and Medicare Advantage and Part D payment policies. Page 37. Available at:

http://www.cms.hhs.gov/MedicareAdvtgSpecRateStats/Downloads/Announcement2010.pdf. Accessed on April 23, 2010.

Drug formularies for Medicare Part D vary from plan to plan.

✔ Beneficiaries must be careful when choosing a Medicare prescription drug plan to ensure that their prescription drugs are covered.

CMS requires that all Medicare prescription drug plans cover at least two drugs in each therapeutic category. There are six categories of drugs that must include almost all drugs in the category because of the importance of the therapeutic class and the need for beneficiaries to have access to all drugs in the class. The six protected drug categories are antipsychotics, antidepressants, antiepileptics, immunosuppressants, cancer, and HIV/AIDS drugs. There are some classes of drugs that are not covered at all by Medicare Part D. These are over-the-counter drugs, benzodiazepines, barbiturates, drugs for weight loss or weight gain, and drugs for erectile dysfunction. Some Part D plans may cover some of these drugs as an added benefit, but they are not required by CMS to do so. Individuals generally pay a higher premium to have a plan with enhanced coverage. If an individual is dual eligible (covered by Medicare and Medicaid), the state Medicaid plan may cover some of the drugs that are not covered by Medicare Part D. This coverage may vary by state.

Like those of any other PBM, Medicare prescription drug plans may use administrative tools to restrict the formulary, such as prior authorization, quantity limits, and step therapy. If a beneficiary has a prescription for a drug that requires prior authorization from the Part D plan, the technician will see a rejection message on the pharmacy system (Prior Authorization Required), in which case the prescribing physician needs to obtain prior authorization for the drug before the claim can be paid. In the meantime, Medicare Part D covers a one-time 30-day supply of the medication to allow sufficient time for the physician to complete the paperwork necessary to obtain the prior authorization. Or the physician can prescribe a different drug that does not require prior authorization. If, however, the drug is not on the formulary of the beneficiary's Part D plan and the physician finds the drug necessary, the beneficiary and prescriber can request an exception to the formulary. The plan will review the request and may allow that drug to be covered. If an exception is not granted by the Part D plan, the beneficiary can submit an appeal. It is important for technicians to know that there are methods available for beneficiaries to attempt to gain access to necessary drugs that may be restricted through their Part D plan through exceptions or appeals. If the technician has problems or questions related to the Part D plan, a call should be placed to the plan's help desk at the number on the prescription ID card.

Processing Medicare Part D prescriptions is similar to processing prescriptions from any other private insurance company or PBM. All Part D claims must contain a National Provider Identifier (NPI). If the prescriber does not have an NPI, or if the pharmacy cannot locate the prescriber's NPI, a non-NPI prescriber ID can be submitted on the claim, if allowed by the payer. If a beneficiary does not have a prescription ID card from the Part D plan, or if the card is not current, the technician can submit an eligibility query in the pharmacy system by performing an E1 transaction. The E1 transaction should return the "4Rx data," RxBIN, RxPCN, RxGrp, and RxID, along with the 800 number of the Part D plan. If the E1 transaction only returns the Part D plan's 800 number, the beneficiary is enrolled in the plan, but the 4Rx data are not yet available. The technician may call the 800 number and obtain the 4Rx information directly. The technician should also give beneficiaries the 800 number so that they can contact the Part D plan and obtain a new card.

As a summary of Medicare Part D, the following are some common questions that beneficiaries might ask technicians, along with brief answers:

- *Am I eligible for Medicare Part D?* You are eligible for Medicare Part D if you are already eligible for Medicare Part A or Part B.
- *When can I join a Medicare Part D plan?* You can join Medicare Part D when you turn 65, when you become eligible for SSI, when you become disabled, or during the open enrollment period from November 15 through December 31.
- *I'm retired and have Medicare, but my prescription coverage is from my former employer. Should I join a Part D plan?* Not if your coverage is creditable. You should contact your current or former employer to find out if your coverage is creditable.
- *What if I don't join a Medicare Part D plan and I don't have creditable coverage?* If and when you decide to enroll in Medicare Part D, you may face a late enrollment penalty.
- *What can I do if my income is so low that I can't afford the premium and copays with Medicare Part D?* You may be eligible for Extra Help. You can sign up for Extra Help by contacting the Social Security Administration at www.ssa.gov or at 1-800-772-1213.
- *How much are my copays?* That varies by plan and by prescription. You can contact the plan, or the copay will be shown when the prescription claim is submitted in the pharmacy system.
- *Will my Part D plan cover all my prescriptions?* That varies by plan and by prescription. You can contact the plan, or the coverage will be shown when the prescription claim is submitted in the pharmacy system.
- *What if I don't have a prescription ID card?* The pharmacy can run an E1 transaction on the pharmacy system and identify your plan information.
- *What if I need a drug, but it's not on the Part D formulary?* You and your physician can submit an exemption. If the exemption is not granted, you can file an appeal.
- *I still don't understand my Part D plan!* You can contact your plan directly or CMS at 1-800-MEDICARE or at www.medicare.gov.

Medicaid. Medicaid is a medical and long-term care program that is jointly funded by the federal and state governments. Participation in Medicaid is optional for states; however, since 1982, all states participate in the Medicaid program.[15] Medicaid covers three main groups of low-income Americans: parents and children, the elderly, and the disabled. State spending on Medicaid is matched by the federal government up to a point (average 57%).[15] The federal government has developed broad guidelines for the Medicaid program that states must follow in order to receive "matching funds"; however, the specific requirements are determined by each state. As a result, there is a wide variation in Medicaid coverage from state to state. Income guidelines are based on federal poverty limits (FPL), which are updated annually. Under health care reform, beginning in 2014, nearly everyone under age 65 with income up to 133% of the FPL will be eligible for Medicaid.[16]

Patients whose incomes exceed the established guidelines for eligibility may qualify for Medicaid if they have medical expenses that exceed a certain threshold. This type of coverage is commonly known as "spend down." As explained previously, the Medicare Prescription Drug benefit, which provides prescription drug coverage for qualified senior citizens, was implemented in January 2006. Medicaid recipients who also qualify for

Medicare are known as "dual eligible." Medicare is usually considered the primary payer for medical benefits for dual eligible patients; however, Medicaid can supplement Medicare benefits by providing coverage for benefits that may not be covered by Medicare and/or providing assistance with copayments for prescription medications. Medicaid functions as the "safety net" or payer of last resort.

States must cover a minimum set of Medicaid benefits for eligible patients. All states provide coverage for prescription drugs that are prescribed by a licensed physician and dispensed by a licensed pharmacist.[15] Additionally, the medication must be recorded on a written prescription; as of April 1, 2008, all Medicaid prescriptions must be electronically prescribed or written/printed on "tamper resistant" paper. Finally, the need for the medication must be supported in the patient's medical record.

In order to be paid for services provided to Medicaid patients, providers (i.e., pharmacies) must sign a contract with the state Medicaid agency. By signing this contract, the provider accepts certain responsibilities. The contract also obligates the provider to accept the payment that Medicaid provides as payment in full. When filling prescriptions for Medicaid patients in the community setting, pharmacy technicians will notice that most prescriptions have low or zero copayments. States may impose **cost sharing** (i.e., copayments for drugs) on services offered through Medicaid; however, certain categories of eligible patients are exempt from cost sharing, including children, pregnant women, and nursing home residents. By law, Medicaid recipients may not be denied services based on their inability to pay the assigned cost sharing.[15] This means that when a Medicaid patient is unable to pay for copayments for prescription drugs, the pharmacy reimbursement is reduced.

✔ In addition to cost sharing, other tools may be utilized to contain the cost of providing medications to Medicaid patients, including formularies or preferred drug lists, quantity limits, prior authorization, and utilization of generic drugs.

Other Public Payers. In addition to Medicare and Medicaid, the government pays for health benefit programs for the Department of Veterans Affairs, Department of Defense, and the Indian Health Service. All veterans of active military service (Army, Navy, Air Force, Marines, and Coast Guard) are potentially eligible for health benefits from the Department of Veterans Affairs (VA).[17] Eligibility is not just for veterans who served in active combat. Beneficiaries do not pay premiums for VA health benefits, but they usually pay copays, depending on their income. Typical copays are $15 for a medical visit and $8 for a 30-day supply of medication.

The VA prescription benefit is considered creditable, meaning that it is at least as good as Medicare Part D. Medicare-eligible veterans can opt out of Medicare Part D and do not incur a late enrollment penalty as long as they continue their VA pharmacy benefits. The VA uses a national drug formulary, and prescriptions and refills are available at VA pharmacies or mail order facilities.[18]

TRICARE is the health benefit program from the Department of Defense. Active military personnel, retirees, and their families are eligible for TRICARE.[19] The TRICARE retail and mail-order prescription benefit is administered by Express Scripts. The prescription benefit is based on a national TRICARE formulary. Like the VA, TRICARE prescription coverage is considered creditable with Medicare Part D.

The Indian Health Service (IHS) provides a comprehensive federal health care delivery system to American Indian and Alaska Native tribes and their descendents.[20]

Claims Processing

There are various payers of pharmacy benefits, and each payer has different policies, procedures, coverage rules, and formulas. Although private insurers pay a large portion of drug costs, Medicare and Medicaid have a significant influence on how drugs are paid for. The next section discusses reimbursement strategies and billing information required to receive payment.

Billing for Drugs and Dispensing Services

Health care insurers process billions of claims each year. In order to process and pay claims in a consistent manner, standardized billing methods are essential. Information needed to submit drug claims depends on the payer and the site of care. Receiving reimbursement or payment for the medications dispensed depends on providing the appropriate information. Billing procedures for the following three main patient care settings are described in this section: inpatient hospital; outpatient hospitals, clinics, and physician offices; and outpatient community settings. Each treatment setting provides various drugs and services, and it is important to understand that each setting has different billing requirements and reimbursement methods.

Inpatient Hospital Setting. In a hospital inpatient setting, per diem and prospective payment are the primary methods of payment. Separate payments are not made for drugs; the drug costs are included in the diagnosis-related groups (DRGs), which are used to determine the payments made to the hospital by insurers. DRGs were introduced in the early 1980s as part of a prospective payment system (PPS) to classify hospital cases based primarily on type of patient, diagnoses, procedures, complications, comorbidities, and resources used.

Patients admitted for a hospital stay are assigned a DRG payment, or reimbursement for inpatient services are often predetermined and are based on this DRG-based prospective payment system. For inpatient claims submitted to Medicare, the steps to determine the PPS payment can be viewed on the CMS Web site (http://www.cms.hhs.gov/AcuteInpatientPPS). Detailed information regarding billing hospital inpatient and/or Medicare Part A claims is beyond the scope of this chapter.

Outpatient Hospitals, Clinics and Physician Offices. In an outpatient hospital, clinic, or physician office setting, physician-administered drugs may either be included as part of the procedure or paid separately. Most drugs given in this setting are considered fee-for-service or separately billable (if the drug exceeds the Medicare packaging threshold). Typically, the fee-for-service formula is based on AWP. Under Medicare Part B, hospital outpatient services are reimbursed using the Outpatient Prospective Payment System (OPPS), which is a predetermined payment system for covered drugs and services. Some drugs are bundled into the ambulatory payment classification (APC). APCs are predetermined outpatient payment categories, similar to inpatient DRGs. As of 2008, drugs and biologicals (pharmaceuticals manufactured using biotechnology methods) with costs exceeding $60 per administration have separate APCs; those at or below the threshold ($60 or less per administration) are bundled or packaged into the APC payment.[21–22]

An example of a bundled service is a procedure to stitch a deep cut. Administering a local anesthetic, such as lidocaine, is an integral part of this procedure, and the cost is less than $60 per administration; therefore, this drug is packaged into the APC payment for the procedure. Drugs that exceed the threshold of $60 per day may receive separate payment that is often equal to average sale price plus 5% (ASP + 5%).[22]

Each drug charge requires the appropriate **Health Care Common Procedure Coding System (HCPCS)** code, and the quantity should be billed in service unit increments. Service units are pre-determined billing increments that may be unrelated to the package size. For example, infliximab (Remicade) injection has a HCPCS code of J1745 and is billed and reimbursed in increments of 10 mg. Darbepoetin alfa (Aranesp) for non-end-stage renal disease (ESRD) has a HCPCS code of J0881 and is billed per 1 mcg.

HCPCS coding is a federal coding system consisting of three levels:

- Level I — Current Procedural Terminology (CPT) codes
- Level II — National Alpha-Numeric codes (CMS)
- Level III — Local Alpha-Numeric codes (local Medicare carriers)

Level II of the HCPCS is a standardized coding system that is used to identify products, supplies, and services not included in the CPT codes (described in the following text). HCPCS codes for drugs are often called J-codes. J-codes are a subset of the Level II code set and are used to identify specific drugs. The term "J-code" refers to a five character alpha-numeric code that often begins with the letter J, although HCPCS codes for drugs may begin with another letter, such as C or Q. HCPCS codes that begin with C or Q are often temporary codes. Examples are C9245 for N-Plate (romiplostim) and Q0481 for epoetin alfa (for patients on dialysis).

The Outpatient Prospective Payment System (OPPS) is based on pre-determined payment rates for products and services. Each HCPCS code is assigned an OPPS status indicator, which identifies whether a product or service is packaged or separately payable. The Medicare OPPS Addendum B lists the products, HCPCS codes, status indicators, and fees.

Key data elements necessary for claim submission include the following:

- Beneficiary name and Health Insurance Claim Number (HICN)
- Date of service
- Health Care Common Procedure Code System (HCPCS) codes
- Common Procedural Terminology (CPT) codes
- International Classification of Diseases, 9th Revision (ICD-9) codes (also known as Diagnosis codes)
- Clinical Modifiers
- National Drug Code (NDC)
- Units of Service (Quantity expressed in service units or billing increments)
- Place of service

Claims may be submitted using paper forms or through an electronic data interchange (see www.cms.hhs.gov/ElectronicBillingEDITrans).

Billing for clinical services requires several of the elements previously listed. CPT codes are used to describe the interaction with the patient and provide information, such as whether the patient is a new or established patient, the nature and complexity of the interaction, and the amount of time spent with the patient. Reimbursement for clinical pharmacy services continues to evolve.

Community Pharmacy Setting. The majority of pharmacy claims are submitted by community pharmacies and reimbursed by a third-party payer. When working in the outpatient care setting, it is essential to understand how drugs are billed and paid. The prescription drug claims **adjudication** process involves the following steps:

- Submitting appropriate information
- Determining eligibility, coverage, and payment
- Communicating reimbursement
- Settling the claim

Historically, prescription medication coverage was limited, and patients often paid cash for drugs. Then, either patients or pharmacies submitted paper claims and receipts for reimbursement. Each insurance company had its own claim form, making the process tedious and time-consuming, particularly for pharmacies. In the late 1970s, a Universal Claim Form was developed by the National Council of Prescription Drug Programs (NCPDP) to provide a consistent format for manual paper pharmacy claim submissions. NCPDP develops standards for information processing for the pharmacy services sector of the health care industry.[7] Billing and reimbursement for prescription medication has since evolved.

An electronic system was implemented in the late 1980s, and the present pharmacy industry uses the NCPDP Telecommunications Standard Format Version 5.1 to adjudicate prescription drug claims through the electronic, online, real-time system. The system was created to standardize the exchange of data for claims submission and adjudication. This format allows communication of claims between pharmacy providers, pharmacy benefit managers, third-party payers, and insurance carriers at the point-of-service. The online claims processing system has become increasingly sophisticated. It provides a consistent format for electronic claims processing and enables pharmacies to perform several functions with immediate response. Pharmacy technicians can verify eligibility, determine formulary coverage status, confirm quantity limits and copay amounts, submit claims, and receive payment information. Proper billing practices rely on several key factors, which are explained in the next section.

Prescription Processing

In order to submit an electronic online claim, key billing elements include the following:

- Prescription Processor (Insurance Company or contracted PBM information on the ID card)
  - BIN (bank identification number)
  - PCN (processor control number)
- Pharmacy Provider Information (specific to each pharmacy)
  - NPI (National Provider Identification): effective May 23, 2008
  - NCPDP or NABP (formerly NPIC = National Pharmacy Identification Code)
- Eligibility (specific to each patient)
  - Member Name and Identification Number (unique identifier)
  - Group Number (insurers have several groups or plans)
  - Relationship (Plan Member, Spouse, Dependent)
- Prescription Information
  - Date of prescription (date when prescription was written and each fill)
  - NDC = National Drug Code (which identifies the manufacturer, drug, strength, dosage form, and package size)
  - Directions for use
  - Quantity dispensed
  - Days Supply
  - Refills (number of refills authorized)
  - Dispense as Written (DAW) or Product Substitution
  - Physician Signature (electronic signature, if permitted), NPI number and DEA number, when required

In addition to processing claims, the present online system provides information such as eligibility information, specific coverage (e.g., whether products are formulary vs. non-formulary items), prompts for prior approval (e.g., process of obtaining authorization to use items that are either restricted, non-formulary, or not initially covered), and copayment amounts. The system sends common claim edits and messages, such as "refill too soon" and "exceeds quantity limits or days supply," and may communicate denials when an item is not covered.

Providing proper billing information is an important task for a pharmacy technician. Reimbursement for prescriptions is dependent on entering and submitting correct and complete information. In a community pharmacy setting, prescription claims are submitted online and adjudicated in real time. Although the computer software offers guidance for correct billing practices, it cannot prevent all errors. Outlined in the following text are basic elements and pharmacy procedures used to enter prescription billing information.

Patients are given an insurance identification card to present at a pharmacy, which contains essential information used to create a patient profile in the pharmacy computer system. A pharmacy may submit prescription drug claims for the eligible person for whom the prescription is written. Eligibility must be assessed and confirmed. Information necessary to file a claim is available on the prescription drug ID card and includes the following:

- Cardholder ID
- Group Number
- Dependent Coverage (relationship codes)
  - 1 = Cardholder or Eligible Primary Person or Subscriber
  - 2 = Spouse of Cardholder
  - 3 = Dependent Child
  - 4 = Other (e.g., Disabled Dependent, Dependent Adult, Dependent Parent, Domestic Partner)
- BIN and PCN Numbers

It is crucial to input and submit prescription information as it is written (as the prescriber wrote it). Prescriptions must be clearly interpreted and translated.

✔ Reimbursement is highly dependent on providing the appropriate information. Failure to provide accurate prescription information can result in serious consequences, such as payment recovery by third-party payers, fines, or termination of pharmacy provider status.

Pharmacies are often subject to audits, which can result in situations in which pharmacies are required to pay back third-party payers. The following are several criteria that can have an impact on reimbursement and are scrutinized during a pharmacy audit:

- Patient Name and Unique Identifier (such as Date of Birth, and Address)
- Date of Prescription: most prescriptions are valid for one year from the date written. Prescriptions for controlled substances are the exception.
- Drug name, strength, package size, and National Drug Code (NDC): this information is essential, and the actual NDC used to fill the prescription must be provided when submitting a claim. The NDC communicates the dosage form, strength, and package size used to fill the prescription.
- Instructions or Directions: the directions must be clear and are used to confirm the quantity and days supply. "Use as directed" is not acceptable because it does not allow for the calculation of quantity and days supply.
- Quantity: the quantity written must be confirmed by translating and calculating the instructions and the days supply. The system may provide a message if the pharmacy attempts to bill for a larger quantity or days supply than allowed by the patient's health plan benefit.
- Days Supply: the quantity dispensed must be translated into the proper number of days. Some health plans limit the quantity and/or days supply. For example, if a physician writes a prescription for Drug X, one tablet to be taken three times a day, and indicates a quantity of 100 tablets, the correct days supply is 33, not 30 days. If the patient's plan only allows a 30-day quantity, the quantity dispensed and submitted for reimbursement must be changed to 90 tablets, and the change must be documented on the face of the prescription.
- Number of Refills: the physician may request refills on most prescription drugs, and this information is entered in the system. The number of refills cannot exceed a 1-year time frame. Refills for controlled substances are more restrictive, and the federal and state laws must be followed.
- DAW (Dispense As Written) codes: if the physician's prescription is written as a generic drug, the technician should attempt to fill the prescription with a generic product. DAW-0 should be the default setting. Entering the appropriate DAW code is important because it communicates information related to product selection. If the physician indicates that the prescription must be filled with a brand-name drug only or "may not substitute" or "no substitution," the claim must be submitted with a DAW-1. Table 20-3 lists DAW codes.

Common reasons for repayment following an audit include the following:

- Incorrect information
  - Dates, drugs, strengths, or directions

Table 20-3. Dispense as Written (DAW) Codes

Code	Description
0	Generic or Single-Source Brand: no product selection
1	Physician DAW: substitution not allowed by provider
2	Patient DAW: substitution allowed; patient requested product dispensed
3	Pharmacist Selected Brand-Name: substitution allowed; pharmacist selected product
4	Generic not in stock: substitution allowed
5	Brand-Name Dispensed at Generic Price: substitution allowed
6	Override
7	Brand-Name Drug Mandated by Law: substitution not allowed
8	Generic Not Available: substitution allowed
9	Other

- Incorrect days supply (quantity ordered and directions should match)
- Overbilled quantity (an amount that exceeds the quantity written)

- Incomplete information
    - No quantity indicated
    - "Use as directed" sig (this is unacceptable: the directions must allow for a calculated days supply)

The following is a case scenario: Mrs. Smith, a new pharmacy customer, presents a prescription for Drug X that is covered by her prescription drug plan. The pharmacy is a provider for her plan, and the processor data (BIN and PCN) are already in the pharmacy's computer system; therefore, the technician does not need to enter this information. What information must be entered to process this prescription?

Aside from entering Mrs. Smith's personal information (e.g., name, address, phone, date of birth, and allergy information) into the computer system, the technician must enter the following information from her insurance card: member identification number, group number, and relationship. The prescription information (drug, dose, directions, quantity, days supply, number of authorized refills, DAW, physician information, etc.) are entered in the computer system and electronically submitted to the third party. An electronic response is received, informing the technician that the prescription was approved. The payment information and copayment amount to collect should be provided. Errors, edits, or comments are communicated as a message. Common messages include eligibility or coverage issues (e.g., patient or drug not covered), quantity limits, or refill too soon.

Understanding the importance of proper claims information is the first part of the process. Another important aspect is how third-party payers pay pharmacies. The success of the pharmacy is dependent on maintaining a profit margin after all expenses are paid.

Rx for Success

Pharmacy technicians play an important role by monitoring payments when processing online prescription claims. If the reimbursement rate is less that the cost of the drug, the pharmacy manager should be alerted in order to further investigate the issue.

Summary

On March 23, 2010, the Patient Protection and Affordable Care Act of 2010 was enacted.[25] This legislation expands health care coverage to people who were previously uninsured or underinsured. As a result, pharmacy billing and reimbursement will continue to evolve. More people will become eligible for Medicaid. More prescriptions will be filled, and commonly used payment benchmarks for prescriptions will change from AWP to AMP. The Medicare Part D coverage gap will close by 2020. Pharmacy technicians play an important role by ensuring that prescriptions contain the appropriate information for proper reimbursement. Common tasks include gathering insurance information, entering it correctly into the pharmacy computer system, and troubleshooting problems based on responses from the third party payer. The challenge for pharmacy technicians is to stay abreast of the changes in billing and reimbursement and understand how these changes impact the pharmacy and the patients they serve.

Self-Assessment Questions

1. Bob Jones is a 48-year-old single male with no children and no known disabilities. His annual income is $15,000. His income does not make him eligible for Medicaid. Bob has no health insurance, and he pays cash for prescriptions. Bob has a prescription for Lipitor, but he is unable to pay for it. A generic form of Lipitor is not currently available. What are Bob's options for obtaining his prescription?
   a. Bob should apply for Medicaid.
   b. Bob should visit www.needymeds.org, because he may be eligible for a drug company-sponsored patient assistance program.
   c. Bob should apply for Medicare Part D.
   d. Bob should not have his Lipitor prescription filled.

2. Which of the following benchmarks is *not* used for prescription drug reimbursement?
   a. AWP
   b. ASP
   c. DMC
   d. MAC

3. ___________ is/are responsible for the greatest portion of prescription drug spending.
   a. Out-of-pocket
   b. Private insurance
   c. Public payers
   d. Patient assistance programs

4. Mr. Simon has been coming into your pharmacy for years and paying cash for his prescriptions. He recently turned 65 years old and has Medicare Part A. Is Mr. Simon eligible for Medicare Part D?
   a. Yes
   b. No

5. Dual eligibles:
   a. are eligible for both Medicaid and Medicare.
   b. are eligible for two types of managed care plans.
   c. have creditable insurance to Medicare Part D.
   d. pay $4 for generic prescriptions.

6. Dual eligibles are responsible for cost sharing for Medicare Part D in the form of:
   a. Premiums
   b. Copays
   c. Coverage gap
   d. Deductibles

7. Greta Jones comes into your pharmacy with a prescription for Ambien 10-mg tablets, Sig: take one tablet daily, Quantity #34. When you enter the information into the pharmacy system, you get a message saying "quantity limit exceeded (30)." You should:
   a. dispense 34 tablets and submit the claim for 30 tablets.
   b. dispense 30 tablets and submit the claim for 30 tablets. Document the change in quantity on the face of the prescription.
   c. not dispense the prescription. Ask Mrs. Jones to obtain a new prescription for 30 tablets.
   d. dispense 34 tablets and submit the claim for 34 tablets.

8. Stanley Simmons has Medicare Part D. He does not qualify for Extra Help. Every month, he has four prescriptions filled. Normally, he pays copayments of $120 for the four prescriptions. This month, the pharmacy system shows that Mr. Simmons's copayments for his prescriptions are $600. You tell Mr. Simmons that:
   a. he is most likely in the donut hole of his Medicare Part D plan and owes $600.
   b. he should ask his physician to obtain prior approvals for the prescriptions.
   c. he should switch to another Medicare Part D plan immediately.
   d. there is an error in the pharmacy system and he only owes $120.

9. A Medicare beneficiary comes into your pharmacy with a new prescription. She enrolled in a Medicare Part D plan three months ago but does not have her prescription ID card. Your pharmacy system does not show any Part D information for her. You
   a. call the major Part D plans and ask if she is a member.
   b. check the Web site www.medicare.gov to determine the name of her plan.

Self-Assessment Questions

c. perform an E1 transaction on the pharmacy system to determine her Part D eligibility information.
d. tell her to go home and look for her card.

10. Mrs. Hernandez is a widow with Medicare Part A and B who receives health care and prescription insurance from her husband's former employer. She received a letter from the employer stating that the prescription drug coverage she has is creditable to Medicare Part D. This letter indicates that Mrs. Hernandez should:
    a. apply for Medicaid.
    b. drop her current coverage since she is a widow.
    c. enroll in Medicare Part D.
    d. remain with her current prescription coverage.
11. A customer comes into your pharmacy with a prescription ID card for a Part D plan. She has a new prescription for Januvid 50 mg tablets. When you enter the information in the pharmacy system, you get a message saying "Item not covered." You tell the customer that the drug is not on the Part D plan's formulary, and she tells you that she must have that particular medication. You
    a. advise the customer to have the physician request an exemption from the Part D plan.
    b. advise the customer to switch Medicare Part D plans immediately.
    c. fill the prescription anyway and charge the normal copayment.
    d. advise the customer to enroll in Medicaid.
12. Mrs. Jones comes into your pharmacy with a new prescription for Aricept and a prescription ID card for Medco Medicare Part D plan. You enter the information into the pharmacy system and get a message that states, "prior authorization required." You tell Mrs. Jones that:
    a. she should switch to a different Medicare Part D plan.
    b. she is entitled to a 30-day supply of medication while her physician completes the paperwork for a prior authorization.
    c. she needs to pay cash for the prescription.
    d. she should try to get the prescription filled in 30 days.
13. Mr. Jones presents a prescription for Lantus 100 units/mL (1 vial = 10 mL) with directions: Inject 20 units QAM and 20 units QPM. Dispense one-month supply with three refills. How many vials or milliliters should be dispensed, and what is the days supply?
    a. 1,000 units (1 vial) for 25 days
    b. 1,000 units (1 vial) for 30 days
    c. 1,200 units (2 vials) for 30 days
    d. 2,000 units (2 vials) for 60 days
14. Ms. Smith presents a prescription for itraconazole 100-mg oral capsules with directions: Take two capsules by mouth twice daily for one week. The prescribing physician signed the prescription, indicating "may substitute." The pharmacy does not have the generic product in stock and only has the brand-name product (Sporanox 100-mg capsules). Which of the following should the pharmacy technician do?
    a. Call another pharmacy to borrow a bottle of itraconazole 100-mg, 28 capsules.
    b. Offer to fill the prescription with the brand-name product. Dispense 28 capsules of Sporanox and process the claim with DAW code 4.
    c. Give the prescription back to Ms. Smith and state that the pharmacy cannot fill the prescription.
    d. Tell Ms. Smith that her prescription will be filled. Dispense 28 capsules of Sporanox and process the claim as itraconazole.

Part 4

Self-Assessment Answers

1) b. Bob can apply for the manufacturers' patient assistance program for Lipitor. Although Bob's income is low, he does not meet the Medicaid criteria, and he is not eligible for Medicare because of his age.
2) c. DMC is not a pricing benchmark. Average Wholesale Price (AWP), Average Sale Price (ASP), Wholesale Acquisition Cost (WAC), and Maximum Allowable Cost (MAC) are all benchmarks used for prescription drug reimbursement.
3) b. In 2008, private insurance paid for 42% of drug costs.
4) a. Yes, Mr. Simon is eligible for Medicare Part D because he is 65 years old and has Medicare Part A coverage.
5) a. Dual eligibles are individuals who are eligible for both Medicaid and Medicare coverage.
6) b. Dual eligibles are responsible only for Medicare Part D prescription copays. Their premiums, deductibles, and coverage gaps are subsidized.
7) b. The quantity written for Greta Jones's prescription exceeds the quantity limit. Rather than delay dispensing her prescription, submit and dispense a quantity of 30 tablets and document the change on the face of the prescription. As a courtesy, call the prescriber and inform the physician of the change.
8) a. Stanley Simmons is most likely in the coverage gap (also known as the donut hole) of his Medicare Part D plan. He must pay all prescription costs until the total prescription spending for the year reaches the catastrophic coverage threshold.
9) c. Pharmacies can perform an E1 transaction on the pharmacy computer system to determine eligibility.
10) d. Although Mrs. Hernandez is eligible to enroll in a Medicare Part D plan, she currently has creditable coverage with her current prescription plan. This letter indicates that she may remain in her current plan and therefore, avoid any penalty from Medicare Part D.
11) a. In order to obtain a medication that is not normally covered under a Part D plan, the *physician* must initiate the request for an exemption. The pharmacy cannot initiate the request.
12) b. When a medication requires prior authorization, the beneficiary is entitled to one 30-day fill while the request for prior authorization is being processed. The patient may request that the physician prescribe a different drug or obtain the necessary documents to process the prior authorization.
13) a. Lantus is available in vials containing 10 mL or 1,000 units, and Mr. Jones's total daily dose equals 40 units. (1,000 units divided by 40 units per day equals 25 days supply). The prescription should be processed for a quantity of 10 mL of Lantus 100 units/mL (1 vial = 10 mL), and the days supply should be 25 days. A 30-day supply is 1,200 units, but, because the product comes in a pre-packaged quantity that cannot be split, the quantity and days supply must be adjusted to accommodate dispensing the package size. If allowed, two vials, or 20 mL, could be dispensed with a 50-day supply.
14) b. The prescribing physician allows for substitution, and, if the customer agrees, the prescription should be processed for a quantity of 28 capsules of the in-stock product for a 7-day supply. The DAW code 4 indicates that the generic product was not in stock. If the customer refuses, the prescription should be returned so that she can fill it elsewhere. A claim should never be processed with a different product (NDC) than what is dispensed.

Resources

Co-Pay Assistance Foundations:
HealthWell Foundation: http://www.healthwellfoundation.org/index.aspx
Chronic Disease Fund: http://www.cdfund.org
Patient Access Network Foundation: http://www.patientaccessnetwork.org
Patient Advocate Foundation: http://www.patientadvocate.org
For additional information on pharmaceutical assistance programs:
http://www.needymeds.com or http://www.rxassist.org

Information on the 340B drug discount program: http://www.hrsa.gov/opa.

Information on Medicare http://www.Medicare.org or http://www.Medicare.gov website.

For more information about Medicare OPPS, refer to the Center for Medicare and Medicaid Services (CMS) Web site (www.cms.hhs.gov).

Visit the OPPS Web site at http://www.cms.hhs.gov/HospitalOutpatientPPS for the most recent Addendum B, which lists the products by HCPCS codes with status indicators.

References

1. Avalere Health. Audioconference on the trends in pharmaceutical pricing and payment: The changing landscape; February 1, 2008. Available at: http://www.avalerehealth.net/conferences/pharmaceutical_pricing.html. Accessed May 14, 2010.
2. AMCP Task Force on Drug Payment Methodologies. AMCP guide to pharmaceutical payment methods. *JMCP.* 2007;13(8),(suppl): S2–S39
3. Hartman M, Martin A, Nuccio O, and the National Health Expenditure Accounts Team. Health spending growth at a historic low in 2008. *Health Aff.* 2010;29(1):147–155.
4. U.S. Census Press Release. Income Climbs, Poverty Stabilizes, Uninsured Rate Increases. Available at http://www.census.gov/Press-Release/www/releases/archives/income_wealth/007419.html. Accessed on May 14, 2010.
5. Richardson J. PBMs: The basics and an overview, The Health Strategies Consultancy. Available at: http://www.ftc.gov/ogc/healthcarehearings/docs/030626richardson.pdf. Accessed May 14, 2010.
6. Academy of Managed Care Pharmacy. Prior authorization and the formulary exception process. Available at: http://www.amcp.org/amcp.ark?p=AAAC630C. Accessed May 14, 2010.
7. National Council for Prescription Drug Programs. Available at: http://www.ncpdp.org/. Accessed May 14, 2010.
8. Centers for Medicare and Medicaid Services. National health expenditures aggregate. Available at: http://www.cms.gov/NationalHealthExpendData/downloads/tables.pdf. Accessed on May 5, 2010.
9. Kaiser Family Foundation. Medicare-A primer. Available at: http://kff.org/medicare/7615.cfm. Accessed on May 14, 2010.
10. Center for Medicare and Medicare Services. Your Medicare coverage. Available at: http://www.medicare.gov/Coverage/Home.asp. Accessed May 14, 2010.
11. Kaiser Family Foundation. Medicare at a glance. Available at: http://www.kff.org/medicare/7067/ataglance.cfm. Accessed on June 20, 2008.
12. Centers for Medicare and Medicaid Services. Medicare and you 2010. Available at: http://www.medicare.gov/Publications/Pubs/pdf/10050.pdf. Accessed on May 14, 2010.
13. DePue R, Stubbings J, Baker DC. Medicare Part D policy update and implications for 2010. *Am J Managed Care.* 2010;16(5):e117–120.
14. Hoadley J, Hargraves E, and Cubanski J. Medicare Part D 2008 data spotlight: Low-income subsidy plan availability. Available at: http://www.kff.org/medicare/7763.cfm. Accessed on June 21, 2008.
15. Kaiser Family Foundation. Medicaid primer book. Available at: http://www.kff.org/medicaid/7334.cfm. Accessed on June 21, 2010.
16. 2010 Poverty Guidelines. Available at: https://www.cms.gov/MedicaidEligibility/Downloads/POV10Combo.pdf. Accessed May 14, 2010.
17. United States Department of Veterans Affairs, VA health care eligibility and enrollment. Available at: http://www.va.gov/healtheligibility/. Accessed on May 14, 2010.
18. United States Department of Veterans Affairs, Pharmacy benefits management strategic health care group. Available at: http://www.pbm.va.gov/NationalFormulary.aspx. Accessed on May 14, 2010.
19. Department of Defense. TRICARE overview. Available at: http://tricare.mil/mybenefit/home/overview. Accessed on May 14, 2010.
20. United States Department of Health and Human Services. Indian health service: a quick look. Available at: http://info.ihs.gov/QuickLook.asp. Accessed on May 14, 2010.
21. MedPAC. Healthcare spending and the Medicare program. Available at: http://www.medpac.gov/documents/Jun08DataBook_Entire_report.pdf. Accessed May 14, 2010.
22. Center for Medicare and Medicare Services. Hospital outpatient prospective payment system; Medicare learning network payment system fact sheet series. Available at: http://www.cms.hhs.gov/MLNProducts/downloads/HospitalOutpaysysfctsht.pdf. Accessed on July, 2008.
25. Kaiser Family Foundation. Summary of new health reform law. Available at: http://kff.org/healthreform/upload/8061.pdf. Accessed April 27, 2010.

Acknowledgment

The authors wish to thank Annexiea Buford, CPhT, for her careful review of this chapter and recommendations.

Appendixes

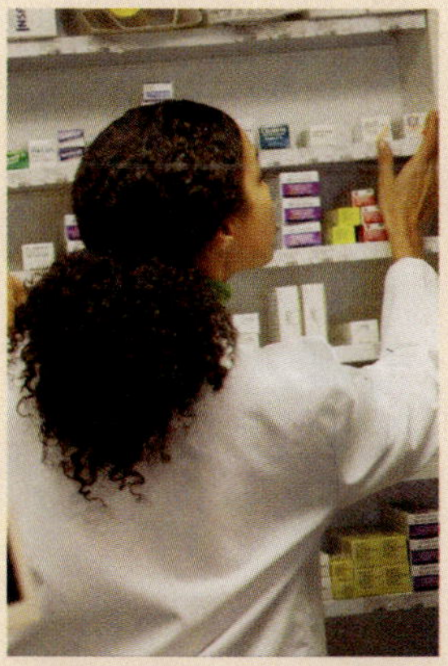

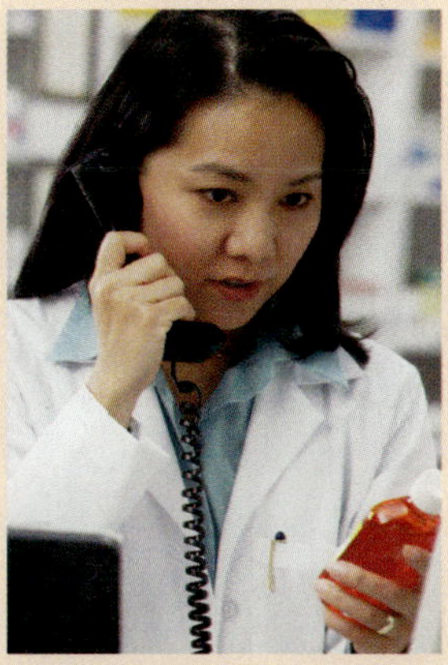

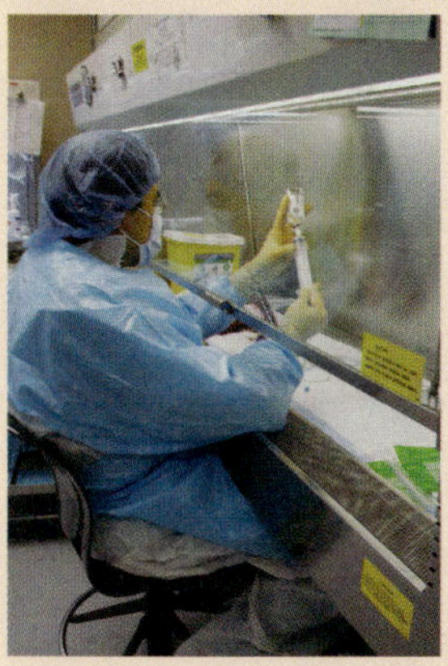

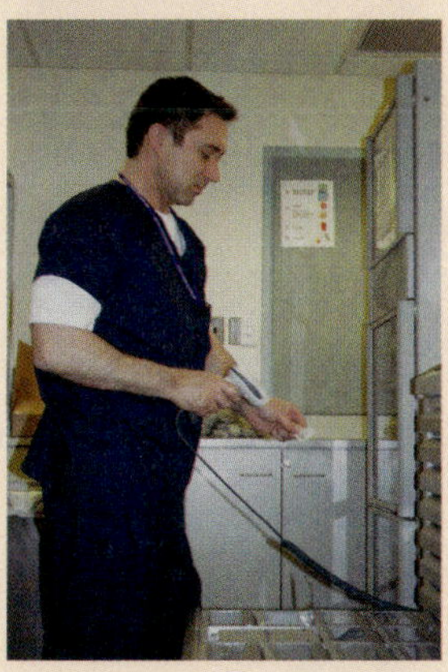

Appendix A

Medical Terminology and Abbreviations

Familiarity with and understanding medical terms and abbreviations is critical to the success of a pharmacy technician because it can help the technician be more helpful and productive.

Learning medical terminology may seem like learning a whole new language. Most medical terms, however, are built from component parts, called word roots, prefixes, and suffixes. The root is the base component of the word, which is modified by the addition of a prefix or suffix. Prefixes are modifying components placed in front of the word root. Examples include pre-, post-, and sub-. Suffixes appear at the end of the word root and are connected to the root by a combining vowel, for example, -ism, -itis, -ous. Combining vowels (most often 'o') are often used to link roots to suffixes and to join roots when a term includes more than one root. These combining vowels are often shown along with the root as a combining form, as in "bronch/o."

The process of defining a medical term starts with identifying and defining the components and then combining those definitions into a coherent whole. For example, consider the word *bronchoscopy*. First, divide the word into its components: "bronch/o" and "-scopy." Then, define each of the parts: *bronch/o* means bronchus, and *-scopy* means the process of viewing. Therefore, bronchoscopy means the process of viewing the bronchus.

What is the definition of *electrocardiogram*? First, break the word into its parts: "electro-," "cardi/o," and "-gram." Second, define each part: *electro-* means electricity, *cardi/o* means heart, and *-gram* means record. Finally, put the definitions together to get the complete definition of the word: recording the electrical activity of the heart.

Tables A-1, A-2, and A-3 include the meanings of many of the most common word roots, prefixes, and suffixes. Familiarity with these components parts will help you understand medical terminology.

After you have reviewed the meanings of component parts, read through the common medical terms by body system. Each term is accompanied by its pronunciation, definition, and an analysis of term structure.

Table A-1. Prefixes

Prefix	Meaning
a-; an-; ana-	no; not; without
ab-	away from
ante-	before; forward
anti-	against
auto-	self
bi-	two; double; both
brady-	slow
carcin-	cancerous
contra-	against; opposite
dys-	difficult; painful
ect-	outside; out
en-	within; in
endo-	within
epi-	above; upon
ex-	out
gynec/o-	woman
hemi-	half
hyper-	above; excessive
hypo-	below; deficient
infra-	below; inferior
inter-	between
intra-	within
iso-	same; equal
macro-	large
mal-	bad; poor; abnormal
meta-	change; after; beyond
micro-	small
multi-	many
neo-	new
non-	not
oligo-	few; less
pan-	all
para-	near; beside
per-	through
peri-	around; surrounding
poly-	many; excessive
post-	after
pre-	before; in front of
primi-	first
retro-	behind; backward; upward

Prefix	Meaning
semi-	half
sub-	below; under
super-	above; over; excess
supra-	above, on top of
sym-	with
syn-	together; with
tachy-	fast
tri-	three
uni-	one
xero-	dry

Table A-2. Suffixes

Suffix	Meaning
-ac; -al; -ar; -ary	pertaining to
-algia	pain
-blast	germ or bud
-cele	hernia; herniation
-centesis	surgical puncture
-crine	to secrete
-crit	to separate
-cyte	cell
-cytosis	condition of cells
-desis	binding together
-ectomy	surgical removal; excision
-emesis	vomit
-emia	blood
-genesis; -genic; -gen	origin; producing; forming
-globin; -globulin	protein
-gram	record
-graph	instrument for recording
-graphy	process of recording
-ia; -iac; -ic	pertaining to
-iasis	formation or presence of
-ism	condition
-itis	inflammation
-ium	structure or tissue
-lepsy	seizure
-lysis; -lytic	break down
-malacia	softening
-megaly	enlargement

Table A-2. Suffixes

Suffix	Meaning
-metry	process of measuring
-oid	resembling; like
-(o)logist	specialist in the study or treatment of
-(o)logy	study of
-oma	tumor
-osis	abnormal condition
-ostomy	creation of an opening
-otomy	incision into
-ous	pertaining to
-paresis	paralysis
-pathy	disease
-penia	decreased number
-pepsia	digestion
-pexy	suspension or fixation
-phagia	eating; swallowing
-phobia	abnormal fear
-phonia	voice; sound
-phoresis	carrying; transmission
-phoria	feeling; mental state
-plasty	surgical repair
-plegia	paralysis
-pnea	breathing
-poiesis	formation
-r/rhage; -r/rhagia	bursting forth
-rrhea	flow; discharge
-rhexis	rupture
-sclerosis	hardening
-scope	instrument for viewing
-scopy	process of viewing
-somnia; somn/o	sleep
-spasm	involuntary contraction or twitch
-stasis	control; stop
-stenosis	narrowing
-therapy	treatment
-thorax	chest; pleural cavity
-tocia; toc/o	labor; birth
-tripsy	crushing
-trophy	growth; development
-tropin	nourish; develop; stimulate

Table A-3. Word Roots

Root	Meaning
abdomin/o	abdomen
aden/o	gland
adip/o	fat
amnio	amnion
andr/o	male; man
angi/o	vessel
aque/o	watery
arteri/o	artery
arteriol/o	arteriole
arthr/o	joint
ather/o	fat; fatty plaque
audi/o	hearing; sound
aur/o	ear
balan/o	glans penis
bili	bile; gall
blephar/o	eyelid
bronch/o	bronchus
bronchiol/o	bronchiole
bucc/o	cheek
burs/o	joint
calc/i	calcium
capnia	carbon dioxide
carcin/o	cancer
cardi/o	heart
carp/o	wrist bones
cephal/o	head
cerebr/o	cerebrum
cirrh/o	yellow
chol/e	bile; gall bladder
cholangi/o	bile duct
cholecyst/o	gall bladder
chondr/o	cartilage
coagul/o	clotting
cochle/o	cochlea
col/o	colon
colp/o	vagina (sheath)
conjuctiv/o	conjunctiva
cor/o; coron/o	heart
corne/o	cornea
cost/o	rib

Table A-3. Word Roots

Root	Meaning
crani/o	cranium; skull
cry/o	cold
cut/o, cuti, cutane/o	skin
cyan/o	blue
cyst/o	bladder, sac
cyt/o	cell
dacry/o	tears
dent	tooth
derm/o, dermat/o	skin
dipl/o	two; double
dips/o	thirst
duoden/o	duodenum
dur/a	dura mater
electr/o	electricity
embry/o	embryo
encephal/o	brain
enter/o	intestines
eosin/o; erythr/o	red
epididym/o	epididymis
episi/o	vulva
esophag/o	esophagus
esthesi/o	sensation
fasci/o	fascia
femor/o	femur
fet/o; fet/i	fetus
fibul/o	fibula
fund/o	fundus
gastr/o	stomach
gingiv/o	gums
glauc/o	silver; gray
gli/o	nerve cell
glomerul/o	glomerulus
gloss/o	tongue
gluc/o, glyc/o	glucose; sugar
gonad/o	sex glands
gravid/a, gravid/o	pregnancy
gyn/o, gyn/e, gynec/o	woman
hemat/o, hem/o	blood
hemangi/o	blood vessel
hepat/o	liver

Table A-3. Word Roots

Root	Meaning
hidr/o	sweat
hormone/o	hormone; an urging on
humer/o	humerus
hydr/o	water; fluid
hyster/o	uterus
ile/o; ili/o	ileum
immune/o	protection
jejun/o	jejunum
kal/i	potassium
kerat/o	cornea
ket/o, keton/o	ketone bodies
kinesi/o	movement
lacrim/o	tears
lact/o	milk
lapar/o	abdominal wall
laryng/o	larynx
ligament/o	ligament
lingua	tongue
lip/o	fat
lith/o	stone
lumb/o	lower back
lymph/o	lymph
mamm/o, mast/o	breast
melan/o	black
men/o	menses; menstruation
mening/o, meningi/o	meninges (membrane)
metacarp/o	hand bones
metatars/o	foot bones
morph/o	form; shape
muc/o	mucus
my/o	muscle
myc/o	fungus
myel/o	bone marrow; spinal cord
myring/o	eardrum
narc/o	sleep
nas/o	nose
nat/o, natal	birth, delivery
nephr/o	kidney
neur/o	nerve
noct/o, nyctal/o	night

Table A-3. Word Roots

Root	Meaning
ocul/o, ophthalm/o,	
opt/o	eye
onych/o	nail
oophor/o	ovary
or/o	mouth
orch/o, orchi/o,	
orchid/o	testis; testicle
orth/o	straight
oste/o	bone
ot/o	ear
ovari/o	ovary
oxi	oxygen
pachy/o	thick
pancreat/o	pancreas
par/o, part/o	bear; labor; childbirth
patell/o	kneecap
pector/o	chest
ped	children
pelv/i	pelvis
perine/o	perineum
peritone/o	peritoneum
phag/o	eat or swallow
phalang/o	finger and toe bones
pharyng/o	pharynx
phleb/o	vein
phot/o	light
phren/o	mind or diaphragm
pil/o	hair
pneum/o	lungs; air
pod/o, podi	foot
presby/o	old age
proct/o	rectum
psych/o, psych/i	mind or soul
pub/o	pubis; pubic bone
pulmon/o	lungs
py/o	pus
pyel/o	renal pelvis
quadr/i	four
radi/o	radius
rect/o	rectum

Table A-3. Word Roots

Root	Meaning
ren/o	kidney
reticul/o	a net
retin/o	retina
rhabdomy/o	skeletal muscle; striated muscle
rheum	watery discharge
rhin/o	nose
salping/o	eustachian or uterine tube
sarc/o	flesh
schiz/o	split
semin/o	semen
septi	bacteria
sial/o	saliva
sinus/o	sinus
somat/o	body
sperm/o, spermat/o	sperm
spher/o	round
sphygm/o	pulse
spir/o	breathe; breath
splen/o	spleen
spondyl/o	vertebra; vertebral column
steth/o	chest
stoma, stomat/o	mouth
synovi/o	joint
tars/o	ankle bones
ten/o; tend/o, tendon/o; tendin/o	tendon
test/o, testicul/o	testis; testicle
thorac/o	chest
thromb/o	clot
thyr/o	thyroid gland
trache/o	trachea
tympan/o	eardrum
urethr/o	urethra
ur/o	urinary tract
vas/o, vascul/o	vessel
ven/o	vein
xanth/o	yellow

Common Medical Terms and Definitions by Body System

Nervous System

Term	Phonetic Spelling	Term Structure	Definition
akinesia	a″kĭ-ne′zhə	a = not, without kinesi/o = movement	Loss of normal muscle movement
cerebrospinal	ser″ə-bro-spi′nəl	cerebr/o = cerebrum spin/o = spine al = pertaining to	Pertaining to the brain and the spinal cord
cerebrovascular	ser″ə-bro-vas′ku-lər	cerebr/o = cerebrum vascul/o = vessel spin/o = spine ar = pertaining to	Pertaining to the brain and blood vessels that supply it
electroencephalogram	e-lek″tro-en-sef′ə-lo-gram″	electr/o = electricity encephal/o = brain gram = record	Record of the electrical activity of the brain
epidural	ep″ĭ-doo′rəl	epi = above, upon dur/a = dura mater al = pertaining to	Pertaining to above the dura mater
epilepsy	ep′ĭ-lep″se	epi = upon lepsy = seizure	A disorder of the central nervous system characterized by recurrent seizures
hemiparesis	hem″ĭ-pə-re′sis	hemi = half paresis = paralysis	Paralysis of one side of the body
hydrocephalus	hi″dro-sef′ə-ləs	hydr/o = water, fluid cephal/o = head	Excess cerebrospinal fluid in the brain
hyperesthesia	hi″pər-es-the′zhə	hyper = above or excessive esthesi/o = sensation ia = condition of	Increased sensitivity to stimulation such as touch, pain, and other sensory stimuli
meningitis	men″in-ji′tis	mening/o = meninges itis = inflammation	Inflammation of the meninges of the brain
myelogram	mi′ə-lo-gram	myel/o = bone marrow or spinal cord gram = record	An x-ray of the spinal cord and nerve roots
neuralgia	nŏŏ-ral′jə	neur/o = nerve algia = pain	Nerve pain
neurologist	nŏŏ-rol′ə-jist	neur/o = nerve logist = specialist in the study or treatment of	A physician who specializes in diseases of the neurological system
paraplegia	par″ə-ple′jə	para = near, beside plegia = paralysis	Paralysis of both lower extremities and, generally, the lower trunk
polyneuritis	pol″e-nŏŏ-ri′tis	poly = many or excessive neur/o = nerve itis = inflammation	Inflammation of two or more nerves
schizophrenia	skiz″o-fre′ne-ə	schiz/o = split phren/o = mind or diaphragm ia = condition of	A type of psychosis in which the mind is said to be split from reality

Common Medical Terms and Definitions by Body System

Cardiovascular System

Term	Phonetic Spelling	Term Structure	Definition
angiography	an″je-og′rə-fe	angi/o = vessel graphy = process of recording	An examination of blood vessels via radiographic study
anoxia	ə-nok′se-ə	an = not, without oxi = oxygen	Without oxygen
arteriogram	ahr-tēr′-e-o-gram	arteri/o = artery gram = record	Record (x-ray) of an artery
arteriosclerosis	ahr-tēr″e-o-sklə-ro′sis	arteri/o = artery scler/o = hard osis = abnormal condition	Thickening, loss of elasticity, and hardening of arterial walls
bradycardia	brad″e-kahr′de-ə	brady = slow cardi/o = heart ia = pertaining to	Pertaining to a slow heart rate
cardiologist	kahr″de-ol′ə-jist	cardi/o = heart logist = specialist in the study or treatment of	A physician who specializes in diseases of the heart
cardiomegaly	kahr″de-o-meg′ə-le	cardi/o = heart megaly = enlargement	Enlarged heart
cardiomyopathy	kahr″de-o-mi-op′ə-the	cardi/o = heart my/o = muscle pathy = disease	Disease of the heart muscle
endarterectomy	end-ahr″tər-ek′tə-me	end/o = within, in arter/o = artery ectomy = surgical removal, excision	Surgical removal of the inside of an artery
endocardium	en″do-kahr′de-um	endo = within, in cardi/o = heart ium = structure, tissue	Membrane lining the cavities of the heart
hypertension	hi″pər-ten′shən	hyper = above or excessive tension	High blood pressure
hypoxemia	hi″pok-se′me-ə	hypo = below or deficient ox/e = oxygen emia = blood	Too little oxygen in the blood
myocarditis	mi″o-kahr-di′tis	my/o = muscle cardi/o = heart itis = inflammation	Inflammation of the heart muscle
myocardium	mi″o-kahr′de-əm	my/o = muscle cardi/o = heart ium = structure, tissue	heart muscle tissue
pericardium	per″ĭ-kahr′de-əm	peri = around, surrounding cardi/o = heart ium = structure, tissue	Lining around the outside of the heart
tachycardia	tak″ĭ-kahr′de-ə	tachy = fast cardi/o = heart ia = pertaining to	Pertaining to a fast heart rate

Common Medical Terms and Definitions by Body System

Respiratory System

Term	Phonetic Spelling	Term Structure	Definition
bronchitis	brong-ki'tis	bronch/o = bronchus itis = inflammation	Inflammation of the bronchi
bronchoscopy	brong-kos'kə-pe	bronch/o = bronchus scopy = process of viewing	Process of viewing the bronchi
dyspnea	disp'ne-ə	dys = difficult, painful pnea = breathing	Difficult, painful, or faulty breathing
hypoxia	hi-pok'se-ə	hypo = deficient or below oxi = oxygen ia = condition of	A condition of deficient oxygen levels
laryngoscope	lə-ring'gə-skōp	laryng/o = larynx scope = instrument for viewing	Instrument for viewing the larynx
laryngospasm	lə-ring'go-spaz"əm	laryng/o = larynx spasm = involuntary contraction or twitch	Contraction of laryngeal muscles, causing constriction
pharyngitis	far"in-ji'tis	pharyng/o = pharynx itis = inflammation	Inflammation of the pharynx
pneumothorax	noo"mo-thor'aks	pneum/o = air or lungs thorax = chest, pleural cavity	Air or gas in the chest cavity
pulmonologist	pool"mə-nol'ə-jist	pulmon/o = lungs logist = specialist in the study or treatment of	Specialist in diseases of the lungs
rhinoplasty	ri'no-plas"te	rhin/o = nose plasty = surgical repair	Surgical repair of the nose
rhinorrhea	ri"no-re'ə	rhin/o = nose rrhea = flow, discharge	Discharge from the nose
spirometry	spi-rom'ə-tre	spir/o = breathe; breath metry = process of measuring	Measurement of breathing
stethoscope	steth'o-skōp	steth/o = chest scope = instrument for viewing	Instrument used to listen to lung and heart sounds through the chest wall
thoracotomy	thor"ə-kot'ə-me	thorac/o = chest otomy = incision into	Incision into the chest
tracheostomy	tra"ke-os'tə-me	trache/o = trachea stomy = creation of an opening	Creation of an opening in the trachea, usually to insert a tube

Common Medical Terms and Definitions by Body System

Musculoskeletal System

Term	Phonetic Spelling	Term Structure	Definition
arthralgia	ahr-thral'jə	arthr/o = joint algia = pain	Joint pain
arthritis	ahr-thri'tis	arthr/o = joint itis = inflammation	Inflammation of the joints
arthroscopy	ahr-thros'kə-pe	arthr/o = joint scopy = process of viewing	Process of viewing a joint
bradykinesia	brad"e-kĭ-ne'zhə	brady = slow kinesi/o= movement	Slow movement
bursitis	bər-si'tis	burs/o = joint itis = inflammation	Inflammation of the bursa, a fluid-filled sac around joints
chondromalacia	kon"dro-mə-la'shə	chondro = cartilage malacia = softening	Softening of the cartilage
craniotomy	kra"ne-ot'ə-me	crani/o = cranium, skull otomy = incision into	Surgical incision of the skull
electromyogram	e-lek"tro-mi'o-gram	electr/o = electricity my/o = muscle gram = record	Record of the electrical activity of a muscle
intercostal	in"tər-kos'təl	inter = between cost/o = rib al = pertaining to	Pertaining to between the ribs
intramuscular	in"trə-mus'ku-lər	intra = within muscul/o = muscle ar = pertaining to	Pertaining to within the muscle
myalgia	mi-al'jə	my/o = muscle algia = pain	Muscle pain
orthopedic	or"tho-pe'dik	orth/o = straight podi = foot ic = pertaining to	Literally, means pertaining to straight foot—pertaining to the study of diseases of the skeletal and muscular system
orthopedist	or"tho-pe'dist	orth/o = straight podi = foot logist = specialist in the study or treatment of	A specialist in the study of diseases of the skeletal and muscular system
osteomyelitis	os"te-o-mi"ə-li'tis	oste/o = bone myel/o = bone marrow or spinal cord itis = inflammation	Inflammation of the bone and bone marrow
patellectomy	pat"ə-lek'tə-me	patell/o = kneecap ectomy = surgical removal, excision	Surgical removal of the kneecap
suprapubic	soo"prə-pu'bik	supra = above, on top of pub/o = pubic bone, pubis ic = pertaining to	Pertaining to above the pubic bone
tendinitis	ten"dĭ-ni'tis	tendin/o = tendon itis = inflammation	Inflammation of the tendon

Common Medical Terms and Definitions by Body System

Endocrine System

Term	Phonetic Spelling	Term Structure	Definition
adenoma	ad″ə-no′mə	aden/o = gland oma = tumor	Tumor of glandular tissue
adrenomegaly	ə-dre″no-meg′ə-le	adren/o = adrenal gland megaly = enlargement	Enlargement of the adrenal gland
andromorphous	an″dro-mor′fəs	andr/o = male morph/o = form, shape ous = pertaining to	Male form or appearance
endocrinology	en″do-krĭ-nol′ə-je	end/o = within, in crine = to secrete logy = study of	Study of the secreting glands that comprise the endocrine system
glucogenic	gloo″ko-jen′ik	gluc/o = glucose, sugar genic = origin, producing, forming	Giving rise to or producing glucose
hormonal	hor-mo′nəl	hormone/o = hormone; an urging on al = pertaining to	Pertaining to hormones
hyperglycemia	hi″pər-gli-se′me-ə	hyper = above or excessive glyc/o = glucose, sugar emia = blood	Too much sugar in the blood
hyperthyroidism	hi″pər-thi′roid-iz-əm	hyper = above or excessive thyr/o = thyroid gland ism = condition	Condition of too much thyroid hormone
hypokalemia	hi″po-kə-le′me-ə	hypo = below or deficient kal/i = potassium emia = blood	Low blood potassium
hyposecretion	hi″po-sə-kre′shən	hypo = below or deficient secretion	Abnormally decreased secretion
ketoacidosis	ke″to-as″ĭ-do′sis	ket/o = ketone bodies acid osis = abnormal condition	Condition of an increased presence of ketone bodies
pancreatitis	pan″kre-ə-ti′tis	pancreat/o = pancreas itis = inflammation	Inflammation of the pancreas
polydipsia	pol″ĭ-dip′se-ə	poly = many or excessive dips/o = thirst ia = condition of	Condition of excessive thirst
thymoma	thi-mo′mə	thym/o = thymus gland oma = tumor	Tumor of thymic tissue
thyroidectomy	thi″roi-dek′tə-me	thyr/o = thyroid gland ectomy = surgical removal, excision	Surgical removal of the thyroid gland

Common Medical Terms and Definitions by Body System

Immune System

Term	Phonetic Spelling	Term Structure	Definition
autoimmune	aw"to-ĭ-mūn'	auto = self immune/o = protection	The disorder characterized by abnormal function of the immune system that causes the body to produce antibodies against itself
immunocompromised	im"u-no-kom'prə-mīzd	immune/o = protection compromised	A condition in which the immune system has been compromised by disease or immunosuppressive agents
leukemia	loo-ke'me-ə	leuk/o = white emia = blood	A malignant blood disease marked by abnormal white blood cells, or leukocytes
lymphadenopathy	lim-fad"ə-nop'ə-the	lymph/o = lymph aden/o = gland pathy = disease	A disease state in which lymph nodes are enlarged
lymphocytopenia	lim"fo-si"to-pe'ne-ə	lymph/o = lymph cyt/o = cell penia = decreased number	An abnormally reduced number of lymphocytes
lymphoma	lim-fo'mə	lymph/o = lymph oma = tumor	A neoplasm of the lymphatic system
macrocytosis	mak"ro-si-to'sis	macro = large cytosis = condition of cells	The presence of large red blood cells
metastasis	mə-tas'tə-sis	meta = beyond, after, or change stasis = stop or control	The spread of cancer cells beyond the original site of the tumor through blood or lymph
pancytopenia	pan"si-to-pe'ne-ə	pan = all cyt/o = cell penia = decreased number	An abnormally reduced number of all types of blood cells
phagocyte	fag'o-sīt	phag/o = eat or swallow cyt/o = cell	A cell that consumes bacteria, foreign particles, and other cells
septicemia	sep"tĭ-se'me-ə	septi =bacteria emia = blood	Bacterial infection of the blood
splenomegaly	sple"no-meg'ə-le	splen/o = spleen megaly = enlargement	An enlarged spleen
thymus	thi'məs	thym/o = thymus gland ectomy = surgical removal, excision	The removal of the thymus gland

Common Medical Terms and Definitions by Body System

Hematologic System

Term	Phonetic Spelling	Term Structure	Definition
anemia	ə-ne′me-ə	an = not, without emia = blood	A blood condition in which there is a reduction in the number of red blood cells, hemoglobin, or the volume of packed red blood cells
hematology	he″mə-tol′ə-je	hemat/o = blood logy = study of	Medical study of the blood
hemocytoblasts	he″mo-si′to-blsts	hem/o = blood cyt/o = cell blast = germ or bud	Primitive cells in the bone marrow that develop into blood cells
hemolysis	he-mol′ə-sis	hem/o = blood lysis = break down	The breakdown of the red blood cell membrane
hematopoiesis	he″mə-to-, hem″ə-to-poi-e′sis	hem/o = blood poiesis = formation	The process of formation and development of various types of blood cells.
leukopenia	loo″ko-pe′ne-ə	leuko = white penia = decreased number	Too few white blood cells
morphology	mor-fol′ə-je	morph/o = form, shape logy = study of	The study of form, including the size and shape of a specimen, such as a blood cell
myeloma	mi″ə-lo′mə	myel/o = bone marrow or spinal cord oma = tumor	Tumor of the bone marrow
myelocyte	mi′ə-lo-sīt	myel/o = bone marrow or spinal cord cyt/o = cell	An immature blood cell in the bone marrow
reticulocyte	rə-tik′u-lo-sīt″	reticul/o = a net cyt/o = cell	Immature red blood cells, or erythrocytes
thrombophlebitis	throm″bo-flə-bi′tis	thromb/o = clot phleb/o = vein itis = inflammation	Inflammation of a vein due to blood clot formation

Common Medical Terms and Definitions by Body System

Gastrointestinal System

Term	Phonetic Spelling	Term Structure	Definition
abdominocentesis	ab-dom"ĭ-no-sen-te'sis	abdomin/o = abdomen centesis = surgical puncture	A puncture of the abdomen for aspiration of abdominal fluid.
cholecystectomy	ko"le-sis-tek'tə-me	cholecyst/o = gall bladder ectomy = surgical removal, excision	Surgical removal of the gall bladder
cirrhosis	sĭ-ro'sis	cirrh/o = yellow osis = abnormal condition	Chronic liver condition that causes yellowing of tissues.
colonoscopy	ko"lon-os'kə-pe	col/o = colon scopy = process of viewing	Process of viewing the colon
dyspepsia	dis-pep'se-ə	dys = difficult, painful pepsia = digestion	The condition of indigestion, or of painful digestion
dysphagia	dis-fa'je-ə	dys = difficult, painful phag/o = eat or swallow ia = pertaining to	Pertaining to difficulty in eating or swallowing
endoscopic	en"do-skop'ik	end/o = within, in scopy = process of viewing ic = pertaining to	Pertaining to the process of viewing within
esophagitis	ə-sof"ə-ji'tis	esophag/o = esophagus itis = inflammation	Inflammation of the esophagus
gastroenterologist	gas"tro-en"tər-ol'ə-jist	gastro = stomach enter/o = intestines ologist = specialist in the study or treatment of	Specialist in the study or treatment of the stomach and intestines
hematemesis	he"mə-tem'ə-sis	hemat/o = blood emesis = vomit	Bloody vomit
hepatomegaly	hep"ə-to-meg'ə-le	hepat/o = liver megaly = enlargement	Enlargement of the liver
nasogastric	na"zo-gas'trik	nas/o = nose gastr/o = stomach ic = pertaining to	Pertaining to the nose and the stomach (e.g., a tube that travels from the nose to the stomach)
pancreatitis	pan"kre-ə-ti'tis	pancreat/o = pancreas itis = inflammation	Inflammation of the pancreas
sublingual	səb-ling'gwəl	sub = below, under lingua = tongue al = pertaining to	Pertaining to under the tongue

Common Medical Terms and Definitions by Body System

Urinary System

Term	Phonetic Spelling	Term Structure	Definition
bacteriuria	bak-tēr″e-u′re-ə	bacteri/o = bacteria ur/o = urinary tract ia = a condition of	The presence of bacteria in the urine
cystoscope	sis′to-skōp″	cyst/o = sac or bladder scope = instrument for viewing	Type of endoscope that is used to examine the bladder
glucosuria	gloo″ko-su′re-ə	gluc/o = glucose, sugar ur/o = urinary tract ia = a condition of	A condition of sugar in the urine
hydronephrosis	hi″dro-nə-fro′sis	hydr/o = water, fluid nephr/o = kidney osis = abnormal condition	A condition of urine pooling in the renal pelvis
ketonuria	ke″to-nu′re-ə	ket/o = ketone bodies ur/o = urinary tract ia = condition of	Condition of ketone bodies in the urine
lithotripsy	lith′o-trip″se	lith/o = stone tripsy = crushing	The crushing of a stone
nephrectomy	nə-frek′tə-me	nephr/o = kidney ectomy = surgical removal, excision	Surgical removal of a kidney
nephrosis	nĕ-fro′sis	nephr/o = kidney osis = abnormal condition	An abnormal condition of the kidney
polyuria	pol″e-u′re-ə	poly = many or excessive ur/o = urinary tract ia = condition of	Condition in which one urinates excessively
pyelonephritis	pi″ə-lo-nə-fri′tis	pyel/o = renal pelvis nephr/o = kidney itis = inflammation	Inflammation of the renal pelvis area of the kidney
ureterolithiasis	u-re″tər-o-lĭ-thi′ə-sis	ureter/o = ureter lith/o = stone iasis = formation of, or presence of	The condition of having a stone form in the ureter
urethralgia	u″re-thral′jə	urethr/o = urethra algia = pain	Pain in the urethra
urologist	u-rol′ə-jist	ur/o = urinary tract logist = a specialist in the study or treatment of	Physician who specializes in conditions of the urinary system
vesicotomy	ves″ĭ-kot′ə-me	vesic/o = sac or bladder otomy = incision into	An incision into the bladder

Common Medical Terms and Definitions by Body System

Other Body Systems

Section I: The Eyes

Term	Phonetic Spelling	Term Structure	Definition
blepharitis	blef"ə-ri'tis	blephar/o = eyelid itis = inflammation	Inflammation of the eyelid
conjunctivitis	kən-junk"tĭ-vi'tis	conjunctiv/o = conjunctiva itis = inflammation	Inflammation of the conjunctiva
exophthalmia	ek"sof-thal'me-ə	ex/o = out ophthalm/o = eye ia = pertaining to	Pertaining to a protuberance of the eye
intraocular	in"trə-ok'u-lər	intra = within ocul/o = eye ar = pertaining to	Pertaining to the inside of the eye
keratoplasty	ker'ə-to-plas"te	kerat/o = cornea plasty = surgical repair	The surgical repair or reconstruction of the cornea
lacrimation	lak"rĭ-ma'shən	lacrim/o = tears ation = a process	The process of secreting tears
ophthalmologist	of"thəl-mol'ə-jist	ophthalm/o = eye ologist = specialist in the study or treatment of	Specialist in diseases of the eye
optometry	op-tom'ə-tre	opt/o = eye metry = process of measuring	Process of measuring the eye
photophobia	fo"to-fo'be-ə	phot/o = light phobia = abnormal fear	Extreme sensitivity and discomfort from light
presbyopia	pres"be-o'pe-ə	presby/o = old age opia – a condition of vision	A vision condition of a reduced ability to focus due to old age
retinitis	ret"ĭ-ni'tis	retin/o = retina itis = inflammation	Inflammation of the retina

Section II: The Ears

Term	Phonetic Spelling	Term Structure	Definition
audiometry	aw"de-om'ə-tre	audi/o = hearing; sound metry = measurement	Measurement of hearing
myringitis	mir"in-ji'tis	myring/o = eardrum itis = inflammation	Inflammation of the tympanic membrane
otorhinolaryngologist	o"to-ri"no-lar"in-gol'ə-jist	ot/o = ear rhin/o = nose laryng/o = larynx ologist = specialist in the study or treatment of	Specialist in diseases of the ear, nose, and throat
otalgia	o-tal'je-ə	ot/o = ear algia = pain	Earache
otitis	o-ti'tis	ot/o = ear itis = inflammation	Inflammation of the ear
otosclerosis	o"to-sklə-ro'sis	ot/o = ear sclerosis = hardening	A condition of hardening of bone tissue in the ear

Term	Phonetic Spelling	Term Structure	Definition
presbyacusis	pres"be-ə-ku'-sis	presby/o = old age acous/o = a hearing condition	Hearing loss due to old age
salpingitis	sal"pin-ji'tis	salping/o = eustachian or uterine tube itis = inflammation	Inflammation of the eustachian tube in the ear or the uterine tube.
tympanometry	tim"pə-nom'ə-tre	tympan/o = eardrum metry = the process of measuring	The process of measuring the compliance and mobility (conductibility) of the tympanic membrane.
tympanoplasty	tim"pə-no-plas'te	tympan/o = eardrum plasty = surgical repair	Surgical repair of the eardrum

Section III: The Dermatologic System

Term	Phonetic Spelling	Term Structure	Definition
dermatitis	der"mə-ti'tis	dermat/o = skin itis = inflammation	Inflammation of the skin
dermatologist	dər"mə-tol'o-jīst	dermat/o = skin ologist = specialist in the study or treatment of	Specialist in the study of diseases of the skin
epidermal	ep"ĭ-dər'məl	epi = on, upon derm/o = skin al = pertaining to	Pertaining to on the skin
histology	his-tol'ə-je	hist/o = tissue logy = study of	The study of tissues
keratosis	ker"ə-to'sis	kerat/o = hard osis = abnormal condition	A condition of thickened epidermis
onychomycosis	on"ĭ-ko-mi-ko'sis	onych/o = nail myc/o = fungus osis = abnormal condition	Fungal infection of the nail
percutaneous	per"ku-ta'ne-əs	per = through cutane/o = skin ous = pertaining to	Through the skin
sarcoma	sahr"ko'mə	sarc/o = flesh oma = tumor	Tumor of the flesh
subcutaneous	sub"ku-ta'ne-əs	sub = below, under cutane/o = skin ous = pertaining to	Pertaining to below the skin
xeroderma	zēr"o-der'mə	xero = dry derm/o = skin	Dry skin

Common Medical Terms and Definitions by Body System

Reproductive System

Term	Phonetic Spelling	Term Structure	Definition
anorchism	an-or′kiz-əm	an = not, without orch/o = testis; testicle ism = condition	The condition in which one or both testes are absent
aspermia	ə-spər′me-ə	a = not, without sperm/o = sperm ia = condition of	The condition in which one is unable to produce or ejaculate sperm
colposcope	kol′po-skōp	colp/o = vagina (sheath) scope = instrument for viewing	A special kind of scope designed to examine the vagina
epididymitis	ep″ĭ-did′ə-mi′tis	epididym/o = epididymis itis = inflammation	Inflammation of the epididymis
episiotomy	ə-piz″e-ot′o-me	episi/o = vulva tomy = incision into	An incision made in the perineum to facilitate childbirth
gynecologist	gi″nə-kol′ə-jist″ə-	gynec/o = woman logist = a specialist in the study or treatment of	A physician who specializes in the reproductive system of women
hydrocele	hi′dro-sēl	hydr/o = water or fluid cele = hernia or herniation	A hernia of fluid in the testis or tubes leading from the testis
hysterectomy	his″tər-ek′tə-me	hyster/o = uterus ectomy = surgical removal, excision	The surgical removal of the uterus
lactogenic	lak″to-jen′ik	lact/o = milk genic = origin, producing, forming	Pertaining to the production of milk
mammogram	mam′ə-gram	mamm/o = breast gram = record	An x-ray of the breast
mastodynia	mas″to-din′e-ə	mast/o = breast dynia = pain	Breast pain
obstetrics	ob-stet′riks	obstetr/o = midwife ic = pertaining to	The specialty pertaining to the care and treatment of mother and fetus throughout pregnancy, childbirth, and the immediate postpartum period
oligospermia	ol″ĭ-go-sper′me-ə	oligo = few or less sperm/o = sperm	Too few sperm in the semen
oophoritis	o″of-ə-ri′tis	oophor/o = ovary itis = inflammation	Inflammation of the ovary
orchiopexy	or″ke-o-pek′se	orchi/o = testis; testicle pexy = suspension or fixation	Surgical treatment of an undescended testicle by freeing it and implanting it into the scrotum
prostatalgia	pros″tə-tal′jə	prostat/o = prostate algia = pain	Painful prostate
vasectomy	və-sek′tə-me	vas/o = vessel ectomy = surgical removal, excision	Excision of part of the vas deferens to produce male sterility

Appendix B

Confused Drug Names

ISMPs List of Confused Drug Names

This list of confused drug names, which includes look-alike and sound-alike name pairs, consists of those name pairs that have been involved in medication errors published in the *ISMP Medication Safety Alert*! and the *ISMP Medication Safety Alert*! Community/Ambulatory Care Edition. The errors involving these medications were reported to ISMP through the ISMP Medication Errors Reporting Program (MERP). This list also contains the names that appear on The Joint Commission's list of look-alike and sound-alike names. The Joint Commission established a National Patient Safety Goal that requires each accredited organization to identify a list of look-alike or sound-alike drugs used in the organization. Those names that appear on The Joint Commission's list have been noted with an asterisk (*) below.

List of Confused Drug Names

Drug Name	Confused Drug Name
Abelcet*	amphotericin B*
Accupril	Aciphex
acetaZOLAMIDE*	acetoHEXAMIDE*
acetic acid for irrigation	glacial acetic acid
acetoH EXAM IDE*	acetaZOLAMIDE*
Aciphex	Accupril
Aciphex	Aricept
Activase	Cathflo Activase
Activase	TNKase
Actonel	Actos
Actos	Actonel
Adacel (Tdap)	Daptacel (DTaP)
Adderall	Inderal
Adderall	Adderall XR
Adderall XR	Adderall
Advair*	Advicor*
Advicor*	Advair*
Advicor	Altocor
Afrin (oxymetazoline)	Afrin (saline)
Afrin (saline)	Afrin (oxymetazoline)
Aggrastat	argatroban
Aldara	Alora
Alkeran	teukeran
Alkeran	Myleran
Allegra	Vlagra
Alora	Aldara
ALPRAZolam*	LORazepam*
Altocor	Advicor
amantadine	amiodarone
Amaryl	Reminyl
Ambisome*	amphotericin B*
Amicar*	Omacor*
Amikin	Kineret
aMILoride	amLODIPine
amiodarone	amantadine
amLQDIPine	aMILoride
amphotericin B*	Abelcet*
amphotericin B*	Ambisome*
Anacin	Anacin-3
Anacin-3	Anacin
antacid	Atacand
Antivert	Axert
Anzemet	Avandamet
Apresoline	Priscoline
argatroban	Aggrastat

Drug Name	Confused Drug Name
argatroban	Orgaran
Aricept	Aciphex
Aricept	Azilect
aripiprazole	proton pump inhibitors
aripiprazole	rabeprazole
Asacol	Os-Cal
Atacand	antacid
Atrovent	Natru-Vent
Avandamet	Anzemet
Avandia	Prandin
Avandia*	Coumadin*
AVINza	INVanz
AVINza*	Evista*
Axert	Antivert
azaCITIDine	azaTHIOprine
azaTHIQprine	azaCITIDine
Azilect	Aricept
B & 0 (belladonna and opium)	Beano
BabyBIG	HBIG (hepatitis B immune globulin)
Bayhep-B	Bayrab
Bayhep-B	Bayrho-D
Bayrab	Bayhep-B
Bayrab	Bayrho-D
Bayrho-D	Bayhep-B
Bayrho-D	Bayrab
Beano	B & 0 (belladonna and opium)
Benadryl	benazepril
benazepril	Benadryl
Benicar	Mevacor
Betadine (with providone-iodine)	Betadine (without providone-iodine)
Betadine (without providone-iodine)	Betadine (with providone-iodine)
Bextra	Zetia
Bicillin C-R	Bicillin t-A
Bicillin t-A	Bicillin C-R
Bicitra	Polycitra
Brethine	Methergjne
Brevibloc	Brevital
Brevital	Brevibloc
buPROPion	busPIRone
busPIRone	buPROPion
Capadex [non-US product]	Kapidex
Capex	Kapidex
Carac	Kuric
captopril	carvedilol
carBAMazepine	OXcarbazepine

List of Confused Drug Names

Drug Name	Confused Drug Name
CARBOplatin	CISplatin
Cardura*	Coumadin*
carvedilol	captopril
Casodex	Kapidex
Cathflo Activase	Activase
Cedax	Cidex
ceFAZolin	cefTRIAXone
cefTRIAXone	ceFAZolin
CeleBREX*	CeleXA*
CeleBREX*	Cerebyx*
CeleXA	ZyPREXA
CeleXA*	CeleBREX*
CeleXA*	Cerebyx*
Cerebyx*	CeleBREX*
Cerebyx*	CeleXA*
cetirizine	sertraline
chlordiazePOXIDE	chlorproMAZINE
chiorproMAZINE	chlordiazePOXIDE
chlorproMAZINE	chlorproPAMIDE
chlorproPAMIDE	chlorproMAZINE
Cidex	Cedax
CISplatin	CARBOplatin
Claritin (loratadine)	Claritin Eye (ketotifen fumarate)
Claritin-D	Claritin-D 24
Claritin-D 24	Claritin-D
Claritin Eye (ketotifen fumarate)	Claritin (loratadine)
Clindesse	Clindets
Clindets	Clindesse
clomiPHENE	clomiPRAMINE
clomiPRAMINE	clomiPHENE
clonazePAM	cloNIDine
clonazePAM	LORazepam
cloNIDine	clonazePAM
cloNIDine*	KlonoPIN*
Clozaril	Colazal
Coagulation factor IX (recombinant)	Factor IX Complex, Vapor Heated
codeine	Iodine
Colace	Cozaar
Colazal	Clozaril
colchicine	Cortrosyn
Comvax	Recombivax HB
Cortrosyn	colchicine
Coumadin*	Avandia*
Coumadin*	Cardura*
Cozaar	Colace

Drug Name	Confused Drug Name
Cozaar	Zocor
cycloSERINE	cycloSPORINE
cycloSPORINE	cycloSERINE
Cymbalta	Symbyax
DACTINomycin	DAPTOmycin
Daptacel (DTaP)	Adacel (Tdap)
DAPTOmycin	DACTINomycin
Darvocet*	Percocet*
Darvon	Diovan
DAUNOrubicin*	DAUNOrubicin citrate liposomal*
DAUNOrubicin*	DOXOrubicin*
DAUNOrubicin*	IDArubicin*
DAUNOrubicin citrate liposomal*	DAUNOrubicin*
Denavir	indinavir
Depakote	Depakote ER
Depakote ER	Depakote
Depo-Medrol	Solu-MEDROL
Depo-Provera	Depo-subQ provera 104
Depo-subQ provera 104	Depo-Provera
desipramine	disopyramide
dexmethylphenidate	methadone
Diabenese	Diamox
Diabeta*	Zebeta*
Diamox	Diabenese
Diflucan*	Diprivan*
Dilacor XR	Pilocar
Dilaudid	Dilaudid-5
Dilaudid-5	Dilaudid
dimenhyDRINATE	diphenhydrAMINE
diphenhydrAMINE	dimenhyDRINATE
Dioval	Diovan
Diovan	Dioval
Diovan	Zyban
Diovan	Darvon
Diprivan*	Diflucan*
Diprivan	Ditropan
disopyramide	desipramine
Ditropan	Diprivan
DOBUTamine	DOPamine
DOPamine	DOBUTamine
Doxil	Paxil
DOXOrubicin*	DAUNOrubicin*
DOXOrubicin*	DOXOrubicin liposomal*
DOXOrubicin*	IDArubicin*
DOXOrubicin liposomal*	DOXOrubicin*

List of Confused Drug Names

Drug Name	Confused Drug Name
Dulcolax (bisacodyl)	Dulcolax (docusate sodium)
Dulcolax (docusate sodium)	Dulcolax (bisacodyl)
DULoxetine	FLUoxetine
Durasal	Durezol
Durezol	Durasal
Duricef	Ultracet
Dynacin	Dynacirc
Dynacirc	Dynacin
edetate calcium disodium	edetate disodium
edetate disodium	edetate calcium disodium
Effexor*	Effexor XR*
EffexorXR*	Effexor*
Enbrel	Levbid
Engerix-B adult	Engerix-B pediatric/adolescent
Engerix-B pediatric/adolescent	Engerix-B adult
Enjuvia	Januvia
ePHEDrine*	EPINEPHrine*
EPINEPHrine*	ePHEDrine*
Estratest	Estratest HS
Estratest HS	Estratest
ethambutol	Ethmozine
Ethmozine	ethambutol
Evista*	AVINza*
Factor IX Complex, Vapor Heated	Coagulation factor IX (recombinant)
Femara	Femhrt
Femhrt	Femara
fentaNYL	SUFentanil
Fioricet	Fiorinai
Fiorinai	Fioricet
flavoxate	fluvoxamine
Flonase	Flovent
Flovent	Flonase
flumazenil	influenza virus vaccine
FLUoxetine	PARoxetine
FLUoxetine	DULoxetine
fluvoxamine	flavoxate
Folex	Foltx
folio acid*	folinic acid (leucovorin calcium)*
folinic acid (leucovorin calcium)*	folic acid*
Foltx	Folex
fomepizole	omeprazole
Foradil	Fortical
Foradil	Toradol
Fortical	Foradil
gentamicin	gentian violet

Drug Name	Confused Drug Name
gentian violet	gBntamicin
glacial acetic acid	acetic acid for irrigation
glipiZIDE	glyBURIDE
glyBURIDE	glipiZIDE
Granulex	Regranex
guaiFENesin	guanFACINE
guanFACINE	guaiFENesin
HBIG (hepatitis 8 immune globulin)	BabyBIG
Healon	Hyalgan
heparin*	Hespan*
Hespan*	heparin*
HMG-CoA Reductase Inhibitors ("statins")	nystatin
HumaLQG*	HumuLIN*
HumaLOG*	NovoLOG*
HumaLDG Mix 75/25	HumuLIN 70/30
Humapen Memoir (for use with HumaLOG)	Humira Pen
Humira Pen	Humapen Memoir (for use with HumaLOG)
HumuLIN*	NovoLIN*
HumuLIN*	HumaLOG*
HumuLIN 70/30	HumaLOG Mix 75/25
Hyalgan	Healon
hydrALAZINE*	hydrOXYzine*
HYDROcodone*	oxyCODONE*
Hydrogesic	hydrOXYzine
HYDROmorphone*	morphine*
hydrOXYzine	Hydrogesic
hydrOXYzine*	hydrALAZINE*
IDArubicin*	DAUNOrubicin*
IDArubicin*	DOXOrubicin*
Inderal	Adderall
indinavir	Denavir
inFLIXimab	riTUXimab
influenza virus vaccine	flumazenil
influenza virus vaccine	tuberculin purified protein derivative (PPD)
Inspra	Spiriva
INVanz	AVINza
iodine	lodine
Isordil	Plendil
isotretinoin	tretinoin
Jantoven	Janumet
Jantoven	Januvia
Janumet	Jantoven

List of Confused Drug Names

Drug Name	Confused Drug Name
Janumet	Januvia
Janumet	Sinemet
Januvia	Enjuvia
Januvia	Jantoven
Januvia	Janumet
K-Phos Neutral	Neutra-Phos-K
Kaopectate (bismuth subsalcylate)	Kaopectate (docusate calcium)
Kaopectate (docusate calcium)	Kaopectate (bismuth subsalcylate)
Kadian	Kapidex
Kaletra	Keppra
Kapidex	Capadex [non-US product]
Kapidex	Capex
Kapidex	Casodex
Kapidex	Kadian
Keflex	Keppra
Keppra	Kaletra
Keppra	Keflex
Ketalar	ketorolac
ketorolac	Ketalar
ketorolac	methadone
Kineret	Amikin
KlonoPIN*	cloMDine*
Kuric	Carac
Kwell	Qwell
LaMICtal	LamISIL
LamISIL	LaMICtal
lamiVUDine*	lamoTRIgine*
lamoTRIgine*	lamiVUDine*
lamoTRIgine	levothyroxine
Lanoxin	levothyroxine
Lanoxin	naloxone
lanthanum carbonate	lithium carbonate
Lantus	Lente
Lariam	Levaquin
Lasix	Luvox
Lente	Lantus
leucovorin calcium*	Leukeran*
Leukeran	Alkeran
Leukeran	Myleran
Leukeran*	leucovorin calcium*
Levaquin	Lariam
Levbid	Enbrel
levetiracetam	levofloxacin
levotloxacin	levetiracetam
levothyroxine	lamoTRIgine
levothyroxine	Lanoxin
Lexapro	Loxitane
Lipitor	Loniten
Lipitor	ZyrTEC
lithium carbonate	lanthanum carbonate
Lodine	codeine
Lodine	iodine
Loniten	Lipitor
Lopressor	Lyrica
LDRazepam*	ALPRAZolam*
LORazepam	clonazePAM
LORazepam	Lovaza
Lotronex	Protonix
Lovaza	LORazepam
Loxitane	Lexapro
Loxitane	Soriatane
Lunesta	Neulasta
Lupron Depot-3 Month	Lupron Depot-Ped
Lupron Depot-Fed	Lupron Depot-3 Month
Luvox	Lasix
Lyrica	Lopressor
Maalox	Maalox Total Stomach Relief
Maalox Total Stomach Relief	Maalox
Matulane	Matema
Materna	Matulane
Maxzide	Microzide
Menactra	Menomune
Menomune	Menactra
Mephyton	methadone
Metadate	methadone
Metadate CD	Metadate ER
Metadate ER	Metadate CD
Metadate ER	methadone
metFORMIN*	metroNIDAZOLE*
methadone	dexmethylphenidate
methadone	ketorolac
methadone	Mephyton
methadone	Metadata
methadone	Metadata ER
methadone	methylphenidate
Methergine	Brethine
methimazole	metolazone
methylphenidate	methadone
metolazone	methimazole
metoprolol succinate	metoprolol tartrate

App B

List of Confused Drug Names

Drug Name	Confused Drug Name
metoprolol tartrate	metoprolol succinate
metroNIDAZOLE*	metFORMIN*
Mevacor	Benicar
Micronase	Microzide
Microzide	Maxzide
Microzide	Micronase
midodrine	Midrin
Midrin	midodrine
mifepristone	misoprostol
Miralax	Mirapex
Mirapex	Miralax
misoprostol	mifepristone
morphine*	HYDROmorphone*
morphine - non-concentrated oral liquid*	morphine - oral liquid concentrate*
morphine - oral liquid concentrate*	morphine - non-concentrated oral liquid*
Motrin	Neurontin
MS Contin*	OxyCONTIN*
Mucinex*	Mucomyst*
Mucinex D	Mucinex DM
Mucinex DM	Mucinex D
Mucomyst*	Mucinex*
Myleran	Alkeran
Myleran	Leukeran
naloxone	Lanoxin
Narcan	Norcuron
Natru-Vent	Atrovent
Navane	Norvasc
Neo-Synephrine (oxymetazoline)	Neo-Synephrine (phenylephrine)
Neo-Synephrine (phenylephrine)	Neo-Synephrine (oxymetazoline)
Neulasta	Lunesta
Neulasta	Neumega
Neumega	Neupogen
Neumega	Neulasta
Neupogen	Neumega
Neurontin	Motrin
Neurontin	Noroxin
Neutra-Phos-K	K-Phos Neutral
NexAVAR	NexIUM
NexIUM	NexAVAR
niCARdipine	NIFEdipine
NIFEdipine	niCARdipine
NIFEdipine	niMODipine
niMODipine	NIFEdipine
Norcuron	Narcan
Normodyne	Norpramin
Noroxin	Neurontin
Norpramin	Normodyne
Norvasc	Navane
NovoLIN*	HumuLIN*
NovoLIN*	NovoLOG*
NovoLIN 70/30*	NovoLOG Mix 70/30*
NovoLOG*	HumaLOG*
NovoLOG*	NovoLIN*
NovoLOG FLEXPEN	NovoLOG Mix 70/30 FLEXPEN
NovoLOG Mix 70/30 FLEXPEN	NovoLOG FLEXPEN
NovoLOG Mix 70/30*	NovoLIN 70/30*
nystatin	HMG-CoA Reductase Inhibitors ("statins")
Occlusal-HP	Dcuflox
Ocuflox	Occlusal-HP
OLANZapine	QUEtiapine
Omacor*	Amicar*
omeprazole	fomepizole
opium tincture*	paregoric (camphorated tincture of opium)*
Oracea	Drencia
Orencia	Oracea
Orgaran	argatroban
Ortho Tri-Cyclen	Ortho Tri-Cyclen LO
Ortho Tri-Cyclen LO	Ortho Tri-Cyclen
Os-Cal	Asacol
OXcarbazepine	carBAMazepine
oxyCODONE*	HYDROcodone*
oxyCODONE*	OxyCOMTIN*
OxyCONTIN*	MS Contin*
OxyCONTIN*	oxyCODONE*
paclitaxel	paclitaxel protein-bound particles
paclitaxel protein-bound particles	paclitaxel
Pamelor	Panlor DC
Pamelor	Tambocor
Panlor DC	Pamelor
paregoric (camphorated tincture of opium)*	opium tincture*
PARoxetine	FLUoxetine
Patanol	Platinol
Pavulon	Peptavlon
Paxil	Doxil
Paxil	Taxol
Paxil	Plavix
pemetrexed	pralatrexate

List of Confused Drug Names

Drug Name	Confused Drug Name
Peptavlon	Pavulon
Percocet*	Darvocet*
Percocet	Procet
PENTobarbital	PHENobarbital
PHENobarbital	PENTobarbital
Pilocar	Dilacor XR
Platinol	Patanol
Plavix	Paxil
Plendil	Isordil
pneumococcal 7-valent vaccine	pneumococcal polyvalent vaccine
pneumococcal polyvalent vaccine	pneumococcal 7-valent vaccine
Polycitra	Bicitra
pralatrexate	pemetrexed
Prandin	Avandia
Precare	Precose
Precose	Precare
prednisoLONE	predniSONE
predniSONE	prednisoLONE
PriLDSEC*	PROzac*
Priscoline	Apresoline
probenecid	Procanbid
Procan SR	Procanbid
Procanbid	probenecid
Procanbid	Procan SR
Procardia XL	Protain XL
Procet	Percocet
Prograf	PROzac
propylthiouracil	Purinethol
Proscar	Provera
Protain XL	Procardia XL
protamine	Protonix
proton pump inhibitors	aripiprazole
Protonix	Lotronex
Protonix	protamine
Provera	Proscar
Provera	PROzac
PROzac	Prograf
PRDzac*	PriLOSEC*
PROzac	Provera
Purinethol	propylthiouracil
QUEtiapine	QLANZapine
quiNIDine	quiNINE
quiNINE	quiNIDine
Qwell	Kwell
rabeprazole	aripiprazole

Drug Name	Confused Drug Name
Razadyne	Rozerem
Recombivax HB	Comvax
Regranex	Granulex
Reminyl	Robinul
Reminyl	Amaryl
Renagel	Renvela
Renvela	Renagel
Reprexain	ZyPREXA
Restoril	Risperdal
Retrovir*	ritonavir*
Rifadin	Rifater
Rifamate	rifampin
rifampin	Rifamate
rifampin	rifaximin
Rifater	Rifadin
rifaximin	rifampin
Risperdal	Restoril
risperidone	ropinirole
Ritalin	ritodrine
Ritalin LA	Ritalin SR
Ritalin SR	Ritalin LA
ritodrine	Ritalin
ritonavir*	Retrovir*
riTUXimab	inFLIXimab
Robinul	Reminyl
ropinirole	risperidone
Roxanol	Roxicodone Intensol
Roxanol	Roxicet
Roxicet	Roxanol
Roxicodone Intensol	Roxanol
Rozerem	Razadyne
Salagen	selegiline
SandIMMUNE	SandoSTATIN
SandoSTATIN	SandIMMUNE
saquinavir	SINEquan
saquinavir (free base)	saquinavir mesylate
saquinavir mesylate	saquinavir (free base)
Sarafem	Serophene
selegiline	Salagen
Serophene	Sarafem
SEROquel	SEROquel XR
SEROquel	Serzone
SEROquel	SINEquan
SEROquel XR	SEROquel
sertraline	cetirizine

App B

List of Confused Drug Names

Drug Name	Confused Drug Name
sertraline	Soriatane
Serzone	SEROquel
Sinemet	Janumet
SINEquan	saquinavir
SINEquan	SEROquel
SINEquan	Singulair
SINEquan	Zonegran
Singulair	SINEquan
sitaGLIPtin	SUMAtriptan
Solu-CORTEF	Solu-MEDROL
Solu-MEDROL	Depo-Medrol
Solu-MEDROL	Solu-CORTEF
Sonata	Soriatane
Soriatane	Loxitane
Soriatane	sertraline
Soriatane	Sonata
sotalol	Sudafed
Spiriva	Inspra
Sudafed	sotalol
Sudafed	Sudafed PE
Sudafed PE	Sudafed
SUFentanil	fentaNYL
sulfADIAZINE	sulfiSOXAZOLE
sulfiSOXAZOLE	sulfADIAZINE
SUMAtriptan	sitaGLIPtin
SUMAtriptan	zolmitriptan
Symbyax	Cymbalta
Tambocor	Pamelor
Taxol	Taxotere
Taxol	Paxil
Taxotere	Taxol
TEGretol	TEGretol XR
TEGretol	Tequin
TEGretol	TRENtal
TEGretol XR	TEGretol
Tequin	TEGretol
Tequin	Ticlid
Testoderm TTS	Testoderm
Testoderm TTS	Testoderm with Adhesive
Testoderm with Adhesive	Testoderm
Testoderm with Adhesive	Testoderm TTS
Testoderm	Testoderm TTS
Testoderm	Testoderm with Adhesive
tetanus diptheria toxoid (Td)	tuberculin purified protein derivative (PPD)

Drug Name	Confused Drug Name
Thalomid	Thiamine
Thiamine	Thalomid
tiaGABine*	tiZANidine*
Tiazac	Ziac
Ticlid	Tequin
tiZANidine*	tiaGABine*
TNKase	Activase
TNKase	t-PA
Tobradex	Tobrex
Tobrex	Tobradex
TOLAZamide	TOLBUTamide
TOLBUTamide	TOLAZamide
Topamax*	Toprol-XL*
Toprol-XL*	Topamax*
Toradol	Foradil
t-PA	TNKase
Tracleer	Tricor
traMADol*	traZODone*
traZODone*	traMADol*
TRENtal	TEGretol
tretinoin	isotretinoin
Tricor	Tracleer
tromethamine	Trophamine
Trophamine	tromethamine
tuberculin purified protein derivative (PPD)	influenza virus vaccine
tuberculin purified protein derivative (PPD)	tetanus diptheria toxoid (Td)
Tylenol	Tylenol PM
Tylenol PM	Tylenol
Ultracet	Duricef
valacyclovir	valganciclovir
Valcyte	Valtrex
valganciclovir	valacyclovir
Valtrex	Valcyte
Varivax	VZIG (varicella-zoster immuneglobulin)
Vesanoid	Vesicare
Vesicare	Vesanoid
Vexol	Vosol
Viagra	Allegra
vinBLAStine*	vinCRIStine*
vinCRIStine*	vinBLAStine*
Viokase	Viokase 8
Viokase 8	Viokase
Vioxx	Zyvox

List of Confused Drug Names

Drug Name	Confused Drug Name
Viracept	Viramune
Viramune	Viracept
Vosol	Vexol
VZIG (varicella-zoster immuneglobulin)	Varivax
Wellbutrin SR*	Wellbutrin XL*
Wellbutrin XL*	Wellbutrin SR*
Xanax*	Zantac*
Xeloda	Xenical
Xenical	Xeloda
Yasmin	Yaz
Yaz	Yasmin
Zantac*	Xanax*
Zantac*	ZyrTEC*
Zebeta*	Diabeta*
Zebeta	Zetia
Zegerid	Zestril
Zelapar (Zydis formulation)	ZyPREXA Zydis
Zestril	Zegerid
Zestril*	Zetia*
Zestril*	ZyPREXA*
Zetia	Bextra
Zetia	Zebeta
Zetia*	Zestril*
Ziac	Tiazac
Zocor	Cozaar
Zocor*	ZyrTEC*
zolmitriptan	SUMAtriptan
Zonegran	SINEquan
Zostrix	Zovirax
Zovirax	Zyvox
Zovirax	Zostrix
Zyban	Diovan
ZyPREXA	CeleXA
ZyPREXA	Reprexain
ZyPREXA*	Zestril*
ZyPREXA*	ZyrTEC*
ZyPREXA Zydis	Zelapar (Zydis formulation)
ZyrTEC	Lipitor
ZyrTEC*	Zantac*
ZyrTEC*	Zocor*
ZyrTEC*	ZyPREXA*
ZyrTEC	ZyrTEC-D
ZyrTEC (cetirizine)	ZyrTEC Itchey Eye Drops (ketotifen fumarate)
ZyrTEC-D	ZyrTEC
ZyrTEC Itchey Eye Drops (ketotifen fumarate)	ZyrTEC (cetirizine)
Zyvox	Vioxx
Zyvox	Zovirax

App B

* *These drug names are included on The Joint Commission's list of look-alike or sound-alike drug names from which an accredited organization creates it own list to satisfy the requirements of the National Patient Safety Goals. Visit http://wwwjointcommission.org for more information about this Joint Commission requirement.*

Institute for Safe
Medication Practices
www.ismp.org

Appendix C

Glossary

Absorption The amount of medication that enters the bloodstream, or systemic circulation.

Accreditation The process of granting recognition or vouching for compliance with established criteria (usually refers to recognition of an institution or program).

Active ingredient Ingredient in the compounded preparation that is responsible for the therapeutic or pharmaceutical action of the medication.

Activity units (mCi) Radiopharmaceuticals are described by activity units, which relate to the number of atoms that give off a radioactive emission per unit of time. The most common activity unit used in the United States is the Curie (Ci). In a nuclear pharmacy, the amount of radioactivity is small, so the millicurie (mCi) unit is mainly used.

Adjudication Prescription claims adjudication refers to the determination of the insurer's payment after the member's insurance benefits are applied to a medical claim.

Adverse reaction A bothersome or unwanted effect that results from the use of a drug, unrelated to the intended effect of the drug.

Aerosol A suspension of very fine liquid or solid particles distributed in a gas, packaged under pressure, and shaken before use, after which medication is released from the container as a spray.

Agranulocytosis A dramatic decrease in white blood cells.

Alligation method A way to help determine how many parts of each strength should be mixed together to prepare the desired strength.

Ambulatory pharmacy A pharmacy generally located within, or in close proximity to a clinic, hospital, or medical center that provides medication services to ambulatory patients.

Aneroid blood pressure monitor Type of monitor that indicates varying blood pressure using a pointer in a gauge.

Antigen A substance that is capable of causing the production of an antibody.

Antiproliferative A substance used to prevent the spread of cells into surrounding tissue.

Apothecary system A system of measurement, originally developed in Greece for use by physicians and pharmacists but now largely replaced by the metric system, including the grain and the dram, the most common apothecary measures seen today.

Aqueous solution A liquid solution that contains purified water as the vehicle.

Arthralgia Joint pain.

Aseptic technique The technique and procedures designed to prevent contamination of drugs, packaging, equipment, or supplies by microorganisms during preparation.

Assay Describes the activity per unit of volume, measured as mCi/mL.

Autoimmunity A misdirected immune response that happens when the body attacks itself.

Automated dispensing technology Electronic storage cabinets or robotics that secure medications and dispense them to nurses or other caregivers when needed.

Automated medication dispensing device A drug storage device or cabinet that contains an inventory of medications that are electronically dispensed so they may be administered to patients in a controlled manner.

Auxiliary prescription label A label affixed to a drug product that alerts users to special handling or administration concerns.

Average manufacturer price (AMP) The average price paid to manufacturers by wholesalers for drugs distributed through retail pharmacies. Includes discounts and other price concessions that are provided by manufacturers.

Average sales price (ASP) Price based on manufacturer-reported selling price data and includes volume discounts and price concessions that are offered to all classes of trade.

Average wholesale price (AWP) A commonly used benchmark for billing drugs that are reimbursed in the community pharmacy setting. The AWP for a drug is set by the manufacturer of the drug.

Avoirdupois system A French system of mass that includes ounces and pounds; the system of mass most commonly utilized in the United States.

Barcode medication administration (BCMA) A process in which the nurse scans a bar code on a patient's ID band and the bar code specific to the medication prior to medication administration. Documentation of the administration is automatically entered into the patient's electronic health record.

Batch record (or batch log) The compounding record for a batch, usually filed by lot number.

Batch repackaging The periodic repackaging of large quantities of medications in unit-dose or single-unit packages.

Beyond-use labeling A date that is given to a medication noting when it should no longer be used, also referred to as the expiration date.

Biennial inventory DEA-registered pharmacies are required by law to take an initial inventory of all controlled substances on hand upon commencing operations or upon changing ownership, with subsequent inventories conducted every two years thereafter.

Bioavailability The percentage of an administered dose of a medication that reaches the bloodstream.

Biological Safety Cabinet A vertical laminar airflow workbench (LAFW) used for the preparation of hazardous medications that confines airflow within the hood.

Biopharmaceutics The study of the manufacture of medications for effective delivery into the body. It includes the relationships between the physical and chemical properties of a drug, the dosage form in which the drug is given, the route of administration, and the effects of properties and dosage on the rate and extent of drug absorption.

Blister packages Often called "bubble packs." Composed of a plastic bubble that forms a cavity for the medication. The package is then sealed with a backing material that also acts as a label.

Body language Body movements or mannerisms that can be interpreted as conveying one's feelings or psychological state of mind.

Body mass index (BMI) A measure of body fat based on height and weight, used to determine if a patient is underweight, of normal weight, overweight, or obese.

Body surface area (BSA) The total surface area of the body, taking the patient's weight and height into account and expressed in m^2.

Brand-name drug A drug that is covered by a patent and is therefore only available from a single manufacturer.

Buccal A solid medication dosage form that is placed in the pocket between the cheek and gum and absorbed through the cheek into the bloodstream.

Case manager Helps determine the location of the therapy. The case manager may work for the insurance company, the hospital, or the home care company. The case manager works to manage the cost of medical care for the patient and may be very influential in steering a patient toward home care.

Centralized dispensing automation Technology that assists in the selection and dispensing of drug products that are located in a central location, such as the pharmacy, and that can include robotics and carousels that use bar code scanning to select and label drug products for patients.

Centralized pharmacy Pharmacy services that are provided from one location (usually centrally located) in the hospital. Pharmacy personnel, resources, and functions primarily reside within this self-contained location.

Certification A voluntary process by which a nongovernmental agency or association grants recognition to an individual who has met certain predetermined qualifications specified by that agency or association. This recognition demonstrates that the certified individual has achieved a certain level of knowledge, skill, or experience.

Chain pharmacy A pharmacy that is part of a large number of corporately owned pharmacies that use the same name and carry similarly branded OTC products.

Child-resistant packaging Child-resistant packaging is special packaging used for hazardous products such as prescription and over-the-counter drugs and household products to reduce the risk of children ingesting dangerous items by adding caps that children will have difficulty opening. Child-resistant packaging must pass federal tests to assure that it meets the federal requirements.

Clearance The total removal of a drug via metabolism and/or excretion. It combines the elimination rate with the flow of a drug through the organs of elimination (i.e., liver and kidneys). It is usually measured in mL/min or L/hr.

CLIA-waived The Clinical Laboratory Improvement Amendment of 1988 established that some clinical tests be exempted from certain laboratory requirements.

Clinical pharmacy services Services provided by a pharmacist focused on patient care. These services vary greatly by facility, but the goal is to ensure that each medication is appropriate, safe, and cost effective (based on the diagnosis of the patient).

Clinic pharmacy An ambulatory pharmacy located in a clinic or medical center to serve the needs of outpatients.

Closed-ended questions Questions that can be answered by a simple "yes" or "no."

Closed formulary A predetermined, specific list of medications approved by the hospital's P&T committee (or equivalent) to be used for the patients it serves.

Coinsurance A percentage charge for a service, such as a prescription or doctor visit.

Colostomy Surgical formation of an artificial anus by connecting the colon to an opening in the abdominal wall.

Communication The transfer of information, knowledge, facts, wishes, or emotions from one source to another.

Community pharmacy Generally a stand-alone pharmacy located within a community that provides medication services to ambulatory patients.

Compliance error An error occurring when patients do not follow their dosing regimen.

Compounding Usually takes place in a pharmacy and includes the preparation, mixing, packaging, and labeling of a small quantity of a drug based on a practitioner's prescription or medication order for a specific patient.

Compounding environment Includes the facilities (i.e., compounding area) and equipment in the pharmacy.

Compounding record The log or record of an actual compounded preparation or batch that was prepared.

Computer physician order entry (CPOE) The entering of patient orders directly into a computer system.

Continuous subcutaneous insulin infusion Delivery of insulin through a pump device that provides the medication 24 hours per day.

Controlled substances Drugs or chemical substances whose possession and use are regulated under the Federal Controlled Substances Act and by state controlled substance laws and regulations. Controlled substances are subject to stricter controls than other prescription and non-prescription drugs.

Control solution A type of solution that mimics blood and that is used to test the accuracy of a blood glucose meter and test strips.

Copayment (copay) The portion of the cost of a prescription that the patient is responsible for paying when a part of the cost is covered by a third-party payer.

Coring Introducing particulate matter in the form of a plastic or rubber "core" or plug into a sterile fluid through the process of penetrating the outer seal of a vial or bag with a needle.

Cost sharing The amount of insurance costs shared by the employee or beneficiary.

Coverage gap Also referred to as the "donut hole." This is a period of no coverage that typically occurs once the individual's total prescription drug spending for the year reaches the initial coverage limit. During the coverage gap, the beneficiary must pay all costs for prescriptions until the total prescription spending for the year reaches the catastrophic coverage threshold.

Cross-sensitivity Sensitivity to one substance that predisposes an individual to sensitivity to other substances that are related in chemical structure.

Cytochrome P450 (CYP) A group of enzymes that metabolize drugs.

Days supply The amount of medication dispensed for a specified time period.

Decentralized pharmacy Pharmacy services that are provided on or near a patient care area. These services are often supported by a central pharmacy. A pharmacy satellite is an example of one form of a decentralized pharmacy service.

Deductible A fixed amount that must be paid each year by the individual before the insurance starts to pay.

Denominator The bottom number of a fraction, representing the total number of parts.

Deteriorated drug error Use of an expired medication or one whose properties have been compromised.

Diagnosis-related group (DRG) A set rate paid for an inpatient procedure based on cost and intensity. Drugs provided during an inpatient stay are not separately reimbursed; they are included in the DRG payment.

Diastole When the heart muscle is relaxed and the chambers are filling with blood; the pressure is at the lowest point in a normal heart.

Digestion The process whereby ingested food is broken up into smaller molecules by chemical or mechanical means.

Direct purchasing Buying directly from a manufacturer. It typically involves the execution of a purchase order from the pharmacy to the manufacturer of the drug.

Disintegration The breakdown of medication from its original solid formulation.

Dispensing The act of preparing a medication for use by a patient as authorized by a prescription.

Dispensing fee The amount paid for dispensing the prescription.

Dissolution The dissolving of medication into solution, usually in the stomach and intestinal tract.

Douche An aqueous solution that is placed into a body cavity or against a part of the body (e.g., the internal vaginal cavity) to clean or disinfect.

Drug distribution services The system(s) used to distribute medications that begins when the medication is received by the pharmacy and ends when the medication is administered to the patient.

Drug Enforcement Administration (DEA) The federal agency that administers and enforces federal laws for controlled substances and illegal substances such as narcotics and other dangerous drugs. The DEA is part of the U.S. Department of Justice.

Drug information request A question regarding a medication.

Drug interaction The impact of a drug or food product on the amount or activity of another drug in the body. This interaction can result in enhanced, reduced, or new activity of the drug in the body.

Drug interactions Effects caused by the combined actions of two or more drugs used simultaneously.

Drug monograph Written information about a drug or class of drugs that contains product details, indications for use, safety information, dosing, administration, and other useful information about the drug(s).

Durable medical equipment Reusable equipment used for the treatment of illness or injury (e.g., wheelchairs, walkers, blood glucose meters).

Elastomeric balloon system An intravenous administration system containing reservoirs that consist of multiple layers of elastomeric (i.e., stretchy, elastic-like) membranes within a hard or soft shell. When the device is filled with diluent and a drug, the elastomeric material expands like a balloon. When tubing is attached to the device and the patient's catheter, the elastic balloon forces the solution through the tubing and into the patient.

Electronic medication administration record (eMAR) A component of the computerized patient medical record in which nurses and other healthcare providers document times and dates when a medication was administered to the patient.

Elimination The removal of a drug from the body, mainly in the urine or feces.

Elixir A clear, sweet, flavored water-and-alcohol (hydroalcoholic) mixture intended for oral use.

Empathy A sharing of or identification with another's feelings or state of mind without actually going through the same experience; the ability to view feelings from the patient's perspective, communicating acceptance or understanding.

Emulsion A mixture of two liquids that normally do not mix, in which one liquid is broken into small droplets (the internal phase) and evenly scattered throughout the other (the external or continuous phase) and an emulsifying agent prevents the internal phase from separating from the external phase.

Endocrine The internal secretion of substances into the systemic circulation (bloodstream).

Endocrine glands Glands that have no ducts; their secretions are absorbed directly into the blood.

Endotracheal Administering a medication into the trachea (windpipe); intratracheal.

Enema A solution that is inserted into the rectum to empty the lower intestinal tract or to treat diseases of that area; often given to relieve severe constipation or to clean the large bowel before surgery.

Excretion The irreversible removal of a drug or metabolite from a body fluid. The most common location of drug excretion in the body is the kidneys; the biliary tract is another important route of excretion.

Expectorate To cough up or spit.

Extemporaneous repackaging Repackaging quantities of medications that will be used within a short period of time.

Extractive A concentrated preparation of material extracted, or removed, from dried plant or animal tissue by soaking it in a solvent, which is then evaporated, leaving behind the tissue parts containing medical activity; examples include extracts, tinctures, and fluidextracts.

Extravasation Leaking of intravenous solutions into areas outside of the vein, resulting in potentially severe tissue damage.

Failure mode and effects analysis (FMEA) A process that evaluates where errors might occur and estimates their potential impact.

Federal upper limit (FUL) The maximum of federal matching funds that the federal government will pay to state Medicaid programs for eligible generic and multisource drugs.

Fee for service A method of payment in which providers bill separately for each patient encounter or service they provide.

First-pass metabolism The metabolism (breaking down) of orally ingested medications by the liver and small intestine before they reach the main bloodstream.

Formulary A specific list of drugs that are included with a given prescription drug plan.

Formulation record An individual record (like a recipe) for a preparation. It includes a listing of the ingredients, compounding equipment, and instructions for preparing the compound. A formulation record may also be referred to as a formula or master formula.

Fraction A part of a whole number, used to express quantities less than one or quantities between two whole numbers.

Free-flow protection A feature that prevents "free-flow" of medication or fluid, which can lead to unintentional overdoses.

Gamma photon Type of radioactive emission. Gamma photons are electromagnetic waves (like x-rays) that have the ability to travel far enough to leave the patient's body and be detected by nuclear medicine imaging equipment.

Generic drug A drug that is no longer covered by a patent and is therefore generally available from multiple manufacturers, usually resulting in a significant reduction in cost.

Geometric dilution Compounding technique used to ensure the uniform mixing when there is a wide discrepancy in amounts of individual ingredients. The preparer starts with the smallest ingredient amount and mixes it with an equal amount (estimated by sight) of the next smallest ingredient amount and continues adding and doubling the size until all ingredients are integrated.

Gonads Reproductive organs; testes in the male, and ovaries in the female. Gonads function to produce reproductive cells and sex hormones.

Graduates Compounding equipment used to measure the volume of liquid ingredients; generally glass or plastic cylinders and conicals.

Group purchasing organization (GPO) An organized group that contracts with manufacturers to purchase pharmaceuticals at discounted prices, in return for a guaranteed minimum purchase volume. Hospitals, independent community pharmacies, and other retail chain pharmacies become members of a GPO to leverage buying power and take advantage of the lower prices that manufacturers offer to the GPOs.

Half-life The amount of time required for one-half of the amount of radioactivity to decay. Also, the time that it takes for 50% of a drug to be eliminated from the body.

Hazardous material Any material that poses a risk to people, animals, property, or the environment.

Healthcare Common Procedure Coding System (HCPCS) A set of medical codes that identifies procedures, equipment, and supplies for claim submission purposes.

Health Insurance Portability and Accountability Act (HIPAA) Federal legislation enacted to establish guidelines for the protection of patients' private health information.

Health literacy The ability to read, understand, and act upon health care information to make appropriate decisions and follow instructions for treatment.

Health system pharmacy The practice of pharmacy in a practice setting that is part of a health-system. A health-system is two or more health-care practice settings (e.g., hospital, home care, ambulatory clinic) that have a working relationship with each other and are managed or owned by the same business entity. Health-systems provide complete health care-related services to the patients they serve.

Hemoglobin A1c Blood test that measures the amount of glucose attached to hemoglobin in red blood cells. Provides an estimate of blood glucose control over the previous 2-3 months.

HEPA Filter A high-efficiency particulate air (HEPA) filter that removes 99.97% of all air particles 0.3 micrometers or larger. It is composed of pleats of filter medium separated by rigid sheets of corrugated paper or aluminum foil that direct the flow of air forced through the filter in a uniform parallel flow.

High alert medications Medications that have a high risk of causing patient harm when used in error.

Home health care Physician-ordered health-care services provided to a patient in the home or other setting in which the patient lives.

Hormone A chemical substance produced in the body that controls and regulates the activity of certain cells or organs. Usually, it is a chemical made by a gland for export to another part of the body; it is not active at its site of synthesis.

Hospital formulary An approved list of medications that are routinely stocked in the hospital pharmacy to treat the types of patients the hospital typically serves.

Household system A system of measurement commonly used in cooking, including the teaspoon, the tablespoon, and the cup.

Ideal body weight (IBW) An estimate of how much a patient should weigh based on his or her height and gender; expressed in kg.

Improper dose error A dose that is greater than or less than that ordered by the prescriber.

Inactive ingredient An ingredient that is necessary to prepare the formulation, but is not intended to cause a pharmacologic response. Inactive ingredients may also be referred to as inert ingredients, added ingredients or substances, or excipients, and include, for example, colorants, flavorants, sweeteners, and wetting agents.

Indemnity A system of health insurance in which the insurer pays for the cost of covered services after care has been given on a fee-for-service basis. It usually defines the maximum amounts covered.

Independent pharmacy A community pharmacy or small group of pharmacies in a limited geographic area that are owned by an individual or small number of individuals.

Inhalant A fine powder or solution of a drug delivered as a mist through the mouth into the respiratory tract.

Initial inventory The inventory a pharmacy takes of its stock of controlled substances upon beginning the dispensing or distribution of controlled substances.

Institutional patient assistance programs (IPAPs) Programs offering assistance to patients in an institution. Bulk medication replacement is provided to the institution (e.g., pharmacy or clinic) instead of to an individual patient. The institution has the obligation of verifying that each patient who receives medications meets the established criteria.

Insulin pen Portable device that contains a prefilled cartridge of insulin.

Intake coordinator The person from the home care company who receives the patient referral. This person is responsible for getting the patient's contact information (address, phone number, etc.), diagnosis, requested home care therapy, pertinent medical data, and insurance information.

Intraarterial Injected directly into an artery and therefore immediately available to act in the body.

Intraarticular Injected directly into the articular (joint) space.

Intracardiac Injected directly into the heart muscle.

Intradermal Injected into the top layers of the skin.

Intramuscular Injected directly into a large muscle mass, such as the upper arm, thigh, or buttock, and absorbed from the muscle tissue into the bloodstream.

Intraperitoneal Administered into the peritoneal space (abdominal cavity).

Intrapleural Administered into the pleural space, which is the sac that surrounds the lungs.

Intrathecal Injected into the space around the spinal cord.

Intratracheal Administered into the trachea (windpipe); endotracheal.

Intrauterine Administered into the uterus.

Intravenous Injected directly into a vein and therefore immediately available to act in the body.

Intraventricular Injected into the brain ventricles or cavities.

Intravesicular Administered into the bladder.

Intravitreal Administered into the vitreous space in the eye; intravitreous.

Intravitreous Administered into the vitreous space in the eye; intravitreal.

Investigational drug services Services provided to support clinical trials involving medications.

Irrigant A solution used to wash or cleanse part of the body, such as the eyes, the urinary bladder, open wounds, or scraped skin.

Jelly A semisolid solution with a high liquid content, usually water.

Just-in-time inventory management An inventory method in which products are ordered and delivered at just the right time—when they are needed for patient care. The goal is minimizing wasted steps, labor, and cost.

Laminar Airflow Workbench (LAFW) A work area (hood) where parenteral products are compounded. Twice-filtered laminar layers of aseptic air continuously sweep the work area inside the hood to prevent the entry of contaminated room air. There are two common types of laminar flow workbenches, horizontal flow and vertical flow.

Lancet A sharp-pointed instrument used to make small incisions, commonly used to obtain blood samples for blood glucose monitoring.

Large Volume Parenteral (LVP) IV solutions greater than 100 mL in volume. LVPs are usually solutions of dilute dextrose and/or sodium chloride with or without drug additives. They are usually given as continuous infusions, but they may be used for intermittent infusions as well.

Legend drug A drug that is required by federal law to be dispensed by prescription only. It is the older term for drugs that are now identified as "Rx Only."

Levigation A compounding method of incorporating a solid (i.e., powder) into an ointment. A small amount of a wetting agent is added to the powder to form a paste, which is then incorporated into the ointment.

Licensure The process by which an agency of the government grants permission to an individual to engage in a given occupation upon finding that the applicant has attained a degree of competency necessary to ensure that public health, safety, and welfare will be protected.

Ligand Chemical substance that will behave in a certain way when injected into the body. For nuclear medicine imaging, a small amount of radioactivity is attached to the ligand, and the ligand "carries" the radioactivity with it as it moves around the body.

Loading dose A larger first dose given to quickly achieve a high drug concentration in the body.

Long-term care Health care provided to a patient in a long-term facility where the patient may stay for an extended period. Long-term care facilities include nursing homes, psychiatric or behavioral health institutions, intermediate-care facilities for mentally disabled patients, and or skilled nursing facilities. Such patients require professional care, but not to the same degree as those who are hospitalized.

Lozenge A hard, disk-shaped solid medication dosage form that contains medication in a sugar base, which is released as the lozenge is held in the mouth and sucked.

Mail-order pharmacy A pharmacy that functions like a warehouse, with pharmacists and technicians who dispense prescriptions that are mailed to (not picked-up by) patients.

Managed Care pharmacy An ambulatory care pharmacy that is owned and operated as part of a managed care system such as a health maintenance organization (HMO).

Manufacturer A company that manufacturers or makes products such as drugs.

Manufacturing Typically occurs in licensed manufacturing facilities and includes the production, conversion, and/or processing of a drug, generally in bulk quantities and without a prescription or medication order.

Material safety data sheets Information sheets provided by manufacturers for chemicals or drugs that may be hazardous in the workplace. They provide information about the specific hazards of the chemicals or drugs used at the worksite, guidelines for their safe use, and recommendations to treat an exposure or clean up a spill.

Maximizing inventory turns An inventory turn occurs when stock is completely depleted and reordered. Ideally, products should not sit on the shelf unused for long periods; they should be purchased and used many times throughout the course of a year. Inventory turns can be calculated by dividing the total purchases in a period by the value of physical inventory taken at a reasonable single point in time.

Maximum allowable cost (MAC) Used for generic or multisource drug reimbursement; usually based on the cost of the lowest available generic equivalent.

Medication administration record (MAR) A component of the paper patient medical record in which nurses and other healthcare providers document times and dates when a medication was administered to the patient.

Medication error Any error occurring in the medication use process.

Medication guides Patient information approved by the FDA to help patients avoid serious adverse effects, inform patients about known serious side effects, and provide directions for use to promote adherence to the treatment. These are available for specific drugs or classes of drugs and must be dispensed with the prescription.

Medication misadventure A general term to describe drug-related incidents.

Medication order A written, electronic, telephone, or verbal request for a patient medication in an inpatient setting.

Medication therapy management (MTM) A service or group of services that optimize therapeutic outcomes for a patient. Such services include: assessment of a patient's health status; formulation of a medication treatment plan; selection, initiation, modification, or administration of medication therapy; monitoring of a patient's response to therapy; review of medications for medication-related problems; documentation and communication of care; provision of patient education and information to increase patient understanding and appropriate use of medications; and coordination and integration of MTM services into the broader health care services provided to the patient.

Medication Use Evaluation (MUE) A performance improvement method that evaluates how medications are being utilized to treat patients in the hospital. The goal is to improve medication use and optimize patient therapy.

Medline A searchable database containing over 16 million references to journal articles and abstracts published in approximately 5,200 biomedical journals.

MedlinePlus An online database sponsored by the government that contains health information for the public on over 500 health conditions.

Message Information, a point of view, or an idea that is being communicated.

Metabolism The breakdown of medication in the body.

Metabolite A breakdown product of a medication that has undergone metabolism.

Metric system The most widely used and accepted system of measurement in the world; based on multiples of ten.

Mnemonic A shorthand name for a drug product that facilitates faster computer data entry.

Monitoring error Failure to review a medication order or associated clinical laboratory values.

Myalgia Muscle pain.

Myelosuppression The suppression of white blood cell and platelet production from the bone marrow.

National Drug Code (NDC) Number A unique number assigned to each drug, strength, and package size for the purpose of identification.

Naturally occurring radioactive material (NORM) Radioactivity that is present naturally in the environment.

Network A group of pharmacies, physicians, hospitals, or other providers who participate in a certain managed care plan.

Nondurable medical equipment Single-use equipment for a medical purpose (e.g., gloves, dressings, syringes and needles).

Non-formulary drug A drug that is not included on the hospital's approved formulary list.

Nonrestricted areas Areas of a nuclear pharmacy where radioactive materials are prohibited.

Nonsterile compounding Compounds prepared in a pharmacy that do not require strict aseptic technique and include preparations such as oral and topical medications.

Nonverbal communication The exchange of messages by using means other than speaking to convey attitudes, beliefs, and emotions.

Nuclear pharmacy A specialty area of pharmacy practice involving the compounding and dispensing of radiopharmaceuticals for diagnostic imaging and therapy.

Numerator The top number of a fraction, representing the number of parts present.

Oil-in-water (O/W) emulsion An emulsion in which small oil droplets (internal phase) are scattered throughout water (external, continuous phase).

Ointment A semisolid medication dosage form, applied to the skin or mucous membranes, which lubricates and softens or is used as a base for drug delivery.

Omission error A scheduled dose that is omitted entirely.

Open-ended questions Questions that require a response other than a simple "yes" or "no"—designed to obtain as much information from an individual as possible.

Open formulary A system in which all medications are available for a prescriber to use on his or her patient.

Orthopedic devices Equipment used for a deformity, disorder, or injury of skeleton and associated structures.

Orthotic Device designed for the support of weak or ineffective joints or muscles.

Ostomy An operation (as a colostomy, ileostomy, or urostomy) to create an artificial passage for bodily elimination.

Over-the-Counter (OTC) drugs Drugs that are available without a prescription.

Package insert A manufacturer's product information sheet that provides general drug information, such as how it works, indications, adverse effects, drug interactions, dosage forms, stability, and dosing information.

Parenteral A route of medication administration that bypasses the gastrointestinal tract, such as intravenous, intramuscular, or subcutaneous administration.

Par-level system An inventory management system in which predetermined stock minimum and maximum quantities to be maintained are established. Once the stocked quantity goes below the par level, more product is ordered.

Pathophysiology Unhealthy function in an individual body system or an organ due to a disease.

Patient assistance programs (PAPs) Programs offering certain free drugs to low-income patients who lack prescription drug coverage and meet certain criteria.

Patient-centered care The responsible provision of drug therapy for the purpose of achieving outcomes that improve a patient's quality of life; focuses on the patient's role and responsibility in his or her medication-taking and health-related behaviors.

Patient-controlled analgesia (PCA) A type of pain management in which the patient receives parenteral narcotics with a basal/continuous rate and/or has the capabilities to give fixed bolus doses to himself or herself using an electronic ambulatory infusion pump. The PCA pump allows one or both of the features to be in use at one time; the clinician may choose to use only the bolus option with lockout periods or only the continuous rate to meet patient needs.

Patient counseling The act of educating a patient, by a pharmacist, regarding the proper use of a prescribed drug, at the time of dispensing.

Patient identification number A unique code number that identifies a given patient (for example, a medical record number) or a patient and specific admission date (for example, an account number).

Patient profile A list of information about a patient, including name, identification number, date of birth, sex, height, weight, lab values, admitting and secondary diagnoses, room and bed number, names of admitting and consulting physicians, allergies, medication history, special considerations, and clinical comments.

Patient service representative Responsible for controlling the patient's inventory of supplies and screening for problems. This person's job is to contact the patient or caregiver weekly or on a routine basis, depending on the anticipated delivery schedule. Often, this individual helps coordinate pickup of supplies and equipment when the patient's therapy is completed.

Pedometer An instrument that records the distance a person covers on foot by responding to the body motion at each step.

Perception The mental process of becoming aware of or recognizing an object or idea.

Percutaneous Through the skin; transdermal.

Peripherally inserted central catheter (PICC) An intravenous catheter that can be inserted at the hospital bedside or at home by specially trained nurses. They are inserted through a vein in the arm, threaded through other veins in the arm, and end up with the tip resting in the superior vena cava.

Peripheral neuropathy Damage of nerves other than the brain and the spinal cord.

Peristalsis Waves of involuntary muscular contractions in the digestive tract. In the stomach, this motion mixes food with gastric juices, turning it into a thin liquid called chyme.

Peristaltic pumps Pumps with a series of roller wheels that press against tubing to force a volume of liquid down the length of the tubing.

Perpetual inventory process An inventory method in which medications, specifically controlled substances, and investigational drugs are inventoried and tracked continuously. Each dose or packaged unit, such as a tablet, vial, or milliliter of fluid volume, is accounted for at all times.

pH The hydrogen ion concentration in a solution/fluid. The lower the pH, the more acidic the solution and the greater the hydrogen ion concentration; a pH of 7.4 is considered to be normal for blood.

Pharmaceutical care Direct, responsible provision of medication-related care that which achieves outcomes that improve a patient's quality of life. Pharmaceutical care involves cooperation between the pharmacist, the patient, and other health care professionals in designing, implementing, and monitoring a therapeutic medication plan. Such a plan serves to identify potential and actual drug-related problems, resolve actual drug-related problems, and prevent potential drug-related problems.

Pharmacist A health care professional licensed by the state to engage in the practice of pharmacy. Pharmacists have advanced training in the pharmaceutical sciences, such as pharmacology (the study of drugs and their actions in the body), pharmacokinetics (the process by which drugs are absorbed, distributed, metabolized, and eliminated in the body), and pharmaceutics (the science of preparing and dispensing drugs).

Pharmacodynamics The study of the relationship between the concentration of a drug in the body and the response or outcome observed or measured in a patient.

Pharmacokinetics The study of the movement of a drug through the body during the following phases: absorption, distribution, metabolism, and excretion.

Pharmacy benefit manager (PBM) An organization that manages pharmacy benefits for managed care organizations, self-insured employers, insurance companies, labor unions, Medicaid and Medicare prescription drug plans, the Federal Employees Health Benefits Program, and other federal, state, and local government entities.

Pharmacy satellite A physical space located in or near a patient care area that can provide a variety of distributive and clinical services.

Physiology The study of how living organisms function normally, including such processes as nutrition, movement, and reproduction.

Positron emission tomography (PET) An advanced nuclear imaging technique that involves the use of short-lived radioactive materials to produce three-dimensional, colored images of those materials functioning in the body.

Practice of pharmacy The practice of pharmacy is regulated by each state through its pharmacy laws and regulations. The state laws and regulations establish the scope of the practice of pharmacy in the particular state, meaning the responsibilities that pharmacists are permitted to perform in the state.

Premium The amount the individual pays to belong to a health plan. Premiums are often paid monthly.

Prescribing error Error occurring during the prescribing process.

Prescription The written or verbal authorization, by an authorized prescriber, for the use of a particular pharmaceutical agent for an individual patient. This term also refers to the physical product dispensed.

Prescription compounding A medication individualized for a specific patient that requires the mixing of ingredients in a pharmacy and is based on a prescription or drug order.

Prescription monitoring programs State prescription drug monitoring programs are programs implemented by the states pursuant to state laws and regulations to collect, review, and analyze information received from pharmacies about controlled substance prescriptions dispensed in the state. The programs provide information that may be reviewed by state law enforcement and regulatory agencies to assist in identifying and investigating potential improper prescribing, dispensing, and use of prescription drugs.

Primary prescription label A label, affixed to a dispensed drug product, that contains legally required information, including pharmacy name and address, patient name, prescriber name, drug name, directions for use, date dispensed, cautionary statements, sequential prescription number, initials or name of dispensing pharmacist, quantity dispensed, number of refills, expiration date, and lot number.

Primary references Original research articles published in scientific journals.

Prime vendor A wholesaler from which a pharmacy purchases 90 to 95% of its pharmaceuticals according to an established arrangement or contract.

Prior authorization Requires the prescriber to receive preapproval from the PBM in order for the drug to be covered by the benefit.

Professional A person who practices an occupation or vocation that requires advanced specialized training.

Professionalism Actively demonstrating the attitudes, qualities and behaviors of a professional while performing the duties of one's profession: "putting the needs of others before your own."

Proportion A combination of two ratios with the same units; a statement of equality between two ratios.

Prospective payment The amount to be paid for drugs is predetermined based on the condition that is being treated. It typically includes all costs associated with treating a particular condition, including medications.

PubMed A Web-based searching system, sponsored by the National Library of Medicine, which can be used to access Medline journal citations.

Purchase order A document executed by a purchaser and forwarded to a supplier that is considered a legal offer to buy products or services.

Quality control A method to check and validate the steps throughout a process to ensure that the final product will be free of defects or medication errors.

Quality improvement A process of systematic steps to achieve desired results with the goal of sustaining and improving medication use processes to reduce the number or variances of medication errors. Quality Improvement (QI) programs describe the desired performance and then identify gaps between the desired and actual performance. QI uses various tools to collect and measure data to identify root causes of variation, implements appropriate improvements to fix the root causes, then measures the impact these changes had in the system.

Quantity limits Set upper limits of an amount of a drug that is covered by the benefit, or the total days of therapy.

Radioactive decay The process of providing stability to an unstable nucleus by removing excess energy. Radiopharmaceutical products essentially become inactive when they have undergone decay.

Radioactivity The emission of radiation that is released from an unstable nucleus.

Radiopharmaceuticals Prescription drugs that contain a radioactive component that are used for diagnostic imaging and therapy.

Rate-restricted IV administration set systems An intravenous administration system used with proprietary fluid reservoirs that are designed specifically for use in the home care setting. The tubing used with these systems is designed to infuse the solution at a set rate. The only way to change the rate of infusion is to change the tubing.

Ratio A representation of the relationship between two items. For example, when calculating a dose, a ratio can be used to show the number of milligrams in the dose per one kilogram of patient weight (mg/kg).

Ratio strengths A ratio expressed as 1:something, where the units are g per mL. The concentrations of weak solutions, such as 1:1000 or 1:10,000 epinephrine, are sometimes expressed this way.

Recall When a product is removed from the market by the manufacturer on its own accord or at the direction of the FDA, for safety or quality reasons, such as mislabeling, contamination, lack of potency, lack of adherence to acceptable Good Manufacturing Practices, or other situations that may present a significant risk to public health.

Receiver The recipient of a message.

Receptor A structure on the surface of a cell (or inside a cell) that selectively receives and binds a specific substance.

Registration The process of making a list or being enrolled in an existing list. A pharmacy technician may be required to be registered with the state board of pharmacy before being able to legally carry out some pharmacy functions.

Regulations (or rules) Regulations (or rules) are issued by an administrative or governmental agency that establish the requirements that must be followed by the regulated persons or entities. For example, a state board of pharmacy issues regulations for pharmacy technicians to establish the qualifications that pharmacy technicians must meet in order to work as a pharmacy technician in a state.

Reimbursement Money that is collected from a third-party payer to cover partial cost or the entire cost of a prescription for a patient.

Requestor The person requesting the information. A requestor could be a nurse, doctor, other health care professional, or a patient.

Response The reaction of a receiver upon receiving a message.

Restricted areas Areas of a nuclear pharmacy where radioactive materials are used and stored.

Retrospective payment Drugs are dispensed and reimbursed later, according to a predetermined formula that is specified in a contract between the pharmacy and the third-party payer, such as the insurance company or pharmacy benefit manager.

Revenue Represents the inflow of funds.

Rhinitis Inflammation of the nasal lining.

Root cause analysis (RCA) A process for retrospectively analyzing an error.

Secondary references Indexing systems such as Medline, which provide a list of journal articles on the topic that is being searched.

Secrete To form and give off.

Sender The individual who conveys a message to a receiver.

Small Volume Parenteral (SVP) Also called an IV piggyback (IVPB). Any IV solution with a total volume of less than or equal to 100 mL.

Smart pumps An infusion pump equipped with IV medication error prevention software. These devices have specific drug libraries, dose calculators, programming limits, and remote communications capabilities.

Specialty pharmacy An area of pharmacy practice that requires very specific knowledge and expertise, such as nuclear or veterinary pharmacy.

Sphygmomanometer An instrument for measuring blood pressure. Sphygmomanometers are available as a mercury column, a gauge with a dial face, and an electronic device with a digital display. A sphygmomanometer consists of a measuring unit attached to a cuff that is wrapped around the upper arm and inflated to constrict the arteries.

Stability Defined in USP-NF as the extent to which a preparation retains, within specified limits and throughout its period of storage and use, the same properties and characteristics that it possessed at the time of compounding.

STAT Abbreviation of the Latin word statim, meaning immediately; commonly used on medication orders to indicate the need for the drug right away.

Step therapy Requiring the use of a recognized first-line drug before a more complex or expensive second-line drug is used. Beneficiaries must try and fail with the first-line drug before a second-line drug can be covered by the benefit.

Sterile compounding Compounds prepared in a pharmacy using strict aseptic technique including preparations such as injections, ophthalmic solutions, and irrigation solutions.

Stock rotation Placing the products that will expire the soonest in the front of the shelf or bin and those with later expiration dates behind them.

Stoma An artificial permanent opening, especially in the abdominal wall, made in surgical procedures.

Subcutaneous Deposited in the tissue just under the skin.

Subgingival Administered via the subgingival space, which is the space between the tooth and gum.

Sublingual Placed under the tongue, where it dissolves and is absorbed into the bloodstream.

Suspension A mixture of fine particles of an undissolved solid spread throughout a liquid or, less commonly, a gas.

Systole When the heart muscle is contracting and ejecting blood from the chambers of the heart; the pressure is at the highest point in a normal heart.

Tall man lettering An error prevention technique used to differentiate look-alike medication names. A portion of the letters are capitalized (e.g., niCARdipine and NIFEdipine).

Technician An individual skilled in the practical or mechanical aspects of a profession. A pharmacy technician assists pharmacists by performing routine, day-to-day functions of the practice of pharmacy that do not require the judgment of a pharmacist.

Tertiary references General references that present documented information in a condensed and compact format, such as textbooks or manuals.

Test strip Specifically designed strip with reagent used to measure blood glucose.

Therapeutic level The blood level at which most patients receive a medication's desired effect with minimal side effects.

Third-party payer An entity other than the patient that is involved in paying partial cost or the entire cost of products and/or services for a patient.

Tolerance A state of unresponsiveness to a specific antigen or group of antigens to which a person is normally responsive. Immune tolerance is achieved under conditions that suppress the immune reaction and is not just the absence of an immune response.

Topical Applied to the skin, mucous membranes, or other external parts of the body, such as fingernails, toenails, and hair.

Total Parenteral Nutrition (TPN) Also known as hyperalimentation, refers to the IV administration of nutrients needed to sustain life.

Transdermal Through the skin; percutaneous.

Transdermal patch A patch that contains a drug in a reservoir in the patch, which is delivered through the patch and absorbed from the skin into the bloodstream.

Transmucosal Administered through, or across, a mucous membrane.

Trituration The act of mixing powders or crushing tablets using a mortar and pestle (i.e., solid is rubbed with mortar and pestle) until a state of fine, evenly sized particles is achieved.

Unauthorized drug error An error occurring when a drug given to or taken by a patient was not ordered by an authorized prescriber.

Unit dose A single or individually packaged medication in a ready-to-administer form for the patient.

Unit dose distribution system A system that provides all or most medications to patients in a unit dose ready-to-administer form.

Unit-dose package A non-reusable container designed to hold a quantity of drug to be administered as a single dose.

Unit-of-use packaging Characterized by a vial, an envelope, or a plastic bag containing several doses of the same medication.

Universal precautions Treating all patients as if they are potentially infectious to prevent employees from exposure to human blood or other potentially infectious material. For example, wearing personal protective equipment (e.g., gloves, masks, gowns), hand washing, and proper handling and disposal of potentially infectious material.

Urostomy An ostomy for the elimination of urine from the body.

Volume of distribution The extent of a medication's outreach to various tissues and spaces throughout the body.

Volumetric pumps Pumps that allow the user to preset a volume to be dispensed into a container on the basis of the draw back setting.

Water-in-oil (W/O) emulsion An emulsion in which small water droplets (internal phase) are spread throughout oil (external, continuous phase).

Wholesale acquisition cost (WAC) Represents the "list price" at which the manufacturer sells the drug to the wholesaler.

Wholesaler A large-scale warehouse with drugs and supplies located in various geographic regions that exist to help bring pharmaceutical products closer to the market.

Wrong administration technique error An error occurring when a medication is given or taken by the wrong route or the use of an improper procedure.

Wrong dose form error Use of the incorrect medication dosage form.

Wrong time error Administration of a medication dose outside of an established scheduled time.

Index

A

D

M

N

O

S

X

Z